AF773287

Metastatic Melanoma: Clinical Advances and Treatments

Metastatic Melanoma: Clinical Advances and Treatments

Edited by **Frederick Nash**

FOSTER ACADEMICS

New Jersey

Published by Foster Academics,
61 Van Reypen Street,
Jersey City, NJ 07306, USA
www.fosteracademics.com

Metastatic Melanoma: Clinical Advances and Treatments
Edited by Frederick Nash

© 2015 Foster Academics

International Standard Book Number: 978-1-63242-276-7 (Hardback)

This book contains information obtained from authentic and highly regarded sources. Copyright for all individual chapters remain with the respective authors as indicated. A wide variety of references are listed. Permission and sources are indicated; for detailed attributions, please refer to the permissions page. Reasonable efforts have been made to publish reliable data and information, but the authors, editors and publisher cannot assume any responsibility for the validity of all materials or the consequences of their use.

The publisher's policy is to use permanent paper from mills that operate a sustainable forestry policy. Furthermore, the publisher ensures that the text paper and cover boards used have met acceptable environmental accreditation standards.

Trademark Notice: Registered trademark of products or corporate names are used only for explanation and identification without intent to infringe.

Printed in China.

Contents

Preface

It is often said that books are a boon to mankind. They document every progress and pass on the knowledge from one generation to the other. They play a crucial role in our lives. Thus I was both excited and nervous while editing this book. I was pleased by the thought of being able to make a mark but I was also nervous to do it right because the future of students depends upon it. Hence, I took a few months to research further into the discipline, revise my knowledge and also explore some more aspects. Post this process, I begun with the editing of this book.

This book presents an overview on latest modalities and advances developed for effectively tackling challenges encountered by physicians in dealing with metastatic melanoma. Surgery continues to be the front-runner treatment option for melanoma confined to the main tumor and/or lymph nodes. Results from randomized regulated trials signify that sentinel node biopsy for the treatment of cutaneous melanoma of average thickness has a significant impact on repetition rates, and adjuvant radiotherapy to the regional lymph node areas following surgical resection decreases loco-regional recurrence in patients under great risk of relapse. Electrochemotherapy, isolated limb perfusion as well as photodynamic remedy remain under assessment for curing stage IV disease. The most promising fact related to novel treatments has been regarding targeted therapies for genetic mutations. Specifically, the assuring outcomes of partial and complete tumor reply in stage IV disease from initial phase trials of the B-RAF kinase inhibitors. This book presents a modern insight into the therapeutic treatment options for patients with metastatic melanoma and is significant for researchers as well as clinicians across the globe. An update on present clinical trials for melanoma treatment has been provided in this book along with informative discussions regarding the treatment of uveal and oral melanoma.

I thank my publisher with all my heart for considering me worthy of this unparalleled opportunity and for showing unwavering faith in my skills. I would also like to thank the editorial team who worked closely with me at every step and contributed immensely towards the successful completion of this book. Last but not the least, I wish to thank my friends and colleagues for their support.

Editor

Part 1

Treatment Options for Cutaneous Melanoma

1

Cutaneous Metastases from Malignant Melanoma: Clinical Features and New Therapeutic Perspectives

Paola Savoia, Paolo Fava and Maria Grazia Bernengo
Department of Biomedical Sciences and Human Oncology, Section of Dermatology, University of Turin, Italy

1. Introduction

In this chapter, cutaneous metastases from malignant melanoma will be analyzed from a clinical and a prognostic point of view.
This non rare condition is often distressing for the patient, as cutaneous lesions increase progressively in number and size and are frequently worsened by ulceration, bleeding and pain.
After a general introduction about the incidence of cutaneous involvement in melanoma natural history, clinical classification of skin metastases will be provided. Then, the impact of cutaneous localizations on prognosis will be evaluated. In the last paragraph, the different therapeutic options for the management of patients with loco-regional or diffused cutaneous metastases will be reviewed.

2. Epidemiology

Skin metastases from solid tumor are not rare. They affect an estimated percentage of patients ranging from 0.7 to 9% in several literature series (Spencer & Helm 1987, Lookingbill, Spangler & Helm 1993, Schwartz 1995, Hu et al. 2008), in the late phases of disease progression or, in more than 7% of patients, as first sign of disseminated disease (Lookingbill, Spangler & Helm 1993, Rosen 1980). Breast cancer is the most commonly involved tumor, accounting for more than 60% of cases of cutaneous spread, followed by colon carcinoma (Krathen, Orengo & Rosen 2003). Moreover, cutaneous metastatic disease is commonly seen with cancer of the lung, kidney and ovary and with sarcoma, lymphoma or leukemia.
As expected, tumor types are differently distributed among the two genders: lung, colon and head and neck tumours together with melanoma account for the majority of skin metastases in males; whereas, breast cancer is the most common neoplasm related to the development of cutaneous secondary lesions in females (Hu et al 2008).
Focusing on melanoma, skin metastases represent a relatively frequent event in the natural history of the disease and can develop in early as well as in late stage of disease. Cutaneous or subcutaneous lesions arise in 10-17% of patients affected by melanoma and almost the 50% of patients with metastatic disease develops skin involvement (Lookingbill, Spangler & Helm 1993, Schwartz 1995, Krathen, Orengo & Rosen 2003).

No specific clinical or histological characteristics were found in patients with cutaneous metastases from melanoma if compared to those with visceral localizations (Savoia et al 2009). However, known risk factors related to prognosis impact on the metastatic melanoma potential.

3. Classification

On the basis of the distance from the primary melanoma, skin metastases are described as local recurrences, in transit disease or distant metastases.

True local recurrences are defined as the reappearance of melanoma in -or contiguous with- an excision scar or a graft and bearing an in situ component (Olsen et al 1970; Brown & Zitelli 1995). The prognosis of local recurrence defined strictly in this way is much better than that associated with in transit disease and 5-year survival rate is related only to the thickness of the primary melanoma. These recurrences are in fact considered as a result of a uncompleted resection of primary melanoma, and are for this reason becoming rare.

In-transit disease (satellitosis) indicates cutaneous or subcutaneous disease between the primary site and the regional lymph nodes. Satellite nodules and in-transit disease are associated with worse prognosis (super imposable to a melanoma with nodal metastases; stage III disease), and the distance of cutaneous deposits from the primary site has no prognostic significance (Balch et al 2009).

Distant cutaneous metastases are defined as tumour lesions that grow in any skin site over the regional lymph nodes. The presence of any distant metastases delineates a stage IV disease, even if patients with sole distant skin metastases (and normal serum LDH levels) have a relatively better prognosis if compared with those of other metastatic patients (Balch et al 2009). Obviously, distant skin melanoma localization can appear together with or in absence of other visceral metastases. Stage and prognosis vary according to AJCC classification as shown in table 1 (Balch et al 2009).

Clinical Staging				**Pathological Staging**			
0	**Tis**	**N0**	**M0**	0	**Tis**	**N0**	**M0**
IA	T1a	N0	M0	**IA**	T1a	N0	M0
IB	T1b	N0	M0	**IB**	T1b	N0	M0
	T2a	N0	M0		T2a	N0	M0
IIA	T2b	N0	M0	**IIA**	T2b	N0	M0
	T3a	N0	M0		T3a	N0	M0
IIB	T3b	N0	M0	**IIB**	T3b	N0	M0
	T4a	N0	M0		T4a	N0	M0
IIC	T4b	N0	M0	**IIC**	T4b	N0	M0
III	any T	N 1-3	M0	**IIIA**	T1-T4a	N1a/2a	M0
				IIIB	T1-T4b	N1a/2a	M0
					T1-T4a	N1b/2b	M0
					T1-T4a/b	N2c	M0
				IIIC	T1-T4b	N1b/2b/2c	M0
					any T	N3	M0
IV	any T	any N	M 1	**IV**	any T	any N	M 1

Table 1. Clinical and pathological staging, AJCC 2009.

4. Clinical features

Skin metastases from melanoma can arise as single or multiple nodules. The most common presentations of cutaneous metastatic disease are brown to black or skin colored papules and nodules, sometimes ulcerated. In the majority of these cases cutaneous metastases were correctly identified by the clinician before the pathologic diagnosis was given; dermoscopy could help in diagnosis, even if skin melanoma metastases have often aspects that are indistinguishable from the characteristic pattern of blue nevi (Carlos-Ortega, de Oca-Monroy & Isyta-Morales 2008). Epidermotropic melanoma metastases are histopatologically characterized by aggregates of atypical melanocytes within the dermis with thinning of the epidermis. Usually there is no lateral extension of atypical melanocytes within the epidermis beyond the concentration of the metastases on the dermis. Metastases differs from primary melanoma by the absence of inflammatory infiltrate and junctional activity, even if a prominent lymphocytic infiltrated can be sometimes observed. In few cases metastatic cells are small and nevoid, with few or any mitoses and differentiation from compound nevi is difficult (Elder E et al, 2005. Tumours and Cysts in dermis and Subcutis, in: *Lever's histopathology of the skin*. Lippincott Williams&Wilkins, Philadelphia).
Less frequently, a wide morphological spectrum of lesions has been described, including erythematous patches or plaques, inflammatory erysipela-like lesions, diffuse sclerodermiform lesions with indurations of the skin ("en cuirasse" metastatic carcinoma), telangiectatic papulovesicles, purpuric plaques mimicking vasculitis, and alopecia aerate-like scalp lesions (Saeed, Keehn & Morgan 2004, Sarya et al 2007). In these cases, clinical diagnosis could be more challenging and metastases can be suspicious for benign entities (Figure 1).

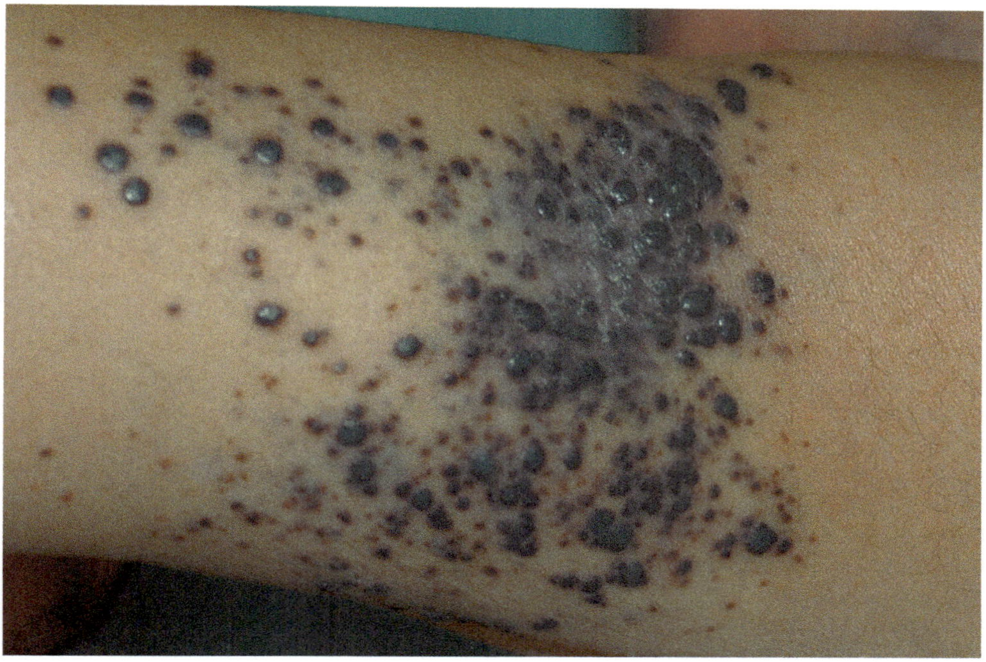

Fig. 1. Clinical features of local recurrences that are defined as the reappearance of melanoma in or contiguous with an excision scar or graft and bearing an *in situ* component.

Moreover, there are also rare cases of so-called zosteriform metastases, with vesicobullous herpetiform lesions or papules and nodules distributed along one or more dermatomes. A previous Varicella Zoster Virus (VZV) infection or widespread lymphatic obstruction by tumor cells can justify the zosteriform pattern (Figure 2).

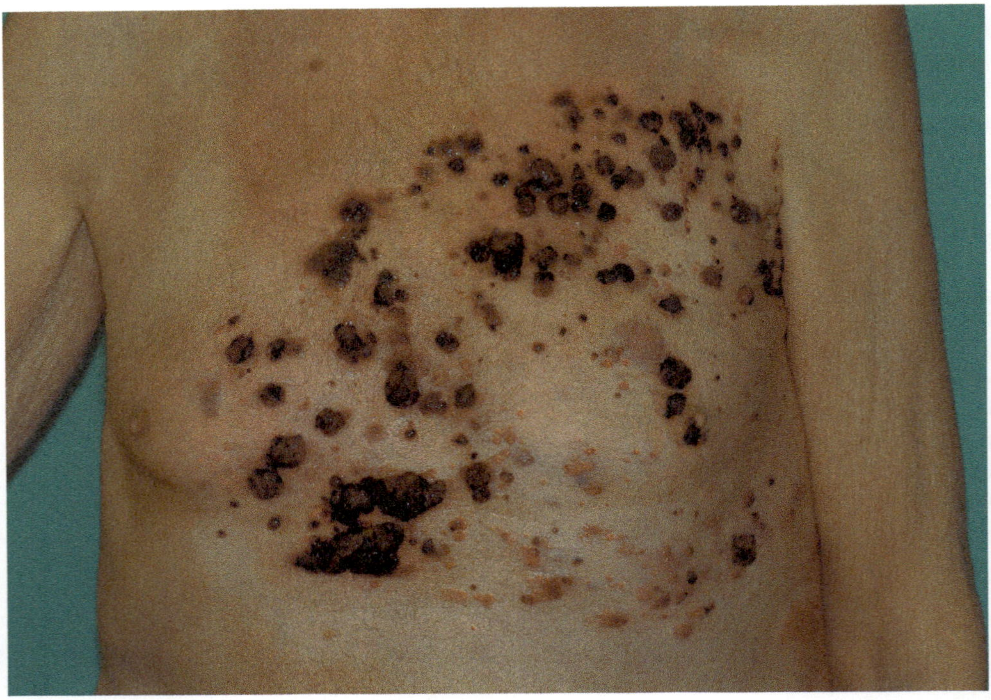

Fig. 2. Zosteriform metastases among thoracic dermatomes.

However, zosteriform metastases, as well as the rare skin metastases occurring on skin graft donor site, could be explained as a Koebner phenomenon (Savoia et al 2009, Marenco et al 2009).

From a clinical point of view, if bleeding and super-infection are not present, superficial skin metastases are usually asymptomatic, even if patients frequently report localized pain and paresthesiae anticipating the onset of clinically evident cutaneous lesions; these symptoms are related to oedema and mechanical stress on the near tissues and usually disappear in a few days. On the other hand, when subcutaneous lesions grow deep infiltrating muscles or nerves become very painful. The management of pain in these cases could be difficult and requires a multidisciplinary approach.

As mentioned earlier, bleeding and super-infections are the most frequent complications of skin metastases and can significantly impact on the patient's quality of life (Kaheler, Egeberts & Hauschild 2010). These complications can also compromise general conditions. Massive bleeding from cutaneous metastases could become life threatening; sepsis related to the bacterial dissemination of infected metastases represents an uncommon but not rare event, that lead to septic shock and death (Figure 3).

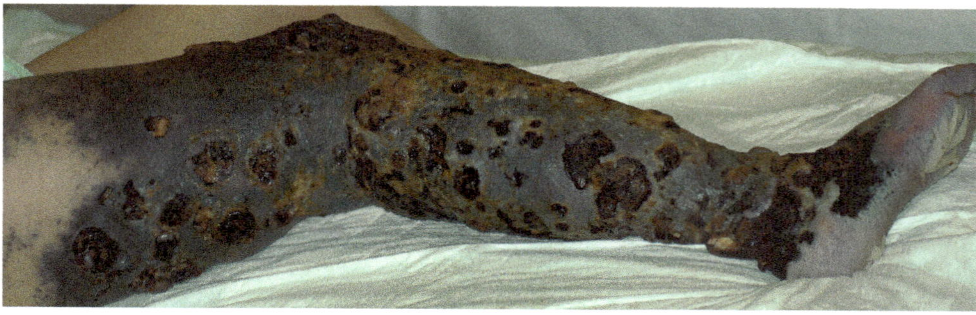

Fig. 3. Infected diffuse metastases from malignant melanoma

5. Pattern of cutaneous localizations

Cutaneous secondary lesions can occur on all anatomic sites, with skin metastases from other solid tumours more frequently found on the head, neck, anterior chest and abdomen, whereas lower extremities are rarely involved (Schwartz, 1995). Conversely, skin metastases from melanoma are more frequently observed on the back in men and on the lower limbs in women. These different patterns of cutaneous localizations among sex can be explained by the fact that in more than 30% of cases, secondary cutaneous localizations occur in the same anatomic area of the primary (Savoia et al 2009).

6. Clinical course and prognosis

In more than half of the cases, skin represents the first site of metastatic involvement after the primary melanoma diagnosis. In about one third of cases, patients develop skin involvement after evidences of regional lymph nodal metastatic disease.

The finding of concomitant distant cutaneous, visceral and nodal metastases account for more than 10% of cases, whereas skin involvement after visceral dissemination is rare, and occurs only in about the 3% of patients (Savoia et al 2009).

Cutaneous metastases are loco regional in nearly 80% of cases, whereas distant metastases were documented in the remaining 20% of patients. A different pattern of cutaneous metastases was related to the time of onset: when cutaneous metastases arise as the first site of relapse, there is a significant higher percentage of locoregional localizations, whereas distant skin involvement was more frequently observed after visceral involvement. No significant differences were found between patients with regional and those with distant metastases regarding to the known risk factors, such as Breslow thickness, Clark level, histotype of the primary melanoma and ulceration (Savoia et al 2009).

It is noteworthy that in patients with distant metastases, primary melanomas arose predominantly at trunk and back, whereas patients with cutaneous loco-regional spreading were affected mainly by primary located at leg and foot. As we know, loco-regional metastases develop as a result of tumour cell embolization in the dermal lymphatic vessels between the primary tumour site and the draining regional lymph node basin; lymphatic stasis to lower limbs consequent to nodal dissection represents an additional risk factor for cutaneous locoregional dissemination.

In contrast, the correlation between disseminated skin lesions and primary melanoma located to the trunk could be explained by the fact that the lymph drainage of this region is

not strictly dependent on a single station, but it could be resulted from more than one lymphatic basin, together with a possible role of haematogenous spreading.
Disease free survival evaluated from the first melanoma diagnosis varies in relation to the first site of metastatization. In our experience, loco regional cutaneous relapses develop early, but show a very late progression to visceral disease. On the contrary, patients with disseminated skin lesions as first site of relapse had a longer disease free interval from the first diagnosis but a shorter time to progression to visceral metastases (Savoia et al 2009).

7. Treatment and clinical management

The choice of the modality of treatment for cutaneous melanoma metastases depends on several factors, including location and number of lesions, presence of systemic involvement, age and general health conditions of patients. Moreover, the prognostic differences between patients with loco-regional and distant skin metastases justify different approaches in their clinical management.
Important therapeutic options including surgery, isolated limb perfusion, local or systemic chemo- and immuno-therapy and radiotherapy are discussed in detail below.

7.1 Surgery

Surgery is the gold standard and represents the most effective treatment for limited in-transit disease, when technically feasible. It is an adequate treatment when the lesions are relatively small and clustered in a reasonable circumscribed area. Primary melanoma should be excised widely with a 1-2 cm margin depending on Breslow thickness, whereas wide surgical margins are unnecessary for the treatment of cutaneous metastases. Usually, metastases are clearly demarcated from the surrounding normal dermis and overlying epidermis and the better approach is the complete macroscopical excision of the lesion. When microscopical involvement of margins is documented, reintervention is not mandatory (Hoekstra, 2008).
If technically possible, direct wound closure is to prefer; the second choice is represented by skin graft, because plastic surgical reconstruction can affect the lymphatic drainage pattern.
Palliative treatment should be considered when results in the control of local complications (e.g. bleeding) and/or in a consistent quality of life improvement.
Amputation should be only considered as palliation for imminent exsanguinating haemorrhage or fungation unacceptable for the patient.

7.2 Isolated limb perfusion

Isolated limb perfusion (ILP) -firstly described by Creech and Krementz in 1958- can deliver high doses of cytotoxic agents to a limb, minimizing systemic toxicity. The dose received regionally can be up to tenfold higher than the systemic mean tolerated dose. Isolated limb perfusion is widely indicated for patients with advanced or recurrent in-transit disease, showing a complete response rate around the 50% in the majority of the published series, with an overall response rate up to 80% (Lens & Dawes 2003, Rossi et al 2010). On the contrary, the role of isolated limb perfusion as adjuvant therapy is still debated (Hoeckstra 2008). The tumour response after perfusion is the only demonstrated prognostic factor affecting local control of the disease and overall survival (Rossi et al 2010).
The usual agent employed is melphalan, with or without tumour necrosis factor (TNF); TNF increases response rate thanks to its selective disruption of the tumour microvasculate, with

a consequent ischemic damage of melanoma cells, even if seems not to influence the long term local control (Di Filippo et al 2006). Dacarbazine is less effective when administered regionally; other combinations of cytostatics (dactinomycin, nitrogen mustard, vindesine, thio-TEPA) have also been proposed but the published series are too small to give absolute conclusions (Daryanani et al 2000, de Wilt et al 2000, Hoeckstra 2008). Hyperthermia, with temperature between 39° to 41° act sinergically with high dose chemotherapy, even if can exacerbate loco regional toxicity (Hoeckstra 2008).

General anesthesia is required. However, age does not represent a contraindication to ILP. Systemic side effects, due to drug releasing into the systemic circulation are rare and mainly represented by nausea, vomiting and mild bone marrow suppression. Local toxic reactions are more frequently described and ranges from mild erythema to deep tissue inflammation; nearly 25% of patients develop neuropathy or pain, whereas chronic edema is usually related to lymphoadenenctomy (Bonifati et al 2000, Rossi et al 2002).

7.3 Electrochemotherapy

Recently, electrochemotherapy (ECT) has been proposed as a new treatment modality for skin metastases of different malignancy, including melanoma. ECT enhances membrane permeability by electric pulses thus permitting a major drug delivery in neoplastic cells and a better cytotoxic effect.

Bleomycin and cisplatin are the drugs more frequently used in ECT with an increased efficacy up to 8.000-fold for bleomicyn, and up to 80-fold for cisplatin (Gaudy et al 2006).

The ECT technique requires only a regional anesthesia or mild general sedation with a lower duration if compared to isolated limb perfusion. With respect to ILP, ECT shows a minimal systemic toxicity; treatment is generally well tolerated; side effects were mainly represented by erythema and edema at the site of treated lesions, superficial erosions, scars and permanent marks from the electrodes (Quaglino et al 2008). Thus ECT can be performed also in patients with major co morbidities.

The first large study about effectiveness of ECT in melanoma treatment, was the multi center European Standard Operating Procedure of Eettrochemoterapy (ESOPE), based on the new Cliniporator™ Elettric Pulse Generator; this study enrolled twenty melanoma patients, with an overall response rate of more than 20% (Marty et al 2008). Several papers recently published confirm these encouraging results of ECT in the control of skin metastases (Campana et al 2009, Moller et al 2009). In our experience, the global response rate was of 79.4, with a percentage of complete remissions of 23.2%(Quaglino et al 2008); complete response was defined in accordance World Health Organiziation (WHO) guidelines as the total clinical disappearance of the tumor (WHO. From *Handbook for Reporting Results of Cancer Treatment, vol 48; pp 22-27.* Geneva, 1997).

The lesion size was the most predictive parameter for response; response rate for larger lesions was significantly lower. Moreover, a second limit is represented by the possible relapse of new lesions on untreated areas: ECT represent in fact a local treatment. However, it is possible to repeat ECT, both on new metastases in untreated areas and on already treated lesions with a previous partial remission or no changes. In our experience, new responses were obtained in about 60% of retreated lesions.

Appropriate dressing should be performed with the aim to control ulceration of cutaneous tumours, local infectious complications and to ensure an acceptable quality of life.

7.4 Radiotherapy

The effectiveness of radiotherapy in the treatment of melanoma metastases is still debated. A poor response was historically observed on in vitro cultures from melanoma cells treated with external-beam radiation (Barranco, Romsdahl & Humphrey 1971). So, radiotherapy was mainly used as palliation when disease was too extensive for surgery and other modalities of treatment were inadvisable or ineffective in stage III and IV melanoma patients. However, a retrospective review (Fenig et al 2009) showed a 52% response rate in stage IV patients who received radiotherapy with palliative intent and others studies (Sause et al 1991; Seegenschmeid et al 1999) demonstrated an overall response rate ranging from 60 to 79% for stage III disease. Moreover, disease-free and overall survival seems to be significant longer in patients who received radiotherapy (Olivier et al, 2007).

7.5 Chemotherapy

Usually, chemotherapy plays a role in the treatment of stage IV melanoma patients with visceral metastases. Regarding cutaneous metastases, chemotherapy can be used in patients with wide spread skin lesions not eligible for local treatments, with or without a concomitant visceral involvement.

Chemotherapy could be used also in stage III, when other loco-regional treatments have failed or are technically not feasable (e.g. cutaneous lesions diffused at trunk or back).

The global response rate is less than 25% for single agent treatment. The gold standard is still represented by Dacarbazine; new molecules as Temozolomide and Fotemustine showed a super imposable disease-free and overall survival, with major toxicity (Middelton et al, 2000). Combination regimens or chemo-immunotherapy give higher response rate but also more severe side effects. However, response to chemo-immunoterapy is not related to statistically significant benefit in term of overall survival when compared with a single-agent treatment.

Recently, Ipilimumab, a human anti-CTLA4 monoclonal antibody showed objective responses or disease stabilization in patients with advanced melanoma (O'Day et al, 2010). No data about the effectiveness of Ipilimumab in the treatment of cutaneous metastases are available, even if several studies are ongoing.

The response rate for in transit metastases treated with dacarbazine is 15-20%; the majority of the responses are partial with a median response duration less than 6 months. Chemoimunotherapy showed also no survival benefit (Hoekstra 2008).

Finally, the clinical efficacy of RAF inhibitors in BRAF mutated melanoma patients are under evaluation after some encouraging preliminary report; a phase I study on patients with both disseminated cutaneous and visceral metastases reported an 81% of clinical responses in patients treated with selective BRAF inhibitor, with a median time to progression of 6-9 months (Flaherty, 2010).

7.6 Others

7.6.1 Laser ablation

Patients with small (<2 cm) and superficial lesions who are not suitable for isolated limb perfusion, ECT or other conventional modalities of treatment can be considered for carbon dioxide (CO_2) laser ablation. This therapy is minimally invasive: only local anesthesia is required and the resultant defect does not require surgical closure but can be covered with a dressing until secondary healing (Lingam & McKay, 1996; Gibson, Byrne & Mc Kay, 2004).

So, can be considered a minimally invasive and effective method of palliation; the role as first line treatment is still debated, in fact the technique can be used to treat only visible and superficial lesions, while deep subcutaneous metastases, large volume lesions and microscopic disease can not be treated with laser ablation (Gimbel, Delman & Zager, 2008).

7.6.2 Cryosurgery

This technique uses temperatures from -50°C to -60°C (with nitrogen spray) to obtain direct tissue destruction. The heat transfer results in vascular stasis, ice crystal and disruption of cell membranes, Ph changes, hypertonic damage and thermal shock that lead to tissue damage and necrosis. Low temperature causes the development of a bulla and a secondary healing with a scar. After the introduction of laser ablation and ECT, cryosurgery is less frequently used in the treatment of cutaneous metastases from melanoma (Hoekstra, 2008).

7.6.3 Intralesional therapy

The intralesional injection of bacillus Calmette-Guérin (BCG) was the first immunotherapy used in the local treatment of cutaneous metastases from melanoma. This procedure was accompanied by sever complications such as ulceration, skin necrosis, and superinfection without significative improvement of lesions treated (Tan & Ho, 1993). Other drugs such as IL-2, INF alpha and dinitrochlorobenzene, with or without sistemic dacarbazine, were more recently used as intralesional therapy (Radny et al, 2003; Strobbe et al, 1997); results are still debating and further investigations are necessary. Encouraging results regarding high-dose intratumoral IL-2 administration in melanoma patients with cutaneous secondarities has been reported (Weide et al, 2010): a complete local response was described in more than 60% of melanoma patients and seemed to be associated with an increased responses to subsequent chemotherapies. Recently, phase I studies confirmed the safety and an enhanced immune response for intralesional injection of Allovectin in metastatic melanoma patients. Unfortunately, phase II studies showed a complete response in only the 3.1% of treated patients, with an overall response rate of 11.8% and a median time-to-progression of 1.6 months (Beidikan et al, 2010).

Rose bengal has been proposed as a possible intralesional treatment, with an objective response rate ranging from 27 to 69%, related to the dose of injection (Thompson, Hersey & Wachter, 2008). Sistemic toxicity is low, even if phototoxic reactions have been described.

An interesting therapeutic option is represented by topical imiquimod. It enhances the immune system activity leading to an induction of melanoma-specific cytotoxic T-cells by cross presentation of melanoma antigen by dendritic cells. Partial remission of locoregional cutaneous metastases treated with imiquimod was demonstrated (Wolf, Richtig, Kopera & Kerl H, 2004).

8. Conclusions

Skin metastases from melanoma are a frequent finding in the natural history of the disease with various clinical, morphological and histopathologic backgrounds. The presence of progressively increasing metastases is often distressing for the patient, and ulceration, bleeding and super-infections can negatively impact on the life-quality. To date, many treatments are available for the clinical management of these lesions. Thus, clinicians should be informed about the prognostic implications and the therapeutic options in order to choose the best cost-effectiveness treatment modality.

9. References

Balch CM, Gershenwald JE, Soong SJ, Thompson JF, Atkins MB, Byrd DR, Buzaid AC, Cochran AJ, Coit DG, Ding S, Eggermont AM, Flaherty KT, Gimotty PA, Kirkwood JM, McMasters KM, Mihm MC Jr, Morton DL, Ross MI, Sober AJ & Sondak VK. Final version of 2009 AJCC melanoma staging and classification. J Clin Oncol. 2009; 27: 6199-6206.

Barranco SC, Romsdahl MM & Humphrey RM. The radiation response of human malignant melanoma cells grown in vitro. Cancer Res. 1971; 31:830-833.

Bedikian A, Richards J, Kharkevitch D, Atkins MB, Whitman E & Gonzalez R. A phase 2 study of high-dose Allovectin-7 in patients with advanced metastatic melanoma. Melanoma Research 2010, 20: 218–226.

Bonifati DM, Ori C, Rossi CR, Caira S, Fanin M & Angelini C. Neuromuscular damage after hyperthermic isolated limb perfusion in patients with melanoma or sarcoma treated with chemotherapeutic agents. Cancer Chemother Pharmacol. 2000; 46: 517-522.

Brown CD, Zitelli JA. The prognosis and treatment of true local cutaneous recurrent malignant melanoma. Dermatol Surg. 1995 Apr;21(4):285-90.

Campana LG, Mocellin S, Basso M,Puccetti O, De Salvo GL, Chiarion-Sileni V, Vecchiato A, Corti L, Rossi CR & Nitti D. Bleomycin-based electrochemotherapy: clinical outcome from a single institution's experience with 52 patients. Ann Surg Oncol. 2009 Jan; 16(1): 191-9.

Carlos-Ortega B, de Oca-Monroy FM & Isyta-Morales A. Dermoscopy findings in malignant skin melanoma with metastases. A case report. Rev Med Inst Mex Seguro Soc. 2009; 47:73-76.

Daryanani D, de Vries EG, Guchelaar HJ, van Weerden TW & Hoekstra HJ. Hyperthermic isolated regional perfusion of the limb with carboplatin. Eur J Surg Oncol. 2000; 26(8): 792-797.

de Wilt JH, Soma G, ten Hagen TL, Kanou J, Takagi K, Nooijen PT, Seynhaevel AL& Eggermont AM. Synergistic antitumour effect of TNF-SAM2 with melphalan and doxorubicin in isolated limb perfusion in rats. Anticancer Res. 2000 Sep- Oct; 20(5B): 3491-3496.

Di Filippo F, Rossi CR, Santinami M, Cavaliere F, Garinei R, Anzà M, Perri P, Botti C, Di Angelo P, Pasqualoni R & Di Filippo S. Hyperthermic isolation limb perfusion with TNFalpha in the treatment of in-transit melanoma metastasis. In Vivo. 2006 Nov-Dec; 20(6A):739-742.

Fenig E, Eidelevich E, Njuguna E, Katz A, Gutman H, Sulkes A & Schechter J. Role of radiation therapy in the management of cutaneous malignant melanoma. Am J Clin Oncol. 1999; 22: 184-186.

Flaherty KT. Narrative review: BRAF opens the door for therapeutic advances in melanoma.Ann Intern Med. 2010 Nov 2;153(9):587-91.

Gaudy C, Richard MA, Folchetti G, Bonerandi JJ & Grob JJ. Randomized controlled study of electrochemotherapy in the local treatment of skin metastases of melanoma. J Cutan Med Surg. 2006 May-Jun; 10(3): 115-121.

Gibson SC, Byrne DS & Mc Kay AJ. Ten-year experience of carbon dioxide laser ablation as treatment for cutaneous recurrence of malignant melanoma. Br J Surg 2004; 91: 893-895.

Gimbel MI, Delman KA & Zager JS. Therapy for unresectable recurrent and in-transit extremity melanoma. Cancer Control. 2008; 15: 225-232.

Hoekstra HJ. The European approach to in-transit melanoma lesions. Int J Hyperthermia. 2008; 24: 227-237.

Hu SC, Chen GS, Lu YW, Wu CS & Lan CC. Cutaneous metastases from different internal malignancies: a clinical and prognostic appraisal. J Eur Acad Dermatol Venereol 2008; 22: 735–740.

Kaheler Kc, Egeberts F& Hauschild A. Electrotherapy in simptomatic melanoma skin metastases: intraindividual comparison with conventional surgery. Dermatol Surg. 2010; 36: 1200-1202.

Krathen RA, Orengo IF & Rosen T. Cutaneous metastasis: a meta-analysis of data. South Med J 2003; 96:164-167.

Lens MB & Dawes M. Isolated limb perfusion with melphalan in the treatment of malignant melanoma of the extremities: a systematic review of randomised controlled trials. Lancet Oncol. 2003 Jun; 4(6): 359-364.

Elder E, Elenitsas R, Johnoson B, Ioffreda M, Miller J & Miller F, 2005. Tumours and Cysts in dermis and Subcutis, in: *Lever's histopathology of the skin*. Lippincott Williams&Wilkins, Philadelphia

Lingam MK & McKay AJ. Carbon dioxide laser ablation as an alternative tratment for cutaneous metastses from malignant melanoma. Br J Surg 1996; 83: 509-512.

Lookingbill DP, Spangler N & Helm KF. Cutaneous metastases in patients with metastatic carcinoma: a retrospective study of 4020 patients. J Am Acad Dermatol 1993; 29: 228–236.

Marenco F, Fava P, Macripò G, Quaglino P, Savoia P & Bernengo MG. Cutaneous melanoma metastases arising on a split-skin graft donor site. Dermatol Surg 2009; 35: 1–4.

Marty M, Sersa G, Garbay JR, Gehl J, Collins CG, Snoj M, Billard V, Geertsen PF, Larkin JO, Miklavcic D, Pavlovic I, Paulin-Kosir SM, Cemazar M, Morsli N, Rudolf Z, Robert C, O'Sullivan GC & Mir LM. Electrochemotherapy–An easy, highly effective and safe treatment of cutaneous and subcutaneous metastases: results of ESOPE (European Standard Operating Procedures of Electrochemotherapy study. Eur J Cancer 2006; 4(Suppl): 3–13.

Middleton MR, Lorigan P, Owen J, Ashcroft L, Lee SM, Harper P & Thatcher N. A randomized phase III study comparing dacarbazine, BCNU, cisplatin and tamoxifen with dacarbazine and interferon in advanced melanoma. Br J Cancer. 2000 Mar; 82(6): 1158-1162.

Möller MG, Salwa S, Soden DM & O'Sullivan GC. Electrochemotherapy as an adjunct or alternative to other treatments for unresectable or in-transit melanoma. Expert Rev Anticancer Ther. 2009 Nov; 9(11): 1611-1630.

O'Day SJ, Maio M, Chiarion-Sileni V,Gajewski V, Pehamberger H, Bondarenko NH, Queirolo P, Lundgren L, Mikhailov M, Roman L, Verschraegen C, Humphrey C, Ibrahim R, de Pril V, Hoos A & Wolchok JD. Efficacy and safety of ipilimumab monotherapy in patients with pretreated advanced melanoma: a multicenter single-arm phase II study. Ann Oncol. 2010 Aug; 21(8): 1712-1717.

Olivier KR, Schild SE, Morris CG, Brown PD & Markovic SN. A higher radiotherapy dose is associated with more durable palliation and longer survival in patients with metastatic melanoma. Cancer 2007; 110: 1791-1795.

Olsen G.Some views on the treatment of melanomas of the skin.Arch Chir Neerl. 1970;22(2):79-90.

Quaglino P, Mortera C, Osella-Abate S, Barberis M, Illengo M, Rissone M, Savoia P & Bernengo MG. Electrochemotherapy with intravenous bleomycin in the local treatment of skin melanoma metastases.Ann Surg Oncol. 2008 Aug;15(8):2215-22. Epub 2008 May 23.

Radny P, Caroli UM, Bauer J, Paul T, Schlegel C, Eigentler TK, Weide B, Schwarz M & Garbe C Phase II trial of intralesional therapy with interleukin-2 in soft-tissue melanoma metastases. Br J Cancer. 2003; 89: 1620-1626

Rosen T. Cutaneous metastases. Med Clin North Am 1980; 64: 885-900.

Rossi CR, Foletto M, Pilati P, Mocellin S & Lise M. Isolated limb perfusion in locally advanced cutaneous melanoma. Semin Oncol. 2002; 29: 400-409.

Rossi CR, Pasquali S, Mocellin S, Vecchiato A, Campana LG, Pilati P, Zanon A & Nitti D. Long-term results of melphalan-based isolated limb perfusion with or without low-dose TNF for in-transit melanoma metastases. Ann Surg Oncol. 2010 Nov; 17(11): 3000-3007. Epub 2010 Apr 29.

Saeed S, Keehn CA & Morgan MB. Cutaneous metastasis: a clinical, pathological, and immunohistochemical appraisal. J Cutan Pathol 2004; 31: 419–430.

Sariya D, Ruth K, Adams-McDonnell R, Cusack C, Xu X, Elenitsas R, Seykora J, Pasha T, Zhang P, Baldassano M, Lessin SR & Wu H. Clinicopathologic correlation of cutaneous metastases: experience from a cancer center. Arch Dermatol 2007; 143:613–620.

Sause WT, Cooper JS, Rush S, Ago CT, Cosmatos D, Coughlin CT, JanJan N & Lipsett J. Fraction size in external beam radiation therapy in the treatment of melanoma. Int J Radiat Oncol Biol Phys. 1991; 20: 429-32.

Savoia P, Fava P, Deboli T, Quaglino P & Bernengo MG. Zosteriform Cutaneous Metastases: A Literature Meta-Analysis and a Clinical Report of Three Melanoma Cases. Dermatol Surg. 2009; 35: 1355-1363.

Savoia P, Fava P, Nardò T, Osella-Abate S, Quaglino P & Bernengo MG. Skin metastases of malignant melanoma: a clinical and prognostic survey. Melanoma Res. 2009; 19: 321–326.

Schwartz RA. Cutaneous metastatic disease. J Am Acad Dermatol 1995; 33: 161–182.

Seegenschmiedt MH, Keilholz L, Altendorf-Hofmann A, Urban A, Schell H, Hohenberger W & Sauer R. Palliative radiotherapy for recurrent and metastatic malignant melanoma: prognostic factors for tumor response and long-term outcome: a 20-year experience. Int J Radiat Oncol Biol Phys. 1999; 44: 607-618.

Spencer PS & Helm TN. Skin metastases in cancer patients. Cutis 1987; 39: 119–121.

Strobbe LJ, Hart AA, Rümke P, Israels SP, Nieweg OE & Kroon BB. Topical dinitrochlorobenzene combined with systemic dacarbazine in the treatment of recurrent melanoma. Melanoma Res. 1997; 7: 507-512.

Tan JK & Ho VC. Pooled analysis of the efficacy of bacille Calmette-Guerin (BCG) immunotherapy in malignant melanoma. J Dermatol Surg Oncol. 1993; 19: 985-990.

Thompson JF, Hersey P & Wachter E. Chemoablation of metastatic melanoma using intralesional Rose Bengal. Melanoma Res. 2008 Dec; 18(6): 405-411.

Weide B, Eigentler TK, Pflugfelder A, Leiter U, Meier F, Bauer J, Schmidt D, Radny P, Pföhler C, Garbe C. Survival after intratumoral interleukin-2 treatment of 72 melanoma patients and response upon the first chemotherapy during follow-up. Cancer Immunol Immunother. 2010; Dec 21.

WHO. From *Handbook for Reporting Results of Cancer Treatment, vol 48;* Geneva, 1997

Wolf IH, Richtig E, Kopera D & Kerl H. Locoregional cutaneous metastases of malignant melanoma and their management. Dermatol Surg. 2004; 30: 244-247.

Part 2

Surgical Treatment of Melanoma

2

Management of Head and Neck Melanoma

James H F Shaw and Michael Fay
Auckland Hospital, Great Mercury Island
New Zealand

1. Introduction

The incidence of melanoma in New Zealand (NZ) is one of the highest in the world: The rate in Caucasians is approximately 50 per 100,000, while the incidence in the NZ Maori population and the NZ Polynesian population is much lower contributing 15% and 7% of the total number of melanoma reported annually (Shaw, 2008). The primary author has twenty-six years' Consultant Surgical experience with melanoma surgery. Our database goes back to 1984 and includes 3,500 patients, of which 550 patients have been managed for head and neck melanoma. We have included all patients with either head and neck primary melanoma or regional melanoma involving cervical regional nodes or parotid nodes managed in the Auckland area 1984-2005. No patients have been excluded. These Head & Neck melanoma (H&NMM) data have never been published in the world literature.
We reviewed our head and neck melanoma data base and this constitutes the basis of this study.

2. Background & methods

The head and neck area is a preferred site for melanoma; 9% of the body's surface area but 15% of the total melanoma distribution(Douglas & Shaw, 1987)
The outcome is probably less favourable in the head and neck area than in limbs or trunk (Douglas & Shaw, 1987) (Fisher & O'Brien, 2002). In addition, some head and neck sites are less favourable than others for example scalp, mucosal lesions tend to be less favourable than facial lesions (Douglas & Shaw, 1987; Fisher & O'Brien, 2002), further it is unclear whether melanomas from the trunk metastasising to cervical lymph nodes are more or less favourable than melanomas spreading to regional nodes with a head and neck primary.
Over the past 20 plus years for lesions < 1 mm in thickness we have used a 1 cm margin for lesions, > 2 mm thickness a 2 cm margin and for lesions between 1 and 2 mm thickness a margin of between 1 and 2 cm. The approach for thin lesions has been based on the work of Umberto Veronessi and colleagues (Veronessi et al, 1998), while our approach for thicker lesions has been validated in a prospective study by Merion Thomas and colleagues (Thomas et al, 2004).
Prior to the advent of sentinel node biopsy regional disease was treated with a therapeutic node dissection after positive fine needle aspirate cytology (FNA). Most commonly this was a selective neck dissection. Since the advent of sentinel node biopsy patients with a positive sentinel node have all been treated with either a selective or modified neck dissection depending upon the site of the primary lesion. After neck dissection virtually all patients

were offered radiotherapy and this was accepted by around half the patients. Nodal disease was classified N0 if no nodes were involved, N1 if one node was positive, N2 if 2-3 nodes were involved, and N3 if 4 or more nodes involved.

Survival was calculated using Kaplan Myer analysis while comparison between patient groups was performed using Chi squared analysis.

Questions asked of our data-base included assessment of :

a. Anatomical-site, sex, and primary thickness on outcome
b. Signficance of local and regional recurrence on outcome
c. Determine extent of neck dissection required as a function of primary anatomical site
d. Determine effect of adjuvant radiation following neck-dissection on regional re-recurrence and survival
e. Assess the outcome for patients with primary site that is:
   i. outside head and neck area
   ii. desmoplastic subtype and
   iii. mucosal subtype

3. Results

3.1 Anatomical distribution and thickness of primary lesions

The commonest H&N primary anatomical site was face (52%), followed by scalp (19%), neck (17%), ear (9%), and mucosal lesions (3 %).

37% of primary lesions were < 0.75 mm thick, 14% were 0.76-1.5 mm thick, 27% were 1.5 - 4.0 mm thick, and 23% were > 4.0 mm thick.

Predictably, as in other parts of the body, the thickness of the primary lesion governed outcome see Figure 1.

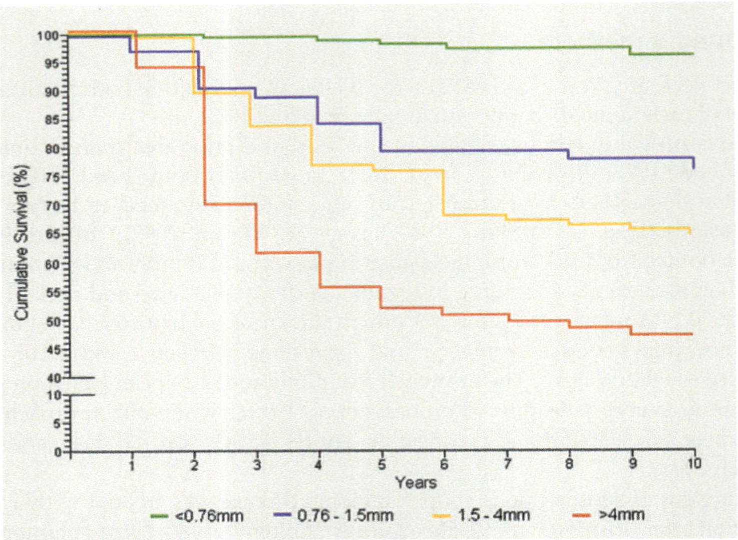

Fig. 1. Effect of Primary Thicknesses on Survival - Auckland

The sex incidence was higher in males than females and is summarised in Table 1:

Trunk primary lesions metastasising to cervical nodes, and scalp lesions, were significantly more common in males (p<0.05, and p<0.03 respectively). Ear lesions were almost twice as common in males as in females.

	Male	Female	Ratio
Face	140	126	1.1
Neck	49	40	1.2
Ear	28	15	1.9
Trunk	15	4	3.8*
Scalp	75	10	7.5 **
Total	307	195	1.6

Table 1. Sex Incidence Head & Neck Melanoma - Auckland

The effect of anatomical site on survival is shown in fig 2. Survival for facial lesions is significantly better than for neck lesions (p<.05) and for Scalp & ear lesions (p<.01).

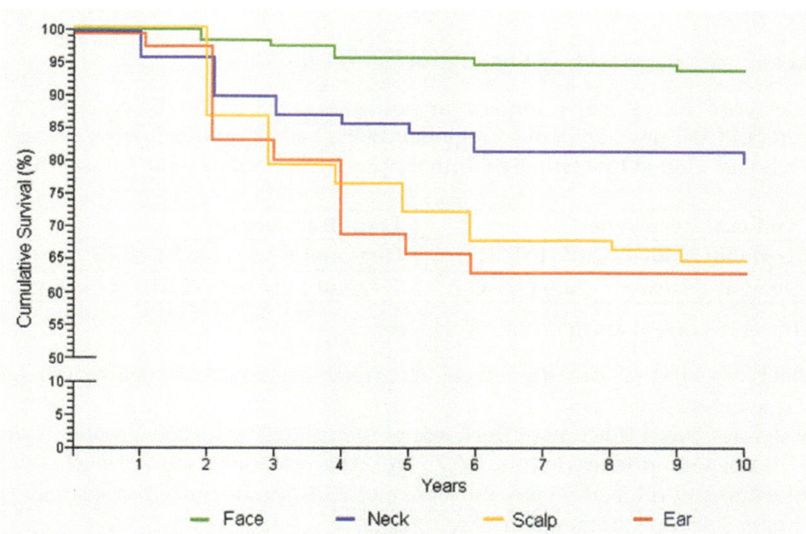

Fig. 2. Effect of Anatomical Site on Survival - Auckland

Local recurrence (LR) occurred in 5% for patients with facial, neck and ear lesions versus 13% for scalp lesions (p < 0.05) and 50% for mucosal lesions (p < 0.01). Local recurrence became progressively more common with increasing thickness of the primary lesion: see Table 2.

Thickness mm	**% Local Recurrence**	**Fraction**
< 0.76	**5%**	8/168
0.76 – 1.5	**11%**	7/62
1.5 – 4.0	**10%**	11/112
> 4	**20%**	20/99
Overall	**10%**	46/441

Table 2. Effect of Thickness on Local Recurrence – Auckland

The pie graph (Fig 3) outlines the most likely reasons for local recurrence and their relative frequencies.

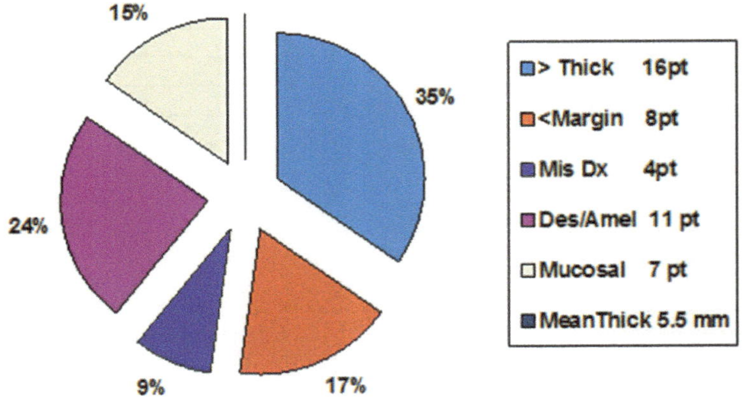

Fig. 3. Factors Associated with 46 Local Recurrences - Auckland

Local recurrence had a major impact on outcome in particular there was a significant increase in both the development of regional disease and also death from disease in those patients who developed LR compared with those who did not develop LR. see Table 3

No Local Recurrence	Local Recurrence
Regional Nodes 26% (97/425)	**Regional** Nodes 46%*21/46***
Dead of Disease 25% (99/425)	**Dead of Disease** 72%*** (33/46)****

Table 3. Local Recurrent & Outcome - Auckland

The impact on survival of either local recurrence or regional recurrence was almost identical: see Figure 3.

Regional disease was a function of thickness of the primary with 5% of patients developing regional disease with primary lesions < 0.75 mm. 25% of patients with primary lesions 0.76 – 1.5 mm thickness developed regional disease and 35% of patients with melanomas over 1.5 mm thickness developed regional disease.

The timing of regional disease was a function of the thickness of the primary melanoma. Patients who had regional disease at initial presentation had a mean primary thickness of over 6 mm, while patients who presented with progressively thinner primary lesions developed regional disease progressively later. see Table 4.

Timing of Nodes	10 Thickness	No of Nodes
@ Diagnosis	**6.2 +/- 1.2 mm**	2.1
@ 1-12 mths	**2.8 +/- 0.4 mm**	3.1
@ 12-48 mths	**1.9 +/- 0.3 mm**	2.8
@ 48 mths +	**1.3 +/- 0.5 mm**	2.2

Table 4. Timing of Nodal Disease v 1^0 Thickness - Auckland

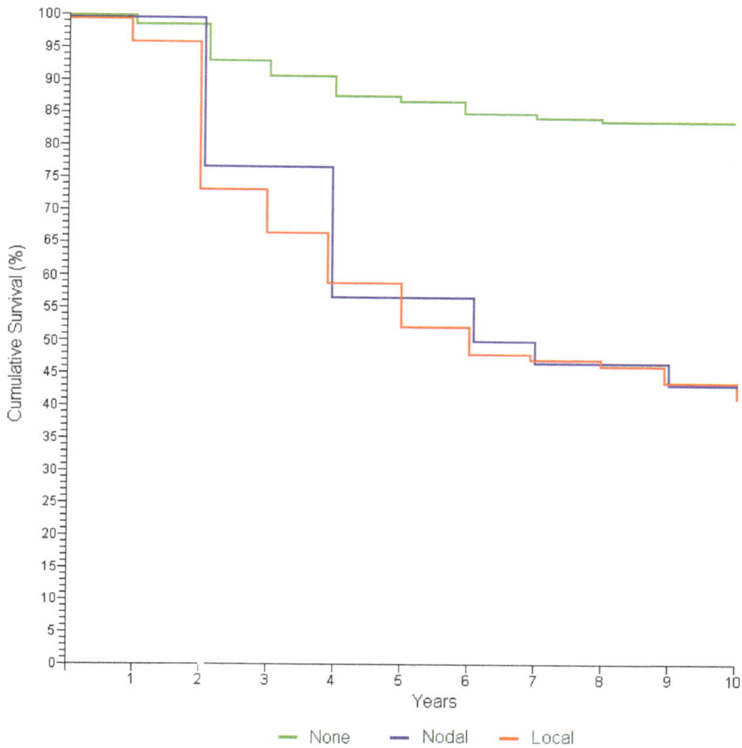

Fig. 3. Influence Local or Regional Recurrence on Survival - Auckland

Survival following the diagnosis of regional disease was not influenced by disease free interval. Although patients who had longer disease free intervals between initial diagnosis and the development of regional disease lived longer overall, once regional disease occurred the survival curves were not significantly different. See fig 4.

The sites of Regional Disease as a Function of anatomical site of the primary lesion are summarised in Table 5. The commonest sites of regional disease were level 2 nodes and parotid nodes.

	Ear n=14	Face n=41	Scalp n=39	Neck n=29	Total n=123
Parotid	**64%**	**46%**	**31%**	**10%**	**38%**
Level 1	-	11%	7%	21%	9%
Level 2	**50%**	**29%**	**30%**	**90%**	**50%**
Level ¾	7%	5%	**20%**	**67%**	**25%**
Level 5	-	5%	**28%**	**67%**	**25%**
Sub-occipital	-	-	**8%**	7%	4%
Post-auricular	-	-	**18%**	7%	6%

Table 5. Regional Disease v Anatomical Site of Melanoma – Auckland

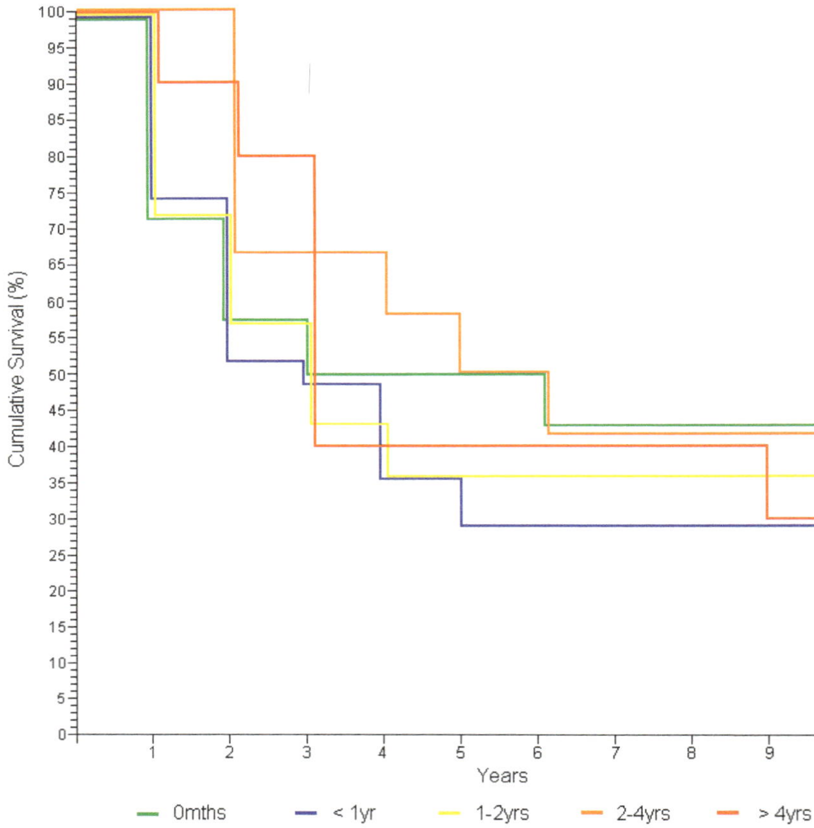

Fig. 4. Survival Node +ve Patients from Onset of Regional Disease - Auckland

3.2 Sentinel node studies

Our Sentinel node data were in general accord with the above data regarding site of regional disease as a function of anatomical site of the primary melanoma with Level 2 and Parotid being the commonest sites of involvement. The unusual findings from these studies were:

1. Bilateral or contralateral sentinel nodes in patients with lesion near the midline.
2. The frequent incidence of multiple sentinel nodes (up to 5)
3. The unpredictability of upper trunk lesions, for example spreading to contralateral Level 1.

See Discussion for detailed analysis of sentinel data with world literature.

3.3 Survival as a function of regional disease

Patients without regional disease (stage No) had 90% 5 year survival. Patients with only one node involved (stage N1), had 70% 5 yr survival, patients with stage N2 disease (2-3 nodes involved) had 57% 5 yr survival, while N3 patients with 4 or more nodes involved had 37% 5 yr survival. See Fig 5

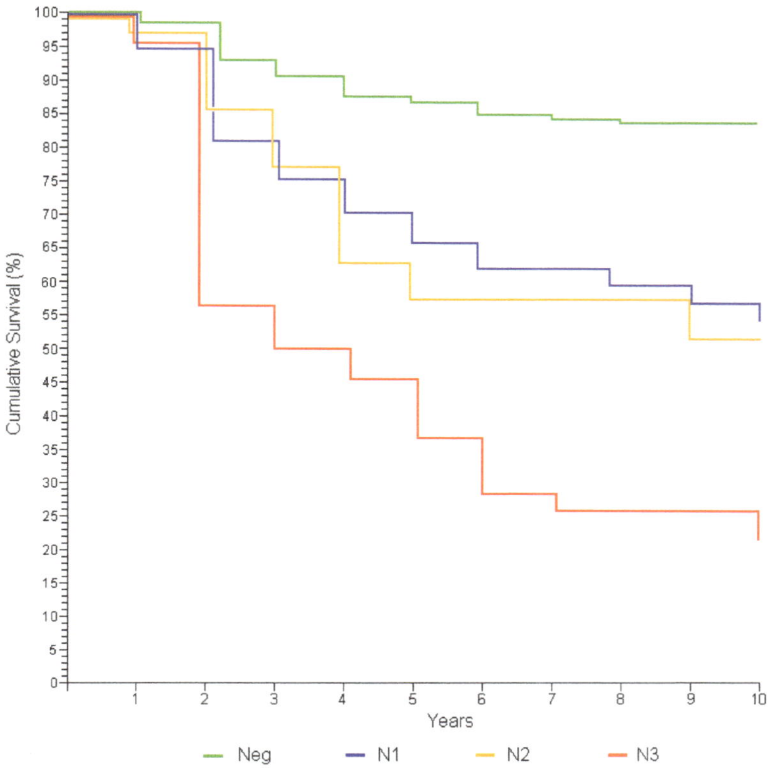

Fig. 5. Stage of Regional Disease & Survival - Auckland

3.4 Regional failure after neck dissection and the impact of radiation

Regional failure was dependent on the N status of the neck. The rate of failure in patients with N1 disease was 5%, N2 disease 17% and N3 disease 22%. These rates of regional failure were all decreased with radiation and these reached statistical significance for patients with N3 disease and for regional disease overall. See Table 6.

	% Failure no RT	% Failure with RT
N1	**11%** 1/19	**3%** 1/31
N2	**25%** 4/16	**9%** 2/22
N3	**38%** 8/21	**10%*** 2/20 $p < .04$
Overall	**28%** 13/46	**7%***** 5/71 $p < .002$

Table 6. Influence of RT on Recurrence after Neck Dissection

Although adjuvant radiation significantly decreased regional recurrence after neck dissection adjuvant radiation had no impact on survival: The Kaplan Meyer curves for survival after neck dissection alone versus neck dissection with radiation the curves were virtually super-imposed. See Fig 6

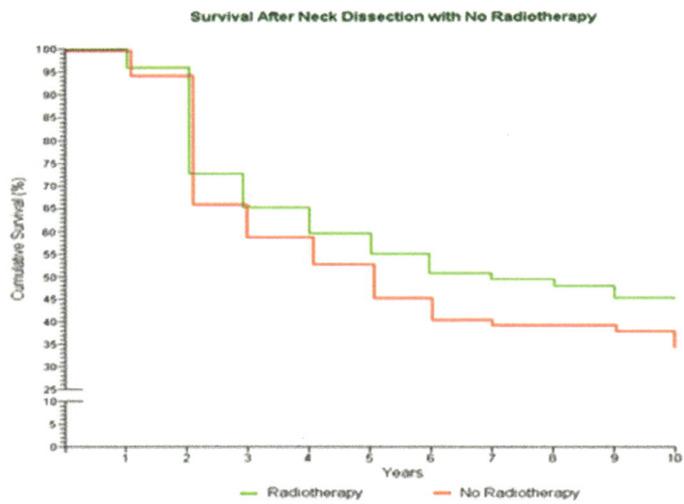

Fig. 6. Survival after neck dissection with and without Adjuvant radiation

3.5 Less common situations

3.5.1 Primary site unknown

There were nine patients in this group all with stage N2 or N3 disease with a 35% 5 year survival which was virtually identical when compared with the 5 year survival for the group of patients with N2 and N3 disease who had a known primary.

3.5.2 Cervical regional disease from primary site on trunk

There were 19 patients in this group, 14 had axillary and neck disease, 5 had neck disease alone. The mean number of nodes involved was was 11 (range 3-48). Neck Levels most commonly involved were:

Level 5: 14 patients
Level 4: 6 patients
Level 3: 4 patients
Level 1 or 2: 4 patients (including 1 patient with contralateral Level 1 disease)
The outcome was very poor with 15/19 patients dead of disease at five years. See Fig 7

3.5.3 Desmoplastic neurotropic melanoma

There were 19 patients in this group. The lesions were thick with a mean thickness of 3.5 mm. When the desmoplastic patient group were compared with patients with equivalent thickness lesions that were not desmoplastic: the local recurrence rate was higher in the desmoplastic group at 26% versus 7% ($p < 0.04$), while regional recurrence was lower in the desmoplastic group at 22% versus 47%. Death from disease was virtually identical in the two groups See Table 7.

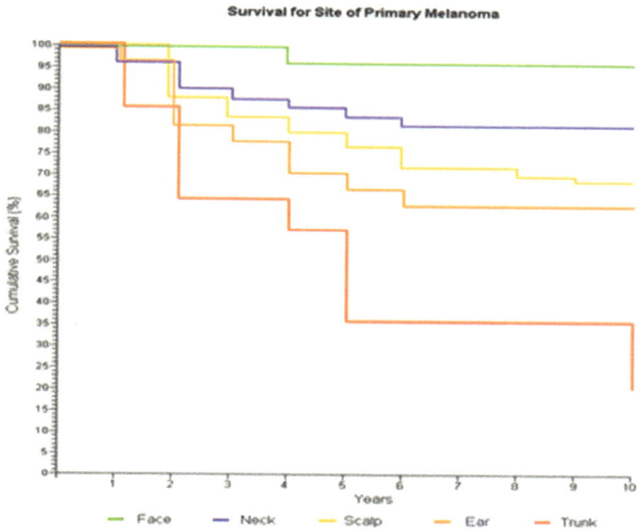

Fig. 7. Survival of Patients with Trunk Primary versus primary lesion in the Head and Neck

	Non Desmoplastic	Desmoplastic
Median Thickness	3.5 mm	4.1 mm
Local Recurrence	7% (20/261)	26%*** (9/19)
Regional Nodes	47%* 107/261)	22%* p.06 (4/19)
Dead of Disease	41% (8/19)	42% (95/261)

Table 7. Desmoplastic v Non-Desmoplastic Melanoma - Auckland - Stratified for Equivalent Thickness

3.5.4 Mucosal melanoma

There were 14 patients in this group. The commonest sites were conjuntival, oral and nasal. There were poor outcomes here even for very thin lesions. Seven of the 14 patients developed local recurrence and 5/14 were dead of disease at 5 years despite a mean thickness of only .3 mm.

4. Discussion

Our study is one of the largest studies of Head & Neck melanoma reported from a single centre. The single greatest experience is however from the Sydney Melanoma Unit (De Wilt et al, 2004; Fisher & O'Brien, 2002; Thompson et al, 2005), and we have compared and contrasted our experience with theirs along with various centres worldwide.

The data from Fisher S.R & O'Brien, C.J., 2002 are similar to ours with respect to anatomical site, sex-incidence. In addition outcome versus anatomical site were similar to reports of others with face and neck lesions having a more favourable outcome than scalp and ear. In addition the reason for these differences is largely explained on the basis of the face & neck lesions being thinner and therefore having a better outcome. Further, although H&NMM

was more common in males the two sites where the incidence was almost the same for males and females (Face and Neck) the outcome was better. We have previously shown that for melanoma overall when all sites are pooled the incidence in males and females is similar (Jones et al, 1999) and that overall males tend to have poorer outcomes than females especially older males (Jones et al, 1999; Shaw, 2008). Trunk and scalp lesions were significantly more common in males in our study: we have previously shown the highest incidence of melanoma in males is on the back (Jones et al, 1999), Scalp melanoma is most common in bald patients and there are more bald men than women (Douglas & Shaw, 1987; Jones et al, 1999).

The outcome for patients with desmoplastic melanoma (DM) is similar to that reported by Quinn and colleagues from the Sydney Melanoma Unit (Quin et al, 1998). In particular DM is associated with a relatively high incidence of LR coupled with a relatively low incidence of regional disease and when compared to non DM melanoma patients a similar risk of death. The relatively low rate of regional disease has some implications when considering the performance of sentinel node studies in patients with DM. Our data indicating that the outcome of patients with regional disease and primary site unknown is similar to patients with regional disease and primary site known when stratified for similar stage of regional disease are in general agreement with the literature (Santini et al, 1985).

Local recurrence (LR) in H&NMM has been reported to be more common than for limb melanomas (Douglas & Shaw, 1987; Jones et al, 1999; Ng et al, 2001). Our current findings are in agreement with this in a general sense, with the pie chart summarising the individual main causative factors, namely thickness of the primary, inadequate margin, unfavourable histological sub-type. We have previously documented the effect of tumour thickness and inadequate margin on local recurrence (Ng et al, 2001). In addition the studies by Balch and colleagues (Balch et al, 2001) have highlighted that tumour thickness is very reliable and an independent predictor of both recurrence and survival.

One sub-group where this rule of thickness being a reliable predictor of outcome is not useful is in patients with mucosal melanoma; the highest incidence of which is in the head and neck region (Tomicic & Wanebo, 2003). In our patients despite the medial thickness being only 1.3 mm the rates of recurrence and death from disease were markedly higher than for non- mucosal lesions of similar thickness. A variety of authors have underlined the poor prognosis associated with mucosal melanoma irrespective of either conservative or radical treatment involving surgery alone or combined with radiation (Tomicic & Wanebo, 2003), but the fact that even very thin lesions tend to recur appears to be relatively under-reported.

The implications of LR are substantial with approximately double the incidence of regional disease and approximately a three- fold risk of dying of melanoma. Further, the impact of LR and regional recurrence on survival were virtually identical. These findings are similar to those reported by O'Brien and colleagues (Fisher & O'Brien, 2002)

The regional nodes of significance when managing H&NMM are outlined in Fig 8. See below: In particular the nodes as classified by Memorial Sloan Kettering Cancer Centre (Shah et al., 1991) involving levels 1-5, along with intra-parotid nodes coupled with the post-auricular nodes and the Sub-occipital nodes highlighted by the SMU (De Wilt et al, 2004). In addition the axillary nodes are important especially for upper trunk lesions and lower neck lesions. The importance of primary lesions from trunk regional to the neck, and neck lesions regional to the axilla(e) has been relatively understudied but following the widespread use of sentinel node studies a far better understanding of H&N regional lymphatics has been developed, especially by Morton and colleagues at the John Wayne Cancer Centre (Morton et al, 2006) and Thomson and colleagues in Sydney Australia (De Wilt et al., 2004; Thompson et al., 2005).

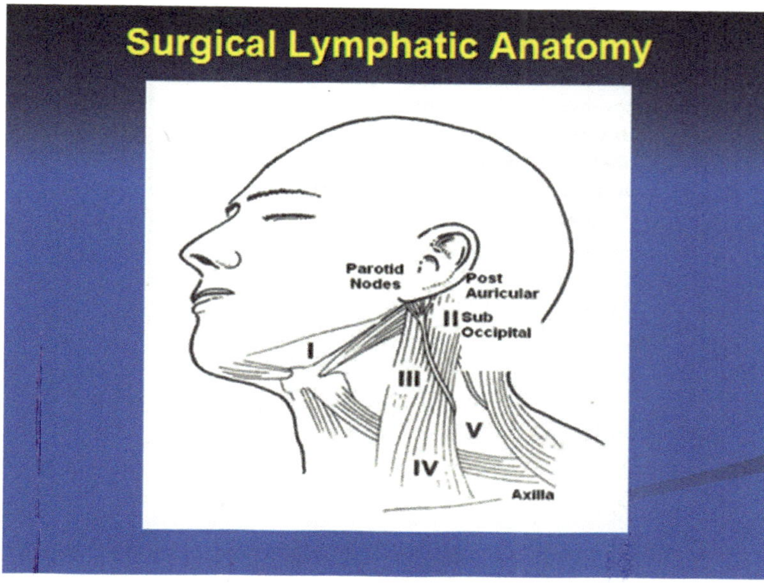

Fig. 8. Surgical Lymphatic Anatomy

Timing of regional failure in our study was a function of primary tumour thickness with patients who had regional disease at initial presentation had a mean primary thickness of over 6 mm, while progressively thinner primary lesions went on to be associated with region disease of several years: 3 mm lesions tending to recur regionally inside 1 yr, 2mm lesions recurring regionally most commonly in 1-4 yrs, and lesions 1-2 mm thick recurring most commonly later than 4 yrs. These findings are similar to those reported by O'Brien and Fischer (Fisher & O'Brien, 2002) and underline the capacity of even relatively thin melanomas to recur many years after initial diagnosis (Thompson et al., 2005). These finding also fit well with the findings of Balch and colleagues in 2001 (Balch et al., 1985). After analysing 10 yr survival data for over 15,000 melanoma patients with lesions in all anatomical sites, the 10 yr mortality increased steadily as a smooth curve as a function of primary thickness from approximately 20% for 1 mm lesions through to 70% mortality for lesions 10 mm thick. See Fig 9 below

For some malignancies disease free interval is an important prognostic factor (Fisher Fisher & O'Brien, 1998), however for melanoma the situation is less clear (Thompson et al., 2005). In our study although patients who developed regional progressively further along the course of their disease had a relative long absolute survival, once regional disease occurred the survival data curves from that time on were not significantly different between the various groups.

One very important but contentious issue in the surgical management of H&NMM patients is the extent of neck dissection which should be performed for regional disease as a function of the anatomical site of the primary melanoma. Shah and colleagues in 1991 (Shah et al., 1991) concluded that virtually all neck nodal levels along with the parotid nodes should be dissected in virtually all patients with H&NMM. Their data were based on therapeutic neck dissections for FNA diagnosed palpable regional disease. Their data are presented in modified format in Table 8

Site of Nodal Involvement v Anatomical Site

Shah et al., Amer J Surg, 1991

	Face	Ant Scalp	Ant Neck	Post Neck	Post Scalp	Ear
Parotid	44%	100%	33%	-	29%	83%
L1	48%	57%	13%	-	47%	27%
L2	48%	65%	50%	50%	60%	73%
L3,4	12%	50%	28%	25%	27%	41%
L5	20%	57%	-	30%	20%	27%

Table 8. Regional H& N Melanoma v Anatomical Site, Shah et al., Amer J Surg 1991

From the Shah data (Shah et al., 1991) one would conclude that virtually all patients with regional H&NMM require a Level 1-5 neck dissection and resection of parotid nodes. The exceptions being that posterior neck does not require parotidectomy (P) or dissection of Level 1, while anterior neck primary while requiring parotidectomy does not require dissection of Level 5 nodes, and only occasionally will level 1 nodes be involved.

Another major study addressing sites of regional disease as a function of anatomical primary melanoma site is that from the Sydney Melanoma Unit (SMU) (De Wilt et al., 2004). Their approach was a different one whereby 918 sentinel nodes were mapped in 362 patients with H&NMM. A modified assessment of their data is presented in Table 9 below.

The conclusions from the Sydney data are in general agreement with those of Shah and colleagues (Shah et al., 1991) whereby:

1. Ear primary requires P, and Levels 2-5 neck dissection, but in contrast to Shah (Shah et al., 1991) level 1 would not require dissection
2. Face primary requires P and Levels 1-4 , but in contrast to Shah (Shah et al., 1991) who found 20% of facial lesions involved L5
3. Anterior scalp requires P and Levels 1-4 and possibly L5 also as 10% chance of involvement at SMU versus 57% involvement at MSKCC.
4. Anterior neck requires Levels 1-5 but not P while Shah (Shah et al., 1991) found 33% had parotid involvement but no L5 disease

918 Sentinel nodes in 362 Melanoma Patients
SMU Ann Surg 2004

	Parotid	L1	L2	L3 / 4	L5	S O	P A	Axilla
Ear	36%	-	90%	12%	27%	-	21%	-
Face	57%	48%	70%	20%	-	-	-	-
P Scalp	14%	-	47%	18%	59%	39%	32%	-
C Scalp	50%	-	70%	10%	30%	20%	50%	-
C Neck	17%	20%	80%	24%	40%	-	-	-
A Scalp	80%	-	90%	-	10%	-	35%	
A low Neck	-	-	28%	21%	77%	-	-	43%
A up Neck	-	13%	63%	38%	25%	-	-	-
P low Neck	-	-	14%	28%	100%	18%	-	23%
P up Neck	11%	-	72%	15%	56%	16%	-	-

Table 9. 918 Sentinel Nodes in 362 Melanoma Partients

5. Posterior neck requires Levels 2-5 neck dissection with P only rarely required, concurring with while Shah (Shah et al., 1991)
6. Posterior scalp requires levels 2-5 neck dissection with only 14% chance of P being required, while Shah (Shah et al., 1991) found level 1 involved in 47% & and Parotid in 29% of patients.

The SMU data (14) also highlight the importance of the post-auricular and the Sub-occipital nodes especially for patients with Ear, Scalp, and posterior neck lesions. These were not assessed in the Shah data (Shah et al., 1991).

Our own data agree with Shah (Shah et al., 1991) that: L1 does not usually require dissection for ear primary

Our data are in agreement with SMU 14(15) :

1. Face does not usually require dissection of L5
2. L1 only rarely involved aside from face and neck primary lesions

Our data are in agreement with both MSKCC and SMU that neck lesions require a L2-5 dissection and occasional inclusion for dissection of L1 and P depending on the site of the neck primary. Our data also highlight the importance of upper trunk lesions spreading to cervical nodes, and the fact that these lesions have an especially bad prognosis as most patients have N2 or N3 disease often with involvement of both cervical nodes and one or more axilla. The importance of trunk lesions involving neck nodes, and the associated bad prognosis has been relatively understudied in the literature. The principal levels involved by trunk primary melanoma are levels 5 followed by levels 4, but occasionally levels 3,2,and 1 are involved. In addition for mid line lesions especially contralateral disease in unexpected sites may occur. In our study the outcome for trunk lesions that metastasised to cervical nodes either alone or in combination with axillary disease is markedly worse than for acral lentigenous melanoma, a known poor prognosis subtype which we have reported on previously (Koea & Shaw, 1988)

In order to provide a guidline for management of the neck in H&NMM we have modified the figure from O'Brien and colleagues (O'Brien, 1999) to provide some general rules regarding extent of neck dissection as a function of primary anatomical site. See Fig 9

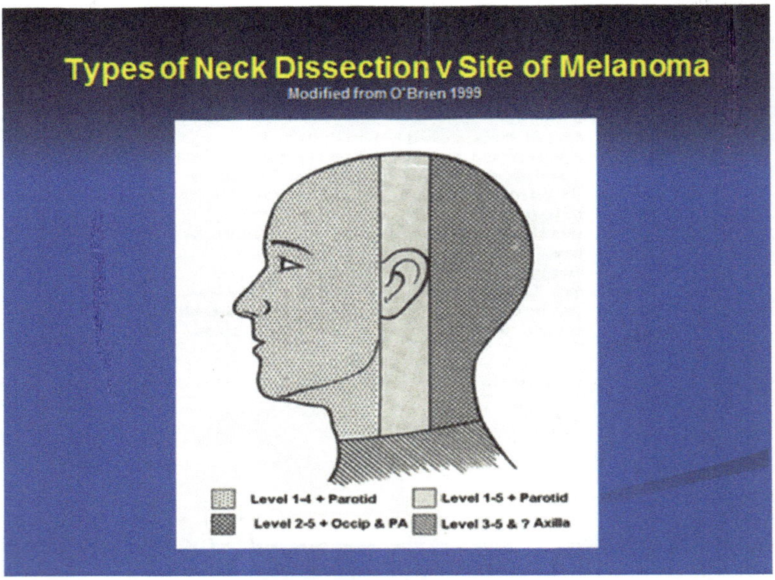

Fig. 9. Types of Neck Dissection v Site of Melanoma

There are a number of provisos to be incorporated with this figure based on our findings and those from SMU (15) and MSKCC (14). These include:

1. The risk of contralateral and bilateral regional disease with primary melanomas close to midline
2. Level 1 is not often involved but occasionally may be involved from as far away as posterior trunk and rarely bilateral
3. Trunk lesions may require dissection of more than levels 4 and 5, and involvement of one or both axillae must be excluded either by sentinel node study or imaging

Results predicting regional disease levels as a function of anatomical site of primary may be different when data from sentinel node studies are compared with studies from therapeutic neck dissection data. Also the extent of the neck dissection performed is also important for example; in our study selective dissection was frequently used in our patients whereas in the Shah (Shah et al., 1991) data many patients underwent either conservative or radical neck dissection. In addition spread of melanoma cells along involved lymphatic channels may be different compared to the distribution of tracer as part of a sentinel node study in a clinically uninvolved neck.

Survival as a function of extent of regional disease in our study is similar to what has been reported by others (Balch et al., 2001; Fisher & O'Brien, 2002; O'Brien, 1999). One common finding across centres is the dramatic drop-off in survival between N1 -N2 disease and N3 disease. The reason for this being that the maximum number of nodes involved in N2 patients is 3 while some patients with N3 disease may have 20 or more nodes involved. See Table 10

Regional Disease 5 yr Survival

	NZ	UAB	SMU	Duke	MDA	Overall
N1	64%	53%	40%	-	39%	50%
N2	57%	48%	-	-	39%	49%
N3	36%	27%	12%		23%	25%
Overall	48%	43%	38%	45%	35%	42%

Table 10. Regional Disease 5y Survival

NZ: New Zealand
UAB: University of Alabama
Duke: Duke University
MDA: MD Anderson Cancer Clinic, Texas
In more detail the results of O'Brien and others (20) are summarised in Table 11 below:

Neck Dissection for Melanoma

O'Brien et al W J Surg 16:222, 1992

- 152 Therapeutic neck dissections
- 28% Re - recurrence in neck
- 34% 10 yr Survival
- 67% if node –ve
- Postoperative RT: multiple nodes or ECS

Table 11. Neck Dissection for Melanoma – (O'Brien et al., 1992)

The role of adjuvant radiation to minimise recurrence after neck disease is debated in the literature. We offered the majority of patients adjuvant radiation while many clinicians offer radiation only for patients with multiple nodes or if extra-nodal spread is present (eg 20).

While the role of adjuvant radiation will only be totally resolved by a prospective randomised study some important findings emerge from our data. Firstly we were able to show a significant reduction in recurrence in patients who received adjuvant radiation, especially those with N3 disease. O'Brien (O'Brien et al., 1997) was also able to demonstrate a reduction in recurrence but this fell short of statistical significance (just). Our overall re-recurrence rate of 28% in patients who did not receive adjuvant radiation is similar to the figure reported by O'Brien et al (O'Brien et al., 1997) and lower than many reports (O'brien et al., 1997). The dramatic decrease in recurrence in our patient both with N3 disease and regional disease overall is in agreement with the findings of Ang and colleagues (Ang et al., 1994) from the MD Anderson unit in Texas. Ang and colleagues (Ang et al., 1994) were able to demonstrate a dramatic reduction in recurrence when neck dissection was followed with adjuvant radiation compared with historic control data where surgery alone was used. Incidently they were also able to demonstrate that adjuvant radiation also reduction in recurrence following excision of prognostically unfavourable primary melanomas. For many years melanoma was considered to not be a radio-responsive tumour but this is now largely refuted (Mendenhall et al., 2008). The fact that adjuvant radiation decreased regional recurrence in our study while not influencing survival makes good sense from the surgical oncology standpoint. Adjuvant radiation is well known to minimise recurrence following neck dissection for squamous cell carcinoma (Fisher & O'Brien, 1998), and adjuvant radiation has been shown to minimise recurrence following anterior resection for rectal cancer (Fisher & O'Brien, 1998), and also minimise recurrence in some patients following surgery for Breast cancer, but in most of these circumstance this decrease in recurrence does not translate into improved survival.

We have not presented data addressing complications in this present study. We have previously presented a comparison between our complications for node dissection in the neck, the axilla, and groin (Shaw & Rumball, 1990). In that study the complication rate following neck dissection and axillary dissection was similar and in both sites was markedly lower than following neck dissection. In addition the complications associated with the addition of adjuvant radiation was lower in the neck than in the two other sites.

5. Conclusions and recommendations

1. The head and neck area is a preferred site for melanoma and has an unfavourable outcome in comparison to the rest of the body with respect to local recurrence and death from disease.
2. There is a complex lymphatic system and both the performance of sentinel node studies in the head and neck area and their analysis is more complex than in the trunk or limbs. Unpredicted sites of sentinel nodes are more common in the head & neck region than in the rest of the body.
3. The timing of regional disease in H&NMM is important. Patients who had palpable regional disease at the time of initial presentation had an average primary thickness over 6 mm. Patients with progressively thinner primary lesions developed regional disease over subsequent years with the general rule being the thicker the primary the more quickly regional disease developed. Many of these patients were assessed prior to the use of sentinel node mapping and this will probably detect patients likely to recur especially in the first year after initial diagnosis of melanoma. Prolonged disease-free interval does not appear to be a favourable prognostic factor once regional disease has occurred.

4. Management of regional disease can often be accomplished using a selective neck dissection, the regional beds requiring resection can be assessed as a function of the primary site of the melanoma. In particular:
   a. For anterior scalp and face parotidectomy plus levels I-IV neck dissection.
   b. For coronal lesions including scalp and ear parotidectomy and levels I-V neck dissection.
   c. For posterior scalp and posterior neck level II-V neck dissection.
   d. For trunk lesions with cervical regional disease Level 4 & 5 neck dissection is appropriate, often in association with one or more axillary dissections.
   e. Recommendations for sites of regional disease that should be resected for various primary melanoma sites are summarised in Fig 7. It is important to note that this is just a guideline as sites of regional disease are unpredictable. In particular upper back lesions involving cervical nodes can occasionally involve as far away as level 1, while primary lesions close to the midline (either head and neck or upper trunk primary) have a tendency to involve either contralateral nodes or bilateral nodes.
   d. The post -auricular nodes and sub- occipital nodes have to be considered in for patients with posterior scalp, coronal scalp and ear lesions and to a lesser extent with patients with posterior neck lesions.
5. Desmoplastic melanoma, mucosal melanoma, and melanoma from trunk metastasising to neck have a relatively poor prognosis. Desmoplastic lesions tend to have relatively low rates of regional disease and relatively high rates of local recurrence resulting in survival similar to non-desmoplastic melanomas. Trunk melanomas metastasising to the neck usually represent N3 disease (occasionally N2) as a result of one or more axillary nodal beds also being involved. In addition trunk lesions, especially those close to the mid-line are one of the least predictable in terms of where they are likely to spread in the neck. Further, while outcome for most melanomas is a function of primary melanoma thickness the exception to this rule is mucosal melanoma where even thin lesions are often lethal.
6. Adjuvant radiation after neck dissection appears to minimises recurrence in the neck but does not appear to impact on survival. A prospective trial would be required to clarify this for certain.

6. References

Ang, K.K., Peters, L.H., Weber, R.S., et al. (1994). Postoperative radiotherapy for cutaneous melanoma of the head and neck region. *International Journal Radiation Oncology Biology Physics*, Vol. 30, pp.(795-798)

Balch, C.M., Soong S.J., Gershenwald, J.E. et al. (2001). Prognostic factors: analysis of 17,600 melanoma patients. *Journal of Clinical Oncology*, Vol. 19, pp.(3622-9)

Douglas, R.G., Shaw J.H.F.(1987). Melanoma of the Head and Neck in Auckland. *New Zealand Medical Journal*, Vol. 100, No. 584-7

De Wilt, J.H., Thompson, J.F., Uren, R.F. et al. (2004) Correlation between preoperative lymphoscintigraphy and metastatic nodal disease sites in 362 patients with cutaneous melanoma of the head and neck, *Annals of Surgery*, Vol. 239, pp.(544-552)

Fisher, S.R., O'Brien, C.J. (2002). *Head and Neck Melanoma. In Cutaneous Melanoma.* 3rd Edition, EdBalch CM, Houghton AN, Sober AJ, Quality Medical Publishing St Louis Missouri.

Jones, W.O., Harman, R., Shaw, J.H.F. (1999). Incidence of malignant melanoma in Auckland New Zealand: highest rates in the world. *World Journal of Surgery*, Vol. 23, pp.(732-5)

Koea, J.B., Shaw, J.H.F. (1988). Acral Lentigenous melanoma in Auckland New Zealand, *British Journal of Surgery*, Vol. 75, pp.(69-72)

Lee, R.J., Gibbs, J.F., Proulx, G.M., et al. (2000). Nodal basin recurrence following lymphadenectomy. *International Journal of Radiation Oncology Biology Physics*, Vol. 48, pp. (1267-1273)

Mendenhall, W.M., Amdur, W.M., Grobmyer, R.J. (2008). Adjuvant radiotherapy for cutaneous melanoma, *Cancer* Vol. 112, pp. (1198-96)

Moffat, F.L., Ketcham, A.S. (2006). Surgery for malignant neoplasia. *In Cancer Surgery* Editor: McKenna, R.J., & Murphy, G.P., pp.(1-20), JB Lippincott, Phil

Morton, D.L., Thompson, J.F., Cochrane, A.J., et al. (2006). Sentinel node biopsy or nodal observation in melanoma, *New England Journal of Medicine*, Vol. 355, pp.(1307-17)

Ng, A.K., Jones, W.O., Shaw, J.H. (2001). Analysis of local recurrence and optimizing excision margins for cutaneous melanoma. *British Journal of Surgery*, Vol. 88, pp. (137-42)

O'Brien, C.J. (1999). *Personal communication*, Royal Australasian college of Surgeons Auckland, New Zealand

O'Brien, C.J., et al. (1992). Neck dissection for melanoma, *World Journal of Surgery*, Vol. 16, pp.(222-229)

O'Brien, C.J., Petersen-Schaefer, K., Stevens, G.N., Bass, P.C., Tew, P., Gebski, V.J., Thompson, J.F., McCarthy, W.H. (1997). *Adjuvant radiotherapy following neck dissection and parotidectomy for metastatic malignant melanoma*. Head & Neck. pp.(589-94)

Quin, M.J., Crotty, K.A., Thompson, J.F., et al. (1998). Desmoplastic and desmoplastic neurotropic melanoma: experience with280 patients. *Cancer* Vol. 83, pp.(1128-1135)

Santini H., Byers, R.M., Wolf, P.F. (1985). Melanoma metastatic to cervical and parotid nodes from an unknown primary site. *American Journal of Surgery*, Vol. 150, pp.(510-52)

Shah, J.P., Kraus, D.H., Dubner, S. (1991) Patterns of regional lymph node metastases from cutaneous melanomas of the head and neck. *American Journal of Surgery*, Vol. 162, pp.(320-324)

Shaw, J.H.F., Rumball, E.M. (1990) Complications and recurrence following lymphadenectomy, *British Journal of Surgery*, Vol. 77, pp.(761-763)

Shaw, J.H.F. (2008). Melanoma in New Zealand: a problem that is not going away. *Journal of the New Zealand Medical Association*, Vol. 121, No: 1279

Tomicic, J., Wanebo, H. (2003). Mucosal melanomas. *Surgical Clinics of North America*. Vol. 83, pp.(237-251)

Thomas, J.M., Newton Bishop, J., Ahern, R. et al (2004) Excision margins in high risk melanoma. *New England Journal of Medicine*, Vol. 27, pp.(350-355)

Thompson, J.F., Scolyer, R.A., Kefford, R.F. (2005) Cutaneous Melanoma, *The Lancet*, Vol. 365, pp.(687-96)

Veronessi, U., Cascinelli N., Adamus, J. et al. (1998), Thin stage 1 primary cutaneous, malignant melanoma: comparison of excision margins of 1 and 3 cm. *New England Journal of Medicine*, Vol. 318, pp.(1159-1162)

3

Impact of Sentinel Node Biopsy on Outcome in Melanoma

Justin Kelly and MJ Kerin
Dept of Academic Surgery, UCHG /NUIG, Galway, Ireland

1. Introduction

The worldwide incidence of malignant melanoma is increasing at an alarming rate. The importance of diagnosing nodal metastatic disease has impacted significantly on the accurate staging and stratification of melanoma patients. As a minimally invasive procedure with low morbidity, sentinel lymph node mapping allows for a detailed histopathologic evaluation involving multiple sections, H&E staining in combination with immunohistochemical staining of the node with the highest chance of containing metastatic foci. Controversy exists regarding the appropriate selection of patients for sentinel lymph node biopsy, particularly among patients with thin melanomas (< 1 mm Breslow thickness), thick melanomas (> 4 mm Breslow thickness), locally recurrent melanoma, nodular melanomas and those affecting the head and neck region. Furthermore, debate continues with regard to false-negative rates, managing in-transit disease, therapeutic benefit and alternatives, such as ultrasound guided biopsy.

In malignant melanoma, no standard systemic adjuvant therapy with confirmed impact on overall survival has been identified thus far for clinically node negative stage I-II patients after excision of the primary, or for clinically node positive stage III patients after lymph node dissection for metastatic regional node involvement. Thus some argue about the initial merits of performing the sentinel node procedure at all.

The aims of this book chapter are

1. to examine the impact of sentinel node biopsy on outcome in melanoma,
2. determine the effect, if any, of stage migration in melanoma
3. to clarify the impact of the different clinical sites on outcome,
4. to ascertain the reasons behind a lack of universal adoption of sentinel node biopsy in melanoma and
5. to critically assess other emerging strategies in the management of melanoma including frozen section analysis of the sentinel node, imprint cytology of the sentinel node, targeted assessment of the regional lymph node basin, the use of risk stratification algorithms of histological factors of the primary tumour and microRNAs.

2. Impact of sentinel node biopsy on outcome in melanoma

The key to survival for patients with melanoma is early detection and treatment of metastatic disease as this may improve disease-free and overall survival rates (Pacifico,

Grover, and Sanders 2004). The status of the regional lymph node basin has been widely shown to be the most important prognostic indicator for patients diagnosed with cutaneous melanoma (Balch et al. 2001). The disease-free survival and overall survival is dependent on the initial disease burden, thus melanomas less than 1mm rarely metastasise while at least 25% of melanomas between 1.5 and 4.0mm and greater than 60% of melanomas greater than 4.0mm thick will have lymph node metastases at presentation (Balch et al. 2001). The disease also depends heavily on the stage at presentation. Patients with early stage disease (i.e. < 1mm thick) achieve long-term survival in more than 90% of cases. However, patients with melanomas greater than 1.0mm thickness have survival rates ranging from 50%-90% (Balch et al. 2001).

The introduction of the sentinel lymph node biopsy (SLNB) technique for the evaluation of patients with truncal and extremity melanoma by Morton et al in 1992 showed that the status of the SLN accurately represented the status of the entire nodal basin from which it was obtained. This study highlighted a novel technique of identifying patients with occult nodal metastasis who warranted possible further therapeutic lymphadenectomy and adjuvant therapy, whilst also sparing the remaining 80% of patients without regional disease the morbidity associated with a formal lymphadenectomy procedure (Morton et al. 1992).

The benefits to performing SLNB versus elective lymphadenectomy are well supported (Pawlik, Ross, and Gershenwald 2004). SLNB is associated with less morbidity and is cheaper to perform (Wrightson et al. 2003). Historically two studies showed a survival benefit in patients who had SLNB performed (Dessureault et al. 2001; Kretschmer et al. 2004). Furthermore a positive sentinel node, Breslow thickness, age and male gender were all independent predictors of overall survival on multivariate analysis (Kretschmer et al. 2004).

The proven benefits for performing SLNB at the time of oncological wide local excision of a primary melanoma in any patient, include both prognostic and staging information, the potential therapeutic impact of a completion lymph node dissection in those with a positive SLN and also has implications of SLN status for adjuvant therapy decisions or entry into pertinent clinical trials. Because the status of the regional lymph nodes is the most single important prognostic factor for patients with melanoma, obtaining this information is essential (Shaw et al. 1985).

The preliminary findings of the MSLT-1 trial (Multicentre Selective Lymphadenectomy Trial) represent the first randomised prospective clinical study to show a potential survival advantage to performing sentinel lymph node biopsy in patients with melanoma (Morton et al. 2006). The study included 1269 patients with intermediate thickness (1.2-3.5mm) primary melanomas randomised to either a wide local excision and observation of regional lymph nodes with lymph node dissection if nodal relapse occurred (n=500) or to a wide local excision and SLNB with immediate regional lymphadenectomy if nodal micrometastases were found (n=769).

There was no difference in overall 5-year melanoma-specific survival rate; 87.1% for the SLNB and 86.6% in the control arm. However, the study did show improved disease-free survival in those patients who underwent the SLNB compared to those in the nodal observation arm group; the 5-year survival rate for node positive melanoma was 72.3 ± 4.6% and 90.2 ± 1.3% in the node negative group (hazard ratio for death, 2.48; 95% confidence interval, 1.54 to 3.98; $P < 0.001$).

The incidence of sentinel-node micrometastases was 16.0% and the rate of nodal relapse in the observation group was 15.6%. The corresponding mean number of tumour-involved

nodes was 1.4 in the biopsy group and 3.3 in the observation group (P<0.001), indicating disease progression during observation. Among patients with nodal metastases, the 5-year survival rate was higher among those who underwent immediate lymphadenectomy than among those in whom lymphadenectomy was delayed (72.3+/-4.6% vs. 52.4+/-5.9%; hazard ratio for death, 0.51; 95% confidence interval, 0.32 to 0.81; P=0.004) (Morton et al. 2006). The study authors concluded that the staging of intermediate-thickness (1.2 to 3.5 mm) primary melanomas according to the results of SLNB provided important prognostic information. However, the study did not show a clear survival advantage associated with SLNB.
Further subset analysis from MSLT-1 comparing patients with a positive SLNB + immediate lymphadenectomy versus those in the nodal observation group showed that there was significant progression to more advanced nodal disease in the nodal observation group and more importantly that there was a significant survival advantage in those undergoing immediate lymphadenectomy.
In order to appreciate the full potential applicability of the results from MSLT-1, it is important to consider the results from the WHO Truncal Melanoma international multicentre randomised trial which examined the use of early elective lymph node dissection (ELND) at the time of WLE of truncal melanomas > 1.5mm versus delayed lymphadenectomy until appearance of regional-node metastases (Balch et al. 2000). Firstly, this trial in addition to one carried out in Europe and published 2 years before (Cascinelli et al. 1998) under the title of WHO Melanoma Programme, did show a trend for improved survival in those patients who had ELND at the time of WLE, however this was not significant. But they did show improved 5-year survival rates in patients with occult regional node metastases 48% versus 27% in patients in whom the regional node dissection was delayed until the time of appearance of regional node metastases, which indeed was significant. The patients with regional nodes that became clinically and histologically positive during follow-up had the poorest prognosis. They concluded that SLNB may become a tool to identify patients with occult node metastases, who could then undergo node dissection (Balch et al. 2000).
These same authors showed that nodal micrometastatic deposits detected by the SLNB will become clinically relevant disease eventually therefore the logic of removing these involved lymph node deposits early may improve patient prognosis (Morton, Cochran, and Thompson 2007). Numerous reasons are cited in an article by Ross et al detailing exactly why the microscopic metastases in sentinel lymph nodes would most likely progress to palpable disease if left intact (Ross and Gershenwald 2008).
Most recently, an international panel comprising a cross section of expert melanoma surgeons who have contributed data and leadership to further investigate the role of SLNB in melanoma recently produced a consensus statement, outlining their overall interpretation of current evidence, as a guide to clinical treatment of patients with clinically localized melanoma. They agreed that SLNB is standard of care in current practice because it is incorporated in staging guidelines from the AJCC, incorporated in the treatment guidelines from the National Comprehensive Cancer Network, and practiced by most specialty surgeons who treat melanoma in the United States, Australia and Western Europe (Balch et al. 2009).

3. Stage migration effect

Oncologically, the prognosis for malignant disease is largely determined by the metastatic potential of the primary tumour. Some authors argue that we cannot alter prognosis by early detection and surgical intervention of involved regional nodes, highlighting the balance between nihilistic pre-determinism and active management. As an oncological community, we have a greater understanding of the mechanisms of action for haematological spread versus lymphatic spread. For many malignancies we know that regional lymphadenectomy improves survival. As to just how far this lymph node dissection is directly therapeutic remains a persistent source of controversy in melanoma.

Many believe that stage-adjusted survival benefit is due in part to the phenomenon of stage migration (*Will Rodgers phenomenon*). In medical stage migration, improved detection of illness (eg when newer technology allows for more sensitive detection of tumour spread) leads to the movement of people from the set of healthy people to the set of unhealthy people. Because these people are not healthy, removing them from the set of healthy people increases the average lifespan of the healthy group. Likewise, the migrated people are healthier than the people already in the unhealthy set, so adding them raises the average lifespan of that group as well. Both lifespan are statistically lengthened, even if early detection of a cancer does not lead to better treatment - because it is detected earlier, more time is lived in the "unhealthy" set of people. It was originally described in 1985 (Feinstein, Sosin, and Wells 1985). Rodgers' original quote -"When the Okies left Oklahoma and moved to California, they raised the average intelligence level in both states" - illustrates the theme. It has been shown that stage migration is responsible at least in part for an apparent improvement in survival for patients with stage III and IV non–small cell lung cancer in the era of PET scanning (Chee et al. 2008). It has also been demonstrated in urological, prostate and laryngeal malignancies (Albertsen et al. 2005; Champion and Piccirillo 2004; Gofrit et al. 2008). A large population-based study assessing the surgical treatment trends for 18449 patients with melanoma in the era of sentinel node biopsy using a SEER database concluded that stage migration is evident with increasing use of SLN biopsy (Cormier et al. 2005).

Furthermore, the theme underlying this phenomenon may no longer be confined to interpreting oncology trials as its' use has been cited in other paramedical arenas including healthcare economics. Young et al studied the measured differences in health care utilisation across an indemnity and managed care plan, finding that apparent increases in utilisation in both plans disappeared when viewed together, reflecting the migration of sicker patients from indemnity to managed care plans (Young et al. 1999).

4. Impact of histological site on outcome

While SLNB has a defined role in cutaneous melanomas of the trunk and extremities, several questions remain unanswered with respect to its application in the head and neck region. These account for up 21% of all melanomas diagnosed annually (Gillgren et al. 2000; Golger et al. 2007; Lachiewicz et al. 2008), have worse outcomes relative to melanomas of the trunk and extremities (Gillgren et al. 2000; Lachiewicz et al. 2008), clinically manifest as thicker lesions at their initial diagnosis and thus present at an advanced stage (Gillgren et al. 2000; Hoersch, Leiter, and Garbe 2006). SLNB for melanomas of the head and neck regions is limited by technical difficulties with specific concern surrounding damage to vital structures such as the facial nerve (Eicher et al. 2002). There is growing concern surrounding the reliability of the SLN to accurately predict the disease status of the entire nodal basin. In the head and neck region, the complexity and variability of the interlacing network of cervical lymphatics was highlight by O'Brien et al who showed a 34% discordance rate between the clinical prediction of lymphatic drainage and lymphoscintigraphy findings in 97 cases of cutaneous melanoma of the head and neck (O'Brien et al. 1995). A recent study from the John Wayne Cancer Institute reported a 'false negative' rate of 8.9%, identifying increasing tumour thickness, the presence of ulceration and head/neck primary tumours as risk factors for the development of recurrence in the presence of a negative node (Gershenwald et al. 1998). A recent study from the Sydney Melanoma Unit showed that up to 30% of patients with lymph node metastases from neck melanomas bypass the nearest node and involve nodes at more distant sites (Pathak et al. 2001), so called "skip metastases".

Numerous studies have evaluated the survival differences between head and neck melanoma versus those of the trunk and extremities and have found that those with melanoma of the head and neck have relatively poorer outcome (Gillgren et al. 2000; Lachiewicz et al. 2008; Thorn et al. 1989).

Specifically in a study involving 51,704 patients with melanoma, 5- and 10-year Kaplan-Meier survival probabilities for scalp/neck melanoma were 83.1% and 76.2%, respectively, compared with 92.1% and 88.7%, respectively, for melanoma of the other sites, including extremities, trunk, face, and ears. They found that patients with melanoma of the scalp/neck had an 84% greater chance of melanoma-related death compared with those with melanomas of the extremity (Lachiewicz et al. 2008). Within this head and neck group, another large population-based study involving 27,097 patients to evaluate tumour location as a prognostic factor in patients with head and neck melanoma (using the Surveillance, Epidemiology, and End Results (SEER) database), showed a 10-year overall survival rate of 56% and a disease free survival rate of 85%, respectively with those patients diagnosed with scalp/neck melanoma having poorer survival versus those with facial melanoma (Tseng and Martinez).

5. Lack of universal adaptation of sentinel node procedure

There has been some international criticism leveled directly at the manner in which MSLT-1 was carried out and the conclusions derived from it (Thomas 2006, 2009). Stated evidence that, tiny sentinel nodal deposits of melanoma have no prognostic relevance and will not progress or disseminate further as determined by the hosts' immune system, is now accruing. Associating a poorer prognosis to these deposits is called prognostic false positivity; which can lead to patients being incorrectly upstaged, undergoing unnecessary completion lymphadenectomy and possibly unnecessary adjuvant therapy (Thomas 2008). The results of the fourth interim analysis of MSLT-I support the hypothesis that prognostic false-positivity is the explanation for the large survival advantage claimed for patients having early lymphadenectomy versus delayed lymphadenectomy. Further detailed analysis of the results of MSLT-1 suggested that the incidence of prognostic false positivity is about 24% in patients with intermediate thickness melanoma and 34% for all patients (Thomas 2008). Further credence is given to this stance from studies confirming that patients with these tiny deposits of nodal melanoma (ie detected by immunohistochemistry alone or <0.1mm in size), have similar prognosis to those who are sentinel node negative (Spanknebel et al. 2005; van Akkooi et al. 2006).

Some believe that a positive sentinel node is likely to be associated with disseminated melanoma deposits elsewhere because they believe that melanoma tumour biology is not predictable. Are these cells released into the circulation, either lymphatic or blood vascular, disseminating widely and beyond? The timing of their manifestation is that which is unpredictable. These disseminated deposits (nodal, in-transit or distant disease) may become clinically apparent at some point in time, in spite of a positive sentinel node (and subsequent regional lymphadenectomy). Thus, assessment histologically of the sentinel node and the extent or number of lymph node deposits does not confer any additional benefit to patients, apart from the fact that they have melanoma deposits outside of their primary site and that in time they are at greater risk of further distant disease.

Some experts argue against the routine use of SLNB as they feel that it is associated with an increased risk of in-transit disease, however this has been readily refuted by evidenced based study who showed that there was no significant difference in the rate of in-transit metastasis between patients who had WLE alone (4.9%) and those who had WLE + SLNB (4.5%) (Pawlik et al. 2005).

Clinicians opposed to the use of the sentinel node will argue that in spite of its' prognostic importance, there is still no clear evidence to support a direct survival advantage from the procedure alone and, that no effective adjuvant therapy (including vaccines, combinations of chemotherapeutic agents, immunostimulants, cytokines and growth factors) has been heretofore discovered and subsequently proven to be of clear benefit (unequivocally prolongs overall survival) in clinical trials to date for these patients (Otley and Zitelli 2000; Thomas and Patocskai 2000; Eggermont and Gore 2007; Sabel and Sondak 2002; Spitler 2002).

Confusion remains whether early completion lymphadenectomy imparts a survival advantage when compared directly to those patients who wait until clinically occult nodal metastatic disease becomes apparent. Some authors site compelling evidence that the assessment of the sentinel node in melanoma is of no benefit whatsoever, does not alter the course of melanoma that has metastasised and should be immediately abandoned from current practice (Medalie and Ackerman 2004). There is growing concern surrounding the reliability of the SLN to accurately predict the disease status of the entire nodal basin. Specific problems have been identified in the head and neck region where the complexity and variability of the interlacing network of cervical lymphatics was highlighted by O'Brien et al who showed a 34% discordance rate between the clinical prediction of lymphatic drainage and lymphoscintigraphy findings in 97 cases of cutaneous melanoma of the head and neck (O'Brien et al. 1995).

Regional nodal failures in melanoma patients following a negative SLNB are not common. Various reasons have been suggested as to why SLNM fails which include (1) when the primary lesion is overlying the draining lymph node basin, (2) learning curve of the performing surgeon / pathologist / nuclear medicine staff, (3) inappropriately high radioactivity level, (4) movement of the dye into the second or non-sentinel lymph node and (5) incorrect injection technique of the dye. It has been suggested that at least a 30 person learning curve be recommended for a surgeon performing these cases (Morton et al. 1999). Patients undergoing SLNM for cutaneous melanoma should be managed via a multi-disciplinary team and the overall success rate of the procedure may be attributable in some part to this.

It is also well recognised that 11–12% (Gadd et al. 1999; Gershenwald et al. 1998) of patients whose sentinel node apparently doesn't harbour cells of melanoma subsequently develop signs of metastatic melanoma disease and conversely patients whose sentinel node does harbour metastatic cells may succumb to their illness in months or they may survive for decades. This high figure does little to add confidence to the therapeutic benefit of sentinel node biopsy.

6. Other emerging strategies

In an ideal oncological world, intra-operative evaluation of the sentinel node for metastatic disease allows a simultaneous completion lymphadenectomy if a positive deposit is immediately identified, preventing the higher costs and additional morbidity associated with a second operation. There is evidence that the sentinel node biopsy procedure is cost-effective compared to wide excision alone (Morton, Howard, and Thompson 2009). Here we discuss some of the emerging strategies addressing this specific issue.

Frozen section analysis of the lymph node was studied in 368 patients with primary cutaneous melanoma ≥1mm or Clarks level IV. 20% (74/368) of sentinel nodes were identified by traditional H&E and immunohistochemical stains, and further frozen sectioning only identified the metastases in 59% (44/74) of these patients (Stojadinovic et al. 2002). The SLN was the only positive lymph node in 86% (64/74) of patients. Additional positive non-SLNs were identified in 10 of 74 patients (14%). This low sensitivity was confirmed in other subsequent studies (Koopal et al. 2000; Tanis et al. 2001). The authors do suggest the potential use of frozen sectioning of a sentinel node found within the parotid gland or neck, thereby reducing the risk of facial and spinal accessory nerve injury during a second operative procedure. Frozen sectioning is a technically difficult procedure to perform and results in freezing artefact of the lymph node, rendering it unsuitable for further analysis.

Another recent development concerning the sentinel node is imprint cytology, which involves bisecting the node, imprinting it and subsequently staining the relevant sections. One study involving 93 patients showed that imprint cytology had a sensitivity and specificity of 38% and 100% respectively (similar figure to that of frozen section) (Creager et al. 2002). Even though it is easier to perform this procedure and without subsequent damage to the lymph node, the low sensitivity severely limits its use in the routine evaluation of the sentinel node. Other algorithms of histological factors concerning the primary tumour have also been developed (vertical growth phase, tumour infiltrating lymphocytes, mitotic rate and thickness) (Kruper et al. 2006). These are able to stratify patients into high and minimal risk for sentinel node disease based on the analysis of their primary lesion, and upon validation, these models could possibly provide a clinically useful tool for making treatment decisions (remove the use of the sentinel node procedure in those with minimal risk), aid in assessing patient risk, and for planning and analyzing clinical trials (Soong et al.).

Some molecular biology techniques for the staging of regional lymph nodes have yielded promising results (Wang et al. 1994). Wang et al, using real-time PCR to identify tyrosine messenger RNA for the detection of micrometastatic lymph node disease, showed that this was a highly sensitive and clinically applicable method to detect micrometastases (tyrosine messenger RNA is found almost exclusively in melanocytes). Furthermore, studies using reverse transcription and polymerase chain reaction to determine tyrosinase mRNA in peripheral blood, (which indicates the presence of circulating melanoma cells), showed that this may be a promising serum marker for melanoma staging and for predicting recurrence, prognosis and response to immune therapy (Brossart et al. 1993). The same group found that the amount of circulating tumour cells correlates with the tumour burden and that in patients with regression of melanoma metastases after immunotherapy, a decrease of the amount of tumour cells in the peripheral blood was observed (Brossart et al. 1995), associating the rate of positivity with stage of the disease.

There is accumulating evidence to support the use of targeted ultrasound assessment of the regional nodal basin at the time of diagnosis of the primary tumour, thus enhancing routine

clinical palpation. It is possible to identify deposits as small as 3-4mm (Bafounta et al. 2004). This does not take into account those nodal deposits below that diameter ie <3mm. Voit et al showed that specific features on preoperative ultrasound (peripheral perfusion, balloon shape and loss of central echoes) and fine needle aspiration cytology can identify 65% of sentinel node metastases and thus reduce the need for surgical procedures on the sentinel node, allowing those patients identified to proceed directly to completion lymphadenectomy (Voit et al.). However these results must be considered with caution. Ultrasound is heavily user-dependent. Given the fact that some patients will present with micrometastatic deposits in their regional nodes that will not be identifiable on ultrasound lowers its' sensitivity. Therefore, a negative ultrasound is not a reliable substitution for biopsy and subsequent histopathological examination of the sentinel node.
MicroRNAs (miRNAs) are non-coding short ribonucleic acid molecules that are post-transcriptional regulators that bind to complementary sequences in the three prime untranslated regions of mRNAs, leading to gene silencing. MiRNAs are present in human plasma in a very stable form that is protected from endogenous RNase activity (Mitchell et al. 2008). There has been a recent surge in reports demonstrating the use of miRNAs as modulators of gene expression and their potential role as both diagnostic and prognostic markers in many malignancies (Iorio and Croce 2009; Osaki, Takeshita, and Ochiya 2008). This is also true for malignant melanoma, where it has been shown that serum levels of miR-221 were significantly increased in melanoma patients, differentiated between in situ and invasive disease, were useful in evaluating tumour progression and monitoring patients during follow-up and that levels of of miR-221 correlated with tumour thickness (Kanemaru et al.).

7. Conclusion

In spite of a lack of definitive evidence associating a positive SLNB result and increased survival rate, the routine use of this novel approach is justified in patients presenting with primary cutaneous malignant melanoma because it provides valid and reliable staging information about the regional nodes using a minimally invasive technique, allows for regional disease control in the presence of a positive sentinel node and increases the potential for cure in patients with at least intermediate thickness disease. Cumulative evidence from MSLT-1, ELND trials and large retrospective trials mentioned above support the view that survival is better for patients with clinically occult sentinel node deposits.

8. References

Albertsen, P. C., J. A. Hanley, G. H. Barrows, D. F. Penson, P. D. Kowalczyk, M. M. Sanders, and J. Fine. 2005. Prostate cancer and the Will Rogers phenomenon. *J Natl Cancer Inst* 97 (17):1248-53.

Bafounta, M. L., A. Beauchet, S. Chagnon, and P. Saiag. 2004. Ultrasonography or palpation for detection of melanoma nodal invasion: a meta-analysis. *Lancet Oncol* 5 (11):673-80.

Balch, C. M., D. L. Morton, J. E. Gershenwald, K. M. McMasters, O. E. Nieweg, B. Powell, M. I. Ross, V. K. Sondak, and J. F. Thompson. 2009. Sentinel node biopsy and standard of care for melanoma. *J Am Acad Dermatol* 60 (5):872-5.

Balch, C. M., S. J. Soong, J. E. Gershenwald, J. F. Thompson, D. S. Reintgen, N. Cascinelli, M. Urist, K. M. McMasters, M. I. Ross, J. M. Kirkwood, M. B. Atkins, J. A. Thompson, D. G. Coit, D. Byrd, R. Desmond, Y. Zhang, P. Y. Liu, G. H. Lyman, and A. Morabito. 2001. Prognostic factors analysis of 17,600 melanoma patients: validation of the American Joint Committee on Cancer melanoma staging system. *J Clin Oncol* 19 (16):3622-34.

Brossart, P., U. Keilholz, M. Willhauck, C. Scheibenbogen, T. Mohler, and W. Hunstein. 1993. Hematogenous spread of malignant melanoma cells in different stages of disease. *J Invest Dermatol* 101 (6):887-9.

Brossart, P., J. W. Schmier, S. Kruger, M. Willhauck, C. Scheibenbogen, T. Mohler, and U. Keilholz. 1995. A polymerase chain reaction-based semiquantitative assessment of malignant melanoma cells in peripheral blood. *Cancer Res* 55 (18):4065-8.

Champion, G. A., and J. F. Piccirillo. 2004. The impact of computed tomography on pretherapeutic staging in patients with laryngeal cancer: demonstration of the Will Rogers' phenomenon. *Head Neck* 26 (11):972-6.

Chee, K. G., D. V. Nguyen, M. Brown, D. R. Gandara, T. Wun, and P. N. Lara, Jr. 2008. Positron emission tomography and improved survival in patients with lung cancer: the Will Rogers phenomenon revisited. *Arch Intern Med* 168 (14):1541-9.

Cormier, J. N., Y. Xing, M. Ding, J. E. Lee, P. F. Mansfield, J. E. Gershenwald, M. I. Ross, and X. L. Du. 2005. Population-based assessment of surgical treatment trends for patients with melanoma in the era of sentinel lymph node biopsy. *J Clin Oncol* 23 (25):6054-62.

Creager, A. J., S. A. Shiver, P. Shen, K. R. Geisinger, and E. A. Levine. 2002. Intraoperative evaluation of sentinel lymph nodes for metastatic melanoma by imprint cytology. *Cancer* 94 (11):3016-22.

Dessureault, S., S. J. Soong, M. I. Ross, J. F. Thompson, J. M. Kirkwood, J. E. Gershenwald, D. G. Coit, K. M. McMasters, C. M. Balch, and D. Reintgen. 2001. Improved staging of node-negative patients with intermediate to thick melanomas (>1 mm) with the use of lymphatic mapping and sentinel lymph node biopsy. *Ann Surg Oncol* 8 (10):766-70.

Eggermont, A. M., and M. Gore. 2007. Randomized adjuvant therapy trials in melanoma: surgical and systemic. *Semin Oncol* 34 (6):509-15.

Eicher, S. A., G. L. Clayman, J. N. Myers, and A. M. Gillenwater. 2002. A prospective study of intraoperative lymphatic mapping for head and neck cutaneous melanoma. *Arch Otolaryngol Head Neck Surg* 128 (3):241-6.

Feinstein, A. R., D. M. Sosin, and C. K. Wells. 1985. The Will Rogers phenomenon. Stage migration and new diagnostic techniques as a source of misleading statistics for survival in cancer. *N Engl J Med* 312 (25):1604-8.

Gadd, M. A., A. B. Cosimi, J. Yu, L. M. Duncan, L. Yu, T. J. Flotte, W. W. Souba, M. J. Ott, L. S. Wong, A. J. Sober, M. C. Mihm, F. G. Haluska, and K. K. Tanabe. 1999. Outcome of patients with melanoma and histologically negative sentinel lymph nodes. *Arch Surg* 134 (4):381-7.

Gershenwald, J. E., M. I. Colome, J. E. Lee, P. F. Mansfield, C. Tseng, J. J. Lee, C. M. Balch, and M. I. Ross. 1998. Patterns of recurrence following a negative sentinel lymph node biopsy in 243 patients with stage I or II melanoma. *J Clin Oncol* 16 (6):2253-60.

Gillgren, P., E. Mansson-Brahme, J. Frisell, H. Johansson, O. Larsson, and U. Ringborg. 2000. A prospective population-based study of cutaneous malignant melanoma of the head and neck. *Laryngoscope* 110 (9):1498-504.

Gofrit, O. N., K. C. Zorn, G. D. Steinberg, G. P. Zagaja, and A. L. Shalhav. 2008. The Will Rogers phenomenon in urological oncology. *J Urol* 179 (1):28-33.

Golger, A., D. S. Young, D. Ghazarian, and P. C. Neligan. 2007. Epidemiological features and prognostic factors of cutaneous head and neck melanoma: a population-based study. *Arch Otolaryngol Head Neck Surg* 133 (5):442-7.

Hoersch, B., U. Leiter, and C. Garbe. 2006. Is head and neck melanoma a distinct entity? A clinical registry-based comparative study in 5702 patients with melanoma. *Br J Dermatol* 155 (4):771-7.

Iorio, M. V., and C. M. Croce. 2009. MicroRNAs in cancer: small molecules with a huge impact. *J Clin Oncol* 27 (34):5848-56.

Kanemaru, H., S. Fukushima, J. Yamashita, N. Honda, R. Oyama, A. Kakimoto, S. Masuguchi, T. Ishihara, Y. Inoue, M. Jinnin, and H. Ihn. The circulating microRNA-221 level in patients with malignant melanoma as a new tumor marker. *J Dermatol Sci* 61 (3):187-93.

Koopal, S. A., A. T. Tiebosch, D. Albertus Piers, J. T. Plukker, H. Schraffordt Koops, and H. J. Hoekstra. 2000. Frozen section analysis of sentinel lymph nodes in melanoma patients. *Cancer* 89 (8):1720-5.

Kretschmer, L., R. Hilgers, M. Mohrle, B. R. Balda, H. Breuninger, B. Konz, C. Kunte, W. C. Marsch, C. Neumann, and H. Starz. 2004. Patients with lymphatic metastasis of cutaneous malignant melanoma benefit from sentinel lymphonodectomy and early excision of their nodal disease. *Eur J Cancer* 40 (2):212-8.

Kruper, L. L., F. R. Spitz, B. J. Czerniecki, D. L. Fraker, A. Blackwood-Chirchir, M. E. Ming, D. E. Elder, R. Elenitsas, D. Guerry, and P. A. Gimotty. 2006. Predicting sentinel node status in AJCC stage I/II primary cutaneous melanoma. *Cancer* 107 (10):2436-45.

Lachiewicz, A. M., M. Berwick, C. L. Wiggins, and N. E. Thomas. 2008. Survival differences between patients with scalp or neck melanoma and those with melanoma of other sites in the Surveillance, Epidemiology, and End Results (SEER) program. *Arch Dermatol* 144 (4):515-21.

Medalie, N., and A. B. Ackerman. 2004. Sentinel node biopsy has no benefit for patients whose primary cutaneous melanoma has metastasized to a lymph node and therefore should be abandoned now. *Br J Dermatol* 151 (2):298-307.

Mitchell, P. S., R. K. Parkin, E. M. Kroh, B. R. Fritz, S. K. Wyman, E. L. Pogosova-Agadjanyan, A. Peterson, J. Noteboom, K. C. O'Briant, A. Allen, D. W. Lin, N. Urban, C. W. Drescher, B. S. Knudsen, D. L. Stirewalt, R. Gentleman, R. L. Vessella, P. S. Nelson, D. B. Martin, and M. Tewari. 2008. Circulating microRNAs as stable blood-based markers for cancer detection. *Proc Natl Acad Sci U S A* 105 (30):10513-8.

Morton, D. L., A. J. Cochran, and J. F. Thompson. 2007. Authors' response to a letter to the editor re: Sentinel node biopsy for early-stage melanoma. *Ann Surg* 245 (5):828-9.

Morton, D. L., J. F. Thompson, A. J. Cochran, N. Mozzillo, R. Elashoff, R. Essner, O. E. Nieweg, D. F. Roses, H. J. Hoekstra, C. P. Karakousis, D. S. Reintgen, B. J. Coventry, E. C. Glass, and H. J. Wang. 2006. Sentinel-node biopsy or nodal observation in melanoma. *N Engl J Med* 355 (13):1307-17.

Morton, D. L., J. F. Thompson, R. Essner, R. Elashoff, S. L. Stern, O. E. Nieweg, D. F. Roses, C. P. Karakousis, N. Mozzillo, D. Reintgen, H. J. Wang, E. C. Glass, and A. J. Cochran. 1999. Validation of the accuracy of intraoperative lymphatic mapping and sentinel lymphadenectomy for early-stage melanoma: a multicenter trial. Multicenter Selective Lymphadenectomy Trial Group. *Ann Surg* 230 (4):453-63; discussion 463-5.

Morton, D. L., D. R. Wen, J. H. Wong, J. S. Economou, L. A. Cagle, F. K. Storm, L. J. Foshag, and A. J. Cochran. 1992. Technical details of intraoperative lymphatic mapping for early stage melanoma. *Arch Surg* 127 (4):392-9.

Morton, R. L., K. Howard, and J. F. Thompson. 2009. The cost-effectiveness of sentinel node biopsy in patients with intermediate thickness primary cutaneous melanoma. *Ann Surg Oncol* 16 (4):929-40.

O'Brien, C. J., R. F. Uren, J. F. Thompson, R. B. Howman-Giles, K. Petersen-Schaefer, H. M. Shaw, M. J. Quinn, and W. H. McCarthy. 1995. Prediction of potential metastatic sites in cutaneous head and neck melanoma using lymphoscintigraphy. *Am J Surg* 170 (5):461-6.

Osaki, M., F. Takeshita, and T. Ochiya. 2008. MicroRNAs as biomarkers and therapeutic drugs in human cancer. *Biomarkers* 13 (7):658-70.

Otley, C. C., and J. A. Zitelli. 2000. Review of sentinel lymph node biopsy and systemic interferon for melanoma: promising but investigational modalities. *Dermatol Surg* 26 (3):177-80.

Pacifico, M. D., R. Grover, and R. Sanders. 2004. Use of an early-detection strategy to improve disease control in melanoma patients. *Br J Plast Surg* 57 (2):105-11.

Pathak, I., C. J. O'Brien, K. Petersen-Schaeffer, E. B. McNeil, J. McMahon, M. J. Quinn, J. F. Thompson, and W. H. McCarthy. 2001. Do nodal metastases from cutaneous melanoma of the head and neck follow a clinically predictable pattern? *Head Neck* 23 (9):785-90.

Pawlik, T. M., M. I. Ross, and J. E. Gershenwald. 2004. Lymphatic mapping in the molecular era. *Ann Surg Oncol* 11 (4):362-74.

Pawlik, T. M., M. I. Ross, J. F. Thompson, A. M. Eggermont, and J. E. Gershenwald. 2005. The risk of in-transit melanoma metastasis depends on tumor biology and not the surgical approach to regional lymph nodes. *J Clin Oncol* 23 (21):4588-90.

Ross, M. I., and J. E. Gershenwald. 2008. How should we view the results of the Multicenter Selective Lymphadenectomy Trial-1 (MSLT-1)? *Ann Surg Oncol* 15 (3):670-3.

Sabel, M. S., and V. K. Sondak. 2002. Tumor vaccines: a role in preventing recurrence in melanoma? *Am J Clin Dermatol* 3 (9):609-16.

Shaw, H. M., C. M. Balch, S. J. Soong, G. W. Milton, and W. H. McCarthy. 1985. Prognostic histopathological factors in malignant melanoma. *Pathology* 17 (2):271-4.

Soong, S. J., S. Ding, D. Coit, C. M. Balch, J. E. Gershenwald, J. F. Thompson, and P. Gimotty. Predicting survival outcome of localized melanoma: an electronic prediction tool based on the AJCC Melanoma Database. *Ann Surg Oncol* 17 (8):2006-14.

Spanknebel, K., D. G. Coit, S. C. Bieligk, M. Gonen, J. Rosai, and D. S. Klimstra. 2005. Characterization of micrometastatic disease in melanoma sentinel lymph nodes by enhanced pathology: recommendations for standardizing pathologic analysis. *Am J Surg Pathol* 29 (3):305-17.

Spitler, L. E. 2002. Adjuvant therapy of melanoma. *Oncology (Williston Park)* 16 (1 Suppl 1):40-8.

Stojadinovic, A., P. J. Allen, B. M. Clary, K. J. Busam, and D. G. Coit. 2002. Value of frozen-section analysis of sentinel lymph nodes for primary cutaneous malignant melanoma. *Ann Surg* 235 (1):92-8.

Tanis, P. J., R. P. Boom, H. S. Koops, I. F. Faneyte, J. L. Peterse, O. E. Nieweg, E. J. Rutgers, A. T. Tiebosch, and B. B. Kroon. 2001. Frozen section investigation of the sentinel node in malignant melanoma and breast cancer. *Ann Surg Oncol* 8 (3):222-6.

Thomas, J. M. 2006. The place of sentinel node biopsy in melanoma after the Multicenter Selective Lymphadenectomy Trial. *ANZ J Surg* 76 (3):98-9.

Thomas, J. M. 2008. Prognostic false-positivity of the sentinel node in melanoma. *Nat Clin Pract Oncol* 5 (1):18-23.

Thomas, J. M. 2008. Sentinel lymph node biopsy in malignant melanoma. *BMJ* 336 (7650):902-3.

Thomas, J. M. 2009. Concerns relating to the conduct and statistical analysis of the Multicenter Selective Lymphadenectomy Trial (MSLT-1) in patients with melanoma. *J Plast Reconstr Aesthet Surg* 62 (4):442-6.

Thomas, J. M., and E. J. Patocskai. 2000. The argument against sentinel node biopsy for malignant melanoma. *BMJ* 321 (7252):3-4.

Thorn, M., H. O. Adami, U. Ringborg, R. Bergstrom, and U. Krusemo. 1989. The association between anatomic site and survival in malignant melanoma. An analysis of 12,353 cases from the Swedish Cancer Registry. *Eur J Cancer Clin Oncol* 25 (3):483-91.

Tseng, W. H., and S. R. Martinez. Tumor Location Predicts Survival in Cutaneous Head and Neck Melanoma. *J Surg Res*.

van Akkooi, A. C., J. H. de Wilt, C. Verhoef, P. I. Schmitz, A. N. van Geel, A. M. Eggermont, and M. Kliffen. 2006. Clinical relevance of melanoma micrometastases (<0.1 mm) in sentinel nodes: are these nodes to be considered negative? *Ann Oncol* 17 (10):1578-85.

Voit, C., A. C. Van Akkooi, G. Schafer-Hesterberg, A. Schoengen, K. Kowalczyk, J. C. Roewert, W. Sterry, and A. M. Eggermont. Ultrasound morphology criteria predict metastatic disease of the sentinel nodes in patients with melanoma. *J Clin Oncol* 28 (5):847-52.

Wang, X., R. Heller, N. VanVoorhis, C. W. Cruse, F. Glass, N. Fenske, C. Berman, J. Leo-Messina, D. Rappaport, K. Wells, and et al. 1994. Detection of submicroscopic lymph node metastases with polymerase chain reaction in patients with malignant melanoma. *Ann Surg* 220 (6):768-74.

Wrightson, W. R., S. L. Wong, M. J. Edwards, C. Chao, D. S. Reintgen, M. I. Ross, R. D. Noyes, V. Viar, P. B. Cerrito, and K. M. McMasters. 2003. Complications associated with sentinel lymph node biopsy for melanoma. *Ann Surg Oncol* 10 (6):676-80.

Young, M. J., J. Lenhart, T. E. Wasser, C. Czerwonka, J. Davidyock, and E. J. Sussman. 1999. Evidence for the Will Rogers phenomenon in migration of employees to managed care plans. *J Gen Intern Med* 14 (9):564-6.

4

Diagnosis and Treatment Options for Brain Metastasis of Melanoma

Khan K. Chaichana and Kaisorn L. Chaichana
Johns Hopkins University School of Medicine, Department of Neurosurgery, Baltimore, USA

1. Introduction

Metastasis to the brain is a devastating and common consequence for patients with malignant melanoma. A significant number of patients with melanoma eventually develop brain metastasis at the time of death. Patients are often symptomatic from their lesions and a large percentage of those with neurological deficits eventually die from the brain metastasis. Diagnosis does not typically occur until late in the disease course, which can preclude many treatment options. Additionally, rapid progression of the disease state and worsening health status magnifies the difficulties of treatment. Currently, contrast-enhanced computer tomography (CT) and magnetic resonance imaging (MRI) remain the main diagnostic modalities. Confirmation is usually achieved with surgical biopsy or resection. After diagnosis, treatment options are somewhat limited - surgical management, radiation therapy, and chemotherapy are most commonly used either alone or in combination.

This chapter provides a description of the common presenting symptoms, diagnostic modalities, and treatment options for patients with metastatic melanoma to the brain. This chapter will also discuss emerging technologies which may have notable impacts on the future of disease management. Ultimately, prompt diagnosis and treatment for patients with brain metastases may have important implications for the duration and quality of life of these patients.

2. Epidemiology and demographics

In general, patients with intracranial metastases significantly outnumber those with primary brain tumors. However, there are a small number of population-based epidemiological studies that address the true incidence of intracranial metastases, and studies devoted primarily to intracranial melanoma metastases are even less common [1]. Along with the limitations inherent to most surveys, such as sampling size and variability, there are several other limiting factors. This includes inadequate reporting, difficulty attaining ante-mortem diagnosis, and greater emphasis cancer databases place on the incidence of primary tumors rather than metastasis [2]. As a result, it is quite likely that current population-based epidemiological studies underestimate the true incidence of cancer metastasizing to the brain [2]. A significant amount of the reported data now originates from clinical, neurosurgical, and autopsy series which are subject to their own limitations as well.

However, as methods of diagnosis and treatment continue to improve, a more accurate picture can be portrayed.

Malignant melanoma is one of the most common systemic cancers to metastasize to the central nervous system (CNS). Following lung and breast carcinoma, melanoma historically has the third highest incidence of metastasis to the brain [3]. One recent study has indicated it may now surpass that of breast carcinoma, most likely a result of increasing rates over time [1]. Of cases with metastasis to the brain, melanoma is the primary tumor for about 5 to 21 percent of these patients [4]. CNS involvement or deficits are the first manifestation of melanoma in 9 to 12 percent of patients [5]. For those that carry a diagnosis of melanoma, between 12 to 60 percent can expect to develop metastases to the brain [6, 7]. However, because it only accounts for 5% of metastatic cancers [8], the total number of cases or individuals is often erroneous [1]. Although melanoma is a less common cancer, it has the highest propensity for metastasis to the brain [1, 9]. An estimated 49 to 73 percent of patients who die from melanoma will have developed brain metastases by the time of death and are found on autopsy [10, 11]. It is responsible for the deaths in an estimated 20 to 55 percent of affected patients, and contributes to death in up to 95 percent of all cases [11-13]. Thus, the impact and consequences of metastatic melanoma are quite detrimental in medicine.

Anyone with a diagnosis of melanoma is at risk for developing CNS metastases. Previous studies have tried to elucidate these factors that increase the risk of CNS metastases. Among the demographic aspects intrinsic to patient demographics, only male gender was found to show greater predominance in patients with brain metastases [14]. Of the characteristics of the primary lesion, melanomas appearing wide, thick, or ulcerated or with acral lentiginous or nodular histological findings were more frequently found in patients who developed brain metastases[14]. Also, primary lesions arising from the mucosal surfaces, skin of the head and neck, or skin of the trunk were more frequently found in this group [14, 15]. Patients with involvement of the lymph nodes or visceral organs, especially the lungs or multiple visceral organs, showed an increased likelihood of metastasizing to the brain [14, 16]. These factors are also associated with shortened overall survival time survival times [14, 16]. Interestingly, with the exception of primary lesions of the head and neck region, these factors did not affect survival after a diagnosis of a brain metastasis [14]. Other factors that were evaluated, such as the patient's race, pigmentation of the primary tumor, and pregnancy at the time of melanoma diagnosis, were not significantly correlated with the development of brain metastases[14]. The average age of presentation of patients with brain metastases is 48 to 53 years old, which is similar to that of patients with extracranial metastases[14, 17].

3. Pathophysiology

Metastases to the brain requires a complex series of steps, each mediated by a combination of intricate molecular mechanisms that are not completely understood. Each of these steps typically involves overcoming various physiological barriers including the blood-brain barrier [2]. Similar to other systemic cancers, as the primary melanoma matures, the process of angiogenesis increases the vascular supply to sustain the metabolic needs of the cancer cells and allows the tumor to grow. It progressively invades the surrounding host tissue and eventually spread hematogenously by invading local venules or lymph channels, which drain into the venous circulation [2]. Because venous circulation returns to the right side of the heart, the first capillary beds the circulating tumor cells encounter are typically found in the lungs. These tumor cells are generally larger than the capillary vessels and may arrest in these pulmonary capillary beds. As a result, patients typically have lung metastases earlier in the time course of melanoma. They may often be identified at the time intracranial metastases are diagnosed. Between about 27 to 68 percent of affected patients may have concurrent lung metastases, which further shortens the survival time [14, 18, 19]. In order to reach arterial circulation and thus the cerebral vasculature, these melanoma cells must reach the left side of the heart either by: (1) metastasizing to the lung and invading the pulmonary venous circulation, (2) traversing the lung capillary bed to the pulmonary venous circulation, or (3) crossing through a patent foramen ovale thus bypassing the pulmonary circulation [2].

When tumor cells reach the left side of the heart and systemic circulation, the most important factors involved in promoting intracranial metastasis are the blood supply and greater preference for brain tissue [2]. The cerebral vasculature receives approximately 15 to 20 percent of the cardiac output in the resting state, which increases the likelihood that circulating tumor cells will reach the brai n[2]. It would be expected to receive a proportional amount as well, however the distribution of metastases based on blood flow, or the mechanical hypothesis, does not account for the high propensity of melanoma to metastasize to the brain compared to other cancers [20]. Instead, the seed and soil hypothesis likely contributes to the metastasis and plays an important role in explaining this phenomenon. This hypothesis postulates that certain genetic alterations in the tumor cells (the seed) influences them to show preference for the brain and find its microenvironment a more favorable place (the soil) to support their growth [20]. These alterations may include increased expression of adhesion molecules that show preferential adhesion to brain endothelial cells [21, 22] and increased production of degradative enzymes enabling tumor cells to penetrate the endothelium and the basement membrane [23]. Locally produced growth factors in the brain may also stimulate growth of the metastatic cells [24].

When tumor cells reach the cerebral vasculature, they may arrest in the capillary beds due to their greater size. In order to form metastases, they must extravasate across the microvasculature of the blood-brain barrier into the brain parenchyma [2]. The blood-brain barrier is a continuous, non-fenestrated endothelium composed of tight junctions and protects against the invasion of microorganisms and also the interaction of most drugs, including chemotherapeutic drugs [25]. However, it provides little protection against the invasion of metastatic cells into the brain parenchyma and may even be altered to a leakier barrier in primary tumors and metastases [26]. The cells adhere to and penetrate the basement membrane and astrocytic foot processes, eventually reaching the parenchyma.

In the end, only about 0.1 percent of the initial circulating tumor cells survive the protective mechanisms of the body to form distant metastases [7]. Additionally, metastasis typically occurs relatively late in the disease course for most patients with malignant melanoma. This may be explained by CNS involvement occurring as a result of a late metastatic event from another distant metastatic site, such as the lungs [7]. It may also be possible that metastasis is actually an early event in the disease course, but relatively slow metastatic growth results in delayed neurological effects and delayed detection [7].

4. Pathology

The histopathology of intracranial metastases mimics that of the primary melanoma. Melanoma can metastasize to virtually any portion of the intracranial cavity. The most common site is the parenchyma, but involvement of any anatomic structure in the CNS can occur, including the dura, leptomeninges, choroid plexus, pituitary, and pineal glands. As with other systemic cancers that metastasize to the brain, the distribution reflects the size and volume of the region and its vasculature. Thus, a significant majority are supratentorial, the most common location being the cerebral hemispheres along the vascular distribution of the border zones (water-shed areas) between the anterior and middle cerebral arteries as well as the middle and posterior cerebral arteries [6, 14]. In total, the parietal lobe is involved in about 26 to 45%, frontal love in 21 to 36%, temporal lobe in 19%, occipital lobe in 11%, cerebellum in 7%, and cerebellum in <1%. The spinal cord is rarely involved [6, 14]. About 75 percent of metastases are found in the gray-white junction, where supplying cerebral vessels are slightly constricted, resulting in reduction of blood flow and thus increased risk of tumor cells arrest [6]. Melanoma is also known to have an increased likelihood of developing multiple metastases. Approximately 16 to 61% of patients will have more than one intracranial lesion at the time of diagnosis [14, 17, 18]. Individual lesions are usually relatively small with the largest typically measuring between 1 to 4 cm in diameter, while few are rarely greater than 4 cm. Larger intracranial lesions are noticeably less common and will most often be solitary [6, 14, 18]. Similar to other systemic cancers, the metastases from melanoma tend to expand as roughly spherical masses and establish well-defined interfaces with the surrounding brain parenchyma. Thus, expansion pushes the normal surrounding tissue aside rather than invading it. This contrasts from most primary brain tumors which often show diffusely infiltrated margins [27].

Metastases from melanoma have the highest risk of hemorrhage as compared to other systemic metastases to the brain. Hemorrhage is found on neuroimaging in 27 to 40% of patients with intracranial lesions, while histopathological evaluation has indicated that 62 to 71% of patients have evidence of a prior hemorrhage [6, 18]. The bleeding may be confined to the intracranial lesion itself, extend into the area surrounding it, or expand into an intracerebral hematoma. When multiple metastases are present, simultaneous hemorrhage usually occurs rather than isolated hemorrhage of individual lesions [28]. This most often results in subacute progression which is characteristic of non-hemorrhagic brain metastases. Occasionally, it can cause significant complications such as hematomas and hydrocephalus from obstruction of cerebrospinal fluid flow [18]. Vasogenic edema surrounding brain metastases is also common and can cause similar effects as hemorrhage.

5. Clinical findings

The clinical presentation of melanoma metastases to the brain does not significantly differ from that of other intracranial metastases or primary brain tumors. The presenting signs and symptoms are dependent on the number and location of the lesions as well as the rate of growth. Regardless of etiology, most CNS lesions produce clinical effects either through compression of surrounding neurological tissue or destruction of neurons. For intracranial metastases, the primary mechanism of action is compression from the local mass effect of tumor expansion or secondary effects from raised intracranial pressure or impediment of cerebrospinal fluid circulation. Most patients present with nonfocal complaints secondary to increased intracranial pressure[19]. Common symptoms of increased intracranial pressure include headaches, mental change, somnolence, and nausea and vomiting. Focal or generalized seizures resulting from irritation of neurons are also common in patients with brain metastases[6]. Patients with a single metastasis often present with additional focal signs and symptoms. This can include such neurological deficits as cranial nerve palsies, visual deficits, hemiparesis, and hemisensory loss[6]. Generally, these nonfocal or focal complaints can present in up 75 percent of patients with brain metastases, whereas the incidence of seizures in patients may be as high 50 percent [6, 14, 29]. Although patients with metastases of melanoma to the brain can present with a range of signs and symptoms, there are still a number of patients who may have few or no obvious indications of an underlying pathology[14, 29]. This may be due insufficient mass effect, however their growth rate compared to primary brain tumors is notably faster. Clinical effects may then be subacute in onset, presenting over weeks rather than months. An acute onset may also occur in such instances as hemorrhagic transformation, dubbed a "tumor TIA". Thus, it is important for physicians to have a high index of suspicion when dealing with patients at risk of developing brain metastases. It is a strong possibility and should be high on the list of differential diagnosis in any patient with a history of melanoma that presents with new neurological signs or symptoms [6].

6. Diagnosis

When there is a high clinical suspicion for metastatic melanoma to the brain based on the history and neurological exam of a patient, neuroimaging is the most important diagnostic modality. Currently, computed tomography (CT) and magnetic resonance imaging (MRI) provide the most beneficial imaging of the CNS. Between these two modalities, MRI with and without gadolinium contrast enhancement is the preferred choice for all systemic metastases. MRI is known to increase the conspicuity of lesions and have increased sensitivity in detecting the presence of additional and smaller metastases to the brain [30, 31]. However, because CT is more readily available in emergent situations, it is often used to image large lesions, hemorrhage, and significant edema, but will be insufficient to definitively rule out intracranial disease [6]. If a single metastasis is found on CT or the scan appears within normal limits, MRI with administration of contrast is warranted because of its improved abilities for detection of lesions [30, 31]. Other radiographic imaging modalities, such as positron emission tomography (PET) with ^{18}F-fluorodeoxyglucose, generally are not useful in the diagnosis or imaging metastatic melanoma of the brain[32].
In the majority of patients, MRI is often the only necessary diagnostic test. However, neuroimaging cannot unequivocally differentiate metastases from other intracranial pathologies. The presence of a lesion on a CT or MRI scan in patient with melanoma or other progressive systemic cancer is not always diagnostic for metastatic spread. The differential diagnosis often includes primary intracranial tumors, cerebral abscess, demyelinating disease, and cerebral infarction or hemorrhage. Each of these etiologies will likely need to be carefully ruled out, however certain characteristics provide for strong evidence of metastases. Brain metastases from melanoma frequently appear bright on T1-weighted images and dark on T2-weighted images. This appearance may be attributed to the production of melanin in the tumor [33, 34]. If hemorrhage occurs, the presence of blood breakdown products can alter the T1-weighted or T2 weighted signal[34, 35]. On CT, brain metastases from melanoma are typically slightly hyperdense compared to the surrounding nervous tissue and exhibit moderate contrast enhancement [6]. Increasing the volume of contrast material injected as well as delaying imaging after the injection of intravenous contrast material may improve detection and conspicuity of lesions on CT examination [36]. When the metastases are small, uniform contrast enhancement is typical, but when larger,

peripheral ring enhancement may occur. This ring is usually thicker in comparison to an abscess and more regular than a primary tumor. As noted previously, metastases are usually found at the gray-white junction in the watershed areas of the brain and are typically spherical in shape with more regular margins and a substantial amount of vasogenic edema surrounding a small tumor nidus [6, 14, 27].

After neuroimaging, confirmatory diagnosis can be accomplished through surgical biopsy or, preferably, excision of the entire mass. This allows for definitive differentiation of metastases originating from melanoma versus metastases from possible systemic cancers and other suspected etiologies. If more than one lesion exists, the largest or most symptomatic one should be addressed first for biopsy or resection. Once a brain metastasis has been discovered either through imaging or biopsy, screening for the primary systemic cancer is necessary if one has not already been diagnosed. In contrast, for those patients who have been diagnosed with malignant melanoma but their neurological exam is within normal limits, routine screening of the CNS with neuroimaging rarely identifies metastases and is thus generally not recommended [37].

7. Survival

The prognosis of patients with disseminated melanoma is particularly poor if the CNS is involved. Currently, no reliably curative treatments are available for patients and most therapeutic trials for melanoma exclude patients with brain metastases [38]. For those with documented brain metastases, the overall median survival time is between 3.8 and 5.2 months, a notably shorter survival time in comparison to patients with other sites of distant metastases. The survival percentages are inversely proportional to the length of time after diagnosis [39-43]. Additionally, the median time between the diagnosis of primary melanoma and the diagnosis of metastatic melanoma to brain is about 3.1 to 3.7 years [13, 14, 41]. Among a number of clinical and pathologic factors that have been analyzed, the disease free-interval (DFI) is one of a few that independently predicts survival after diagnosis of AJCC stage IV melanoma. Significant survival benefit occurs when the DFI is greater than 12 months. The anatomical site of the primary melanoma has also been shown to have predictive value. There is an almost fourfold difference between sites associated with highest survival and lowest survival rate. Melanomas with primary metastasis from the skin and lymph nodes have a median survival of about 15 months, whereas those from the brain and liver have a median survival of about 4 months. The third factor that independently predicts survival is the preceding stage of disease before the patient is diagnosed with stage IV melanoma. Patients experience significant survival benefit if they develop stage IV melanoma without progressing through stage III and have a DFI greater than or equal to 72 months, or if they progress through stage III to stage IV and have a DFI greater than or equal to 18 months. Other factors such as gender, age, Breslow depth, Clark level, year of diagnosis, and number of metastatic sites have not shown predictive value[39].

8. Supportive therapy

Several approaches can be taken to provide patients with supportive measures until more definitive treatment can be considered and administered. This primarily involves the medical management of cerebral edema and the resulting increased intracranial pressure, the control of seizures, and the prevention of other associated complications and conditions.

These are generally the most common medical problems in patients with metastasis of melanoma to the brain as well as most other brain tumor. The overall survival in patients with brain metastases treated with only supportive care is approximately 1 to 2 months[14].

8.1 Steroids

The vasogenic edema that is characteristic of metastases is a significant factor in the morbidity of patients. It occurs as a result of BBB break down, allowing sodium and water to leak into and accumulate in the extracellular space of the brain parenchyma[44, 45]. Corticosteroids have been shown to adequately manage this vasogenic edema and can dramatically improve a patient's condition[46, 47]. The beneficial effects are often noticeable within 6 to 24 hours after the first dose and reach maximum effect within 3 to 7 days[48]. Its mechanism of action is quite complex and not completely understood. The antiedema effect may be contributed to stabilization and reduction of the permeability of tumor capillaries through endothelial cell interactions[44, 45]. Corticosteroids are usually indicated in any patient who is symptomatic from the metastatic edema and during the course of definitive treatment with radiation or surgery, but it is typically not necessary in asymptomatic patients with small metastases unless treatment with radiation or surgery is expected[49, 50]. Dexamethasone is administered most commonly because it has minimal mineralocorticoid activity and may have a lower risk of complications compared to other corticosteroids[47]. Long-term use of corticosteroids can result in such significant adverse effects as myopathy, osteoporosis and avascular bone necrosis, diabetes mellitus, cognitive dysfunction, gastrointestinal (GI) hemorrhage, bowel perforation, and opportunistic infections, such as Pneumocystis jirovecci pneumonitis and oropharyngeal candidiasis[51].
In instances of significant mass effect or acute decompensation of brain metastases, the onset of effects of corticosteroids is not quick enough and thus the approach to medical management changes[45]. Acute decompensation can be due to a number of causes such as intratumoral hemorrhage, obstructive hydrocephalus, seizures, or hyponatremia. The resulting acutely increased intracranial pressure should be addressed immediately in order to minimize the risk of herniation or worse[47]. This involves stabilization of the BBB, minimization of the vasogenic edema, and emergent intervention with surgical debulking or irradiation. Elevation of the head of the bed, hyperventilation, mannitol, diuretics and are all rapid onset measures that can provide support until steroids take effect and should precede any neuroimaging[49, 52].

8.2 Antiepileptics

Seizures are a common occurrence in patients with brain metastases. The likelihood of seizures is highest in patients with melanoma compared to other cancers including lung and breast carcinoma[51]. Those who present with seizures should generally be treated with antiepileptic drugs (AED)[49]. The use of prophylaxis is often based on individual preference of the treating physician rather than supporting clinical evidence[45]. No significant benefit has been shown with anticonvulsant prophylaxis using phenobarbital, phenytoin, or valproic acid in patients who had no history of seizures[45]. In addition to the lack of efficacy, the risk of potential side effects has been shown to be increased in patients with brain tumors[53]. Overall, almost 25 percent of patients diagnosed with either a primary or metastatic brain tumor and are taking AEDs experience side effects severe enough to warrant a change in or discontinuation of therapy [53]. Thus, it is recommended that prophylactic anticonvulsants should not be routinely used in patients with newly diagnosed brain tumors[53]. However, because there is a high risk of recurrence, long-term treatment with AEDs is indicated after a patient with melanoma metastases to the brain has suffered their first seizure[51]. Phenytoin has historically been the mainstay of anticonvulsant therapy because it is generally effective and well tolerated. Selection of the particular AEDs to administer requires careful consideration of the treatment the patient is receiving. This is because important interactions can occur with other drugs commonly used in treatment for brain metastases, such as antineoplastic agents and dexamethasone, often from activation of hepatic metabolism through the cytochrome P450 enzyme system[49]. Newer AEDs, including levetiracetam and topiramate, typically do not affect cytochrome P450 and have shown greater reduced seizure frequency and fewer side effects[54].

Anticonvulsant prophylaxis after supratentorial surgery is generally recommended for patients, including those undergoing resection of brain metastases. AEDs have been shown to be beneficial in preventing early seizures postoperatively[45]. However, there is not strong evidence to support the use of long-term treatment to reduce the incidence of late seizures after supratentorial surgery. Thus, in those patients with brain metastases from melanoma who have not had a seizure, the recommended plan for antiepileptic therapy is to gradually taper and discontinue AEDs after the first postoperative week. This is especially appropriate for patients who are medically stable and are experiencing notable side effects from their anticonvulsant medication[53].

8.3 Anticoagulants

Patients with any systemic cancer are known to be in a hypercoagulable state, increasing their risk for deep venous thrombosis (DVTs) and venous thromboembolisms (VTEs). This is especially true for brain metastases for which thromboembolic disease contributes significantly to morbidity and mortality[55]. The risk is often greatest in hemiplegic patients and in the postoperative period since patients are often immobile. In order to prevent DVTs and VTEs from occurring after craniotomy, adequate prophylaxis is often necessary. However, this can be difficult due to the possibility of intratumoral hemorrhage and intracranial bleeding with anticoagulation therapy. Current methods of prophylaxis include mechanical and/or pharmacological interventions, however no optimal one has been identified and current recommendations remain controversial[56]. Unfractionated heparin (UFH) and low-molecular-weight heparin (LMWH) are the main pharmacological anticoagulants which inhibit formation of thrombi. Mechanical methods attempt to minimize venous stasis and enhance fibrinolysis. This includes early ambulation, compression stocking, intermittent external pneumatic compression devices, and electrical calf muscle stimulation. In general, both approaches are effective in preventing DVTs and VTEs[57], but heparin may be more effective although at a greater risk of intracranial hemorrhage[45]. Mechanical prophylaxis with concomitant anticoagulation therapy during the postoperative period is not only safe but also protects patients more so than either approach does alone[57].

In patients that have developed a DVT, treatment is necessary to prevent a pulmonary embolism (PE), restore lower limb circulation, and resolve other associated problems. Pharmacological treatment with UFH and LMWH are the mainstays of therapy, with LMWH showing better outcomes including fewer bleeding complications. Patients who have strict contraindications against anticoagulation can be treated with placement of an inferior vena cava (IVC) filter[49]. However, these should generally not be the first line of treatment because it has a higher complication rate and are less effective in prevent PE in comparison to anticoagulation. One retrospective study of IVC filter complications occurring in patients with brain tumors and DVT found that there was a complication rate of 62 percent and PE still occurred in 12 percent of cases despite proper placement of the IVC filter[58]. Thus, IVC filters should be reserved for patients that have had recent craniotomy, are at increased risk for intracranial hemorrhage, are poorly compliant with medications, or will have prolonged thrombocytopenia from chemotherapy.

9. Definitive treatment

After receiving supportive measures, patients diagnosed with melanoma that has metastasized to the central nervous system must be evaluated for the possibility and type of definitive treatment. Current options available to physicians include whole brain radiation therapy (WBRT), stereotactic surgery, conventional surgical resection, or chemotherapy. These can frequently be used alone or in combination with one other. However, for the majority of patients, these are largely palliative measures. Determining the optimal modality is dependent on a number of factors including the size, number, location, and sensitivity of the lesion, the overall status of the malignant melanoma, the neurological status as measured by the Karnofsky Performance Scale (KPS), general condition of the patient, and the preferences of the patient and his or her family. It can thus be difficult to decide on a course of treatment given the number of issues that need to be considered.

9.1 Whole brain radiation therapy

The first use of external beam WBRT for treatment of brain metastases was reported in 1954 by Chao et al[59] and again later in 1961 by Chu et al[60]. It has since become an important treatment modality for brain metastases. One of the fundamental benefits of WBRT is that it is a noninvasive means in which to treat the entire brain and provide palliation of symptoms. Thus, it allows for relatively simple targeting of any and all lesions in the brain with radiation including microscopic ones, micrometastases, which are not detected on neuroimaging. This has been demonstrated in studies which showed that prophylactic and postoperative irradiation of the brain decreases subsequent development of intracranial metastases. This effect is most likely due to elimination of micrometastases that were present at the time[61, 62]. External WBRT is thus advantageous and typically considered the mainstay of treatment for most patients with multiple metastatic deposits from melanoma in the brain[38, 63, 64]. More localized treatment modalities would be less beneficial in such situations because it would require targeting of each lesion individually. However, solitary metastases that are too large for either surgical resection or stereotactic surgery or those that impinge on sensitive areas of the brain are often treated with WBRT[63, 65].

The broad application of radiation to the brain can also be an important disadvantage. This is because it not only affects the malignant tissue, but the normal tissue is also exposed to the harmful effects of ionizing radiation. Side effects are typically dependent on the total dosage, dosing interval, and fraction size. Acute side effects of external WBRT include memory loss, fatigue, headaches, temporary hair loss, scalp rash or desquamation, hyperpigmentation, otitis media, and cerebral edema[63, 66]. Somnolence syndrome is a set of symptoms, often seen in children, involving lethargy, anorexia, and irritability that present 1 to 4 months after treatment. There are generally no focal neurological deficits with this syndrome[66-68]. If the patient survives long-term, late side effects may occur which include cerebral edema, atrophy, focal radiation necrosis, white matter demyelination, leukoencephalopathy, endocrinopathy, and progressive cognitive dysfunction[69-71]. A recent randomized controlled trial found that patients suffered significantly greater decline in learning and memory functions after receiving WBRT compared to patients only receiving stereotactic radiosurgery[72]. These consequences should be considered if the patient has the potential to survive for a prolonged amount of time following radiation treatment. Another issue that is important when considering external WBRT for treatment of metastatic melanoma to the brain is the significant resistance melanoma has to this mode of radiation therapy. Of all the primary tumor types, malignant melanoma is considered to be one of the most radioresistant to WBRT[73]. Larger fractions may be necessary in order to achieve desired effect, increasing the likelihood for negative side effects[74]. However, because there are few other effective modalities for treatment of multiple metastases in the brain, it is still commonly used in these patients.

The Radiation Therapy Oncology Group (RTOG) conducted several extensive phase III randomized trials to evaluate the efficacy of various treatment schedules. The results of which indicated that 30 Gy administered in 10 fractions of 3 Gy over a period of 2 weeks results in palliative results and survival time equivalent to more protracted and higher-dose schedules[75, 76]. This has since become the most commonly used external WBRT schedule in the United States for brain metastases in general. Although this is often inadequate for long-term tumor control except in the most radiosensitive histologies, it allows for minimization of toxicity and negative side effects of irradiation. The median survival after administration of WBRT to patients with brain metastases is typically improved to about 3 to 6 months but is dependent on the number of lesions, the radiosensitivity of the metastases, and the status of the underlying cancer. Despite its known general resistance to radiation therapy, studies have shown local tumor response of melanoma metastases to the brain after administration of WBRT[77, 78]. Many fractionation schemes have been devised with larger doses per fraction in an attempt to enhance this tumor response. However, a review of several retrospective series has revealed that no scheme is better than the current standard of 30 Gy in 10 fractions[38]. Improved clinical outcomes may occur after WBRT, showing mildly increased median survival times to about 2.0 to 6.1 months[79-82]. When patients are stratified according to the RTOG recursive partitioning analysis (RPA), the effect of WBRT can be better extrapolated. The RPA separates patients into three prognostic groups according to their KPS, extracranial disease, and patient age. Those in RPA class 1 frequently have the best prognosis due to younger age (<65 years) and higher KPS scores (>70) whereas RPA class 3 often have the worst prognosis due to lower KPS scores (<70). The survival times after WBRT expectedly correlate with RPA class. Those with brain metastases originating from melanoma had median survival times of about 7.1 to 10.5 for patients in class 1, 4.2 to 5.9 for patients in class 2, and 1.8 to 2.3 for patients in class 3[82, 83]. Despite only having minimal effects on the survival time, using external WBRT and supportive management in patients with metastatic melanoma of the brain has demonstrated palliation of symptoms[79]. Symptomatic improvement is an important effect that can enhance the quality of life given the bleak prognosis despite all treatment modalities. Patients often have improvement of headaches, weakness, and mental status. There are some who question its ability to reverse neurological symptoms and suggest omitting WRBT melanoma metastases are fewer than four[72]. However, WBRT still currently remains the mainstay of treatment for patients with multiple brain metastases but is not typically first-line in solitary metastases [65]. It is a viable adjuvant therapy in addition to serving as an option for primary therapy. In cases of single brain metastases, surgical resection or stereotactic radiosurgery are usually the preferable option for primary therapy unless both are contraindicated. Patients that additionally have advanced systemic disease or conditions that preclude surgery or radiosurgery in addition to a solitary lesion would likely be better suited for WBRT.

9.2 Surgical resection

Surgical resection was first reported for use in the treatment of brain metastases in 1926 by Grant[84]. As noted earlier, metastatic brain tumors characteristically form well-circumscribed and rounded masses at the junction of the gray and white matter. This renders them highly amenable to surgical resection. Additionally, with modern neurosurgical techniques and the available new technologies such as functional mapping, intraoperative ultrasonography, and computer assisted stereotaxy, surgical resection can be accomplished with increased precision and control. It has become a mainstay of treatment despite the development of newer methods including WBRT or stereotactic radiosurgery. This is because it offers several advantages over both. Surgery **(Figure 1)** provides immediate palliative action and relief of symptoms with removal of the lesion, which decreases the intracranial pressure, alleviates compression and mass effect on the surrounding parenchyma, prevents or stops hemorrhage and edema into the intracranial space, and restores CSF flow if obstruction has occurred. No other treatment modality can provide this immediate effect which is critical in emergent situations such as impending herniation or posterior fossa tumors. Removal of the tumor with surgical resection additionally provides diagnostic advantages. It is the only modality that allows for physical extraction of the mass in order to determine a histological and pathological diagnosis. This is important in patients in which the etiology of the lesion is uncertain or the primary cancer has not been identified. Studies have demonstrated that up to approximately 11 percent of suspected cranial metastases are actually found to be nonmetastatic lesions, such as cerebral abscesses or primary tumors, on pathological evaluation[85]. Surgical resection also avoids some of the prominent drawbacks of WBRT, most notably the resistance of melanoma metastases to radiation therapy and the negative effects of diffuse radiation on normal neurological tissue. Instead, it circumvents the use of radiation and surgically localizes the area of the metastases, minimizing damage to the rest of the unaffected brain parenchyma and avoiding the acute and long-term side effects depicted in WBRT. Surgical resection is thus most advantageous for solitary or a limited number of metastases to brain where diffuse involvement does not occur. However, there is still significant morbidity and mortality associated with surgical resection given its invasive nature. These risks continue to gradually improve with the advancement of available procedures and tools, as was seen with the utilization of CT and MRI neuroimaging. Several recent studies have shown the risk of mortality to be between 0 to 14.2 percent during the postoperative period [14, 18, 86, 87] which is compared to earlier reports of mortality in up to 22 percent of patients[87].

Given the limited survival time of patients harboring metastatic melanoma of the brain, postoperative neurological deficits and prolonged recovery times are best avoided if possible. Patient selection is important in minimizing poor outcomes and maximizing the response to treatment. In general, surgical resection is most appropriate for patients with a

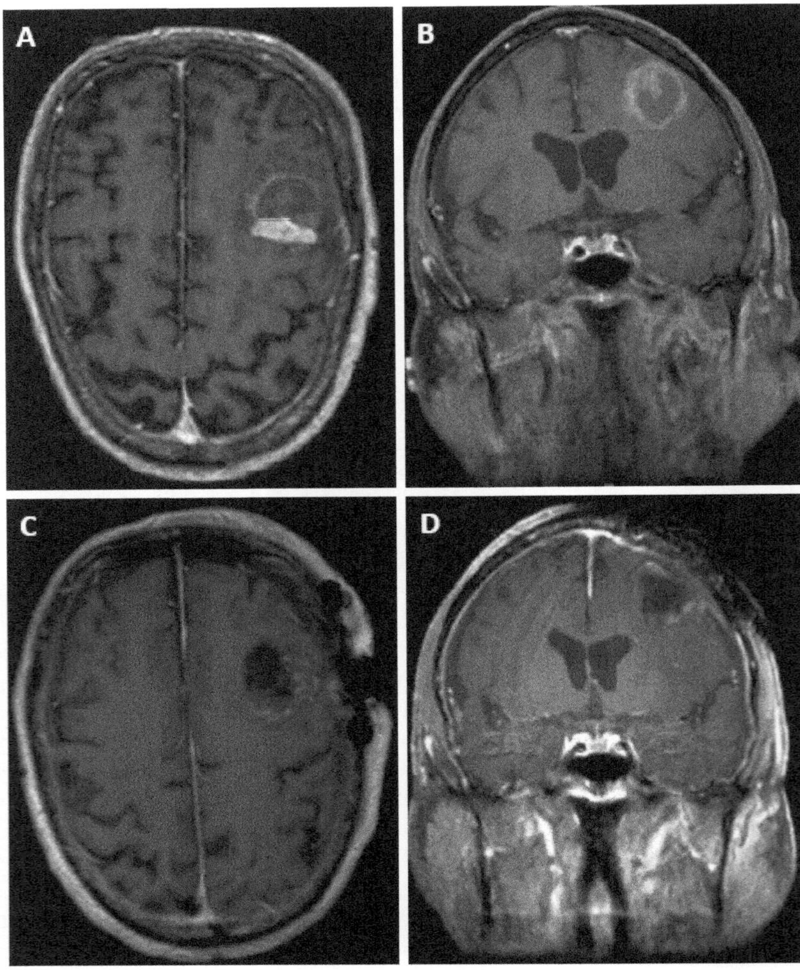

Fig. 1. Representative patient with intracranial metastatic melanoma who underwent surgical resection. **A,** pre-operative contrast-enhanced axial and **B,** coronal T1 magnetic resonance image (MRI) demonstrating left frontal metastasis with intratumoral hemorrhage. **C,** post-operative contrast-enhanced axial and **D,** coronal T1 MRI demonstrating gross total resection of the metastasis.

single brain metastasis, limited systemic disease, and favorable KPS score (>70). Metastases greater than 3 cm in diameter should be preferentially treated with surgery because large tumors typically have minimal response to the other modalities[88]. Selection of patients with multiple metastases to the brain remains somewhat controversial. Several retrospective studies have examined the efficacy of surgical resection alone in the treatment of brain metastases from melanoma. It is clear that surgical resection of a single melanoma metastases greater extends the survival time in comparison WBRT alone or supportive therapy alone. In these studies, the median survival time after surgery varies between 5 and 22 months with the more recent ones showing a median survival time between 8 and 16 months[87-89]. In contrast to solitary metastasis, the role of surgical intervention in cases of multiple brain metastases remains controversial due to lack of randomized control trials[63]. Previously, this was typically a contraindication, but one retrospective study challenged this notion. Bindel et al[90] compared patients with single and multiple brain metastases that were treated with surgical resection. Patients that underwent partial resection of multiple metastases, complete resection of multiple metastases, and resection of a single metastasis all had similar rates of surgical morbidity and mortality of approximately 8 to 9 percent and 0 to 4 percent, respectively. However, those patients that underwent only a partial resection demonstrated a median survival time of about 6 months, whereas those that were treated with complete resection were found to have a longer median survival time of about 14 months. This provided evidence that total surgical resection of multiple metastases was comparable to resection of a solitary metastasis in efficacy. Several ensuing studies showed similar support for the use of surgical resection in the presence of multiple metastases[91, 92]. Thus, surgical resection of multiple metastases can be supported, although the general recommendation limits the number to less than 3 lesions in patients that have limited or controlled systemic disease.

A regimen that has been frequently discussed in the treatment of brain metastases is the combination of surgery plus external WBRT. Several studies have been conducted to compare the value of surgical resection followed by WBRT to that of either modality alone. Patchell et al[85] and Vecht et al[93] both demonstrated that those patients who were treated with the combination regimen had longer median survival times that those patients who received only WBRT. In contrast, Mintz et al[94] found that there was no survival advantage or improved quality of life with the administration of WBRT after surgery. This finding may be due to the overall lower patient performance status and greater prevalence of patients with more severe extracranial disease in their study. Patchell et al[85] actually demonstrated that patients with active systemic disease had a poorer prognosis when treated with surgical resection and WBRT. Studies comparing surgery alone with the adjunctive WBRT have also shown mixed results. Dosoretz et al[95] found that WBRT at a total dose of 30 Gy showed no survival advantages after surgical resection of a solitary metastasis. DeAngelis et al[70] and Hagen et al[96] also reported no effect on survival time, but noted WBRT postoperatively may reduce the risk of recurrence and thus recommend its use in patients after surgical resection for a single metastasis. Patchell et al has also further investigated the advantages of this combination regimen. In this prospective trial, patients were randomized to treatment with external WBRT or observation after surgery for a solitary brain metastasis. The results showed that patients who received the WBRT postoperatively had improved tumor control as seen by lower recurrence of metastases anywhere in the brain as well as at the site of resection. As with DeAngelis et al[70] and Hagen et al[96], this trial did not demonstrate prolonged survival time in patients receiving the adjunctive WBRT and did not slow the functional decline of patients, as measured by their KPS scores. Other studies have specifically addressed its use in melanoma metastases and have shown similar nonsignificant affect on prolonging survival times.

9.3 Stereotactic radiosurgery

Stereotactic surgery (SRS), also known as Gamma Knife, was first introduced in 1951 by Leksell[97]. Since then, it has developed into a sophisticated system that has the ability to accurately target an intracranial lesion and administer focal, collimated beams of ionizing radiation produced from a linear accelerator (linacs) or cobalt-60 sources. The radiation dose is administered in a single fraction via numerous crossfiring of beams of radiation that converge onto the targeted sight. The crossfiring of these beams from numerous directions allows for rapid radiation falloff in the surrounding tissue and thus minimize extraneous exposure. The advantage of SRS lies in its ability to administer localized treatment while sparing the rest of the normal brain parenchyma from the diffuse irradiation that occurs in WBRT. Moreover, the mechanism of action of SRS is thought to be different than WBRT and may instead affect the tumor vasculature, which would increase its effectiveness against the typically radioresistant cancers including malignant melanoma[98]. The advantage of SRS **(Figure 2)** over surgical resection is attributed to its ability to reach small, deep metastases in the brain without significant disruption to the rest of the brain parenchyma. Thus, it avoids the prolonged recovery time, increased length of hospital stay, and high costs that occur with an invasive surgery and instead only requires the administration of a single-fraction of radiation. Although it generally avoids these immediate side effects of surgical resection, delayed complications from SRS can occur which typically resemble other radiation-induced side effects such as radiation necrosis. This occurs in less than 10 percent of patients and is dependent on the volume treated and dose administered.

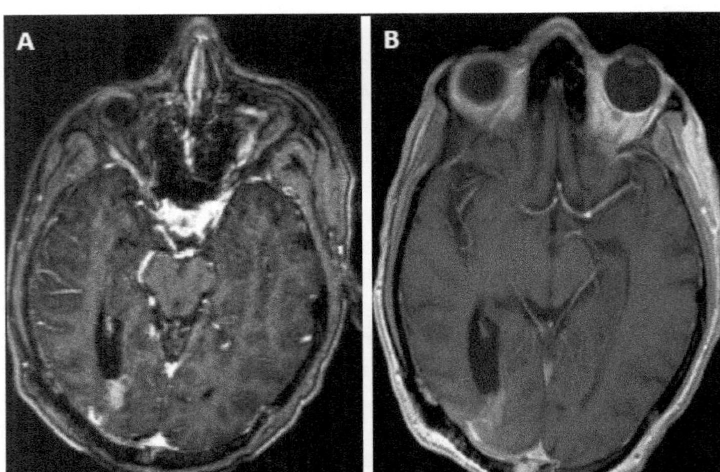

Fig. 2. Representative patient with intracranial metastatic melanoma who underwent stereotactic radiosurgery. **A,** pre-radiation contrast-enhanced axial T1 magnetic resonance image (MRI) demonstrating right occipital lobe metastatic melanoma. **B,** post-radiation contrast-enhanced axial T1 MRI.

There are a few disadvantages of SRS in comparison to the other treatment modalities. In comparison to surgery, its minimally invasive approach cannot provide immediate treatment effects which are often important in critical or life-threatening situations such as impending herniation. The inability to remove metastases also prevents a definitive histological diagnosis, and given the chance a suspected cranial metastases may actually be a nonmetastatic lesions, pathological diagnosis can be of great importance[85]. Also, increased risks in treating large metastases have hindered its use for those tumors that are larger than 3 cm in diameter. This is due to the limited conformity that can be achieved for large tumors, resulting in decreased response with increasing tumor size and increased radiation doses to the surrounding brain parenchyma[99]. Mehta et al[100] noted that tumors less than 2 cm^3 in volume showed a total response rate of 78 percent whereas as tumors greater than 10 cm^3 in volume demonstrated a total response rate less than 50 percent. Thus, SRS is typically recommended for patients with lesions less than 3 cm on neuroimaging, patients with lesions that are surgically inaccessible, patients that are asymptomatic, or patients that cannot tolerate surgery.

Multiple studies examining the efficacy of SRS have shown generally positive results. For all types of metastatic histologies, the local control rate after treatment with SRS ranges between 85 and 90 percent at one year[101-103]. For metastatic melanoma to the brain, the local control rate was shown to be approximately 90 to 97 percent[103-105]. Clinically, stabilization or improvement of neurological symptoms after treatment was noted in about 78 to 100 percent of patients[104, 106]. Patients also demonstrated a median survival time comparable to that of surgical resection which was found to be about 5 to 14 months[106-110]. However, as with the other treatment modalities, patient factors and selection affects outcome. Those with minimal extracranial disease typically fared better than their counterparts more extrcranial disease. This is also true for patients with overall better performance status, as measured by the KPS, compared to those with lower performance status. Patients with solitary brain lesions additionally demonstrated longer survival times than those patients with multiple brain lesions. However, an increased number of metastases should not be a reason to withhold SRS treatment[106-110].

Combination therapy has been studied and utilized in the treatment of metastatic melanoma to the brain. A landmark RTOG-sponsored study[111] compared the treatment of brain metastases using WBRT alone and SRS plus WBRT. Patients were first stratified according to the number of brain metastases and the extent of their extracranial disease and then randomized to treatment with WBRT only and SRS plus WBRT. There was a significant survival advantage for those harboring a solitary lesion treated with the combination therapy. There was no survival advantage for patients with multiple metastases treated with the combination approach. However, patients treated with WBRT and SRS were more likely to have improved or stable performance status and also decreased need for steroid use after therapy. There was no difference in mental status change and no increase in toxicity with the SRS and WBRT administration. The authors thus concluded that the combination approach of SRS plus WBRT should be the standard treatment for patients with a single unresectable brain metastasis. For patients with two to three bran metastases, despite the survival advantage the combination treatment should be considered because it results in improvement in the overall performance status.

To date, there are no prospective, randomized control trials comparing SRS with surgical resection. However, a few retrospective studies have provided insight into a comparison between the two treatment modalities. Auchter et al[112] designed a multi-institutional retrospective analysis comparing the outcome of patients treated with surgery and SRS and found no difference in the overall survival, functional independence, or recurrence rate. O'Neill et al[113] conducted a similar comparison and found no difference in median survival time after treatment with either approach. However, there was a significant difference in local tumor control, with no recurrence occurring after administration of SRS and about 58 percent recurrence after surgical resection. Bindel et al[114] conducted a smaller study in which patients undergoing SRS or surgical resection were matched on the basis of age, sex, primary tumor histology, extent of systemic disease, pretreatment KPS score, time to diagnosis of brain metastases, and number of brain metastases. The results demonstrated an overall survival advantage for surgical resection with a median survival time of 16.4 months compared to 7.5 months in the SRS treated group. Surgical resection also showed superiority to SRS in terms of local recurrence and morbidity. Thus, they favored the use of surgery over SRS for the treatment of solitary brain metastases. Cho et al[115] conducted a more encompassing study analyzing the treatment of solitary brain metastases with WBRT only, surgery plus WBRT, or SRS plus WBRT. The results demonstrated that the actuarial survival time was the same for the combination surgery group and the SRS surgery group, and both had longer survival times than patients receiving WBRT alone. Cho et al thus concluded that SRS is a reasonable and potentially more attractive alternative than surgical resection for single brain metastases. There are still several ongoing trials that include SRS in the treatment plan for brain metastases.

9.4 Chemotherapy

The use of chemotherapy for the treatment of extracranial melanoma has generally shown a poor response. Thus, it is not surprising that the response of melanoma metastases to the brain is also poor. The effect of cisplatin and etoposide has been shown to have a 0 percent response rate while other common metastatic cancers such as NSCLC and breast carcinoma have shown up to a 39 percent response. A significant obstacle for chemotherapeutic action on intracranial metastases is the BBB which limits the passage of large molecules into the brain parenchyma. Even after penetrating the BBB, some agents are rapidly eliminated and only have a transient effect. Attempts have been made to identify agents that can adequately cross the BBB to have tumorcidal effects. Fotemustine, a nitrosurea with high penetrations, has been shown to have response rates ranging from 12 to 25 percent in phase II European trials but is not available in the United States[116, 117]. Temozolamide, a dacarbazine analogue with high penetration, was approved for use by the FDA for use in primary brain tumors and was found to have a modest response rate of 7 percent for metastatic melanoma[118]. Combination chemotherapy has also been explored for increased effectiveness. A combination regimen of temozolomide and thalidomide, an antiangiogenic agent, has been explored because of its action against the vascularization of the tumor. Although the response was slightly better, this was at the expense of increased toxicity. A combination of chemotherapy and external WBRT is also being actively explored. Mornex et al[119] compared fotemustine alone versus fotemustine and WBRT and found that the response rates and survival times were not significantly different. Similarly, a phase III trial comparing WBRT alone and temozolomide plus WBRT demonstrated improved response rate but no prolonged survival time[120]. In general, current evidence does not support routinely administering chemotherapeutic agents for the treatment of cerebral metastases from melanoma.

9.5 Immunotherapy

Melanoma is a highly immunogenic tumor and treatment with immunotherapy has been attempted to halt the metastatic process. Predominantly from case studies, the overall response has not been optimal. Traditionally, the diagnosis of brain metastases has been an exclusionary criterion for receiving immunotherapy in patients with melanoma. However, biological response modifiers (BRMs) and cellular immunotherapy have been able to induce infrequent responses from brain metastases. One case report noted the near complete response in a patient with brain metastases after a treatment regimen of interleukin-2 (IL-2), interferon (IFN), and 5-fluorouracil[121]. Anecdotal cases of partial or complete responses have also been reported after ipilimumab therapy for metastatic melanoma to the brain which was treated earlier by surgery or SRS[122]. Another case report identified a patient with brain metastasis refractory to IL-2 and chemotherapy was responsive to lymphodepletion followed by infusion with autologous MART-reactive tumor infiltrating lymphocytes (TILs) and high doses of IL-2[123]. Hong et al[124] investigated the response rate and response duration of melanoma brain metastases to adoptive cell therapy (ACT) with autologous antitumor lymphocytes plus IL-2 following a lymphodepleting preparative regimen. They found that greater than 50 percent of patients had complete or partial response to the treatment regimen with rare occurrence of negative side effects. Majer et al[125] conducted a study of 70 patients with or without brain metastases treated with temozolomide or DTIC plus the BRMs IL-2 and IFN-α 2B. They demonstrated that patients with brain metastases who were treated previously with SRS had a prolonged median survival time of 15.8 months versus 11.1 months in patients without brain involvement. Overall, there have been limited studies and trials into the use of immunotherapy and additional investigation into its efficacy is needed.

10. Conclusions

Metastasis to the brain is a devastating and common consequence for patients with malignant melanoma. A significant number of patients with melanoma eventually develop brain metastasis at the time of death. Current treatment options typically include surgery and radiation therapy for brain metastases but the number of options is increasing. Prolonged survival depends on prompt diagnosis and treatment for patients harboring these lesions.

11. References

[1] Barnholtz-Sloan, J.S., et al., *Incidence Proportions of Brain Metastases in Patients Diagnosed (1973 to 2001) in the Metropolitan Detroit Cancer Surveillance System*. J Clin Oncol, 2004. 22(14): p. 2865-72.

[2] Gavrilovic, I.T. and J.B. Posner, *Brain metastases: epidemiology and pathophysiology*. J Neurooncz, 2005. 75(1): p. 5-14.

[3] Johnson, J.D. and B. Young, *Demographics of brain metastasis*. Neurosurg Clin N Am, 1996. 7(3): p. 337-44.

[4] Suki, D., *The epidemiology of brain metastasis*, in *Intracranial Metastases: current management strategies*, R. Sawaya, Editor. 2004, Wiley-Blackwell: Malden, MA. p. 20-34.

[5] Coit, D.G., *Role of surgery for metastatic malignant melanoma: a review*. Semin Surg Oncol, 1993. 9(3): p. 239-45.
[6] Ewend, M.G., L.A. Carey, and H. Brem, *Treatment of melanoma metastases in the brain.* Semin Surg Oncol, 1996. 12(6): p. 429-35.
[7] Fidler, I.J., et al., *The biology of melanoma brain metastasis.* Cancer Metastasis Rev, 1999. 18(3): p. 387-400.
[8] Ahmedin, J., et al., *Cancer statistics, 2010.* CA Cancer J Clin, 2010. 60(5): p. 277-300.
[9] Chason, J.L., F.B. Walker, and J.B. Landers, *Metastatic carcinoma in the central nervous system and dorsal root ganglia.* Cancer, 1963. 16(6): p. 781-7.
[10] del la Monte, S., G.W. Moore, and G.M. Hutchins, *Patterned distribution of metastses from malignant melanoma in humans.* Cancer Res, 1983. 43(7): p. 3427-33.
[11] Patel, K.J., et al., *Metastatic pattern of malignant melanome: a study of 216 autopsy cases.* Am J Surg, 1978. 135(6): p. 807-10.
[12] Skibber, J.M., et al., *Cranial irradiation after surgical excision of brain metastases in melanoma patients.* Ann Surg Oncol, 1996. 3(2): p. 118-23.
[13] Bryne, T.N., T.L. Cascino, and J.B. Posner, *Brain metastasis from melanoma.* J Neuroonc, 1983. 1(4): p. 313-7.
[14] Sampson, J.H., et al., *Demographics, prognosis, and therapy in 702 patients with brain metastases from malignant melanoma.* J Neurosurg, 1998. 1998(88): p. 1.
[15] Daryanani, D., et al., *Increased incidence of brain metastases in cutaneous head and neck melanoma.* Melanoma Res, 2005. 15(2): p. 119-24.
[16] Ballo, M.T., et al., *Combined-modality therapy for patients with regional nodal metastases from melanoma.* Int J Radiat Oncol Biol Phys, 2006. 64(1): p. 106-13.
[17] Stevens, G., I. Firth, and A. Coates, *Cerebral metastases from malignant melanoma.* Radiother Oncol, 1992. 23(3): p. 185-91.
[18] Wronski, M. and E. Arbit, *Surgical treatment of brain metastases from melanoma: a retrospective study of 91 patients.* J Neurosurg, 2000. 93(1): p. 9-18.
[19] Choi, K.N., H.R. Withers, and M. Rotman, *Intracranial metastases from melanoma.* Cancer, 1985. 56(1): p. 1-9.
[20] Fidler, I.J., *The pathogenesis of cancer metastasis: the 'seed and soil' hypothesis revisited.* Nat Rev Cancer, 2003. 3(6): p. 453-8.
[21] Nicolson, G.L., *Cancer metastasis: tumor cell and host organ properties important in metastasis to specific secondary sites.* Biochem Biophys Acta, 1988. 948(2): p. 175-224.
[22] Nicolson, G.L., *Organ specificity of tumor metastasis: role of preferential adhesion, invasion and growth of malignant cells at specific secondary sites.* Cancer Metastasis Rev, 1988. 7(2): p. 143-88.
[23] Liotta, L.A., P.S. Steeg, and W.G. Stetler-Stevenson, *Cancer metastasis and angiogenesis: an imbalance of positive and negative regulation.* Cell, 1991. 64(2): p. 327-36.
[24] Yung, W.K.A., et al., *Intracranial metastases*, in *Cancer in the Nervous System*, V.A. Levin, Editor. 2002, Oxford University Press: New York. p. 321-40.
[25] Shapiro, W.R. and J.R. Shapiro, *Principles of brain tumor chemotherapy.* Semin Oncol, 1986. 13(1): p. 56-69.

[26] Stewart, P.A., et al., *Quantative study of microvessel ultrastructure in human peritumoral brain tissue. Evidence for a blood-brain barrier defect.* J Neurosurg, 1987. 67(5): p. 697-705.

[27] Loeffler, J.S., et al., *The treatment of recurrent brain metastases with stereotactic radiosurgery.* J Clin Oncol, 1990. 8(4): p. 576-82.

[28] Graus, F., L.R. Rogers, and J.B. Posner, *Cerebrovascular complications in patients with cancer.* Medicine, 1985. 64(1): p. 16-35.

[29] Brega, K., et al., *Surgical treatment of brain metastases.* Cancer, 1990. 66(10): p. 2105-10.

[30] Schellinger, P.D., H.M. Meinck, and A. Thron, *Diagnostic accuracy of MRI compared to CCT in patients with brain metastases.* J Neuroonc, 1999. 44(3): p. 275-81.

[31] Sze, G., et al., *Detection fo brain metastases: comparison of contrast-enhanced MR with unenhanced MR and enhanced CT.* AJNR Am J Neuroradiol, 1990. 11(4): p. 785-91.

[32] Tyler, D.S., et al., *Positiron emission tomography scanning in malignant melanoma.* Cancer, 2000. 89(5): p. 1019-25.

[33] Dewulf, P., et al., *Cerebral metastatic malignant melanoma: CT and MR findings with pathological correlation.* J Belge Radiol, 1993. 76(5): p. 318-9.

[34] Isiklar, I., et al., *Intracranial metastatic melanoma: correlation between MR imaging characteristics and melanin content.* AJR, 1995. 165(6): p. 1503-12.

[35] Woodruff, W.W., et al., *Intracerebral malignant melanom: high-field-strength MR imaging.* Radiology, 1987. 165(1): p. 209-13.

[36] Davis, P.C., et al., *Diagnosis of cerebral metastases: double-dose delated CT vs contrast-enhanced MR imaging.* AJNR Am J Neuroradiol, 1991. 12(2): p. 292-300.

[37] Miranda, E.P., et al., *Routing imaging of asymptomatic melanoma patients with metastasis to sentinael lymph nodes rarely identifies systemic disease.* Arch Surg, 2004. 139(8): p. 831-7.

[38] McWilliams, R.R., et al., *Treatment of brain metastases from melanoma.* Mayo Clin Proc, 2003. 78(12): p. 1529-36.

[39] Barth, A., L.A. Wanek, and D.L. Morton, *Prognostic factors in 1,521 melanoma patients with distant metastases.* J Am Coll Surg, 1995. 181(3): p. 193-201.

[40] Davies, M.A., et al. (2010) *Prognostic factors for survival in melanoma patients with brain metastases.* Cancer.

[41] Fife, K.M., et al., *Determinants of outcome in melanoma patients with cerebral metastases.* J Clin Oncol, 2004. 22(7): p. 1293-1300.

[42] Staudt, M., et al., *Determinant of survival in patients with brain metastases from cutaneous melanoma.* Br J Cancer, 2010. 102(8): p. 1213-8.

[43] Raizer, J.J., et al., *Brain and leptomeningeal metastases from cutanous melanoma: survival outcomes based on clinical features.* Neuro Oncol, 2008. 10(2): p. 199-207.

[44] Papadopoulos, M.C., et al., *Molecular mechanisms of brain tumor edema.* Neuroscience, 2004. 129(4): p. 1011-20.

[45] Drappatz, J., et al., *Medical management of brain tumor patients.* Neurol Clin, 2007. 25(4): p. 1035-71.

[46] Kaal, E.C. and C.J. Vecht, *The management of brain edema in brain tumors.* Curr Opin Oncol, 2004. 16(6): p. 593-600.

[47] Ryken, T.C., et al., *The role of steroids in the management of brain metastases: a systematic review and evidence-based clinical practice guideline.* J Neurooonc, 2010. 96(1): p. 103-14.

[48] Gutin, P.H., *Corticosteroid therapy in patients with cerebral tumor: benefits, mechanims, problems, practicalities.* Semin Oncol, 1975. 2(1): p. 274-81.

[49] Wen, P.Y., et al., *Medical management of patients with brain tumors.* J Neurooonc, 2006. 80(3): p. 313-32.

[50] Koehler, P.J., *Use of corticosteroids in neuro-oncology.* Anticancer Drugs, 1995. 6(1): p. 19-33.

[51] Kamar, F.G. and J.B. Posner, *Brain metastases.* Semin Neurol, 2010. 30(3): p. 217-35.

[52] Layton, A.J. and A. Gabrielli, *Elevated intracranial pressure*, in *Textbook of neurointensive care*, A.J. Layton, A. Gabrielli, and W.A. Friedman, Editors. 2004, Saunders: Philadelphia. p. 709-32.

[53] Glantz, M.J., et al., *Practice paramenter: anticonvulsant prophylaxis in patients with newly diagnosed brain tumors.* Neurology, 2000. 54(10): p. 1886-93.

[54] Maschio, M., et al., *Antiepileptics in brain metastases: safety, efficacy, and impact on life expectancy.* J Neurooonc, 2009. 98(1): p. 109-16.

[55] Schiff, D. and L.M. Deangelis, *Therapy of venous thromboembolism in patients with brain metastases.* Cancer, 1994. 73(2): p. 493-8.

[56] Browd, S.R., et al., *Prophylaxis for deep venous thrombosis in neurosurgery: a review of the literature.* Neurosurg Focus, 2004. 17(4): p. E1.

[57] Auguste, K.I., A. Quinones-Hinojosa, and M.S. Berger, *Efficacy of mechanical prophylaxis for venous thromboembolism in patients with brain tumors.* Neurosurg Focus, 2004. 17(4): p. E3.

[58] Levin, J.M., et al., *Complications of therapy for venous thromboembolic disease in patients with brain tumors.* Neurology, 1993. 43(6): p. 1111.

[59] Chao, J.H., R. Phillips, and J. Nickson, *Roentgen-ray therapy of cerebral metastases.* Cancer, 1954. 7(4): p. 682-9.

[60] Chu, F.C.H. and B.B. Hilaris, *Value of radiation therapy in the management of intracranial metastases.* Cancer, 1961. 14(3): p. 577081.

[61] Patchell, R.A., et al., *Postoperative radiotherapy in the treatment of single metastases to the brain.* JAMA, 1998. 280(17): p. 1485-9.

[62] Raizer, J., *Radiosurgery and whole-brain radiation therapy for brain metastases.* JAMA, 2006. 295(21): p. 2535-36.

[63] Peacock, K.H. and G.J. Lesser, *Current therapeutic approaches in patients with brain metastases.* Curr Treat Options Oncol, 2006. 7(6): p. 479-89.

[64] Fogarty, G., et al., *Whole brain radiotherapy after local treatment of brain metastases in melanoma patients - a randomised phase III trial.* BMC Cancer, 2011. 11(142).

[65] Khuntia, D., et al., *Whole-brain radiotherapy in the managment of brain metastases.* J Clin Oncol, 2006. 24(8): p. 1295-1304.

[66] Butler, J.M., S.R. Rapp, and E.G. Shaw, *Managing the cognitive effects of brain tumor radiation therapy.* Curr Treat Options Oncol, 2006. 7(6): p. 517-23.

[67] Littman, P., et al., *The somnolence syndrome in leukemic children following reduced daily dose fractions of cranial radiation.* Int J Radiat Oncol Biol Phys, 1984. 10(10): p. 1851-3.

[68] Faithfull, S. and M. Brada, *Somnolence syndrome in adults following cranial irradiation for primary brain tumors.* Clin Oncol (R Coll Radiol), 1998. 10(4): p. 250-4.

[69] DeAngelis, L.M., J.Y. Delattre, and J.B. Posner, *Radiation-induced dementia in patients cured of brain metastases.* Neurology, 1989. 39(6): p. 789-96.

[70] DeAngelis, L.M., et al., *The role of postoperative radiotherapy after resection of a single brain metastases.* Neurosurgery, 1989. 24(6): p. 798-805.

[71] Lee, Y.Y., C. Nauert, and J.P. Glass, *Treatment-related white matter changes in cancer patients.* Cancer, 1986. 57(8): p. 1473-82.

[72] Chang, E.L., et al., *Neurocognition in patients with brain metastases treated with radiosurgery or radiosurgery plus whole-brain irradiation: a randomised controlled trial.* Lancet Oncol, 2009. 10(11): p. 1037-44.

[73] Barranco, S.C., M.M. Romsdahl, and R.M. Humphreys, *The radiation response of human malignant melanoma cells grown in vitro.* Cancer Res, 1971. 31(6): p. 830-3.

[74] Overgaard, J., *The role of radiotherapy in recurrent and metastatic malignant melanoma: a clinical and radiobiological study.* Int J Radiat Oncol Biol Phys, 1986. 12(6): p. 867-72.

[75] Borgelt, B., et al., *The palliation of brain metastases: final results of the first two studes by the Radiation Therapy Oncology Group.* Int J Radiat Oncol Biol Phys, 1981. 6(1): p. 1-9.

[76] Kurtz, J.M., et al., *The palliation of brain metastases in a favorable patient population: a randomized clinical trial by the Radiation Therapy Oncology Group.* Int J Radiat Oncol Biol Phys, 1981. 7(7): p. 891-5.

[77] Rate, W., L. Solin, and A. Turrisi, *Palliative radiotherapy for metastatic malignant melanoma: brain metastases, bone metastases, and spinal cord compression.* Int J Radiat Oncol Biol Phys, 1988. 15(4): p. 859-64.

[78] Doss, L. and M. Memula, *The radioresponsiveness of melanoma.* Int J Radiat Oncol Biol Phys, 1982. 8(7): p. 1131-4.

[79] Carella, R.J., et al., *Value of radiation therapy in the management of patients with cerebral metastases from malignant melanoma: Radiation Therapy Oncology Group Brain Metastases Study I and II.* Cancer, 1980. 45(4): p. 679-83.

[80] Stridslev, I.C., S. Hagen, and O. Klepp, *Radiation therapy for brain metastases from malignant melanoma.* Acta Radiol Oncol, 1984. 23(4): p. 231-5.

[81] Ellerhorst, J., et al., *Whole brain irradiation for patients with metastatic melanoma: a review of 87 cases.* Int J Radiat Oncol Biol Phys, 2001. 49(1): p. 93-7.

[82] Buchsbaum, J.C., et al., *Survival by radiation therapy oncology group recursive partitioning analysis class and treatment modality in patients with brain metastases from malignant melanoma: a retrospective study.* Cancer, 2002. 94(8): p. 2265-72.

[83] Gaspar, L., et al., *Recursive partitionaing analysis (RPA) of prognostic factors in three Radiation Therapy Oncology Group (RTOG) brain metastases trials.* Int J Radiat Oncol Biol Phys, 1997. 37(4): p. 745-51.

[84] Grant, F.C., *Concerning intracranial malignant metastases: their frequency and the value of surgery in their treatment.* Ann Surg, 1926. 84(5): p. 635-46.

[85] Patchell, R.A., et al., *A randomized trial of surgery in the treatment of single metastases to the brain.* N Engl J Med, 1990. 322(8): p. 494-500.

[86] Brega, K., et al., *Surgical treatment of brain metastases in malignant melanoma.* Cancer, 1990. 66(10): p. 2105-10.

[87] Zacest, A.C., et al., *Surgical management of cerebral metastases from melanoma: outcome in 147 patients treated at a single institution over two decades.* J Neurosurg, 2002. 96(3): p. 552-8.
[88] Al-Shamy, G. and R. Sawaya, *Management of brain metases: the indispensable role of surgery.* J Neurooonc, 2009. 92(3): p. 275-82.
[89] McWilliams, R.R., et al., *Melanoma-induced brain metastases.* Expert Rev Anticancer Ther, 2008. 8(5): p. 742-55.
[90] Bindal, R.K., et al., *Surgical treatment of multiple brain metastases.* J Neurosurg, 1993. 79(2): p. 210-6.
[91] Iwadate, Y., H. Namba, and A. Yamaura, *Significance of surgical resection for the treatment of multiple brain metastasis.* Anticancer Res, 2000. 20(1B): p. 573-7.
[92] Paek, S.H., et al., *Reevaluation of surgery for the treatment of brain metastases: review of 208 patients with single or multiple brain metastases treated at one institution with modern neurosurgical techniques.* Neurosurgery, 2005. 56(5): p. 1021-34.
[93] Vecht, C.J., et al., *Treatment of single brain metastasis: radiotherapy alone or combined with neurosurgery?* Ann Neurol, 1993. 33(6): p. 583-90.
[94] Mintz, A.H., et al., *A randomized trial to assess the efficacy of surgery in addition to radiotherapy in patients with a single cerebral metastasis.* Cancer, 1996. 78(7): p. 1470-6.
[95] Dosoretz, D.E., et al., *Management of solitary metastasis to the brain: the role of elective brain irradiation following complete surgical resection.* Int J Radiat Oncol Biol Phys, 1980. 6(12): p. 1727-30.
[96] Hagan, N.A., et al., *The role of radiation therapy following resection of single brain metastasis from melanoma.* Neurology, 1990. 40(1): p. 158-60.
[97] Leksell, L., *The stereotaxic method and radiosurgery of the brain.* Acta Chir Scand, 1951. 102(4): p. 316-9.
[98] Niranjan, A., et al., *Experimental radiobiological investigations into radiosurgery: present understanding and future directions.* Neurosurgery, 2004. 55(3): p. 495-504.
[99] Smith, M.L. and J.Y. Lee, *Stereotactic radiosurgery in the management of brain metastases.* Neurosurg Focus, 2007. 22(3): p. E5.
[100] Mehta, M.P., et al., *Defining the role of radiosurgery in the management of brain metastases.* Int J Radiat Oncol Biol Phys, 1992. 24(4): p. 619-25.
[101] Flickinger, J.C., et al., *Radiosurgery: Its role in brain metastasis management.* Neurosurg Clin N Am, 1996. 7(3): p. 497-504.
[102] Young, R.F., *Radiosurgery for the treetment of brain metastases.* Semin Surg Oncol, 1998. 14(1): p. 70-8.
[103] Douglas, J.G. and K. Margolin, *The treatment of brain metastases from malignant melanoma.* Semin Oncol, 2002. 29(5): p. 518-24.
[104] Mori, Y., et al., *Stereotactic radiosurgery for cerebral metastatic melanoma: factors affecting local disease control and survival.* Int J Radiat Oncol Biol Phys, 1998. 42(3): p. 581-9.
[105] Somaza, S., et al., *Stereotactic radiosurgery for cerebral metastatic melanoma.* J Neurosurg, 1993. 79(5): p. 661-6.
[106] Lavine, S.D., et al., *Gamma knife radiosurgery for metastatic melanoma: an analysis of survival, outcome, and complications.* Neurosurgery, 1999. 44(1): p. 59-64.

[107] Brown, P.D., et al., *Stereotactic radiosurgery for patients with "radioresistant" brain metastases.* Neurosurgery, 2002. 51(3): p. 656-65.
[108] Mathieu, D., et al., *Gamm knife radiosurgery in the management of malignant melanoma brain metastases.* Neurosurgery, 2007. 80(3): p. 471-81.
[109] Mingione, V., et al., *Gamma surgery for melanoma metastases in the brain.* J Neurosurg, 2002. 96(3): p. 544-51.
[110] Nam, T.K., et al., *Gamma knife surgery for brain metastases in patients harboring four or more lesions: survival and prognostic factors.* J Neurosurg, 2005. 102(Suppl): p. 147-50.
[111] Andrews, D.W., et al., *Whole brain radiation therapy with or without stereotactic radiosurgery boost for patients with one to three brain metastases: phase III results of the RTOG 9508 randomised trial.* Lancet, 2004. 363(9422): p. 1665-72.
[112] Auchter, R.M., et al., *A multiinstituional outcome and prognostic factor anaylsis of radiosurgery for resectable single brain metastasis.* Int J Radiat Oncol Biol Phys, 1996. 35(1): p. 27-35.
[113] O'Neill, B.P., et al., *A comparison of surgical resection and stereotactic radiosurgery in the treatment of solitary brain metastases.* Int J Radiat Oncol Biol Phys, 2003. 55(5): p. 1169-76.
[114] Bindal, A.K., et al., *Surgery versus radiosurgery in the treatment of brain metastasis.* J Neurosurg, 1996. 84(5): p. 748-54.
[115] Cho, K.H., et al., *Stereotactic radiosurgery for patients with single brain metastasis.* J Radiosurgol, 1998. 1(2): p. 79-85.
[116] Kleeberg, U.R., et al., *Palliative therapy of melanoma patients with fotemustine. Inverse relationship between tumour load and treamtnet effectiveness. A mutlicentre phase II trial of the EORTC-Melanoma Cooperative Group (MCG).* Melanoma Res, 1995. 5(3): p. 195-200.
[117] Jacquillat, C., et al., *Final report of the French multicenter phase II study of the nitrosurea fotemustine in 153 evaluable patients with disseminated malignant melanoma including patients with cerebral metastases.* Cancer, 1990. 66(9): p. 1873-8.
[118] Siena, S., G. Landonio, and E. Baietta, *Temozolomide for the treatment of brain metastases associated with metastatic melanoma: a phase II study.* J Clin Oncol, 2003. 22(11): p. 2101-7.
[119] Mornex, F., et al., *Randomized phase III trial of fotemustine versus fotemustine plus whole brain irradiation in cerebral metastases of melanoma [in French].* Cancer Radiother, 2003. 7(1): p. 1-8.
[120] Antonadou, D., et al., *Phase II randomized trial of temozolomide and concurrent radiotherapy in patients with brain metastases.* J Clin Oncol, 2002. 20(17): p. 3644-50.
[121] Savas, B., et al., *Multidrug resistant malignant melanom with intracranial metastasis responding to immunotherapy.* Anti-cancer Res, 1999. 19(5C): p. 4413-20.
[122] Schartz, N.E.C., et al., *Complete regression of a previously untreated melanoma brain metastasis with ipilimumab.* Melanoma Res, 2010. 20(3): p. 247-50.
[123] Dudley, M.E., et al., *Adoptive cell transfer therapy following non-myeloablative but lymphodepleting chemotherapy for the treatment of patients with refractory metastatic melanoma.* J Clin Oncol, 2005. 23(10): p. 2346-57.

[124] Hong, J.J., et al., *Succesful treatment of melanoma brain metastases with adoptive cell therapy.* Clin Cancer Res, 2010. 16(19): p. 4892-8.
[125] Majer, M., et al., *Biochemotherapy of metastatic melanoma in patients with or without recently diagnosed brain metastases.* Cancer, 2007. 110(6): p. 1329-37.

Part 3

Targeted Chemotherapy and Immunotherapy

5

Chemotherapy

Aylin Türel Ermertcan, Ferdi Öztürk and Kamer Gündüz
Celal Bayar University, Faculty of Medicine, Department of Dermatology
Turkey

1. Introduction

The number of melanoma cases worldwide is increasing faster than any other cancer. Although early detection, appropriate surgery, and adjuvant therapy have improved outcomes, the prognosis of metastatic melanoma remains very poor. Advanced melanoma is still associated with an extremely poor median survival, ranging from 2 to 8 months, with only 5% surviving more than 5 years and remains one of the most treatment-refractory malignancies. Many agents have been investigated for antitumor activity in melanoma but the current treatment options for patients with metastatic disease are limited and non-curative in the majority of cases (Mouawad et al, 2010).

The treatment of a patient with metastatic melanoma depends on multiple factors including the overall condition and age of the patient, the sites and number of metastases, pace of the disease, and the patient's wishes for treatment. Currently, the goals of treatment are directed toward palliation of symptoms, particularly if the improvement in the symptoms related to the disease exceeds the side effects associated with the therapy (Green & Schuchter, 1998).

In advanced melanoma, single agent chemotherapy, combination chemotherapy, biochemotherapy (chemoimmunotherapy), targeted therapy, Toll-like receptor agonists and antiangiogenic therapies have been used (Bhatia et al., 2009; Chowdhury, 1999; Cohen & Falkson, 1998; Jilaveanu et al., 2009; Lutzky, 2010; O'Day et al, 2002; Tarhini & Agarwala, 2006; Treisman & Garlie, 2010).

In this chapter, classical chemotherapeutic agents, regimens and new chemotherapeutics, such as targeted therapies for melanoma treatment have been reviewed.

2. Chemotherapy

Melanoma is considered a chemotherapy-resistant disease, and systemic chemotherapy has failed to significantly improve the survival of patients with nonresectable metastatic melanoma. The disease frequently becomes refractory to the agents even after initial responses are observed. Despite the lack of curative effect for the patient with advanced metastatic disease, chemotherapy continues to play a role in palliation of the disease. Although many agents have been used for melanoma treatment, single agent chemotherapy has generally been considered ineffective. Despite the poor overall outcome with these agents, they are still in common use in the clinic (Treisman & Garlie, 2010).

For stage IV melanoma, palliative systemic chemotherapy is the mainstay of treatment and is associated with median survival durations with combination regimens of 6-9 months and

5-year survival rates of approximately 6%, which are not influenced significantly by any therapy yet tested in rigorous multicentre cooperative group trials (Eggermont & Kirkwood, 2004).

2.1 Single agent chemotherapy

A large number of clinical trials have tested different single drugs like alkylating agents, nitrosureas, vinca alkaloids, platinum drugs, taxanes, topoisomerase inhibitors and anthracyclines, but few have shown an objective response rate (<20%) or an increase in progression-free and overall survival rates (Mouawad et al, 2010).

2.1.1 Alkylating agents

Dacarbazine (DTIC) is the first US Food and Drug Administration (FDA) approved chemotherapeutic agent for the treatment of metastatic melanoma (Green & Schuchter, 1998; Mouawad et al, 2010). The response rates with dacarbazine were 15-25%, with median response durations of 5-6 months, but less than 5% of complete responses. Long-term follow-up of patients treated with DTIC alone shows that less than 2% of the patients could survive for 6 years (Mouawad et al, 2010, Sasse et al., 2009). DTIC is a prodrug of the alkylating agent 5-(3-methyltriazen-1-yl) imidazole-4-carboximide (MTIC). The drug is generally well tolerated, with nausea as its major side effect, which can be controlled with antiemetic therapy (Treisman & Garlie, 2010). Doses and schedules of DTIC vary widely, with no data suggest that response rates are influenced by these variables. The most commonly used regimen is 850-1000 mg/m^2 intravenously, on day 1 only, repeated every 3 weeks (Green & Schuchter, 1998). It can be applied 200 mg/m^2 intravenously daily for 5 days every 3 weeks (Jilaveanu et al., 2009). It is more effective for subcutaneous, lymph node, and pulmonary metastases (Jilaveanu et al., 2009), but it is ineffective in brain metastases (Marsden et al., 2010). DTIC has been used as a standard for comparing the efficacy of new regimens (Coit et al., 2011; Marsden et al., 2010).

Temozolomide (TMZ), an imidazotetrazine derivative of dacarbazine, is another cytotoxic alkylating agent and has the same active metabolite as dacarbazine. It is usually used to treat solid tumors, such as brain tumors, due to its ability to cross the blood-brain barrier, and might therefore constitute an alternative to DTIC in treating brain metastases, for which dacarbazine is ineffective (Jilaveanu et al., 2009; Treisman & Garlie, 2010).

TMZ was shown to have an objective response rate of 21% (12 of 56 patients) in a phase II study, with a median survival time of 5.5 months (Treisman & Garlie, 2010). Temolozomide was equivalent to dacarbazine in treating metastatic melanoma in a large randomized trial of melanoma patients with incipient metastatic disease. It was administered orally to one group at a dose of 200 mg/m^2 for 5 days every 4 weeks and compared with dacarbazine administered iv at 250 mg/m^2 for 5 days every 3 weeks. The median overall survival was 7.7 months for patients treated with TMZ and 6.4 for those treated with DTIC. The 6-month overall survival rate was 61% and 51%, respectively; the overall survival was not statistically significant. The median progression-free survival was significantly longer in patients treated with temozolomide (1.9 months versus 1.5 months). No big differences were observed in toxicity between the two drugs (Jilaveanu et al., 2009). The results of another multicentre phase III trial that randomized 859 patients to receive DTIC vs an extended dosing schedule of TMZ (150 mg/m^2/d on 7 consecutive days every 14 days) were recently reported. The investigators found no significant differences between DTIC and TMZ in objective response rate, progression-free survival, or overall survival (Bhatia et al., 2009).

Although temozolomide administered as a single agent might have some advantages in a select group of patients, it has not been FDA-approved for advanced stage melanoma; however, it is widely used in the United States. Temozolomide and dacarbazine are being studied in combination with other therapies (Jilaveanu et al., 2009). The addition of IFN to TMZ resulted in higher response rates; however, survival was similar for both treatments and the combination was associated with higher toxicity. TMZ has shown promising results in the treatment of brain metastases from melanoma and may be a reasonable option if surgery or radiation is not appropriate (Quirt et al., 2007).

In a randomized phase III study, Middleton et al. compared dacarbazine and temozolomide in 305 patients with advanced melanoma. They found that median survival time was 7.7 months for patients treated with temozolomide and 6.4 months for those treated with DTIC. Median progression-free survival was significantly longer in the temozolomide-treated group (1.9 months) than in the DTIC-treated group (1.5 months) ($p=0.012$). No major difference in drug safety was observed. Temozolomide therapy improved health-related quality of life; more patients showed improvement or maintenance of physical functioning at week 12. They concluded that temozolomide demonstrated efficacy equal to that of DTIC and was an oral alternative for patients with advanced metastatic melanoma (Middleton et al., 2000).

2.1.2 Antimicrotubular agents

Microtubular toxins and microtubular disassembly inhibitors have both been used in patients with metastatic melanoma. The vinca alkaloids especially vinblastine and vindesine, based on their modest activities and limited toxicities, have primarily been used in combination therapy (Mouawad et al., 2010; Treisman & Garlie, 2010). They are not effective as monotherapy. Vinflunine ditartrate and vinorelbine are the other vinca alkaloid agents that have been used in phase II trials (Jilaveanu et al., 2009).

Paclitaxel and docetaxel, taxanes, are microtubule disassembly inhibitors with antitumor activity in a variety of neoplastic diseases. Paclitaxel has been evaluated in several phase I and II studies, and has demonstrated an approximately 12% to 16% response rate in previously untreated patients. Paclitaxel is commonly used in combination with carboplatin in other malignancies, and was similarly tested in melanoma (Treisman & Garlie, 2010). Weekly administration of paclitaxel at a dose of 80 to 100 mg/m^2 (on days 1, 8, and 15 every 4 weeks) is well tolerated by most patients. Alternatively, a higher dose can be administered once every 3 to 4 weeks (Bhatia et al., 2009). A phase II docetaxel study showed a 12.5% response rate in melanoma with one of the patients having a durable complete response, and it still being actively studied in other combinations, with some benefit (Treisman & Garlie, 2010). Several studies have evaluated docetaxel, at a dose of 100 mg/m^2 administered intravenously over 1 hour every 21 days, with response rates ranging from 15% to 19% (Green & Schuchter, 1998).

Associated toxicities include fatique, alopecia, myelosuppression, neuropathy, myalgias, and hypersensitivity reactions (Bhatia et al., 2009).

2.1.3 Platinum analogs

Cisplatin and carboplatin have modest activity in patients with metastatic melanoma. Single agent cisplatin given at conventional doses yields a response rate of less than 10%. However, a phase II study that used a higher dose (150 mg/m^2) of cisplatin in combination with amifostine reported an objective response rate of 53%, although the responses were shortlived. A response rate of 19% was observed with carboplatin in a phase II study in chemotherapy-naive patients with metastatic melanoma. Carboplatin has also been used in combination with paclitaxel in previously treated patients (Bhatia et al., 2009).

2.1.4 Nitrosoureas

The nitrosoureas are a group of alkylating agents that act by cross-linking DNA (Treisman & Garlie, 2010). Carmustine (BCNU), lomustine (CCNU) and fotemustine have single-agent activity comparable to dacarbazine, although they cause more myelosuppression and alopecia. A chloroethyl nitrosourea, fotemustine rapidly crosses the blood-brain barrier and has been found to have encouraging activity in patients with brain metastases. When compared to dacarbazine in a phase III trial involving 229 patients with metastatic melanoma, fotemustine was associated with a higher objective response rate (15% vs 7%, respectively) and a trend toward improved survival (7.3 vs 5.6 months, respectively). In patients without brain metastases at inclusion, the median time to development of brain metastases was 22.7 months in the fotemustine arm vs 7.2 months in the dacarbazine arm. Fotemustine has not been approved by the FDA but is available in Europe (Bhatia et al., 2009).

In clinical practice, these agents have a limited role as single agents, but have been used in combination chemotherapy (Treisman & Garlie, 2010).

2.1.5 Tamoxifen

The identification of estrogen receptors in melanoma led to initial trials of hormonal therapy for the diseases, and tamoxifen, an estrogen receptor antagonist, might be considered one of the first targeted agents used for the therapy for melanoma. Tamoxifen was initially used as a single agent and then in combination with various chemotherapeutic regimens. Although initial studies suggested a benefit for tamoxifen as a single agent in the treatment of metastatic melanoma, subsequent studies showed a response rate of only 5%. In addition, evaluation of samples using immunostaining failed to demonstrate estrogen receptors. Tamoxifen could have several other effects including effects on angiogenesis, synergic effects with chemotherapy, and reversal of multidrug resistance. More recently, preclinical studies have shown that tamoxifen potentiates the cytotoxic action of chemotherapeutic agents, specifically DTIC and cisplatin (Green & Schuchter, 1998). Several randomized clinical trials have been conducted to assess the therapeutic benefit of tamoxifen in combination chemotherapy regimens. Cocconi et al of the Group of Italian Investigators For Cancer Research (GOIRC) compared DTIC alone to DTIC plus tamoxifen in a study of 117 patients. They found a statistically significant survival advantage to tamoxifen (48 weeks versus 29 weeks) and a higher response rate in patients receiving DTIC and tamoxifen compared with DTIC alone (Cocconi & Bella et al., 1992). In another randomized clinical trial, Rusthoven et al of the National Cancer Institute of Canada (NCIC) conducted a double-blind, placebo-controlled trial comparing response rates and survival of 200 patients receiving the Dartmouth regimen with and without tamoxifen. There was no statistically significant difference between the two groups in either overall response rate or survival (Rusthoven & Quirt et al., 1996).

In a metaanalysis of published randomized controlled trials involved 912 patients, it has been demonstrated that tamoxifen does not improve the overall response rate, complete

response rate, or survival rate when administered along with combined chemotherapy or biochemotherapy regimens (Lens et al., 2003).
Single drugs used in metastatic melanoma have been summarized in table 1.

Drugs	Abbreviation	Number of patients	Dose	Overall response	References
Dacarbazine	DTIC	1868	250 mg/m^2/day x 5 d	15-25%	Hill 2nd et al., 1979
Temozolomide	TMZ	305	150-200 mg/m^2/day x 5 d	14%	Bleehen et al., 1995; Newlands et al., 1992
Carmustine	BCNU	122	75-110 mg/m^2	13-18%	Ahmann et al., 1976
Semustine	MET-CCNU	347	130 mg/m^2	16%	Ahmann et al., 1976
Fotemustine	FTMU	153	100 mg/m^2/week x 3 w	20-25%	Jacquillat et al., 1990
Cisplatin	CDDP	114	60-150 mg/m^2	15%	Glover et al., 1987
Carboplatin	CBDCA	30	400 mg/m^2 iv every 4 weeks	19%	Evans et al., 1987
Vindezine	VDS	273	3 mg/m^2 slow iv (7-14 day intervals)	14%	Quagliana et al., 1984
Vinblastine	VLB	62	6-8 mg/m^2 slow iv 1/week	13%	Quagliana et al., 1984
Docetaxel	TXT	43	100 mg/m^2 iv every 21 days	14%	Aamdal et al., 1994
Paclitaxel	TXL	34	125-275 mg/m^2	15%	Einzig AI et al., 1991
Tamoxifen	TAM	172	20 mg/day orally	7%	Rumke et al., 1992

Table 1. Single drugs used in metastatic melanoma

2.2 Combination chemotherapy

The role of combination chemotherapy in the treatment of metastatic melanoma remains uncertain. Historically there have been suggestions of improved activity with combination regimens, but reports of high response rates have generally emerged from single institution studies, and when large multicentre trials have been performed they have not confirmed these improvements (Chowdhury et al., 1999). There are a numerous combinations of chemotherapy for melanoma that have been are being developed and studied. These regimens have generally employed DTIC or, more recently, TMZ. Larger multiinstitution studies and results of randomized clinical trials strongly suggest that DTIC alone is as good as any of the combination regimens. Various combinations of DTIC, nitrosoureas, and cisplatin with other chemotherapeutic agents have been extensively evaluated in phase II clinical trials, with response rates ranging from 20% to 40%. The more commonly tested combinations are presented in table 2.

A four-drug combination referred to as the BOLD regimen which includes bleomycin, vincristine, CCNU and DTIC was first studied regimen. Initial studies produced a response rate of 40%, with a 9% complete response rate. Follow-up phase II studies failed to confirm these results, with subsequent response rates falling to 4% to 20%. Another chemotherapeutic regimen extensively evaluated is the combination of vinblastine, cisplatin, and DTIC (CVD regimen), which was developed by Legha and colleagues. The response rates with this three-drug regimen range from 24% to 45% (Green & Schuchter, 1998). The Dartmouth regimen (CDBT) (McClay regimen) is a combination of cisplatin, carmustine, DTIC, and tamoxifen (NCCN Guidelines Version 2011 Melanoma, Treisman & Garlie, 2010).

Regimen	Doses	Response rate
BOLD	Bleomycin, 15 U day 1,4 Vincristine, 1mg/m^2 day 1,4 CCNU, 80 mg/m^2 day 1 DTIC, 200 mg/m^2 day 1-5 28-day cycles	9%-40%
CVD	Cisplatin, 20 mg/m^2 day 2-5 Vinblastine, 1.6 mg/m^2 day 1-5 DTIC, 800 mg/m^2 day 1 21-day cycles	24%-45%
CBDT (Dartmouth)	Cisplatin, 25 mg/m^2 day 1-3 BCNU, 150 mg/m^2 day 1 (given every other cycle) DTIC, 220 mg/m^2 day 1-3 Tamoxifen, 20 mg/day 21-day cycles	19%-55%

Table 2. Combination chemotherapy regimens in metastatic melanoma

In a large phase III study comparing the CVD regimen to DTIC alone, there was a trend toward improved response and survival. The Dartmouth regimen originally resulted in a 55% response rate in the initial series of 20 patients with metastatic melanoma (Treisman & Garlie, 2010). A phase III multicentre trial that randomized 240 patients to the Dartmouth regimen vs dacarbazine monotherapy did not show a statistically significant benefit in favor of the combination. Despite a modest difference in objective response rate in favor of CDBT over DTIC (16.8% and 9.9%, respectively; p=.13), there was no significant difference in overall survival (7.7 and 6.3 months, respectively; p=.52). Myelosuppression, fatique, nausea, and vomiting were significantly higher in the CDBT arm (Chapman et al., 1999).

Sileni et al. compared the activity and toxicity of the combination of dacarbazine, carmustine, cisplatin and tamoxifen (DBDT regimen) versus DTIC alone in patients with metastatic melanoma. Sixty patients were randomly assigned to receive BCNU 150 mg/m^2 intravenously on day 1, cisplatin 25 mg/m^2 iv. daily on days 1 to 3, DTIC 220 mg/m^2 iv daily on days 1 to 3 and tamoxifen 160 mg orally daily for 7 days prior to chemotherapy (DBDT arm). Treatment cycles were repeated every 28 days, while BCNU was given every two cycles. The DTIC arm patients received DTIC alone 1200 mg/m^2 iv on day 1, repeated every 21 days. The overall response rate was 26% in the DBDT arm and 5% in the DTIC arm. Complete responses were 2.5% for DBDT and 0% for DTIC. The median progression-free survival and median survival were 4 and 9 months, respectively for DBDT, and 2 and 7 months for DTIC. DBDT was associated with significant haematological toxicity: 33% of the patients experienced a grade III or IV neutropenia and 28% a grade III or IV thrombocytopenia. The overall response rate obtained with DBDT was greater than that obtained with DTIC alone; however, this combination increased toxicity (Sileni et al., 2001).

The combination of paclitaxel and carboplatin (PC) has been reported to have antitumor activity in patients with metastatic melanoma, including patients who have received prior chemotherapy (Bhatia et al., 2009).

Zimpfer-Rechner et al. performed a randomized, multicentre, second-line clinical phase II study of paclitaxel either as monotherapy or combined with carboplatin given on an outpatient basis. In arm A, paclitaxel was administered at a dose of 100 mg/m^2 intravenously on day 1 each week for 6 weeks. In arm B, paclitaxel was administered at a dose of 80 mg/m^2 intravenously followed by carboplatin 200 mg/m^2 on day 1 each week for 6 weeks. The next cycle was administered after a 2 week intermission. The study was stopped after 40 patients because the overall response rate was below 10% in both arms. The median survival time after initiation of second-line treatment was 209 days for patients treated with paclitaxel only, and 218 days for those treated with paclitaxel/carboplatin. The median time to progression was around 56 days in both arms. Paclitaxel with or without carboplatin had only limited efficacy, and the combination of these drugs adds significantly to haematological toxicity without improving response or survival rates (Zimpfer-Rechner et al., 2003).

Rao et al. published their results with the combination of paclitaxel and carboplatin in 31 patients with metastatic melanoma. These patients had a median of two previous therapies, with the majority (29; 94%) having failed prior temozolomide or dacarbazine therapy. The most commonly used regimen was weekly paclitaxel (at a dose of 100 mg/m^2) and carboplatin administered on days 1,8, and 15 of a 28-day cycle. An objective partial response was noted in 8 patients (26%) with an additional 6 patients (19%) having stable disease; a clinical benefit was noted in 45% of those patients treated. The median time to disease progression was 3 months (range, 0-7 mos), with a median overall survival of 7.8 months (range, 1-14 mos). They concluded that the combination of paclitaxel and carboplatin appeared to have definite and clinically meaningful activity when used as second-line therapy after temozolomide or dacarbazine (Rao et al., 2006).

In a report on synthesis of randomized trials, 48 studies having 111 active treatment arms (24 with dacarbazine monotherapy, n=1390; 75 with dacarbazine combinations, n=4962; 12 with non-dacarbazine treatments, n=783) treating 7135 patients were examined. Response to dacarbazine monotherapy ranged between 5.3% and 28% (average 15.3%). Partial responses comprised 73% of successes. Only adding interferons improved response rates but survival duration was not significantly longer. All other treatments alone or in combination were ineffective (Lui et al., 2007).

A listing of major randomized studies evaluating DTIC versus drug combination is summarized in table 3.

Control arm dacarbazine dose/schedule	Study arm drugs (dose/schedule)	No. of randomised patients	Overall response (%)	Overall survival (months)	Study by
2 mg/kg/day (iv) × 10 days	Carmustine 150 mg/m^2 (iv) + vincristine 2 mg/m^2 (iv) on day 1 only	50	22 vs 25	NA	Bellet et al., 1976
250 mg/m^2 (iv) on days 1-5 every 3 weeks	Cisplatin 20 mg/m^2/day for 4 days starting on day 2 + vinblastine 1.6 mg/m^2/day × 5 days + dacarbazine 800 mg/m^2 (iv) on day 1	104	11 vs 24	5 vs 6	Buzaid et al., 1993
1000 mg/m^2 bid short iv infusion every 3 weeks	Tamoxifen 10 mg twice daily by mouth 1 week before chemotherapy +carmustine 150 mg/m^2 on day 1+dacarbazine 220 mg/m^2 (iv)+cicplatin 25 mg/m^2/days 1-3	240	10.2 vs 18.5	6.3 vs 7.7	Chapman et al., 1999
250 mg/m^2 (iv) for 4 days every 3 weeks	Dacarbazine 250 mg/m^2 (iv) days 1-4 every 3 weeks + detorubicin 120 mg/m^2 iv every 3 weeks	51	15 vs 36	5 vs 6	Chauvergne et al., 1982
1200 mg/m^2 day 1 every 3 weeks	Carmustine 150 mg/m^2 (iv) on day 1 + cisplatin 25 mg/m^2 (iv)/day on days 1-3 + dacarbazine 220 mg/m^2 (iv)/day on days 1-3 + tamoxifen 160 mg orally/day × 7 days prior to chemotherapy. Treatment cycles repeated every 28 days, BCNU every 2 cycles	60	6 vs 26	7 vs 9	Chiarion Sileni et al., 2001
2.5 mg/m^2 (I.V.) injection on days 1-4 every 4 weeks	Dacarbazine 2.5 mg/m^2 (iv) by means of bolus injection on days 1-4 every 4 weeks + corynebacterium parvum 7 mg (im) 1 week before starting DTIC and at 4-week intervals thereafter	49	22 vs 27	5 vs 5	Clunie et al., 1980
250 mg/m^2 on days 1-5 every 3 weeks	Dacarbazine 250 mg/m^2 (iv) × 5 days, every 3-weeks + tamoxifen 20 mg/m^2 orally daily	117	12 vs 28	11.8 vs 7.25	Cocconi et al., 1992

Control arm dacarbazine dose/schedule	Study arm drugs (dose/schedule)	No. of randomised patients	Overall response (%)	Overall survival (months)	Study by
200 mg/m² (iv) for 5 days repeated every 3 weeks	po methyl-CCNU 200 mg/m² once every 6 weeks Dacarbazine 150 mg/m² (iv) × 5 days/3 weeks + po methyl-CCNU 130 mg/m²1/6 weeks	415	15 vs 15 15 vs 14	4.0 vs 4.2 4.0 vs 4.0	Costanza et al., 1977
250 mg/m² (iv) on days 1–5 every 3 weeks	Dacarbazine 250 mg/m² (iv)/day on days 1–5 + epirubicin 90 mg/m² on day 1 every 3 weeks	42	9 vs 21	NA	Lopez et al., 1984
250 mg/m² (iv) on days 1–10 every 4 weeks	Vinblastine 6 mg/m²/day (iv) on days 1–2 + 24-h infusion of bleomycin 15 units/m² from days 1–5 + cisplatin 50 mg/m² 1 h (iv) infusion on day 5. After four courses, vinblastine and cisplatin were given alone. Courses repeated on a cycle of 4 weeks	77	14 vs 10	4.1 vs 3.42	Luikart et al., 1984
300 mg/m²/day × 6 days every month days.	Dacarbazine 100 mg/m²/8 h × 6 days every month days Carmustine 150 mg/m² + vincristine 2 mg/m² every 30 days	120	32 vs 29 32 vs 24	8.5 vs 8.4 8.5 vs 6.5	Moon et al., 1975
250 mg/m²/day (iv) for 5 days every 4 weeks	Dacarbazine 250 mg/m²/day (iv) × 5 days every 4 weeks + vindesine 3 mg/m²/week	119	18 vs 25	4.1 vs 5.7	Ringborg et al., 1989
220 mg/m² on days 1–3, q 21 days	Dacarbazine 220 mg/m² on day 1–3 + carboplatine AUC 5, day 1, q 21 days	148	11.7 vs 21.3	7 vs 9	Babovic et al., 2008
200 mg/m²/day (iv) for 5 days every 28 days	Arm 2: (I.V.) IFN-α 15 MU/m²/day days 1–5 × 3 weeks, then (sc) 10 MU/m² 3×/week + dacarbazine 200 mg/m² daily (iv) days 1–5 starting on day 22, every 28 days Arm 3: orally tamoxifen 20 mg/day starting day 1 + dacarbazine 200 mg/m²/day	280	15 vs 21 15 vs 18 15 vs 19	9.99 vs 9.33 9.99 vs 7.97 9.99 vs 9.54	Falkson et al., 1998

Control arm dacarbazine dose/schedule	Study arm drugs (dose/schedule)	No. of randomised patients	Overall response (%)	Overall survival (months)	Study by
	(iv) days 1–5 every 28 days Arm 4: (iv) IFN-α 15 MU/m²/day days 1–5 × 3 weeks, then (sc) 10 MU/m² 3×/week + orally tamoxifen 20 mg/day starting day 1 + dacarbazine 200 mg/m²/day (iv) days 1–5/28 days				
800 mg/m² (iv) on days 1 and 21	Dacarbazine 800 mg/m² (iv) days 1 and 21 + daily (im) INF-α 3 MIU at days 1–3, 6 MIU days 4–6, and 9 MIU daily thereafter. Started concomitantly Dacarbazine 800 mg/m² (iv) days 1 and 21 + (IM) INF-α 3 MIU 3×/week. Started concomitantly	266	20 vs 28 20 vs 23	11 vs 13 11 vs 11	Bajetta et al., 1994
800 mg/m² (iv) every 3 weeks	Dacarbazine (iv) escalating dose 200 mg/m², 400 mg/m², 800 mg/m²/3 weeks; sc IFN-α starting at 3 MU/day on days 1–3, 9 MU/day on days 4–70, then 9 MU 3×/week	170	17 vs 21	7.36 vs 6.27	Thomson et al., 1993

Table 3. Key randomized studies evaluating dacarbazine (DTIC) vs drug combination

2.3 Biochemotherapy

Biochemotherapy, the combination of chemotherapy and biologic response modifiers, was developed in the early 1990s to improve response rates and durable remissions in metastatic melanoma. The initial regimens were given sequentially (chemotherapy followed by biologic response modifiers) because of concern of toxicity if all the drugs were given simultaneously. Paradoxically, sequential regimens were highly toxic because of the duration of treatment (10 to 14 days) and the combined and non-overlapping toxicities of chemotherapy and biologic response modifiers (O'day et al., 2002). An outpatient biochemotherapy regimen (carmustine, cisplatin, dacarbazine, tamoxifen, IL-2 and interferon with lower dose subcutaneous IL-2 and interferon) was developed by Thompson et al (Thompson et al., 1997). The first concurrent inpatient biochemotherapy regimen was developed by Legha et al. „Legha regimen" combined cisplatin, vinblastine and dacarbazine (CVD) chemotherapy with continuous infusion IL-2 (9 MU/m² per day) for 4 days and 5 days of subcutaneous interferon alfa (5 MU/m^2 per day) at 21-day intervals. The results were encouraging with an overall response rate of 64%, a complete response rate of 21%, median survival of 12 months, and a 2-year survival rate of 10%. Efficacy was comparable to the inpatient sequential regimens, but the regimen was significantly less toxic. Fever/neutropenia occured in 64% of patients and was the most significant reversible toxicity (Legha et al., 1998; O'day et al., 2002). The Legha regimen was subsequently modified by McDermott et al. to reduce toxicity. The modifications included reduction in the vinblastine dose, empiric granulocyte colony-stimulating factor (G-CSF) posttreatment, routine 5-HT3 antagonist anti-emetic therapy, prophylactic antibiotics, frequent changes in central lines, dose reductions for toxicity, and limitation of treatment to a maximum of 4 cycles of therapy (McDermott et al., 2000). In a phase II trial with these modifications, toxicity was improved and the response rate was 48%, the complete remission rate was 20%, and the median survival was 11 months. Fever/neutropenia was not observed. G-CSF has now become a standard component of concurrent biochemotherapy regimens. Further modifications of the Legha regimen have been published with decrescendo dosing of continuous infusion IL-2. The rationale for decrescendo dosing of IL-2 is based on improved clinical response and reduced cumulative IL-2 toxicity (O'day et al., 2002).

Ridolfi et al conducted a multicenter prospective randomized clinical trial in outpatients with metastatic melanoma to compare chemotherapy with biochemotherapy using immunomodulant doses of IL-2 and IFNα-2b. They randomized 176 patients with advanced melanoma to receive chemotherapy (cisplatin and dacarbazine with or without carmustine every 21 days) or biochemotherapy comprising the same chemotherapy regimen followed by low-dose subcutaneous IL-2 for 8 days and IFNα-2b three times a week, both for six cycles. At a median follow-up of 18 (chemotherapy) and 16 (biochemotherapy) months, median overall survival was 9.5 versus 11.0 months ($p=.51$), respectively. Treatment-related toxicity was fairly similar in both groups. They concluded that the addition of low-dose immunotherapy did not produce a significant advantage in overall survival, time to progression, or overall response (Ridolfi et al., 2002).

Bajetta et al. investigated the effects of additional cytokines to chemotherapy in 151 untreated metastatic melanoma patients. 75 patients received cisplatin 30 mg/m^2 on days 1-3, vindesine 2.5 mg/m^2 on day 1 and dacarbazine 250 mg/m^2 on days 1-3. 76 patients received same CVD scheme plus interferon-α2b on days 1-5 and interleukin-2 on days 1-5 and 8-15, both administered subcutaneously, either recycled every 3 weeks. 10% of the patients were alive at a median of 52 months from start of therapy. They observed a response rate of 21% on arm A versus 33% on arm B; three patients (4%) given biochemotherapy had complete responses. Median time to progression was identical; median overall survival time was 12 months on arm A and 11 months on arm B. They also concluded that biochemotherapy was not better than chemotherapy alone, therefore biochemotherapy can not be recommended as standard first-line therapy for metastatic melanoma (Bajetta et al., 2006).

3. Novel targeted agents

The mitogen-activated protein kinase pathway plays a key role in melanoma development and is an important therapeutic target. Disregulation of this pathway may result in increased signalling activity leading to proliferation, invasion, metastasis, migration, survival and angiogenesis. Activating mutations in the BRAF and NRAS genes have been found to be relatively frequent in melanoma, occurring in approximately 50-60% and 15% of tumors, respectively (Lutzky, 2010). It has been shown that mutations in the KIT gene are more frequent in patients with melanomas arising from mucosal, acral and sun-damaged skin primary sites. NRAS and BRAF mutated melanomas are more commonly derived from non sun-damaged skin (Curtin et al., 2005; Curtin et al., 2006).

Recent reports describing major responses in KIT-mutated melanomas treated with imatinib mesylate and other drugs that inhibit KIT tyrosine kinase have led to larger trials of imatinib mesylate in mutation enriched populations, in an attempt to confirm that mutated KIT is a clinically important target in this small subpopulation of patients with melanoma. The most common BRAF mutation in melanoma (in 90% of BRAF-mutated melanomas) is the V600E mutation, which activates BRAF 500-fold. Sorafenib inhibits the BRAF serine/threonine kinase as well as various receptor tyrosine kinases, with significant activity in the VEGFR. Two randomized clinical trials testing sorafenib in combination with chemotherapy in melanoma produced negative results. The most likely explanation is that sorafenib is not very active against V600E mutated BRAF kinase. More specific BRAF-targeting drugs have been developed are under investigation. In a phase I trial recently published, PLX4032, an oral, selective inhibitor of oncogenic V600E BRAF kinase, induced complete or partial tumor regression in 81% of patients who had melanoma with the V600E BRAF mutation, with responses being observed in all sites of disease. Cutaneous side effects, fatigue and arthralgia were the most common side effects (Lutzky, 2010).

In a phase II study evaluating the effects of sorafenib in advanced melanoma, a total of 101 patients received placebo plus dacarbazine (n=50) or sorafenib plus dacarbazine (n=51). On day 1 of a 21-day cycle, patients received intravenous dacarbazine 1000 mg/m^2 for a maximum of 16 cycles. Oral sorafenib 400 mg or placebo was administered twice a day continuously. Median progression-free survival in the sorafenib plus dacarbazine arm was 21.1 weeks versus 11.7 weeks in the placebo plus dacarbazine arm (p=0.068). There were statistically significant improvements in progression-free survival rates at 6 and 9 months, and in time to progression in favour of the sorafenib plus dacarbazine arm. No difference in overall survival was observed. Sorafenib plus dacarbazine was well tolerated in patients with advanced melanoma and yielded an encouraging improvement in progression-free survival (McDermott et al., 2008). Hauschild et al reported a phase III randomized, placebo-controlled study on the efficacy and safety of sorafenib with carboplatin and paclitaxel in advanced melanoma who had progressed on a dacarbazine-or temozolomide-containing regimen. A total of 270 patients were randomly assigned to receive intravenous paclitaxel 225 mg/m^2 plus intravenous carboplatin at area under curve 6 (AUC 6) on day 1 of a 21-day cycle followed by either placebo (n=135) or oral sorafenib 400 mg (n=135) twice daily on days 2 to 19. The median progression-free time was 17.9 weeks for the placebo plus carboplatin arm and 17.4 weeks for the sorafenib plus carboplatin arm (p=.49). Response rate was 11% with placebo versus 12% with sorafenib. Grade III thrombocytopenia, diarrhea, and fatigue were more common in patients treated with sorafenib plus carboplatin versus placebo plus carboplatin. The addition of sorafenib to carboplatin did not improve any of the end points over placebo plus carboplatin in this study (Hauschild et al., 2009).

BAY 43-9006 is a novel RAF inhibitor that inhibits B-RAF and C-RAF. It is orally available and has been shown to be well tolerated. In a phase I/II trial of BAY 43-9006 in combination with carboplatin and paclitaxel, 35 melanoma patients were treated for at least 6 weeks. Among 32 evaluable patients, 11 (34%) had partial responses, including 10 ongoing at 3-16 months. Nineteen patients had stable disease as best response. The combination demonstrated activity in melanoma and had a favourable safety profile and no apparent pharmacokinetic interactions (Tarhini & Agarwala, 2006).
Angiogenesis and signalling through the ref/mitogen-activated protein/extracellular signal-regulated kinase/extracellular signal-regulated kinase cascade have been reported to play important roles in melanoma. Ref/mitogen-activated protein/extracellular signal-regulated kinase inhibitor AZD6244 is a new targeted agent for advanced melanoma (Friday & Adjei, 2008). Other important molecular pathways have been found to be altered in melanoma, opening new avenues for therapeutic intervention. These include the phosphatidylinositol-3-kinase, microphtalmia-associated transcription factor, cyclin-dependent kinases, notch-1 and iNOS pathways. Early clinical trials with drugs that are active in these pathways are being conducted (Lutzky, 2010).

4. Conclusion

Metastatic melanoma has remained refractory to systemic treatment for decades. Single-agent or combination chemotherapy or biologic response modifiers alone have not resulted in response rates of durable remissions that are high enough to affect median survival. In the past decade, biochemotherapy regimens have been developed that appear to produce systemic response in approximately 50% patients and durable remissions in 10% to 20%. Modified concurrent biochemotherapy regimens have preserved efficacy and reduced toxicity, thus allowing for larger community-based clinical trials that are currently ongoing. These trials will determine the role of biochemotherapy as first-line treatment for metastatic disease. Further understanding of the molecular and immunologic mechanisms that promote survival of melanoma tumor cells will undoubtedly lead to the development of better, more specific and perhaps less toxic agents.

5. References

Aamdal, S.; Wolff, I. & Kaplan, S. (1994). Docetaxel (Taxotere) in Advanced Malignant Melanoma: A Phase II Study of the EORTC Early Clinical Trials Group. *Eur J Cancer,* Vol. 30, pp. 1061-1064.

Ahmann DL. (1976). Nitrosoureas in the Management of Disseminated Malignant Melanoma. *Cancer Treat Rep,* Vol. 60, pp. 747-751.

Babovic, N.; Matkovic, S.; Ursulovic, T.; Kreacic, M.; Milosavljevic, M. & Jelic, M. (2008). Randomized Phase II Study of Dacarbazine (DTIC) with or without Carboplatin (CBDCA) in patients with Stage IV Cutaneous Melanoma. *Annals of Oncology,* Vol. 19, pp. 239-246.

Bajetta, E.; Di Leo, A. & Zampino, MG. (1994). Multicenter Randomized Trial of Dacarbazine Alone or in Combination with Two Different Doses and Schedules of Interferon alpha-2a in the Treatment of Advanced Melanoma. *J Clin Oncol,* Vol. 12, pp. 806-811.

Bajetta, E.; Vecchio, MD.; Nova, P.; Fusi, A.; Daponte, A.; Sertoli, MR.; Queirolo, P.; Taveggia, P.; Bernengo, MG.; Legha, SS.; Formisano, B. & Cascinelli, N. (2006). Multicenter Phase III Randomized Trial of Polychemotherapy (CVD Regimen) versus The Same Chemotherapy (CT) Plus Subcutaneous Interleukin-2 and Interferon-α2b in Metastatic Melanoma. *Annals of Oncology,* Vol. 17, pp. 571-577.

Bellett, RE.; Mastrangelo, MJ.; Laucius, JF. & Bodurtha, AJ. (1976). Randomized Prospective Trial of DTIC (NSC-45388) Alone versus BCNU (NSC-409962) plus Vincristine (NSC-67574) in the Treatment of Metastatic Malignant Melanoma. *Cancer Treat Rep,* Vol. 60, pp. 595-600.

Bhatia, S.; Tykodi, SS. & Thompson JA. (2009). Treatment of Metastatic Melanoma: An Overview. *Oncology,* Vol. 23, pp. 488-496.

Bleehen, NM.; Newlands, ES. & Lee, SM. (1995). Cancer Research Campaign Phase II Trial of Temozolomide in Metastatic Melanoma. *J Clin Oncol,* Vol. 13, pp. 910-913.

Buzaid, AC.; Legha, SS.; Winn, R.; Belt, R.; Pollock, T. & Wiseman C. (1993). Cisplatin, Vinblastine and Dacarbazine (CVD) versus Dacarbazine Alone in Metastatic Melanoma: Preliminary Results of A Phase II Cancer Community Oncology Program (CCOP) Trial. *J Clin Oncol,* Vol. 12, pp. 389.

Chapman, PB.; Einhorn, LH.; Meyers, ML.; Saxman, S.; Destro, AN.; Panageas, KS.; Begg, CB.; Agarwala, SS.; Schuchter, LM.; Ernstoff, MS.; Houghton, AN. & Kirkwood, JM. (1999). Phase III Multicenter Randomized Trial of the Dartmouth Regimen versus Dacarbazine in Patients with Metastatic Melanoma. *J Clin Oncol,* Vol. 17, pp. 2745-2751.

Chauvergne, J. ;Bui, NB. & Cappelaere, P. (1982). Chemotherapy in Advanced Malignant Melanoma. Results of A Controlled Trial Comparing A Combination of Dacarbazine (DTIC) and Detorubicin with Dacarbazine Alone. *Sem Hop,* Vol. 58, pp. 2697-2701.

Chiarion Sileni, V.; Nortilli, R. & Aversa, SM. (2001). Phase II Randomized Study of Dacarbazine, Carmustine, Cisplatin and Tamoxifen versus Dacarbazine Alone in Advanced Melanoma Patients. *Melanoma Res,* Vol. 11, pp. 189-196.

Chowdhury, S.; Vaughan, MM. & Gore, ME. (1999). New Approaches to the Systemic Treatment of Melanoma. *Cancer Treatment Reviews,* Vol. 25, pp. 259-270.

Clunie, GJ.; Gough, IR.; Dury, M.; Furnival, CM. & Bolton, PM. (1980). A Trial of Imidazole Carboxamide and Corynebacterium parvum in Disseminated Melanoma: Clinical and Immunologic Results. *Cancer,* Vol. 46, pp. 475-479.

Cocconi, G.; Bella, M. & Calabresi, F. (1992). Treatment of Metastatic Malignant Melanoma with Dacarbazine plus Tamoxifen. *N Engl J Med,* Vol. 327, pp. 516-523.

Cohen, GL. & Falkson, CI. (1998). Current Treatment Options for Malignant Melanoma. *Drugs,* Vol.55, No. 6, pp. 791-799.

Costanza, ME.; Nathanson, L. & Schoenfeld D. (1977). Results with methyl-CCNU and DTIC in Metastatic Melanoma. *Cancer,* Vol. 40, pp. 1010-1015.

Curtin, JA.; Fridlyand, J. & Kageshita, T. (2005). Distinc Sets of Genetic Alterations in Melanoma. *N Engl J Med,* Vol. 353, pp. 2135-2147.

Curtin, JA.; Busam, K. & Pinkel, D. (2006). Somatic Activation of KIT in Distinct Subtypes of Melanoma. *J Clin Oncol,* Vol. 24, pp. 4340-4346.

Eggermont, AMM. & Kirkwood, JM. (2004). Re-evaluating the Role of Dacarbazine in Metastatic Melanoma: What have we learned in 30 years? *European Journal of Cancer,* Vol. 40, pp. 1825-1836.

Einzig, AI.; Hochster, H. & Wiernik, PH. (1991). A Phase II Study of Taxol in Patients with Malignant Melanoma. *Invest New Drugs,* Vol. 9, pp. 59-64.

Evans, LM. ; Casper, ES. & Rosenbluth, R. (1987). Phase II Trial of Carboplatin in Advanced Malignant Melanoma. *Cancer Treat Rep,* Vol. 71, pp. 171-172.

Falkson, CI.; Ibrahim, J.; Kirkwood, JM.; Coates, AS.; Atkins, MB. & Blum, RH. (1998). Phase III Trial of Dacarbazine versus Dacarbazine with Interferon alpha-2b versus Dacarbazine with Tamoxifen versus Dacarbazine with Interferon alpha-2b and Tamoxifen in Patients with Metastatic Malignant Melanoma: An Eastern Cooperative Oncology Group Study. *J Clin Oncol,* Vol. 16, pp. 1743-1751.

Friday, BB. & Adjei, AA. (2008). Advances in Targeting the ras/Raf/MEK/Erk Mitogen-activated Protein Kinase Cascade with MEK Inhibitors for Cancer Therapy. *Clin Cancer Res,* Vol. 14, pp. 342-346.

Glover, D.; Glick, JH.; Weiler, C.; Fox, K. & Guerry, D. (1987). WR-2721 and High-dose Cisplatin : An Active Combination in the Treatment of Metastatic Melanoma. *J Clin Oncol,* Vol. 5, pp. 574-578.

Green, RJ. & Schuchter, LM. (1998). Systemic Treatment of Metastatic Melanoma with Chemotherapy. *Hematology/Oncology Clinics of North America,* Vol. 12, pp.863-875.

Hauschild, A.; Agarwala, SS.; Trefzer, U.; Hogg, D.; Robert, C.; Hersey, P.; Eggermont, A.; Grabbe, S.; Gonzalez, G.; Gille, J.; Peschel, C.; Schadendorf, D.; Garbe, C.; O'day, S.; Daud, A.; White, JM.; Xia, C.; Patel, K.; Kirkwood, JM. & Keilholz, U. (2009). Results of a Phase III, Randomized, Placebo-Controlled Study of Sorafenib in Combination With Carboplatin and Paclitaxel As Second-Line Treatment in Patients With Unresectable Stage III or Stage IV Melanoma. *J Clin Oncol,* Vol. 27, pp. 2823-2830.

Hill 2nd, GJ.; Metter, GE. & Krementz, ET. (1979). DTIC and Combination Therapy for Melanoma. II. Escalating Schedules of DTIC with BCNU, CCNU, and Vincristine. *Cancer Treat Rep,* Vol. 63, pp. 1989-1992.

Jacquillat, C.; Khayat, D. & Banzet, P. (1990). Final Report of the French Multicenter Phase II Study of the Nitrosourea Fotemustine in 153 Evaluable Patients with Disseminated Malignant Melanoma Including Patients with Cerebral Metastases. *Cancer,* Vol.66, pp. 1873-1878.

Jilaveanu, LB.; Aziz, SA. & Kluger HM. (2009). Chemotherapy and Biologic Therapies for Melanoma: Do They Work? *Clin Dermatol,* Vol. 27, pp. 614-625.

Legha, SS. ; Ring, S. & Eton, O. (1998). Development of a Biochemotherapy Regimen with Concurrent Administration of Cisplatin, Vinblastine, Dacarbazine, Interferon alpha, and Interleukin-2 for Patients with Metastatic Melanoma. *J Clin Oncol,* Vol. 16, 1752-1759.

Lens, MB.; Reiman, T. & Husain, AF. (2003). Use of Tamoxifen in the Treatment of Malignant Melanoma. *Cancer,* Vol. 98, pp. 1355-1361.

Lopez, M.; Perno, CF.; Di Lauro, L.; Papaldo, P.; Ganzina, F. & Barduagni, A. (1984). Controlled Study of DTIC versus DTIC plus Epirubicin in Metastatic Malignant Melanoma. *Invest New Drugs,* Vol. 2, pp. 319-322.

Lui, P. ; Cashin, R. ; Machado, M. ; Hemels, M. ; Corey-Lisle, PK. & Einarson TR. Treatments for Metastatic Melanoma : Synthesis of Evidence From Randomized Trials. *Cancer Treatment Reviews,* Vol. 33, pp. 665-680.

Luikart, SD.; Kennealey, GT. & Kirkwood, JM. (1984). Randomized Phase III Trial of Vinblastine, Bleomycin, and cis-dichlorodiammine-platinum versus Dacarbazine in Malignant Melanoma. *J Clin Oncol,* Vol. 2, pp. 164-168.

Lutzky, J. (2010). New Therapeutic Options in the Medical Management of Advanced Melanoma. *Semin Cutan Med Surg,* Vol. 29, pp. 249-257.

Marsden, JR.; Newton-Bishop, JA.; Burrows, L.; Cook, M.; Corrie, PG.; Cox, NH.; Gor, ME.; Lorigan, P.; MacKie, R.; Nathan, P.; Peach, H.; Powell, B. & Walker, C. (2010). Revised UK Guidelines for the Management of Cutaneous Melanoma 2010. *Journal of Plastic, Reconstructive & Aesthetic Surgery,* Vol. 63, pp. 1401-1419.

McDermott, DF. ; Mier, JW. & Lawrence, DP. (2000). A Phase II Pilot Trial of Concurrent Biochemotherapy with Cisplatin, Vinblastine, Dacarbazine, Interleukin 2, and Interferon alpha-2b in Patients with Metastatic Melanoma. *Clin Cancer Res,* Vol. 6, pp. 2201-2208.

McDermott, DF.; Sosman, JA.; Gonzalez, R.; Hodi, FS.; Linette GP.; Richards, J.; Jakub, JW.; Beeram, M.; Tarantolo, S.; Agarwala, S.; Frenette, G.; Puzanov, I.; Cranmer, L.; Lewis, K.; Kirkwood, J.; White, JM.; Xia, C.; Patel, K. & Hersh, E. (2008). Double-Blind Randomized Phase II Study of the Combination of Sorafenib and Dacarbazine in Patients With Advanced Melanoma: A Report From the 11715 Study Group. *J Clin Oncol,* Vol. 26, pp. 2178-2185.

Middleton, MR.; Grob, JJ.; Aaronson, N.; Fierlbeck, G.; Tilgen, W.; Seiter, S.; Gore, M.; Aamdal, S.; Cebon, J.; Coates, A.; Dreno, B.; Henz, M.; Schadendorf, D.; Kapp, A.; Weiss, J.; Fraass, U.; Statkevich, P.; Muller, M. & Thatcher, N. (2000). Randomized Phase III Study of Temozolomide versus Dacarbazine in the Treatment of Patients with Advanced Metastatic Malignant Melanoma. *J Clin Oncol,* Vol. 18, pp. 158-166.

Moon, JH.; Gailani, S. & Cooper, MR. (1975). Comparison of the Combination of 1,3-bis(2-chloroethyl)-1-nitrosourea (BCNU) and Vincristine with Two Dose Schedules of 5-(3,3-dimethyl-1-triazino) Imidazole 4-carboxamide (DTIC) in the Treatment of Disseminated Malignant Melanoma. *Cancer,* Vol. 35, pp. 368-371.

Mouawad, R.; Sebert, M.; Michels, J.; Bloch, J.; Spano, JP. & Khayat D. (2010). Treatment for Metastatic Malignant Melanoma: Old Drugs and New Strategies. *Critical Reviews in Oncology/Hematology,* Vol.74, pp. 27-39.

NCCN Guidelines Version 1.2011 Panel Members. (2011). Melanoma. NCCN Guidelines Panel Disclosures.

Newlands, ES.; Blackledge, GR. & Slack JA. Phase I Trial of Temozolomide (CCRG 81045: M&B 39831: NSC 362856). *Br J Cancer,* Vol. 65, pp. 287-291.

O'day, SJ.; Kim, CJ. & Reintgen, DS. (2002). Metastatic Melanoma: Chemotherapy to Biochemotherapy. *Cancer Control,* Vol. 9, No. 1, pp. 31-38.

Quagliana, JM.; Stephens, RL.; Baker, LH. & Costanzi, JJ. (1984). *J Clin Oncol*, Vol. 2, pp. 316-319.

Quirt, I.; Verma, S.; Petrella, T.; Bak, K. & Charette, M. (2007). Temozolomide for the Treatment of Metastatic Melanoma: A Systematic Review. *The Oncologist*, Vol.12, pp. 1114-1123.

Rao, RD. ; Holtan, SG. ; Ingle, JN. ; Croghan, GA. ; Kottschade, LA. ; Creagan, ET. ; Kaur, JS. ; Pitot, HC. & Markovic, SN. (2006). Combination of Paclitaxel and Carboplatin as Second-Line Therapy for Patients with Metastatic Melanoma. *Cancer*, Vol. 106, pp. 375-382.

Ridolfi, R. ; Chiarion-Sileni, V. ; Guida, M. ; Romanini, A. ; Labianca, R. ; Freschi, A. ; Lo Re, G. ; Nortilli, R. ; Brugnara, S. ; Vitali, P. & Nanni, O. (2002). Cisplatin, Dacarbazine with or without Subcutaneous Interleukin-2, and Interferon Alfa-2b in Advanced Melanoma Outpatients : Results From An Italian Multicenter Phase III Randomized Clinical Trial. *J Clin Oncol*, Vol. 20, pp. 1600-1607.

Ringborg, U.; Rudenstam, CM.; Hansson, J.; Hafstrom, L.; Stenstam, B. & Strander, H. (1989). Dacarbazine versus Dacarbazine-Vindesine in Disseminated Malignant Melanoma : A Randomized Phase II Study. *Med Oncol Tumor Pharmacother*, Vol. 6, pp. 285-289.

Rumke, P.; Kleeberg, UR. & MacKie, RM. (1992). Tamoxifen As a Single Agent for Advanced Melanoma in Postmenopausal Women. A Phase II Study of the EORTC Malignant Melanoma Cooperative Group. *Melanoma Res*, Vol. 2, pp. 153-156.

Rusthoven, RJ. & Quirt IC. (1996). Randomized, double-blind, placebo-controlled trial comparing the response rates of carmustine, dacarbazine and cisplatin with and without tamoxifen in patients with metastatic melanoma. *J Clin Oncol*, Vol.14, pp. 2083-2090.

Sasse, AD.; Sasse, EC.; Clark, LGO.; Ulloa, L. & Clark, OAC. (2009). Chemoimmunotherapy versus Chemotherapy for Metastatic Malignant Melanoma (Review). *The Cochrane Library*, Vol.1, pp. 1-47.

Sileni, VC. ; Nortilli, R. ; Aversa, SML. ; Paccagnella, A. ; Medici, M. ; Corti, L. ; Favaretto, AG. ; Cetto, GL. & Monfardini, S. (2001). Phase II Randomized Study of Dacarbazine, Carmustine, Cisplatin and Tamoxifen versus Dacarbazine Alone in Advanced Melanoma Patients. *Melanoma Research*, Vol. 11, pp. 189-196.

Tarhini, AA. & Agarwala, SS. (2006). Cutaneous Melanoma: Available Therapy for Metastatic Disease. *Dermatologic Therapy*, Vol. 19, pp. 19-25.

Thompson, JA. ; Gold, PJ. & Fefer, A. (1997). Outpatient Chemoimmunotherapy for the Treatment of Metastatic Melanoma. *Semin Oncol*, Vol. 24, pp. 44-48.

Thomson, DB.; Adena, M. & McLeod, GR. (1993). Interferon-alpha 2a Does Not Improve Response or Survival When Combined with Dacarbazine in Metastatic Malignant Melanoma : Results of A Multi-institutional Australian Randomized Trial. *Melanoma Res*, Vol. 3, pp. 133-138.

Treisman, J. & Garlie, N. (2010). Systemic Therapy for Cutaneous Melanoma. *Clin Plastic Surg*, Vol. 37, pp. 127-146.

Zimpfer-Rechner, C.; Hofmann, U.; Figl, R.; Becker, JC.; Trefzer, U.; Keller, I.; Hauschild, A. & Schadendorf, D. (2003). Randomized Phase II Study of Weekly Paclitaxel versus

Paclitaxel and Carboplatin as Second-Line Therapy in Disseminated Melanoma: A Multicentre Trial of the Dermatologic Co-operative Oncology Group (DeCOG). *Melanoma Res,* Vol. 13, pp. 531-536.

6

Chemocentric Chemoimmunotherapy: A New Concept in Melanoma Immunotherapy

Paul Howell[1], Soroosh Radfar[2], Yixiang Wang[3] and Hung Khong[1]
[1]*Mitchell Cancer Institute, University of South Alabama, Mobile*
[2]*Dana-Farber Cancer Institute, Boston*
[3]*Central Laboratory, Peking University School and Hospital of Stomatology, Beijing*
[1,2]*United States of America*
[3]*China*

1. Introduction

According to the American Cancer Society, 68,130 new cases of melanoma and 8,700 deaths were predicted for 2010 (Jemal et al., 2010). Although melanoma comprises only 5% of all skin cancers, it is by far the deadliest, responsible for 75% of skin cancer-related deaths, and its incidence is steadily increasing worldwide. Primary cutaneous melanoma has an excellent outcome with early surgical intervention, but regional and distant metastatic disease have a much more dismal prognosis. Current five-year survival rates equal 91% for all disease sites, including 98% for local disease, 62% for regional disease (including regional lymph node involvement), and only 15% for those with distant metastasis (median survival is only 7.5 months). Unfortunately, for those patients who will develop locally advanced and metastatic melanoma, current treatment options are limited in scope and effectiveness; thus, the overall poor mortality rates for these patients emphasize the need for better treatment modalities, methods of relapse prevention and earlier recognition of pre-neoplastic and neoplastic cells (Atallah & Flaherty, 2006; Balch et al., 2001a, 2001b; Blesa et al., 2011).

Currently, there are no curative therapies for metastatic melanoma. Until March 25, 2011, the U.S. Food and Drug Administration (FDA) had only approved two drugs for the treatment of metastatic melanoma, the DNA alkylating agent dacarbazine and high-dose Interleukin-2 (IL-2). Dacarbazine alkylates and crosslinks DNA in all phases of the cell cycle, impairing DNA function, inducing cell-cycle arrest and apoptosis (Bajetta et al., 2002), and is a common chemotherapeutic option for multiple cancers (Seam et al., 2009; Yang & Chapman, 2009). IL-2 activates endogenous anti-tumor-reactive T cells and natural killer (NK) cells. Notably, circulating NK cells from stage IV melanoma patients were recently shown to exhibit a unique phenotypic and functional character toward melanoma cells, and this unique character was altered in patients after treatment with chemotherapy (Fregni et al., 2011). Dacarbazine induces objective tumor regression in 15-20% of metastatic melanoma patients with a median survival of only 8-9 months and a 2-3% complete response rate, and single agent bolus IL-2, while providing a 20-30% objective response rate, creates significant long-term response in only 5% of patients treated, is fraught with toxicity and costly. Combination low-dose IL-2 and chemotherapy and single-agent high-dose IL-2 produce a similarly low complete response (Atkins et al., 2000; Tsao et al., 2004). Other cytotoxic compounds have resulted in poor response rates and significant adverse effects, including temozolomide, cisplatin, carboplatin, vinca alkaloids, taxanes, and nitrosoureas (Bafaloukos et al., 2002; Bajetta et al., 2002; Blesa et al., 2011; Khayat et al., 2002; Middleton et al., 2000). Notable agents of promise currently undergoing testing are anti-CD40, anti-PD-1L, 1-MT (1-methyl-D-tryptophan), and the BRAF-inhibitor PLX4032 (Bollag et al., 2010; Comin-Anduix; Flaherty et al., 2010; Fonsatti et al., 2010). On March 25, 2011, the U. S. Food and Drug Administration approved ipilimumab (Yervoy™, Bristol-Myers Squibb Company, New York, NY, USA), a monoclonal antibody against the inhibitory lymphocyte receptor, CTLA4, as an injection for the treatment of unresectable or metastatic melanoma (Hodi et al., 2010).

Advanced melanomas are infamously resistant to chemotherapy, principally due to the presence of inherent primary anti-apoptotic and acquired cellular chemoresistance mechanisms (Serrone & Hersey, 1999). Of note, a recent study by Rosner et al. (Rosner et al., 2011) described a means to circumvent such apoptosis resistance. Without activating the apoptosis signaling cascade or utilizing other apoptotic nucleases, recombinant deoxyribonuclease I (DNaseI), engineered with a nuclear localization signal and mutated actin-binding site to avoid entering its inactive bound form, was effective in inducing apoptosis in an apoptosis-resistant melanoma cell model with 70-100% killing efficiency, emphasizing its potential application in many of the known apoptosis-resistant cancers.

Surgical resection of primary and known metastatic lesions is still the most effective means of improving overall survival of melanoma patients, though palliative care is standard for patients with metastases after first-line dacarbazine or other physician-preferred therapy, as survival is very rare (Rass et al., 2008; Tagawa et al., 2006; Yang et al., 2006). Surgery in partnership with radiation is standard for locoregional control, while additional chemical-, cell- or antibody- based therapies, or some combination thereof, are commonly attempted for systemic eradication of tumor cells in the blood or at unspecified sites in the body to combat current disease and prevent relapse and metastatic implantation. Melanoma has attracted a lot of interest from immunologists due to a heightened frequency over other solid tumors to display fast, spontaneous, complete tumor regression associated with a specific cellular immune response (Kadison & Morton, 2003). Chemoimmunotherapy, tumor vaccines and other chemotherapeutic combinations have shown improvement in objective response rates for melanoma patients, but they have not yet been able to show significant survival benefits (Bajetta et al., 2006; Eton et al., 2002; Kaufmann et al., 2005). Indeed, a recent meta-analysis of 18 studies comprising 2,625 participants revealed improved objective response rates in metastatic melanoma patients treated with chemoimmunotherapy compared with chemotherapy, but no improvement was noted in overall survival benefit (Sasse et al., 2007). Additionally, hematological and non-hematological toxicities were greatest in those undergoing chemoimmunotherapy.

While the historic chemoimmunotherapeutic approach has been to sensitize tumor cells to immunotherapy with administration of chemotherapeutic compounds, we have described a high degree of chemosensitization with pre-treatment of non-tumor-Ag-specific CD4+ T cells (Radfar et al., 2009), our termed 'chemocentric chemoimmunotherapy' strategy. This technique may provide a basis for development of novel methods of selectively reducing the chemoresistance of virtually all tumor cell types, given the lack of requirement for tumor-Ag-specific T cells. We will present an overview of conventional chemoimmunotherapy development for melanoma and examine the functional significance of chemocentric chemoimmunotherapy for melanoma and other cancers.

2. Background

It has long been part of the clinical canon that chemotherapy drugs negatively affect immunological systems, inhibiting anti-tumor immune activity by a variety of related mechanisms. However, the intricacies of the chemo-immuno interaction provide areas of opportunity for utilizing chemo drugs to enhance the immune response. These cytotoxic drugs tend to target dividing lymphocytes, necessary for development of an immune response, but they also deplete CD4+/CD25+ regulatory T cells (T reg), potentially enhancing the response. Again, conversely, lymphodepletion triggers homeostatic T cell reconstitution which proceeds to create T cells recognizing tumor as self. Opportunities arise during the depletion of T reg and the heightened formation of T cells, allowing an avenue to both infuse the patient with tumor-reactive T cells which are now not impeded by T reg and the potential to create within the patient a large quantity of T cells reactive to some tumor antigen(s).

Conventional cancer chemotherapy is capable of inducing the death of immunologically sensitive tumor cells by utilizing the host innate and adaptive immune responses, e.g. through the induction of immunoregulatory cytokines (Bracci et al., 2007), and some of these drugs can alter cellular pathways of immune suppression and tolerance in a dose- and time-dependent manner, e.g. inducing homeostatic proliferation (Bracci et al., 2007; Proietti et al., 1998), or modulate the extracellular release of certain proteins upon cell death, e.g. HMGB1 release and subsequent tumor survival/metastasis-promoting inflammation is inhibited by oxaliplatin (Dong et al., 2007). Additionally, some chemo drugs can modulate the expression of tumor antigens and antigen processing/presentation machinery on tumor cells. For example, 5-Fluorouracil (5-FU) has been shown to induce carcinoembryonic antigen (CEA) expression in colon and breast cancer cells (Correale et al., 2003) while 5-aza-2′-deoxycytidine can induce the expression of cancer testis antigens and the cell surface MHC class I complex in melanoma and other cancers (Adair & Hogan, 2009; Coral et al., 2002; Fonsatti et al., 2007; Natsume et al., 2008). Notably, direct intralesional injection of the MHC class I complex, which allows tumor immune evasion when defective in numerous cancers (Lampen & van Hall, 2011; Maleno et al., 2011), via high-dose Allovectin-7® (Vical Inc., San Diego, CA, USA), a cationic lipid-formulated bicistronic plasmid encoding MHC-I components β-2 microglobulin and HLA-B7, in 127 recurrent or previously unresponsive to chemotherapy stage III and IV melanoma patients tested for efficacy in a recent phase II dose escalation study produced an objective response of 11.8% with median duration of response of 13.8 months (Bedikian et al., 2010). Tissue from two responding patients was noted for the absence of melanoma upon histological analysis, and the therapy was well tolerated.

Drugs of complementary activity and dissimilar toxicities are routinely combined to enhance individual anti-tumor effects. In the 1960s, effective combination antibiotic therapy for tuberculosis influenced the combination treatment strategy of acute lymphocytic leukemia and lymphoma. A number of significant combination chemotherapeutic regimens were developed in the 1980s, including CVD (cisplatin, vinblastine, and dacarbazine) and the Dartmouth regimen (cisplatin, carmustine, dacarbazine, and tamoxifen) (Del Prete et al., 1984; Legha et al., 1989). Notably, according to two independent clinical trials of the 1990s, CVD and Dartmouth were not shown to significantly increase overall survival relative to dacarbazine alone (Buzaid et al., 1993; Chapman et al., 1999). Although dacarbazine and cisplatin-based combination chemotherapy/biochemotherapy regimens combining IFN and/or IL-2 are now recommended by the National Comprehensive Cancer Network (NCCN) Clinical Practice Guidelines in Oncology for Melanoma for stage III and IV melanomas, promising increases in response rates notwithstanding (Riker & Howell, 2010a, 2010b), significant improvement in long-term responses has yet to be seen.

Early efforts to combine chemotherapy with immunomodulators, particularly cancer vaccines, were discounted given the understood detrimental myelosuppressive properties of many chemotherapeutic compounds (Emens, 2008). This suppression was purported to be short-lived and reversible, as the replenishing of leukocytes following chemotherapy would show, by Harris et al. in 1976 (Harris et al., 1976). As reviewed by Sinkovics and Horvath (Sinkovics & Horvath, 2006), around this time, the M.D. Anderson Hospital Melanoma-Sarcoma Service submitted multiple grant applications to the NCI for combination chemoimmunotherapeutic intervention strategies for patients with metastatic melanomas and sarcomas. Despite NCI rejection, clinical trials began, utilizing the findings of Lindenmann and Klein (Lindenmann & Klein, 1967) from nearly a decade earlier which showed an acquired immunity to tumor formation in mice injected with the cell culture lysates of oncolytic myxo- or paramyxovirus-infected tumor cells. Sinkovics et al. further adapted this strategy for the post-chemotherapy administration of cultured tumor cell lysates infected with oncolytic, attenuated PR8 influenza A virus. PR8 viral oncosylates, the immunotherapeutic suspension, were comprised of UV-irradiated, endotoxin-free tumor cell cultures with low levels of live PR8 virus. 'Tumor-specific active immunization' with viral oncosylates two-to-three weeks post-chemotherapy resulted in heightened rates of remission with moderate, occasionally significant increases in survival.

Early phase clinical trials have been able to show response rates of up to 50% for chemoimmunotherapies (Atkins et al., 2003; Eton et al., 2002; Keilholz et al., 1997; Rosenberg et al., 1999); however, the duration of responses has been limited in most cases to less than a year. Importantly, systemic toxicities and adverse side effects tend to be heightened with chemoimmunotherapeutic interventions in relation to chemotherapy or immunotherapy alone. Furthermore, many of the most common chemotherapies were not inherently designed to take into account the entire tumor-host microenvironment and the effects of such therapies in conjunction with locally and systemically active immunological mechanisms. Designing treatment course strategy according to the character of the tumor-host microenvironment milieu is vital for its long-term efficacy (Formenti, 2010; Pages et al., 2009; Zitvogel et al., 2008). Today, thirty years after the first modern chemoimmunotherapy clinical trials were initiated, the impasse that is melanoma chemoresistance has continued to stymie significant, clinically-applicable advancement in this therapeutic field. Given the recurring roadblocks of current treatment strategies, traditional methods of chemotherapy and immunotherapy use are being radically adjusted to achieve a better overall clinical outcome.

3. Conventional chemoimmunotherapy for the treatment of melanoma

Immunotherapy can play an important role in the treatment of cancer, and combinations of chemotherapy and immunotherapy have been investigated in many clinical trials. Although some phase III trials have shown mixed results regarding duration of survival, meta-analyses have found no improvement in overall survival (Allen et al., 1998; Ives et al., 2007; Keilholz et al., 1998; Sasse et al., 2007). Chemoimmunotherapy, or biochemotherapy, has been extensively studied in melanoma. Conventional chemoimmunotherapeutic strategies include two major categories. The first category uses cytokines such as IL-2 and/or IFN-α in combination with chemotherapy. This experimental strategy was not supported by strong preclinical evidence and has not been shown to be superior to chemotherapy alone (Atkins et al., 2003; Eton et al., 2002; Keilholz et al., 1997, 2005; Rosenberg et al., 1999). The second category is a strategy that we have termed 'immunocentric chemoimmunotherapy'. In this approach, the primary or central focus is on immunotherapy, with chemotherapy playing a peripheral role in immunomodulation. Using this approach, melanoma patients have been successfully treated with non-myeloablative, lymphodepleting chemotherapy and adoptive cell transfer with tumor-Ag specific lymphocytes and high dose IL-2 (Dudley et al., 2002, 2005). Although this strategy is promising, it is not widely applicable to non-melanoma cancers due to the difficulty in generating large numbers of tumor-Ag specific tumor-infiltrating lymphocytes. To date, there have been no studies using chemoimmunotherapy that have shown a significant improvement in overall survival (Atkins et al., 2003, 2008; Bajetta et al., 2006; Eton et al., 2002; Kielholz et al., 1997, 1998, 2005; Middleton et al., 2007; Punt et al., 2006; Ridolofi et al., 2002; Rosenberg et al., 1999), and the development of immunotherapy for the treatment of a broad range of cancer types is still lacking. Given the proven capacity of many already developed and thoroughly tested, well characterized chemotherapeutic agents to have significant, specific and intricate influence over global and localized immune response, adjustments to the multitudes of chemoimmunotherapeutic strategic fronts are currently being made in anticipation of a clinically relevant breakthrough.

3.1 Cytokines and chemotherapy

Activated T cells amplify cytokines that are essential for an effective immune response (Szabo et al., 2003). These include IL-2, TNF-α, IL-21 (by activated CD4+ T cells), GM-CSF, IFN-γ, and other as yet unidentified cytokines. In addition to their immunomodulatory activities, some cytokines can also have direct effects on tumor cells and/or tumor vasculature. TNF-α is known to induce hemorrhagic necrosis in tumors (Carswell et al., 1975; Old, 1985) and has also been shown to induce apoptotic and necrotic tumor cell death *in vitro* (Helson et al., 1975; Laster et al., 1988; Rubin et al., 1988; Sugarman et al., 1985). The hemorrhagic necrotic effect of TNF-α has been shown to be more potent when used in combination with chemotherapy in a rat sarcoma model (Manusama et al., 1996). However, in these studies, TNF-α had no direct activity against tumor cell lines *in vitro* and demonstrated no synergy with chemotherapy, acting instead on the tumor vasculature (van Horssen et al., 2006; Watanabe et al., 1988). The IFNs can exert direct effects on the proliferation, differentiation, and apoptosis of tumor cells (Chawla-Sarkar et al., 2001, 2003; Detjen et al., 2001; Gooch et al, 2000; Pfeffer et al., 1998). However, the response to the IFNs varies considerably, depending on the tumor histology, and resistance to the IFNs has been reported in several tumor types (Burke et al., 1999; Harvat & Jetten, 1996; Kaplan et al., 1998; Phan-Bich et al., 1997).

Several early-phase trials of cytokines combined with cisplatin-based therapies have shown an overall response rate of ~50%, though such responses are of very short duration and often complicated by a high degree of systemic toxicity and adverse side effects. Over the past 15 years, numerous cisplatin-based cytokine combination regimens have been assessed (Atkins et al., 2002, 2003; Atzpodien et al., 2002; Buzaid et al., 1993; Flaherty et al., 2001; Legha et al., 1989, 1998; McDermott et al., 2000; Pejcic et al., 2010; Rosenberg et al., 1999,

2011; Thompson et al., 1997). Notably, in a phase II trial from 1997, Thompson et al. describe the development and utility of an outpatient chemoimmunotherapy treatment regimen of monthly cycles of intravenous cisplatin, carmustine, dacarbazine, and tamoxifen plus self-administered subcutaneous recombinant IL-2 and IFN-α for 32 metastatic melanoma patients, 30 assessed for clinical response (Thompson et al., 1997). After three months, they note a complete response rate of 13% and a 30% partial response, and toxicity was primarily restricted to minor fever and nausea with only a few instances of hospitalization for toxicity management.

Rosenberg et al. (Rosenberg et al., 1999) reported in 1999 on their phase II clinical trial testing tamoxifen, cisplatin, and dacarbazine in 52 metastatic melanoma patients, while the 50 patients in the other arm received the same therapy followed by IL-2 and IFN-α2b. The chemoimmunotherapy arm exhibited 44% total response rate while the chemotherapy arm was 27%; however, of the seven complete responders, only three received the cytokines, indicating no significant impact of cytokines on complete response, and median duration of response was less than six months. Even more disappointing, most of the toxicities were reported for the chemoimmunotherapy group. Median duration of survival was 10.7 months for those receiving cytokines compared to 15.8 months for those without. A regimen of concurrent treatment with CVD chemotherapy, IL-2 and low-dose IFN-α has shown to be better tolerated and more practical than sequential treatment of CVD followed by IL-2/IFN-α (Atkins et al., 2002; Eton et al., 2002; Legha et al., 1998), though randomized phase III trials of this CVD/IL-2/IFN-α combination show no improvement in response or survival over CVD and modified CVD chemotherapy regimens alone (Atkins et al., 2003; Keilholz et al., 2005). In regard to pre-treatment of a chemoimmunotherapeutic regimen with chemotherapy, Punt et al. (Punt et al., 2006) reported on a randomized, phase II clinical trial of metastatic melanoma patients receiving either dacarbazine, cisplatin, IFN-α and IL-2 or the same combination after an initial treatment of two cycles of dacarbazine, finding no difference between the two groups in terms of median overall survival.

O'Day et al. (O'Day et al., 2009) treated 133 chemotherapy-naïve metastatic melanoma patients with CVD, decrescendo IL-2, and IFN-α2b with granulocyte-macrophage colony-stimulating factor (GM-CSF) cytokine support. Maintenance biotherapy with low-dose IL-2 and GM-CSF followed by intermittent pulses of decrescendo IL-2 over 12 months was provided for those without disease progression. The overall response rate was 44% with 8% complete response and 36% partial response. Stable disease was noted for 29% of patients; median progression-free survival was 9 months, and median survival was 13.5 months with 12-month and 24-month survival rates at 57% and 23%, respectively, providing evidence of above average long-term survival rates for these patients. Further randomized trials need to be carried out.

A recent multicenter phase II chemoimmunotherapy trial of the Dermatologic Cooperative Oncology Group (DeCOG) testing the multi-kinase inhibitor sorafenib in combination with pegylated-IFN-α2b (PEG-IFN-α2b) in 55 patients with metastatic melanoma resulted in two patients with partial response and 14 with stable disease (29.1% disease control rate in intent-to-treat population) (Egberts et al., 2011). Median progression-free survival was 2.5 months, and toxicities were primarily hematological, including one treatment-related bleeding complication leading to death. A smaller study of 22 metastatic melanoma patients receiving a regimen of CVD with PEG-IFN-α2b, subcutaneous IL-2 and oral 13-cis-retinoic acid, with maintenance biotherapy for those with clinical response after six courses, provided 12 objective responses with seven maintenance-receiving patients having stable disease after six months (Recchia et al., 2008). Median progression-free and overall survivals were 23.3 and 45.7 months, respectively, with mostly hematological toxicities and 21% of patients exhibiting grade 2 autoimmune reactions.

3.2 Immunocentric chemoimmunotherapy

Another conventional strategy is one that we have termed 'immunocentric chemoimmunotherapy'. This strategy is an immunotherapy-focused approach which uses chemotherapy as an immunomodulator to enhance the effect of cancer vaccines or adoptive cell transfer therapy. Based on this approach, recent studies using chemotherapy to prepare the host before the infusion of *ex vivo* activated, melanoma Ag-specific tumor-infiltrating lymphocytes and high dose IL-2 have resulted in impressive response rates.

3.2.1 Cancer vaccines

Cancer vaccines are promising for their abilities to elicit both humoral (antibody) and cellular (T cell) immune responses (Finn, 2008; Schoenfeld et al., 2010) specifically against tumor cells, as well as for their minimal side effects and the potential for development of immunologic memory allowing for a long-term, durable response to treatment without the need for continuous therapy (Yannelli & Wroblewski, 2004). The presence of cell surface antigens and receptors, capable of activating a myriad of intracellular biochemical pathways, makes possible the development of cancer vaccines with highly stringent criteria for target tumor cell selection and may assist in the focused delivery and activity of chemotherapeutic agents. The recent FDA-approval of sipuleucel-T (Provenge®; Dendreon Inc., Seattle, WA, USA), the first personalized therapeutic cancer vaccine, for the treatment of advanced prostate cancer, has opened the doors for novel vaccine development for other cancers, contributing to the heightened interest in targeted immune-based study of cancer systems.

Nistico et al. (Nistico et al., 2009) recently reported on their phase I/II pilot study testing 36 HLA-A2+ disease-free, stage II to IV melanoma patients with standard-dose dacarbazine administered one day before vaccination with HLA-A2 restricted melanoma antigen A (melan-A/MART-1) and gp100 melanoma peptide vaccination compared with vaccination alone. Dacarbazine significantly increased the numbers of peptide-specific CD8+ effector memory T cells which recognize and lyse HLA-A2+/melan-A+ tumor cells, indicating the enhancement of effective CD8+ T cell recognition of vaccine peptides after treatment with a chemotherapy drug in patients with melanoma. Another more recent pilot clinical trial (Palermo et al., 2010) by the Nistico group examined the role of dacarbazine again as pre-treatment to this vaccine therapy, noting a progressive widening of the T cell receptor repertoire diversity with concomitant high avidity and tumor reactivity in melan-A–specific T cell clones of patients treated with this chemoimmunotherapy and a trend toward longer survival. Alternatively, patients receiving vaccine alone exhibited a tendency to narrowing the T cell receptor repertoire diversity and a decrease of tumor lytic activity in one patient.

3.2.2 Adoptive cell transfer

One of the most exciting avenues for melanoma therapy is adoptive cell transfer of tumor-reactive T cells harvested from the tumor itself, expanded and activated *ex vivo* using various methods (e.g., high concentrations of IL-2) and then transferred back into the patient. The success of adoptive cell transfer depends on the specificity of T cells for the tumor and their ability to survive and proliferate in the environment. Notably, intratumoral injection of toll-like receptor agonists were found to enhance the potency of activated adoptive cell transfer against a murine model with established subcutaneous melanoma tumors, acting to enhance IFN-γ production and subsequent killing of the now more immunogenic tumor cells by adoptively transferred T cells (Amos et al., 2011). Metastatic melanoma patients have benefited in certain settings with adoptive cell transfer of tumor-infiltrating lymphocytes in combination with chemotherapeutic lymphodepletion, with an impressive objective response rate of 50-70% (Dudley & Rosenberg, 2007; Gattinoni et al., 2006; Hershkovitz et al., 2010; Khattar et al., 2009; Rosenberg et al., 2008, 2011; Rosenberg & Dudley, 2009). Given the promising results of adoptive cell transfer strategies in melanoma and other cancers, many notable contributions are being made toward a more discrete understanding of this field.

During expansion of tumor-infiltrating lymphocytes for infusion, CD8+ T cells are driven to differentiate into effector cells, losing key costimulatory molecules such as CD28 and CD27. Costimulation with CD137/4-1BB was recently shown to significantly increase lymphocyte survival during melanoma adoptive cell transfer and improve the anti-tumor response (Hernandez-Chacon et al., 2011). Inozume et al. (Inozume et al., 2010) reported on the recovery of function of PD-1 cell surface receptor protein on CD8+ T cells in melanoma digests after *ex vivo* conditioning with IL-2, leading to the production of much more tumor-specific IFN-γ compared with PD-1^{-} T cells and the proposal of PD-1 functional operation or presence being a capable biomarker for selecting tumor-specific lymphocytes from melanomas. As a common practice in adoptive cell transfer prior to infusion of these lymphocytes, patient lymphodepletion of T reg and other lymphocytes in competition for cytokines allows for a much more potent response to activated tumor-specific T cells (Dudley et al., 2002, Wrzesiniski et al., 2010). Adoptive cell transfer with autologous tumor-infiltrating lymphocytes, conditioned with cyclophosphamide and fludarabine, and IL-2 tested in 50 metastatic melanoma patients selected to receive either 2-Gy (non-myeloablative) or 12-Gy (myeloablative) of total body irradiation resulted in response rates of 49%, 52% and 72% for patients not receiving radiation and those receiving either 2- or 12-Gy, respectively (Dudley et al., 2008). The authors note the possibility for increased tumor-infiltrating lymphocyte activity, proliferation, and/or persistence in the body and at the tumor site as a result of rising cytokine availability following irradiation, having seen a significant increase of IL-7 and IL-15 in the serum following the myeloablative regimen. This trial is part of three whose combined and complete results were recently published by Rosenberg et al. (Rosenberg et al. 2011), providing impressive objective response and overall survival rates. In a panel of 93 heavily pretreated metastatic melanoma patients (86% with visceral metastases and 95% recurring after prior therapy), they found adoptive cell transfer of autologous lymphocytes plus high-dose IL-2, administered within one day following a lymphodepletion regimen of cyclophosphamide and fludarabine or either 2- or 12-Gy of total body irradiation, to produce 52 objective responses (56%) with 20 (22%) complete responses, 19 of which lasted a span of three to seven years.

Other clinical studies have utilized genetically engineered peripheral T cells in place of tumor-infiltrating lymphocytes. Due to limitations in generating tumor-specific T cells for adoptive cell transfer, Morgan et al. (Morgan et al., 2006) reported on the specific conference of tumor recognition by autologous lymphocytes from peripheral blood of 15 metastatic melanoma patients using a retrovirus that encodes a T cell receptor recognizing a tumor antigen. Adoptive cell transfer of these transduced cells after lymphodepletion resulted in durable engraftment of more than 10% of peripheral blood lymphocyte levels for over two months after infusion. In two patients demonstrating objective regression of metastatic melanoma lesions, circulating engineered cells were maintained at high levels at one year after infusion.

Such viral T cell receptor engineering is currently being studied for advanced melanoma and general (Chinnasamy et al., 2010) cancer therapy by Dr. Steven A. Rosenberg's group and colleagues in The National Cancer Institute's Surgery Branch (Rosenberg & Dudley, 2009). Indeed, they have recently described the selective delivery of IL-12, noted for its limited immunostimulatory clinical application due to toxicity, into the tumor microenvironment upon tumor-Ag recognition by T cell receptors on genetically engineered lymphocytes, enhancing *in vivo* melanoma tumor regression without toxicity (Zhang et al., 2011). Another recent report from this group describes adoptive cell transfer of autologous T cells with a T cell receptor against the NY-ESO-1 cancer/testis antigen, expressed in ~25% of patients with melanoma and other epithelial cancers, resulting in an objective response in five of 11 patients with NY-ESO-1-expressing tumors, with two complete responses of greater than one year (Robbins et al., 2011).

3.3 Cyclophosphamide for melanoma immunocentric chemoimmunotherapy

Cyclophosphamide has been an invaluable chemotherapeutic agent in studying immunocentric methodology and application. Numerous reports have shown the synergistic capabilities of cyclophosphamide in combination with immunotherapeutics, describing its ability to induce cytokine expression, type I IFNs and homeostatic proliferation of B and T cells and to deplete the T reg population from the tumor site, increasing the possibility of CD8+ T cell-mediated targeting and destruction of tumor cells (Berd et al., 1986, 1990, 2004; Bracci et al., 2007; Dummer et al., 2002; Ercolini et al., 2005; Ghiringhelli et al., 2004; Livingston et al., 1987, 1994; Maine & Mule, 2002; North, 1982; Nowak et al., 2006; Proietti et al., 1998; Schiavoni et al., 2000; Turk & Parker, 1982; Zitvogel et al., 2008). An important study in 2005 showed non-myeloablative lymphodepleting chemotherapy with cyclophosphamide and fludarabine conditioning of tumor-infiltrating lymphocytes followed by infusion and subsequent high-dose IL-2 treatment to produce a 51% overall response rate in 35 metastatic melanoma patients previously having received IL-2 therapy, all but one being refractory to IL-2 (Dudley et al., 2005).

A surge of recent studies have expounded on the role of cyclophosphamide in T reg modulation and immune therapies that can take advantage of the T reg depleted tumor environment. Combination cyclophosphamide and an agonist antibody against the co-stimulatory CD4+ Foxp3+ T reg cell receptor OX40 has recently been shown to induce apoptosis of the tumor T reg population and induce the influx of CD8+ T cells resulting in a potent anti-tumor response in an *in vivo* B16 melanoma model (Hirschhorn-Cymerman et al., 2009). Furthermore, Kohlmeyer et al. (Kohlmeyer et al., 2009) reported chemotherapeutic preconditioning with cyclophosphamide prior to adoptive cell transfer and viral vaccination followed by adjuvant peritumoral injections of immunostimulatory nucleic acids to be a highly effective chemoimmunotherapeutic regimen, resulting in complete regression of primary and lung metastatic lesions in the normally adoptive cell transfer-resistant genetically engineered Hgf-Cdk4R24C metastatic melanoma mouse model.

In following the combination of chemotherapy and adoptive cell transfer with immune-enhancing cytokines, such as IL-2 (Dudley et al., 2002, 2005; Dudley & Rosenberg, 2007;

Mihalyo et al., 2004), and the recent characterization of IL-21 with adoptive cell transfer by Hinrichs et al. (Hinrichs et al., 2008), another study describes the boosting of immunocentric therapeutic efficacy with IL-21 (Petersen et al., 2010), an immune-enhancing cytokine that, unlike IL-2, does not support proliferation of activated T reg nor activation-induced cell death (Spolski & Leonard, 2008; Waldmann, 2006). As collective data would indicate, IL-21 likely enhances the T reg-depleting capabilities of cyclophosphamide by abrogating T reg development, via the inhibition of IL-2 secretion, and function (Elsaesser et al., 2009; Fantini et al., 2007; Hinrichs et al., 2008; Peluso et al., 2007; Piao et al., 2008; Yi et al., 2009). Mice with established tumors, subsequently treated with cyclophosphamide and adoptive cell transfer and/or daily injections of IL-21, exhibited better early tumor growth inhibition up to five days after the last (day 7) IL-21 injection and increased circulating tumor-specific T cells with the IL-21 administration. The authors note the potential for continued tumor growth stunting with continued IL-21 injection as well as the importance of timing considerations for this particular design (Skak et al., 2009). A similar study by Salem et al. (Salem et al., 2007) showed a more pronounced effect using peptide vaccination and naïve T cells, possibly a more effective option than pre-primed cells for adoptive cell transfer (Hinrichs et al., 2008).

4. Chemocentric chemoimmunotherapy

We have developed a third strategy for combining chemo- and immunotherapy, termed 'chemocentric chemoimmunotherapy' (Radfar et al., 2009). In this model, chemotherapy plays the central effector role, while immunotherapy is used to sensitize the tumor and its microenvironment to the cytotoxic effect of chemotherapy. This strategy employs the use of nonspecifically activated CD4+ T lymphocytes (aCD4) as a chemosensitizer of tumor cells followed by treatment with chemotherapeutic drugs. The rationale for this strategy is based on the known ability of activated T cells to secrete multiple cytokines that can regulate proliferation and/or apoptosis of tumor cells and the ability of activated T cells to exert direct activity on tumor cells through apoptotic pathways such as the Fas/Fas ligand pathway; for instance, tumor cell apoptosis is initiated when the Fas ligand, present on activated T cells, binds the Fas receptor, present on tumor cells. This model does not depend on Ag-specific activation of T cells and is, therefore, potentially applicable to a wide variety of tumor types and patients regardless of their HLA status. Indeed, preclinical studies examining the role of chemocentric chemoimmunotherapy in melanoma, breast, colon and prostate cancer cell lines have shown a dramatic enhancement of induced tumor-cell apoptosis. With the added advantage of ease of use and cost effectiveness in the clinic, chemocentric chemoimmunotherapy is a promising future methodology that is widely applicable, in terms of patient character schema, cost and basic technical utility, in the clinical setting.

4.1 Chemosensitization with nonspecifically activated CD4+ T cells

According to conventional wisdom, it is counterintuitive to administer chemotherapy immediately after cell therapy because the transferred immune cells will be eliminated by chemotherapy. Although this may be true in the setting of conventional immunocentric chemoimmunotherapy, where immunotherapy plays the major effector role and chemotherapy is used to prepare the host, this approach is rational in the context of chemocentric chemoimmunotherapy, where chemotherapy exerts the principal effector function and immunotherapy is used transiently for the purpose of presensitization.

We have recently demonstrated that presensitization of tumor cells with nonspecifically activated CD4+ T cells (aCD4) greatly enhanced the cytotoxic effect of chemotherapy in both *in vitro* and *in vivo* models (Radfar et al., 2009). This activity was observed for all seven tumor cell lines as well as all four chemotherapeutic agents tested. Soluble factors secreted from the activated CD4+ T cells were found to be responsible for the observed effect, with IFN-γ playing a major role in the chemosensitization of tumor cells. IFN-γ by itself, however, was consistently inferior to activated CD4+ T cells in the chemosensitization of tumor cells.

For three human metastatic melanoma, two human breast, one prostate and one colon cancer cell line, treated with 5-FU, temozolomide (TMZ), carboplatin (Carbo), or paclitaxel, chemosensitization with aCD4 had a dramatic impact on tumor cell viability and *in vivo* tumor formation. TMZ, the oral imidazotetrazine derivative of dacarbazine that is also capable of crossing the blood-brain barrier, ultimately produces the same dacarbazine compound after intake and has been shown in clinical trial to be similarly effective in treating metastatic melanoma as dacarbazine (Middleton et al., 2000). Treatment of the A375 melanoma cell line with TMZ after presensitization with aCD4 resulted in near complete cell death, with residual cell viability as low as 5%, compared to 67% viability for cells treated with TMZ that were not presensitized with aCD4. Similar study of two more melanoma cell lines provided comparable results. Further tests using Carbo, a drug with minimal activity against melanoma, resulted in a decrease of melanoma cell viability of ~83% at the optimal aCD4 concentration, compared with no change in viability after Carbo treatment alone. Non-melanoma cell lines treated with paclitaxel, Carbo or 5-FU all gave similar results.

Presensitization was found to be mediated in large part via cytokines, principally IFN-γ, and not through cell-cell contact. aCD4 supernatants were screened for 13 common Th1 and Th2 pro- and anti-inflammatory cytokines. IL-1b, IL-5, and IL-12p70 levels were negative or minimally expressed. The remaining 10 were tested for in combination against aCD4 alone for their chemosensitizing ability, assessed based on viability after TMZ treatment. There was no increase in chemosensitizing ability of combination IL-2/-4 over cells without cytokine addition, and combinations IL-6/-8 and IL-10/-12p40/-13 produced enhanced activity of 7% and 8%, respectively. Combination IFN-γ/TNF-α/GM-CSF significantly enhanced the cytotoxic activity of TMZ by 17%. While most individual cytokines provided little to no enhancement of TMZ cytotoxicity, IFN-γ in combination with other cytokines consistently provided the greatest impact on chemosensitization, and IFN-γ combinations showed no improvement over IFN-γ itself; however, the effects of IFN-γ by itself or in combination lagged the single combination of all 10 tested cytokines. Administration of aCD4 alone prior to TMZ treatment as a positive control yielded the best results, showing significant enhancement of TMZ cytotoxic cell killing over the 10-cytokine combination.

Lysates from A375 cells presensitized with aCD4 followed by treatment with TMZ were analyzed via a transwell system for cytoplasmic histone-associated DNA fragments as a measure of apoptosis. Melanoma cells treated with TMZ alone or aCD4 alone resulted in slightly higher levels of DNA fragments, ~49 arbitrary units (AU) and 54 AU, respectively, as compared 23 AU for nontreated cells. However, when A375 cells were presensitized with aCD4 and treated with TMZ, the level of DNA fragments detected, 1041 AU, was more than 21-fold over that of the TMZ alone group, 19-fold over the aCD4 alone group, and 45-fold over the nontreatment control. In addition, a significantly higher level of caspase-8 activity, ~2300 RFU, was detected in cells in the experimental group compared with the control groups, i.e., no treatment (524.4 $\pm$ 3.5 RFU), TMZ treatment only (508.6 $\pm$ 28.3 RFU), or aCD4 treatment only (392.7 $\pm$ 4.0 RFU). A reduction in the relative expression of Bcl-2 protein was also detected in A375 cells treated with aCD4 alone or the combination of aCD4 followed by TMZ, but not in cells treated with TMZ alone. These data demonstrated that presensitization of tumor cells with aCD4 led to a decrease in Bcl-2, and that treatment with aCD4 and TMZ together resulted in enhanced caspase-8 activity, resulting in significant reduction in cell viability through an increase in apoptosis. The combination of aCD4 and chemotherapy yielded dramatic results at 24 hours in viability experiments. To evaluate true pro-apoptotic potential of aCD4 presensitization, apoptosis assays were performed at earlier time points, 12 hours instead of 24 hours after treatment with chemotherapy. For caspase-8 activity, chemotherapy treatment was stopped after 5 to 6 hours. Even at these early time points when aCD4 alone or chemotherapy alone had no discernable effects, the combination of aCD4 and chemotherapy resulted in a dramatic increase in apoptosis and caspase-8 activity.

Two human tumor xenograft models provided evidence of significant tumor growth delay for melanoma and breast cancer after presensitization with aCD4 and subsequent treatment with TMZ or paclitaxel, respectively. The melanoma xenograft also displayed significant growth inhibition. In the first model, injections of aCD4 were made intratumorally, followed 48 hours later with intraperitoneal administration of TMZ, to athymic nude mice bearing human melanoma A375 xenograft. There was a significantly pronounced delay in tumor growth compared with mice receiving no treatment or either treatment alone. Similarly, mice bearing aggressive MDA-MB-231 human breast tumors treated with aCD4 followed by paclitaxel had significant delay in tumor growth compared with each of the control groups. The difference between aCD4 plus paclitaxel versus paclitaxel alone was statistically significant. Interestingly, aCD4 alone had a significant growth inhibition effect on the melanoma xenograft but not on the breast cancer xenograft. This was consistent with the known immuno sensitivity of melanoma compared with other solid tumors. To assess toxicity resulting from the experimental treatment, animal weights were measured and recorded during the course of the study. No statistically significant difference in weight was found between the experimental group and control groups up to day 30 after initiation of treatment.

Some recent studies may help shed light onto the possible mechanisms that underlie the dramatic chemosensitizing effect of aCD4. Inflammation and inflammatory cytokines, as represented by a mixture of IL-1β, TNF-α, and IFN-γ, were shown to generate nitric oxide through the induction of nitric oxide synthase, resulting in global inhibition of DNA repair activity in cholangiocarcinoma cells (Jaiswal et al., 2000). Perrotta et al. (Perrotta et al., 2007) further described chemosensitization through dendritic-cell-mediated intratumoral administration of nitric oxide in a B16 mouse melanoma model. Other studies demonstrated that IFN-β or IL-24 could overcome TMZ resistance in neuroblastoma and melanoma, respectively, through down-regulation of the DNA repair enzyme O6-methylguanine-DNA methyltransferase expression and activity (Rosati et al., 2008; Zheng et al., 2008). Additionally, several recent clinical studies have reported improved response rates and survival with salvage chemotherapy in patients who previously received cancer vaccination and developed an immune response (Antonia et al., 2006; Arlen et al., 2006; Gribben et al., 2005; Schlom et al., 2007; Wheeler et al., 2004). Our model may provide a plausible mechanism to explain these observations as well as to facilitate further understanding, design, and development of improved methods for chemoimmunotherapy in cancer.

5. Conclusion

Despite intense research efforts, scientists are still struggling with the simplest principles of tumor cell proliferation, cell cycle kinetics and the genetic basis of malignant transformation and tumor progression. In particular, treatment options for melanoma are few, and those with metastatic disease have been afforded only meager therapeutic options in the past, maintaining a disappointing 15% five-year survival rate. In somewhat of a contradiction, melanoma is now at the forefront of targeted and immunological therapeutic study, evident by the surging number of relevant publications and the recent addition of ipilimumab to a short list of FDA-approved therapies for metastatic melanoma patients. One of the most popular and theoretically promising of these directions currently being studied is combination chemoimmunotherapy.

While many chemoimmunotherapeutic regimens have resulted in lackluster responses, our novel adaptation of this methodology for melanoma and other cancers, utilizing non-tumor-specific activation of CD4+ T cells as a chemosensitizer, has provided exciting results. We have shown dramatic increases in the efficacies of four functionally unique chemotherapeutic drugs in seven cell lines comprising four different cancer types with our 'chemocentric chemoimmunotherapeutic' strategy. After presensitization with aCD4, cytotoxicity was greatly enhanced for all chemo drugs, both *in vitro* and *in vivo*, against all cell types tested. In addition, we recently described the presensitization of tumor cells with aCD4 prior to gamma-irradiation to significantly enhance cancer cell growth inhibition (Wang et al., 2010). Soluble factors released by aCD4, particularly IFN-γ, were primarily responsible for the observed activity, and TNF-α, though inactive by itself, significantly augmented the radiosensitizing activity of IFN-γ.

Not only are the time and monetary costs of producing non-tumor-specific activated CD4+ T cells far and away less than the current standard of activating against a specific set of patient tumor cell antigens, but, as our data shows, aCD4 may also be applied in patients with a variety of cancer types in synergistic conjunction with the most currently effective and applicable chemotherapy for the individual patient. Regardless of the cell line used or its sensitivity or resistance to a particular chemotherapeutic drug, in all our tested cases, presensitization with aCD4 greatly enhanced the cytotoxicity of the drugs, resulting in near complete cell death. Therefore, patients with a typically chemoresistant cancer, such as metastatic melanoma, may be able to benefit from enhanced chemotherapeutic efficacy with aCD4 presensitization. Additionally, utilization of a much broader range of chemotherapeutic agents may be possible for patients who might normally have only a small number of available options, specific for their tumor type and physical condition. Patients may thus be able to receive treatment sooner, accessing the readily available wealth of well-studied chemotherapeutic drugs without the need to await new drug development and testing. To this end, drug selection may ultimately be better tailored to patient tolerance, creating a therapeutic strategy with greater anti-tumor activity, therefore, less time for development of chemoresistance, and better tolerance which will allow more patients to remain on their particular regimen for its appropriate duration. Indeed, the utilization of this novel technique may be able to provide a more effective and efficient means to combat melanoma and other cancers.

6. References

Adair, S.J. & Hogan, K.T. (2009). Treatment of Ovarian Cancer Cell Lines with 5-Aza-2'-Deoxycytidine Upregulates the Expression of Cancer-Testis Antigens and Class I

Major Histocompatibility Complex-Encoded Molecules, *Cancer Immunol Immunother*, Vol. 58, No. 4, pp. 589-601, 1432-0851

Allen, I.; Kupelnick, B.; Kumashiro, M.; et al. (1998). Efficacy of Interleukin-2 in the Treatment of Metastatic Melanoma-Systematic Review and Meta-Analysis. *Sel Cancer Ther,* Vol. 1, pp. 168–173

Amos, S.M.; Pegram, H.J.; Westwood, J.A., et al. (2011). Adoptive Immunotherapy Combined with Intratumoral TLR Agonist Delivery Eradicates Established Melanoma in Mice, *Cancer Immunol Immunother*, Vol. 60, No. 5, pp. 671-683, 1432-0851

Antonia, S.J.; Mirza, N.; Fricke, I., et al. (2006). Combination of P53 Cancer Vaccine with Chemotherapy in Patients with Extensive Stage Small Cell Lung Cancer, *Clin Cancer Res*, Vol. 12, No. 3 Pt 1, pp. 878-887, 1078-0432

Arlen, P.M.; Gulley, J.L.; Parker, C., et al. (2006). A Randomized Phase Ii Study of Concurrent Docetaxel Plus Vaccine Versus Vaccine Alone in Metastatic Androgen-Independent Prostate Cancer, *Clin Cancer Res*, Vol. 12, No. 4, pp. 1260-1269, 1078-0432

Atallah, E. & Flaherty, L. (2005). Treatment of Metastatic Malignant Melanoma, *Curr Treat Options Oncol*, Vol. 6, No. 3, pp. 185-193, 1527-2729

Atkins, M.B.; Kunkel, L.; Sznol, M., et al. (2000). High-Dose Recombinant Interleukin-2 Therapy in Patients with Metastatic Melanoma: Long-Term Survival Update, *Cancer J Sci Am*, Vol. 6 Suppl 1, pp. S11-14, 1081-4442

Atkins, M.B.; Gollob, J.A.; Sosman, J.A., et al. (2002). A Phase II Pilot Trial of Concurrent Biochemotherapy with Cisplatin, Vinblastine, Temozolomide, Interleukin 2, and IFN-Alpha 2b in Patients with Metastatic Melanoma, *Clin Cancer Res*, Vol. 8, No. 10, pp. 3075-3081, 1078-0432

Atkins, M.B.; Lee, S.; Flaherty, L.E.; et al. (2003) A Prospective Randomized Phase III Trial of Concurrent Biochemotherapy (BCT) with Cisplatin, Vinblastine, Dacarbazine (CVD), IL-2, and Interferon α-2b (IFN) Versus CVD Alone in Patients with Metastatic Melanoma (E3695): An ECOG-Coordinated Intergroup Trial. In: *Program and abstracts of the American Society of Clinical Oncology Annual Meeting,* Chicago, IL, May 31-June 3, p. 708a

Atkins, M.B.; Hsu, J.; Lee, S., et al. (2008). Phase III Trial Comparing Concurrent Biochemotherapy with Cisplatin, Vinblastine, Dacarbazine, Interleukin-2, and Interferon Alfa-2b with Cisplatin, Vinblastine, and Dacarbazine Alone in Patients with Metastatic Malignant Melanoma (E3695): A Trial Coordinated by the Eastern Cooperative Oncology Group, *J Clin Oncol*, Vol. 26, No. 35, pp. 5748-5754, 1527-7755

Atzpodien, J.; Neuber, K.; Kamanabrou, D., et al. (2002). Combination Chemotherapy with or without s.c. IL-2 and IFN-Alpha: Results of a Prospectively Randomized Trial of the Cooperative Advanced Malignant Melanoma Chemoimmunotherapy Group (Acimm), *Br J Cancer*, Vol. 86, No. 2, pp. 179-184, 0007-0920

Bafaloukos, D.; Aravantinos, G.; Fountzilas, G., et al. (2002). Docetaxel in Combination with Dacarbazine in Patients with Advanced Melanoma, *Oncology*, Vol. 63, No. 4, pp. 333-337, 0030-2414

Bajetta, E.; Del Vecchio, M.; Bernard-Marty, C., et al. (2002). Metastatic Melanoma: Chemotherapy, *Semin Oncol*, Vol. 29, No. 5, pp. 427-445, 0093-7754

Bajetta, E.; Del Vecchio, M.; Nova, P., et al. (2006). Multicenter Phase III Randomized Trial of Polychemotherapy (CVD Regimen) Versus the Same Chemotherapy (Ct) Plus Subcutaneous Interleukin-2 and Interferon-Alpha2b in Metastatic Melanoma, *Ann Oncol*, Vol. 17, No. 4, pp. 571-577, 0923-7534

Balch, C.M.; Buzaid, A.C.; Soong, S.J., et al. (2001). Final Version of the American Joint Committee on Cancer Staging System for Cutaneous Melanoma, *J Clin Oncol*, Vol. 19, No. 16, pp. 3635-3648, 0732-183X

Balch, C.M.; Soong, S.J.; Gershenwald, J.E., et al. (2001). Prognostic Factors Analysis of 17,600 Melanoma Patients: Validation of the American Joint Committee on Cancer Melanoma Staging System, *J Clin Oncol*, Vol. 19, No. 16, pp. 3622-3634, 0732-183X

Bedikian, A.Y.; Richards, J.; Kharkevitch, D., et al. (2010). A Phase 2 Study of High-Dose Allovectin-7 in Patients with Advanced Metastatic Melanoma, *Melanoma Res*, Vol. 20, No. 3, pp. 218-226, 1473-5636

Berd, D.; Maguire, H.C., Jr. & Mastrangelo, M.J. (1986). Induction of Cell-Mediated Immunity to Autologous Melanoma Cells and Regression of Metastases after Treatment with a Melanoma Cell Vaccine Preceded by Cyclophosphamide, *Cancer Res*, Vol. 46, No. 5, pp. 2572-2577, 0008-5472

Berd, D.; Maguire, H.C., Jr.; Mccue, P., et al. (1990). Treatment of Metastatic Melanoma with an Autologous Tumor-Cell Vaccine: Clinical and Immunologic Results in 64 Patients, *J Clin Oncol*, Vol. 8, No. 11, pp. 1858-1867, 0732-183X

Berd, D.; Sato, T.; Maguire, H.C., Jr., et al. (2004). Immunopharmacologic Analysis of an Autologous, Hapten-Modified Human Melanoma Vaccine, *J Clin Oncol*, Vol. 22, No. 3, pp. 403-415, 0732-183X

Blesa, J.M.; Pulido, E.G.; Candel, V.A., et al. (2011). Melanoma: From Darkness to Promise, *Am J Clin Oncol*, Vol. 34, No. 2, pp. 179-187, 1537-453X

Bollag, G.; Hirth, P.; Tsai, J., et al. (2010). Clinical Efficacy of a Raf Inhibitor Needs Broad Target Blockade in BRAF-Mutant Melanoma, *Nature*, Vol. 467, No. 7315, pp. 596-599, 1476-4687

Bracci, L.; Moschella, F.; Sestili, P., et al. (2007). Cyclophosphamide Enhances the Antitumor Efficacy of Adoptively Transferred Immune Cells through the Induction of Cytokine Expression, B-Cell and T-Cell Homeostatic Proliferation, and Specific Tumor Infiltration, *Clin Cancer Res*, Vol. 13, No. 2 Pt 1, pp. 644-653, 1078-0432

Burke, F.; Smith, P.D.; Crompton, M.R., et al. (1999). Cytotoxic Response of Ovarian Cancer Cell Lines to IFN-Gamma Is Associated with Sustained Induction of IRF-1 and P21 mRNA, *Br J Cancer*, Vol. 80, No. 8, pp. 1236-1244, 0007-0920

Buzaid, A.C.; Legha, S.S.; Winn, R.; et al. (1993) Cisplatin (C), Vinblastine (V), Dacarbazine (D) (CVD) Versus Dacarbazine Alone in Metastatic Melanoma: Preliminary Results Phase III Cancer Community Oncology Program (CCOP). *Proc Annu Meet Am Soc Clin Oncol*, Vol. 12, p. 1328

Carswell, E.A.; Old, L.J.; Kassel, R.L., et al. (1975). An Endotoxin-Induced Serum Factor That Causes Necrosis of Tumors, *Proc Natl Acad Sci U S A*, Vol. 72, No. 9, pp. 3666-3670, 0027-8424

Chapman, P.B.; Einhorn, L.H.; Meyers, M.L., et al. (1999). Phase III Multicenter Randomized Trial of the Dartmouth Regimen Versus Dacarbazine in Patients with Metastatic Melanoma, *J Clin Oncol*, Vol. 17, No. 9, pp. 2745-2751, 0732-183X

Chawla-Sarkar, M.; Leaman, D.W. & Borden, E.C. (2001). Preferential Induction of Apoptosis by Interferon (IFN)-Beta Compared with IFN-Alpha2: Correlation with Trail/Apo2l Induction in Melanoma Cell Lines, *Clin Cancer Res*, Vol. 7, No. 6, pp. 1821-1831, 1078-0432

Chawla-Sarkar, M.; Lindner, D.J.; Liu, Y.F., et al. (2003). Apoptosis and Interferons: Role of Interferon-Stimulated Genes as Mediators of Apoptosis, *Apoptosis*, Vol. 8, No. 3, pp. 237-249, 1360-8185

Chinnasamy, D.; Yu, Z.; Theoret, M.R., et al. (2010). Gene Therapy Using Genetically Modified Lymphocytes Targeting VEGFR-2 Inhibits the Growth of Vascularized Syngenic Tumors in Mice, *J Clin Invest*, Vol. 120, No. 11, pp. 3953-3968, 1558-8238

Comin-Anduix, B.; Chodon, T.; Sazegar, H., et al. (2010). The Oncogenic BRAF Kinase Inhibitor Plx4032/Rg7204 Does Not Affect the Viability or Function of Human Lymphocytes across a Wide Range of Concentrations, *Clin Cancer Res*, Vol. 16, No. 24, pp. 6040-6048, 1078-0432

Coral, S.; Sigalotti, L.; Altomonte, M., et al. (2002). 5-Aza-2'-Deoxycytidine-Induced Expression of Functional Cancer Testis Antigens in Human Renal Cell Carcinoma: Immunotherapeutic Implications, *Clin Cancer Res*, Vol. 8, No. 8, pp. 2690-2695, 1078-0432

Correale, P.; Aquino, A.; Giuliani, A., et al. (2003). Treatment of Colon and Breast Carcinoma Cells with 5-Fluorouracil Enhances Expression of Carcinoembryonic Antigen and Susceptibility to Hla-a(*)02.01 Restricted, CEA-Peptide-Specific Cytotoxic T Cells in Vitro, *Int J Cancer*, Vol. 104, No. 4, pp. 437-445, 0020-7136

Del Prete, S.A.; Maurer, L.H.; O'donnell, J., et al. (1984). Combination Chemotherapy with Cisplatin, Carmustine, Dacarbazine, and Tamoxifen in Metastatic Melanoma, *Cancer Treat Rep*, Vol. 68, No. 11, pp. 1403-1405, 0361-5960

Detjen, K.M.; Farwig, K.; Welzel, M., et al. (2001). Interferon Gamma Inhibits Growth of Human Pancreatic Carcinoma Cells Via Caspase-1 Dependent Induction of Apoptosis, *Gut*, Vol. 49, No. 2, pp. 251-262, 0017-5749

Dong Xda, E.; Ito, N.; Lotze, M.T., et al. (2007). High Mobility Group Box I (HMGB1) Release from Tumor Cells after Treatment: Implications for Development of Targeted Chemoimmunotherapy, *J Immunother*, Vol. 30, No. 6, pp. 596-606, 1524-9557

Dudley, M.E.; Wunderlich, J.R.; Robbins, P.F., et al. (2002). Cancer Regression and Autoimmunity in Patients after Clonal Repopulation with Antitumor Lymphocytes, *Science*, Vol. 298, No. 5594, pp. 850-854, 1095-9203

Dudley, M.E.; Wunderlich, J.R.; Yang, J.C., et al. (2005). Adoptive Cell Transfer Therapy Following Non-Myeloablative but Lymphodepleting Chemotherapy for the Treatment of Patients with Refractory Metastatic Melanoma, *J Clin Oncol*, Vol. 23, No. 10, pp. 2346-2357, 0732-183X

Dudley, M.E. & Rosenberg, S.A. (2007). Adoptive Cell Transfer Therapy, *Semin Oncol*, Vol. 34, No. 6, pp. 524-531, 0093-7754

Dudley, M.E.; Yang, J.C.; Sherry, R., et al. (2008). Adoptive Cell Therapy for Patients with Metastatic Melanoma: Evaluation of Intensive Myeloablative Chemoradiation Preparative Regimens, *J Clin Oncol*, Vol. 26, No. 32, pp. 5233-5239, 1527-7755

Dummer, W.; Niethammer, A.G.; Baccala, R., et al. (2002). T Cell Homeostatic Proliferation Elicits Effective Antitumor Autoimmunity, *J Clin Invest*, Vol. 110, No. 2, pp. 185-192, 0021-9738

Egberts, F.; Gutzmer, R.; Ugurel, S., et al. (2011). Sorafenib and Pegylated Interferon-{Alpha}2b in Advanced Metastatic Melanoma: A Multicenter Phase II Decog Trial, *Ann Oncol*, 1569-8041

Elsaesser, H.; Sauer, K. & Brooks, D.G. (2009). Il-21 Is Required to Control Chronic Viral Infection, *Science*, Vol. 324, No. 5934, pp. 1569-1572, 1095-9203

Emens, L.A. (2008). Chemotherapy and Tumor Immunity: An Unexpected Collaboration, *Front Biosci*, Vol. 13, pp. 249-257, 1093-4715

Ercolini, A.M.; Ladle, B.H.; Manning, E.A., et al. (2005). Recruitment of Latent Pools of High-Avidity Cd8(+) T Cells to the Antitumor Immune Response, *J Exp Med*, Vol. 201, No. 10, pp. 1591-1602, 0022-1007

Eton, O.; Legha, S.S.; Bedikian, A.Y., et al. (2002). Sequential Biochemotherapy Versus Chemotherapy for Metastatic Melanoma: Results from a Phase III Randomized Trial, *J Clin Oncol*, Vol. 20, No. 8, pp. 2045-2052, 0732-183X

Fantini, M.C.; Rizzo, A.; Fina, D., et al. (2007). Il-21 Regulates Experimental Colitis by Modulating the Balance between Treg and Th17 Cells, *Eur J Immunol*, Vol. 37, No. 11, pp. 3155-3163, 0014-2980

Finn, O.J. (2008). Cancer Immunology, *N Engl J Med*, Vol. 358, No. 25, pp. 2704-2715, 1533-4406

Flaherty, L.E.; Atkins, M.; Sosman, J., et al. (2001). Outpatient Biochemotherapy with Interleukin-2 and Interferon Alfa-2b in Patients with Metastatic Malignant Melanoma: Results of Two Phase II Cytokine Working Group Trials, *J Clin Oncol*, Vol. 19, No. 13, pp. 3194-3202, 0732-183X

Flaherty, K.T.; Puzanov, I.; Kim, K.B., et al. (2010). Inhibition of Mutated, Activated BRAF in Metastatic Melanoma, *N Engl J Med*, Vol. 363, No. 9, pp. 809-819, 1533-4406

Fonsatti, E.; Nicolay, H.J.; Sigalotti, L., et al. (2007). Functional up-Regulation of Human Leukocyte Antigen Class I Antigens Expression by 5-Aza-2'-Deoxycytidine in Cutaneous Melanoma: Immunotherapeutic Implications, *Clin Cancer Res*, Vol. 13, No. 11, pp. 3333-3338, 1078-0432

Fonsatti, E.; Maio, M.; Altomonte, M., et al. (2010). Biology and Clinical Applications of CD40 in Cancer Treatment, *Semin Oncol*, Vol. 37, No. 5, pp. 517-523, 1532-8708

Formenti, S.C. (2010). Immunological Aspects of Local Radiotherapy: Clinical Relevance, *Discov Med*, Vol. 9, No. 45, pp. 119-124, 1944-7930

Fregni, G.; Perier, A.; Pittari, G.; et al. (2011) Unique Functional Status of Natural Killer Cells in Metastatic Stage IV Melanoma Patients and Its Modulation by Chemotherapy. *Clin Cancer Res*, Vol. 17, No. 9, pp. 2628-2637

Gattinoni, L.; Powell, D.J., Jr.; Rosenberg, S.A., et al. (2006). Adoptive Immunotherapy for Cancer: Building on Success, *Nat Rev Immunol*, Vol. 6, No. 5, pp. 383-393, 1474-1733

Ghiringhelli, F.; Larmonier, N.; Schmitt, E., et al. (2004). Cd4+Cd25+ Regulatory T Cells Suppress Tumor Immunity but Are Sensitive to Cyclophosphamide Which Allows Immunotherapy of Established Tumors to Be Curative, *Eur J Immunol*, Vol. 34, No. 2, pp. 336-344, 0014-2980

Gooch, J.L.; Herrera, R.E. & Yee, D. (2000). The Role of P21 in Interferon Gamma-Mediated Growth Inhibition of Human Breast Cancer Cells, *Cell Growth Differ*, Vol. 11, No. 6, pp. 335-342, 1044-9523

Gribben, J.G.; Ryan, D.P.; Boyajian, R., et al. (2005). Unexpected Association Between Induction of Immunity to the Universal Tumor Antigen CYP1B1 and Response to Next Therapy, *Clin Cancer Res*, Vol. 11, No. 12, pp. 4430-4436, 1078-0432

Harris, J.; Sengar, D.; Stewart, T., et al. (1976). The Effect of Immunosuppressive Chemotherapy on Immune Function in Patients with Malignant Disease, *Cancer*, Vol. 37, No. 2 Suppl, pp. 1058-1069, 0008-543X

Harvat, B.L. & Jetten, A.M. (1996). Gamma-Interferon Induces an Irreversible Growth Arrest in Mid-G1 in Mammary Epithelial Cells Which Correlates with a Block in Hyperphosphorylation of Retinoblastoma, *Cell Growth Differ*, Vol. 7, No. 3, pp. 289-300, 1044-9523

Helson, L.; Green, S.; Carswell, E., et al. (1975). Effect of Tumour Necrosis Factor on Cultured Human Melanoma Cells, *Nature*, Vol. 258, No. 5537, pp. 731-732, 0028-0836

Hernandez-Chacon, J.A.; Li, Y.; Wu, R.C., et al. (2011). Costimulation Through the CD137/4-1bb Pathway Protects Human Melanoma Tumor-Infiltrating Lymphocytes from Activation-Induced Cell Death and Enhances Antitumor Effector Function, *J Immunother*, Vol. 34, No. 3, pp. 236-250, 1537-4513

Hershkovitz, L.; Schachter, J.; Treves, A.J., et al. (2010). Focus on Adoptive T Cell Transfer Trials in Melanoma, *Clin Dev Immunol*, Vol. 2010, No. 260267

Hinrichs, C.S.; Spolski, R.; Paulos, C.M., et al. (2008). Il-2 and Il-21 Confer Opposing Differentiation Programs to Cd8+ T Cells for Adoptive Immunotherapy, *Blood*, Vol. 111, No. 11, pp. 5326-5333, 1528-0020

Hirschhorn-Cymerman, D.; Rizzuto, G.A.; Merghoub, T.; et al. (2011) OX40 engagement and chemotherapy combination provides potent antitumor immunity with concomitant regulatory T cell apoptosis. *J Exp Med*, Vol. 206, No. 5, pp. 1103-1116

Hodi, F.S.; O'day, S.J.; Mcdermott, D.F., et al. (2010). Improved Survival with Ipilimumab in Patients with Metastatic Melanoma, *N Engl J Med*, Vol. 363, No. 8, pp. 711-723, 1533-4406

Inozume, T.; Hanada, K.; Wang, Q.J., et al. (2010). Selection of Cd8+Pd-1+ Lymphocytes in Fresh Human Melanomas Enriches for Tumor-Reactive T Cells, *J Immunother*, Vol. 33, No. 9, pp. 956-964, 1537-4513

Ives, N.J.; Stowe, R.L.; Lorigan, P., et al. (2007). Chemotherapy Compared with Biochemotherapy for the Treatment of Metastatic Melanoma: A Meta-Analysis of 18 Trials Involving 2,621 Patients, *J Clin Oncol*, Vol. 25, No. 34, pp. 5426-5434, 1527-7755

Jaiswal, M.; Larusso, N.F.; Burgart, L.J., et al. (2000). Inflammatory Cytokines Induce DNA Damage and Inhibit DNA Repair in Cholangiocarcinoma Cells by a Nitric Oxide-Dependent Mechanism, *Cancer Res*, Vol. 60, No. 1, pp. 184-190, 0008-5472

Jemal, A.; Siegel, R.; Xu, J., et al. (2010). Cancer Statistics, 2010, *CA Cancer J Clin*, Vol. 60, No. 5, pp. 277-300, 1542-4863

Kadison, A.S. & Morton, D.L. (2003). Immunotherapy of Malignant Melanoma, *Surg Clin North Am*, Vol. 83, No. 2, pp. 343-370, 0039-6109

Kaplan, D.H.; Shankaran, V.; Dighe, A.S., et al. (1998). Demonstration of an Interferon Gamma-Dependent Tumor Surveillance System in Immunocompetent Mice, *Proc Natl Acad Sci U S A*, Vol. 95, No. 13, pp. 7556-7561, 0027-8424

Kaufmann, R.; Spieth, K.; Leiter, U., et al. (2005). Temozolomide in Combination with Interferon-Alfa Versus Temozolomide Alone in Patients with Advanced Metastatic Melanoma: A Randomized, Phase III, Multicenter Study from the Dermatologic Cooperative Oncology Group, *J Clin Oncol*, Vol. 23, No. 35, pp. 9001-9007, 0732-183X

Keilholz, U.; Goey, S.H.; Punt, C.J., et al. (1997). Interferon Alfa-2a and Interleukin-2 with or without Cisplatin in Metastatic Melanoma: A Randomized Trial of the European Organization for Research and Treatment of Cancer Melanoma Cooperative Group, *J Clin Oncol*, Vol. 15, No. 7, pp. 2579-2588, 0732-183X

Keilholz, U.; Conradt, C.; Legha, S.S., et al. (1998). Results of Interleukin-2-Based Treatment in Advanced Melanoma: A Case Record-Based Analysis of 631 Patients, *J Clin Oncol*, Vol. 16, No. 9, pp. 2921-2929, 0732-183X

Keilholz, U.; Punt, C.J.; Gore, M., et al. (2005). Dacarbazine, Cisplatin, and Interferon-Alfa-2b with or without Interleukin-2 in Metastatic Melanoma: A Randomized Phase III Trial (18951) of the European Organisation for Research and Treatment of Cancer Melanoma Group, *J Clin Oncol*, Vol. 23, No. 27, pp. 6747-6755, 0732-183X

Khattar, M.; Chen, W. & Stepkowski, S.M. (2009). Expanding and Converting Regulatory T Cells: A Horizon for Immunotherapy, *Arch Immunol Ther Exp (Warsz)*, Vol. 57, No. 3, pp. 199-204, 1661-4917

Khayat, D.; Bernard-Marty, C.; Meric, J.B., et al. (2002). Biochemotherapy for Advanced Melanoma: Maybe It Is Real, *J Clin Oncol*, Vol. 20, No. 10, pp. 2411-2414, 0732-183X

Kohlmeyer, J.; Cron, M.; Landsberg, J., et al. (2009). Complete Regression of Advanced Primary and Metastatic Mouse Melanomas Following Combination Chemoimmunotherapy, *Cancer Res*, Vol. 69, No. 15, pp. 6265-6274, 1538-7445

Lampen, M.H. & Van Hall, T. (2011). Strategies to Counteract MHC-I Defects in Tumors, *Curr Opin Immunol*, Vol. 23, No. 2, pp. 293-298, 1879-0372

Laster, S.M.; Wood, J.G. & Gooding, L.R. (1988). Tumor Necrosis Factor Can Induce Both Apoptic and Necrotic Forms of Cell Lysis, *J Immunol*, Vol. 141, No. 8, pp. 2629-2634, 0022-1767

Legha, S.S.; Ring, S.; Papadopoulos, N., et al. (1989). A Prospective Evaluation of a Triple-Drug Regimen Containing Cisplatin, Vinblastine, and Dacarbazine (CVD) for Metastatic Melanoma, *Cancer*, Vol. 64, No. 10, pp. 2024-2029, 0008-543X

Legha, S.S.; Ring, S.; Eton, O., et al. (1998). Development of a Biochemotherapy Regimen with Concurrent Administration of Cisplatin, Vinblastine, Dacarbazine, Interferon Alfa, and Interleukin-2 for Patients with Metastatic Melanoma, *J Clin Oncol*, Vol. 16, No. 5, pp. 1752-1759, 0732-183X

Lindenmann, J. & Klein, P.A. (1967). Viral Oncolysis: Increased Immunogenicity of Host Cell Antigen Associated with Influenza Virus, *J Exp Med*, Vol. 126, No. 1, pp. 93-108, 0022-1007

Livingston, P.O.; Cunningham-Rundles, S.; Marfleet, G., et al. (1987). Inhibition of Suppressor-Cell Activity by Cyclophosphamide in Patients with Malignant Melanoma, *J Biol Response Mod*, Vol. 6, No. 4, pp. 392-403, 0732-6580

Livingston, P.O.; Wong, G.Y.; Adluri, S., et al. (1994). Improved Survival in Stage III Melanoma Patients with Gm2 Antibodies: A Randomized Trial of Adjuvant Vaccination with Gm2 Ganglioside, *J Clin Oncol*, Vol. 12, No. 5, pp. 1036-1044, 0732-183X

Maine, G.N. & Mule, J.J. (2002). Making Room for T Cells, *J Clin Invest*, Vol. 110, No. 2, pp. 157-159, 0021-9738

Maleno, I.; Aptsiauri, N.; Cabrera, T., et al. (2011). Frequent Loss of Heterozygosity in the Beta2-Microglobulin Region of Chromosome 15 in Primary Human Tumors, *Immunogenetics*, Vol. 63, No. 2, pp. 65-71, 1432-1211

Manusama, E.R.; Nooijen, P.T.; Stavast, J., et al. (1996). Synergistic Antitumour Effect of Recombinant Human Tumour Necrosis Factor Alpha with Melphalan in Isolated Limb Perfusion in the Rat, *Br J Surg*, Vol. 83, No. 4, pp. 551-555, 0007-1323

McDermott, D.F.; Mier, J.W.; Lawrence, D.P., et al. (2000). A Phase II Pilot Trial of Concurrent Biochemotherapy with Cisplatin, Vinblastine, Dacarbazine, Interleukin 2, and Interferon Alpha-2b in Patients with Metastatic Melanoma, *Clin Cancer Res*, Vol. 6, No. 6, pp. 2201-2208, 1078-0432

Middleton, M.R.; Grob, J.J.; Aaronson, N., et al. (2000). Randomized Phase III Study of Temozolomide Versus Dacarbazine in the Treatment of Patients with Advanced Metastatic Malignant Melanoma, *J Clin Oncol*, Vol. 18, No. 1, pp. 158-166, 0732-183X

Middleton, M.; Hauschild, A.; Thomson, D., et al. (2007). Results of a Multicenter Randomized Study to Evaluate the Safety and Efficacy of Combined Immunotherapy with Interleukin-2, Interferon-{Alpha}2b and Histamine Dihydrochloride Versus Dacarbazine in Patients with Stage IV Melanoma, *Ann Oncol*, Vol. 18, No. 10, pp. 1691-1697, 1569-8041

Mihalyo, M.A.; Doody, A.D.; Mcaleer, J.P., et al. (2004). In Vivo Cyclophosphamide and IL-2 Treatment Impedes Self-Antigen-Induced Effector CD4 Cell Tolerization: Implications for Adoptive Immunotherapy, *J Immunol*, Vol. 172, No. 9, pp. 5338-5345, 0022-1767

Morgan, R.A.; Dudley, M.E.; Wunderlich, J.R., et al. (2006). Cancer Regression in Patients after Transfer of Genetically Engineered Lymphocytes, *Science*, Vol. 314, No. 5796, pp. 126-129, 1095-9203

Natsume, A.; Wakabayashi, T.; Tsujimura, K., et al. (2008). The DNA Demethylating Agent 5-Aza-2'-Deoxycytidine Activates NY-ESO-1 Antigenicity in Orthotopic Human Glioma, *Int J Cancer*, Vol. 122, No. 11, pp. 2542-2553, 1097-0215

Nistico, P.; Capone, I.; Palermo, B., et al. (2009). Chemotherapy Enhances Vaccine-Induced Antitumor Immunity in Melanoma Patients, *Int J Cancer*, Vol. 124, No. 1, pp. 130-139, 1097-0215

North, R.J. (1982). Cyclophosphamide-Facilitated Adoptive Immunotherapy of an Established Tumor Depends on Elimination of Tumor-Induced Suppressor T Cells, *J Exp Med*, Vol. 155, No. 4, pp. 1063-1074, 0022-1007

Nowak, A.K.; Lake, R.A. & Robinson, B.W. (2006). Combined Chemoimmunotherapy of Solid Tumours: Improving Vaccines?, *Adv Drug Deliv Rev*, Vol. 58, No. 8, pp. 975-990, 0169-409X

O'day, S.J.; Atkins, M.B.; Boasberg, P., et al. (2009). Phase II Multicenter Trial of Maintenance Biotherapy after Induction Concurrent Biochemotherapy for Patients with Metastatic Melanoma, *J Clin Oncol*, Vol. 27, No. 36, pp. 6207-6212, 1527-7755

Old, L.J. (1985). Tumor Necrosis Factor (TNFf), *Science*, Vol. 230, No. 4726, pp. 630-632, 0036-8075

Pages, F.; Galon, J.; Dieu-Nosjean, M.C., et al. (2009). Immune Infiltration in Human Tumors: A Prognostic Factor That Should Not Be Ignored, *Oncogene*, Vol. 29, No. 8, pp. 1093-1102, 1476-5594

Palermo, B.; Del Bello, D.; Sottini, A., et al. (2010). Dacarbazine Treatment before Peptide Vaccination Enlarges T-Cell Repertoire Diversity of Melan-A-Specific, Tumor-Reactive CTL in Melanoma Patients, *Cancer Res*, Vol. 70, No. 18, pp. 7084-7092, 1538-7445

Pejcic, I.; Vrbic, S.; Filipovic, S., et al. (2010). Concurrent Chemoimmunotherapy: Is It Still the Best Option for the Treatment of Metastatic Melanoma in Patients with Good Performance Status?, *J Buon*, Vol. 15, No. 3, pp. 470-474, 1107-0625

Peluso, I.; Fantini, M.C.; Fina, D., et al. (2007). IL-21 Counteracts the Regulatory T Cell-Mediated Suppression of Human CD4+ T Lymphocytes, *J Immunol*, Vol. 178, No. 2, pp. 732-739, 0022-1767

Perrotta, C.; Bizzozero, L.; Falcone, S., et al. (2007). Nitric Oxide Boosts Chemoimmunotherapy Via Inhibition of Acid Sphingomyelinase in a Mouse Model of Melanoma, *Cancer Res*, Vol. 67, No. 16, pp. 7559-7564, 0008-5472

Petersen, C.C.; Diernaes, J.E.; Skovbo, A., et al. (2010). Interleukin-21 Restrains Tumor Growth and Induces a Substantial Increase in the Number of Circulating Tumor-Specific T Cells in a Murine Model of Malignant Melanoma, *Cytokine*, Vol. 49, No. 1, pp. 80-88, 1096-0023

Pfeffer, L.M.; Dinarello, C.A.; Herberman, R.B., et al. (1998). Biological Properties of Recombinant Alpha-Interferons: 40th Anniversary of the Discovery of Interferons, *Cancer Res*, Vol. 58, No. 12, pp. 2489-2499, 0008-5472

Phan-Bich, L.; Buard, A.; Petit, J.F., et al. (1997). Differential Responsiveness of Human and Rat Mesothelioma Cell Lines to Recombinant Interferon-Gamma, *Am J Respir Cell Mol Biol*, Vol. 16, No. 2, pp. 178-186, 1044-1549

Piao, W.H.; Jee, Y.H.; Liu, R.L., et al. (2008). IL-21 Modulates CD4+ CD25+ Regulatory T-Cell Homeostasis in Experimental Autoimmune Encephalomyelitis, *Scand J Immunol*, Vol. 67, No. 1, pp. 37-46, 1365-3083

Proietti, E.; Greco, G.; Garrone, B., et al. (1998). Importance of Cyclophosphamide-Induced Bystander Effect on T Cells for a Successful Tumor Eradication in Response to Adoptive Immunotherapy in Mice, *J Clin Invest*, Vol. 101, No. 2, pp. 429-441, 0021-9738

Punt, C.J.; Suciu, S.; Gore, M.A., et al. (2006). Chemoimmunotherapy with Dacarbazine, Cisplatin, Interferon-Alpha2b and Interleukin-2 Versus Two Cycles of Dacarbazine Followed by Chemoimmunotherapy in Patients with Metastatic Melanoma: A Randomised Phase II Study of the European Organization for Research and Treatment of Cancer Melanoma Group, *Eur J Cancer*, Vol. 42, No. 17, pp. 2991-2995, 0959-8049

Radfar, S.; Wang, Y. & Khong, H.T. (2009). Activated CD4+ T Cells Dramatically Enhance Chemotherapeutic Tumor Responses in Vitro and in Vivo, *J Immunol*, Vol. 183, No. 10, pp. 6800-6807, 1550-6606

Rass, K. & Tilgen, W. (2008). Treatment of Melanoma and Nonmelanoma Skin Cancer, *Adv Exp Med Biol*, Vol. 624, pp. 296-318, 0065-2598

Recchia, F.; Candeloro, G.; Necozione, S., et al. (2008). Multicenter Phase II Study of Chemoimmunotherapy in the Treatment of Metastatic Melanoma, *Anticancer Drugs*, Vol. 19, No. 2, pp. 201-207, 0959-4973

Ridolfi, R.; Chiarion-Sileni, V.; Guida, M., et al. (2002). Cisplatin, Dacarbazine with or without Subcutaneous Interleukin-2, and Interferon Alpha-2b in Advanced Melanoma Outpatients: Results from an Italian Multicenter Phase III Randomized Clinical Trial, *J Clin Oncol*, Vol. 20, No. 6, pp. 1600-1607, 0732-183X

Riker, A.I. & Howell, P.M. (June 2010). Treatment Options for Patients with Stage III & IV Melanoma: Part I: A Look at Existing Neoadjuvant and Adjuvant Treatments, In: *Contemporary Oncology*, 16.06.2010, Available from http://www.hcplive.com/publications/contemporary_oncology/2009/Contemporary_Oncology_Fall_2009/Stage_III_IV_Melanoma_fall_2009

Riker, A.I. & Howell, P.M. (June 2010). Treatment Options for Patients with Stage III & IV Melanoma: Part II: Experimental Treatments for Stage III/IV or Refractory/Recurrent Melanoma, In: *Contemporary Oncology*, 03.06.2010, Available from http://www.hcplive.com/publications/contemporary_oncology/2009/Contemporary_Oncology_Fall_2009/Stage_III_IV_Melanoma_fall_2009

Robbins, P.F.; Morgan, R.A.; Feldman, S.A., et al. (2011). Tumor Regression in Patients with Metastatic Synovial Cell Sarcoma and Melanoma Using Genetically Engineered Lymphocytes Reactive with NY-ESO-1, *J Clin Oncol*, Vol. 29, No. 7, pp. 917-924, 1527-7755

Rosati, S.F.; Williams, R.F.; Nunnally, L.C., et al. (2008). Ifn-Beta Sensitizes Neuroblastoma to the Antitumor Activity of Temozolomide by Modulating O6-Methylguanine DNA Methyltransferase Expression, *Mol Cancer Ther*, Vol. 7, No. 12, pp. 3852-3858, 1535-7163

Rosenberg, S.A.; Yang, J.C.; Schwartzentruber, D.J., et al. (1999). Prospective Randomized Trial of the Treatment of Patients with Metastatic Melanoma Using Chemotherapy with Cisplatin, Dacarbazine, and Tamoxifen Alone or in Combination with Interleukin-2 and Interferon Alfa-2b, *J Clin Oncol*, Vol. 17, No. 3, pp. 968-975, 0732-183X

Rosenberg, S.A.; Restifo, N.P.; Yang, J.C., et al. (2008). Adoptive Cell Transfer: A Clinical Path to Effective Cancer Immunotherapy, *Nat Rev Cancer*, Vol. 8, No. 4, pp. 299-308, 1474-1768

Rosenberg, S.A. & Dudley, M.E. (2009). Adoptive Cell Therapy for the Treatment of Patients with Metastatic Melanoma, *Curr Opin Immunol*, Vol. 21, No. 2, pp. 233-240, 1879-0372

Rosenberg, S.A.; Yang, J.C.; Sherry, R.M., et al. (2011). Durable Complete Responses in Heavily Pretreted Patients with Metastatic Melanoma Using T Cell Transfer Immunotherapy, *Clin Cancer Res*, 1078-0432

Rosner, K.; Kasprzak, M.F.; Horenstein, A.C., et al. (2011). Engineering a Waste Management Enzyme to Overcome Cancer Resistance to Apoptosis: Adding Dnase1 to the Anti-Cancer Toolbox, *Cancer Gene Ther*, Vol. 18, No. 5, pp. 346-357, 1476-5500

Rubin, B.Y.; Smith, L.J.; Hellermann, G.R., et al. (1988). Correlation between the Anticellular and DNA Fragmenting Activities of Tumor Necrosis Factor, *Cancer Res*, Vol. 48, No. 21, pp. 6006-6010, 0008-5472

Salem, M.L.; Kadima, A.N.; El-Naggar, S.A., et al. (2007). Defining the Ability of Cyclophosphamide Preconditioning to Enhance the Antigen-Specific CD8+ T-Cell Response to Peptide Vaccination: Creation of a Beneficial Host Microenvironment Involving Type I IFNs and Myeloid Cells, *J Immunother*, Vol. 30, No. 1, pp. 40-53, 1524-9557

Sasse, A.D.; Sasse, E.C.; Clark, L.G., et al. (2007). Chemoimmunotherapy Versus Chemotherapy for Metastatic Malignant Melanoma, *Cochrane Database Syst Rev*, No. 1, pp. CD005413, 1469-493X

Schiavoni, G.; Mattei, F.; Di Pucchio, T., et al. (2000). Cyclophosphamide Induces Type I Interferon and Augments the Number of CD44(hi) T Lymphocytes in Mice: Implications for Strategies of Chemoimmunotherapy of Cancer, *Blood*, Vol. 95, No. 6, pp. 2024-2030, 0006-4971

Schlom, J.; Arlen, P.M. & Gulley, J.L. (2007). Cancer Vaccines: Moving Beyond Current Paradigms, *Clin Cancer Res*, Vol. 13, No. 13, pp. 3776-3782, 1078-0432

Schoenfeld, J.; Jinushi, M.; Nakazaki, Y., et al. (2010). Active Immunotherapy Induces Antibody Responses That Target Tumor Angiogenesis, *Cancer Res*, Vol. 70, No. 24, pp. 10150-10160, 1538-7445

Seam, P.; Janik, J.E.; Longo, D.L., et al. (2009). Role of Chemotherapy in Hodgkin's Lymphoma, *Cancer J*, Vol. 15, No. 2, pp. 150-154, 1528-9117

Serrone, L. & Hersey, P. (1999). The Chemoresistance of Human Malignant Melanoma: An Update, *Melanoma Res*, Vol. 9, No. 1, pp. 51-58, 0960-8931

Sinkovics, J.G. & Horvath, J.C. (2006). Evidence Accumulating in Support of Cancer Vaccines Combined with Chemotherapy: A Pragmatic Review of Past and Present Efforts, *Int J Oncol*, Vol. 29, No. 4, pp. 765-777, 1019-6439

Skak, K.; Sondergaard, H.; Frederiksen, K.S., et al. (2009). In Vivo Antitumor Efficacy of Interleukin-21 in Combination with Chemotherapeutics, *Cytokine*, Vol. 48, No. 3, pp. 231-238, 1096-0023

Spolski, R. & Leonard, W.J. (2008). Interleukin-21: Basic Biology and Implications for Cancer and Autoimmunity, *Annu Rev Immunol*, Vol. 26, pp. 57-79, 0732-0582

Sugarman, B.J.; Aggarwal, B.B.; Hass, P.E., et al. (1985). Recombinant Human Tumor Necrosis Factor-Alpha: Effects on Proliferation of Normal and Transformed Cells in Vitro, *Science*, Vol. 230, No. 4728, pp. 943-945, 0036-8075

Szabo, S.J.; Sullivan, B.M.; Peng, S.L., et al. (2003). Molecular Mechanisms Regulating Th1 Immune Responses, *Annu Rev Immunol*, Vol. 21, pp. 713-758, 0732-0582

Tagawa, S.T.; Cheung, E.; Banta, W., et al. (2006). Survival Analysis after Resection of Metastatic Disease Followed by Peptide Vaccines in Patients with Stage IV Melanoma, *Cancer*, Vol. 106, No. 6, pp. 1353-1357, 0008-543X

Thompson, J.A.; Gold, P.J. & Fefer, A. (1997). Outpatient Chemoimmunotherapy for the Treatment of Metastatic Melanoma, *Semin Oncol*, Vol. 24, No. 1 Suppl 4, pp. S44-48, 0093-7754

Tsao, H.; Atkins, M.B. & Sober, A.J. (2004). Management of Cutaneous Melanoma, *N Engl J Med*, Vol. 351, No. 10, pp. 998-1012, 1533-4406

Turk, J.L. & Parker, D. (1982). Effect of Cyclophosphamide on Immunological Control Mechanisms, *Immunol Rev*, Vol. 65, pp. 99-113, 0105-2896

Van Horssen, R.; Ten Hagen, T.L. & Eggermont, A.M. (2006). TNF-Alpha in Cancer Treatment: Molecular Insights, Antitumor Effects, and Clinical Utility, *Oncologist*, Vol. 11, No. 4, pp. 397-408, 1083-7159

Waldmann, T.A. (2006). The Biology of Interleukin-2 and Interleukin-15: Implications for Cancer Therapy and Vaccine Design, *Nat Rev Immunol*, Vol. 6, No. 8, pp. 595-601, 1474-1733

Wang, Y.; Radfar, S. & Khong, H.T. (2010). Activated CD4+ T Cells Enhance Radiation Effect through the Cooperation of Interferon-Gamma and TNF-Alpha, *BMC Cancer*, Vol. 10, p. 60, 1471-2407

Watanabe, N.; Niitsu, Y.; Umeno, H., et al. (1988). Toxic Effect of Tumor Necrosis Factor on Tumor Vasculature in Mice, *Cancer Res*, Vol. 48, No. 8, pp. 2179-2183, 0008-5472

Wheeler, C.J.; Das, A.; Liu, G., et al. (2004). Clinical Responsiveness of Glioblastoma Multiforme to Chemotherapy after Vaccination, *Clin Cancer Res*, Vol. 10, No. 16, pp. 5316-5326, 1078-0432

Wrzesinski, C.; Paulos, C.M.; Kaiser, A., et al. (2010). Increased Intensity Lymphodepletion Enhances Tumor Treatment Efficacy of Adoptively Transferred Tumor-Specific T Cells, *J Immunother*, Vol. 33, No. 1, pp. 1-7, 1537-4513

Yang, A.S. & Chapman, P.B. (2009). The History and Future of Chemotherapy for Melanoma, *Hematol Oncol Clin North Am*, Vol. 23, No. 3, pp. 583-597, 1558-1977

Yang, H.G.; Hu, B.L.; Xiao, L., et al. (2011). Dendritic Cell-Directed Lentivector Vaccine Induces Antigen-Specific Immune Responses against Murine Melanoma, *Cancer Gene Ther*, Vol. 18, No. 5, pp. 370-380, 1476-5500

Yannelli, J.R. & Wroblewski, J.M. (2004). On the Road to a Tumor Cell Vaccine: 20 Years of Cellular Immunotherapy, *Vaccine*, Vol. 23, No. 1, pp. 97-113, 0264-410X

Yi, J.S.; Du, M. & Zajac, A.J. (2009). A Vital Role for Interleukin-21 in the Control of a Chronic Viral Infection, *Science*, Vol. 324, No. 5934, pp. 1572-1576, 1095-9203

Zhang, L.; Kerkar, S.P.; Yu, Z., et al. (2011). Improving Adoptive T Cell Therapy by Targeting and Controlling Il-12 Expression to the Tumor Environment, *Mol Ther*, Vol. 19, No. 4, pp. 751-759, 1525-0024

Zheng, M.; Bocangel, D.; Ramesh, R., et al. (2008). Interleukin-24 Overcomes Temozolomide Resistance and Enhances Cell Death by Down-Regulation of O6-Methylguanine-DNA Methyltransferase in Human Melanoma Cells, *Mol Cancer Ther*, Vol. 7, No. 12, pp. 3842-3851, 1535-7163

Zitvogel, L.; Apetoh, L.; Ghiringhelli, F., et al. (2008). Immunological Aspects of Cancer Chemotherapy, *Nat Rev Immunol*, Vol. 8, No. 1, pp. 59-73, 1474-1741

7

Simultaneous Knockdown of Mutant BRAF and Expression of INK4A in Melanoma Cells Leads to Potent Growth Inhibition and Apoptosis

Jianli Dong and Chet L. Schwab
University of Texas Medical Branch, Galveston Texas
USA

1. Introduction

Melanoma is the eighth most common cancer in the United States and incidence is increasing at a rate greater than all other cancers. Estimates indicate that in 2010 there were 68,130 new cases of melanoma in the United States and 8,700 deaths from the disease. Overall, the lifetime risk of developing melanoma is about 2% (1 in 50) for Caucasians, 0.5% (1 in 200) for Hispanics, and 0.1% (1 in 1,000) for African Americans (American Cancer Society). Malignant melanoma results from transformation of melanocytes with progression through histologically recognizable sequential steps including radial growth phase (RGP), vertical growth phase (VGP), and metastasis (Elder, 1999). In RGP, neoplastic cells are confined to the epidermis or with microinvasion into the dermis. In more advanced VGP, cancer cells expand in the dermis and generate tumor nodules and have a high potential for metastatic spread. In the metastatic phase, cancer cells disseminate to lymph nodes or distant organs (Clark & Tucker, 1998; Elder, 1999). Optimal treatment varies based on stage of disease. For the early diagnosed and localized melanomas, surgery is the treatment of choice and may be curative provided the lesion is excised completely. However, for invasive and metastatic melanomas, there is no effective treatment and many patients die within 6-8 months after diagnosis. The aggressive growth of melanoma cells and their intrinsic resistance to standard modalities of cancer treatment account for the dismal prognosis (Poulikakos & Rosen, 2011; Tawbi & Buch, 2010). Therefore, the ability to inhibit growth and overcome drug resistance is central to the effective treatment of melanomas.

Treatment options for advanced melanoma are currently limited to immunotherapy, single agent cytotoxic chemotherapies, and surgery. Recently, Yervoy (Ipilimumab), an inhibitor of cytotoxic T-lymphocyte antigen 4 (CTLA-4) gained Food and Drug Administration (FDA) approval to treat metastatic melanomas. It is the first drug shown to prolong the lives of patients with advanced melanoma (Weber, 2011). However, its effect is limited. Patients with metastatic melanoma treated with Yervoy lived a median of approximately 10 months compared with 6.4 months for patients in a control group. Treatment with interferon Alpha 2B has shown improvement in disease free survival although overall survival benefit results are conflicting (American Cancer Society, http://www.cancer.org/). Interleukin 2 has also shown activity against metastatic melanoma although patient populations are limited by severe toxicity. Dacarbazine is the most studied of single agent cytotoxic agents for malignant melanoma and is considered gold standard for comparison of systemic chemotherapy. However, no survival benefit has been shown in randomized controlled trials. Complete response rates are 3-5%, and long term remission rates are less than 2% under systemic treatments for metastatic cutaneous melanoma. Combination chemotherapy involving dacarbazine increases toxicity without improvement in median survival compared to dacarbazine alone. Metastatic melanoma can sometimes be treated with surgery. Patients can achieve prolonged overall survival after complete resection of tumors. Unfortunately, beneficiary outcome of surgical resection is limited to single or solitary melanoma metastases compared with patients with disseminated disease (Sosman et al., 2011).

Results of the recent phase I clinical trial with PLX4032, a specific inhibitor of mutant BRAF, have generated great excitement because approximately 80% of BRAF mutant metastatic melanomas regressed in response to PLX4032 treatment. Though this trial was considered a true victory in the fight against melanomas, attention has been drawn to the fact that regressed tumors resurge more aggressively within 8 months after the start of therapy. Constitutive deregulation of BRAF-MEK-ERK and p16-CDK4-RB pathways occur at high frequencies in melanomas. We have shown that suppression of either BRAF-MEK or CDK4 activity inhibits cell growth, and that simultaneous inhibition of both BRAF-MEK and CDK4 activities compounds this effect and triggers significant apoptosis in melanoma cells. Our data suggest BRAF-MEK-ERK and p16-CDK4-RB pathways may act additively or synergistically in the malignant growth of melanoma cells, and could be jointly targeted for treatment of melanoma. We have recently reported that the expression of K type human endogenous retrovirus (HERV-K) correlates with ERK activation and p16 loss in melanoma cells and can be inhibited by MEK and CDK4 inhibitors, especially in combination. Given that HERV-K may drive malignant growth downstream of BRAF-MEK and CDK4, we hypothesize cells with activated HERV-K may escape the therapeutic effects of MEK and CDK4 blockers, and that triple inhibition of BRAF-MEK, CDK4, and HERV-K should be more effective than single or double inhibition.

2. Mutational activation of NRAS-BRAF-MEK-ERK pathway in melanoma cells

In a systematic genome-wide screen for gene mutations, Davies et al. (Davies et al., 2002) identified BRAF mutations in 70% of human malignant melanomas. A T1799A transversion in exon 15, resulting in a V600E substitution in the BRAF kinase domain, accounts for over 90% of BRAF mutations detected in melanoma samples. In addition to melanomas, BRAF mutations have been identified in several other tumor types including thyroid, ovarian, colorectal, and lung (Davies et al., 2002). BRAF, one of three members of the RAF family (ARAF, BRAF, CRAF), is a component of the RAS-RAF-mitogen activated protein kinase/ERK kinase (MEK)-extracellular signal regulated kinase (ERK) signaling pathway. RAF gene encodes cytoplasmic serine/threonine kinases that transduces regulatory signals from RAS to MEK-ERK (Mercer & Pritchard, 2003). RAF genes are differentially expressed with CRAF being ubiquitously expressed; ARAF predominantly found in urogenital tissue, and BRAF having highest expression in neural and testes (Mercer & Pritchard, 2003). Mutant BRAF has increased kinase activity causing intrinsic ERK activation in cultured NIH3T3, COS, and human melanocytes, and leads to elevated transforming activity of cultured NIH3T3 and human melanocytes (Davies et al., 2002; Dong et al., 2003; Satyamoorthy et al., 2003; Wellbrock et al., 2004). Suppression of mutant BRAF expression has been reported to cause inhibition of melanoma cell proliferation and survival *in vitro* and *in vivo* (Hingorani et al., 2003; Karasarides et al., 2004; Rotolo et al., 2005; Sumimoto et al., 2004).

In addition to BRAF mutation, NRAS mutation occurs in about 10% of melanomas (Davies et al., 2002; Dong et al., 2003; Michaloglou et al., 2008) that can also lead to constitutive activation of the MEK-ERK pathway. Apart from NRAS and BRAF mutation, other factors have been identified leading to constitutive activation of the ERK signaling. For example, amplification and somatic mutations of KIT and constitutive expression of growth factors HGF and FGF (Fecher et al., 2008; Panka et al., 2006a). The RAF-MEK-ERK pathway conveys extra- and intracellular signals to transcription regulators that control gene expression in response to these signals. The pathway impinges on all the functional hallmarks of cancer cells including immortalization, growth factor independent proliferation, loss of responsiveness to cell cycle checkpoint signals, evasion of apoptosis; insensitivity to growth inhibitory signals, ability to invade and metastasize, and ability to attract blood vessels (Chang et al., 2003; Kolch, 2000; Pearson et al., 2001) and represents rich druggable targets for drug development (Fig. 1, http://clinicaltrials.gov/) (Fecher et al., 2008; Panka et al., 2006a).

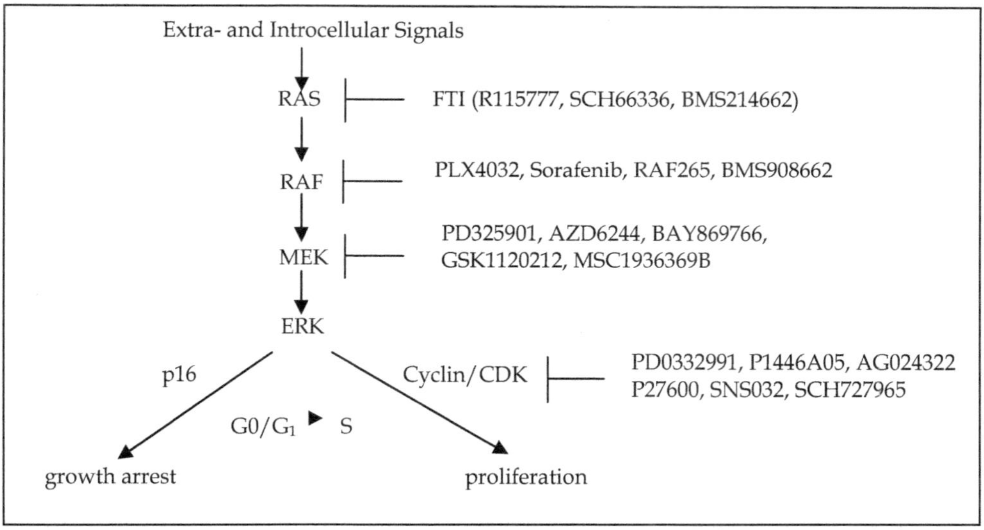

Fig. 1. RAS-RAF-MEK-ERK signaling pathway and specific inhibitors. RAF relays RAS signals through MEK to ERK. The activation of this pathway has multiple effects on cell proliferation, differentiation, and survival depending on the cellular contexts. Also shown are inhibitors to components of the pathway that are in active clinical trials (http://clinicaltrials.gov/). FTI, farnesyl transferase inhibitor.

3. Detection and specific inhibition of mutant BRAF

We performed research and validation studies to detect BRAF codon 600 mutations (Dong et al., 2003; Rotolo et al., 2005). As shown in Figure 2, a PCR and Sanger sequencing assay is used to detect BRAF codon 600 mutations. The common T1799A transversion changes wild-type GTG (valine) to GAG (glutamate) at codon 600 (V600E). In addition, a two-nucleotide substitution, GTG to AAG (lysine), V600K, is occasionally identified in melanoma cells (Fig. 2A; Dong, 2003). BRAF proteins harboring V600E or V600K mutations, but not wild-type BRAF, are specifically inhibited by mutant specific BRAF inhibitor PLX4032 (Bollag et al., 2010; Flaherty et al., 2010; Rubinstein et al., 2010; Solit & Rosen, 2011). It is interesting to note that although most BRAF mutant alleles co-exist with wild-type copies, some melanoma cells show loss of the wild-type allele (Fig. 2A, A1799 LOH, AA1798-1799 LOH). Although rare, these cases suggest that loss of wild-type allele may offer growth advantage to cancer cells. We developed a PCR and restriction fragment length polymorphism (RFLP) assay (PCR-RFLP) to detect the common T1799A BRAF mutation (Fig. 2B). We designed a PCR forward primer (5'-GTA AAA ATA GGT GAT TTT GGT CTA GCT GAA G-3') to create, when the mutant A1799 follows in the DNA template, an MboII restriction site [GAAG**A**(N8)↓]. The reverse primer also has an MboII site for enzyme digestion and size control. PCR products are digested with MboII and restriction fragments separated by electrophoresis (Fig. 2B). The method is validated by direct sequencing of PCR products. Using this method, we identified melanoma cell lines that are wild-type (1363Mel), heterozygous (624Mel, WM35) or show LOH (A375) for the T1796A mutation (Rotolo et al., 2005).

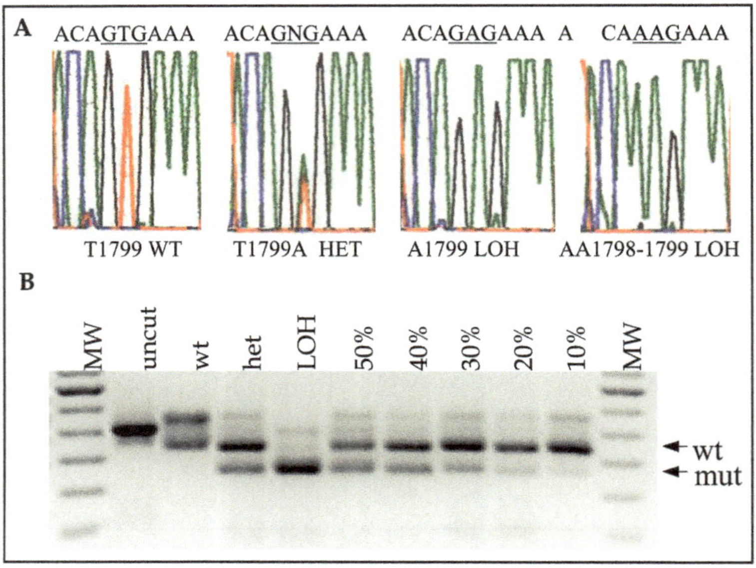

Fig. 2. BRAF codon 600 mutation analysis. (A) Wild-type (wt) and mutant (mut) alleles are detected by Sanger sequencing. The heterozygous (HET) sequence showed approximately 50:50 ratio of wt vs. mut alleles. Samples with no detectable wild-type allele are called loss of heterozygosity (LOH). A two-nucleotide substitution, GTG to AAG, is occasionally identified in melanoma specimens. (B) PCR-RFLP assay to increase sensitivity of detecting mutant allele (10% vs 30% by Sanger sequencing). Control and enzyme digested PCR amplicons are separated by electrophoresis on a 3% agarose or 10% polyacrylamide gel. The undigested PCR amplicon, digested wt and mut bands are 255, 218, and 178 bps, respectively. Serial dilutions containing 50%, 40%, 30%, 20%, and 10% of mutant alleles are used to determine assay sensitivity. Various heteroduplex bands are visible. MW, 50 bp molecular weight marker.

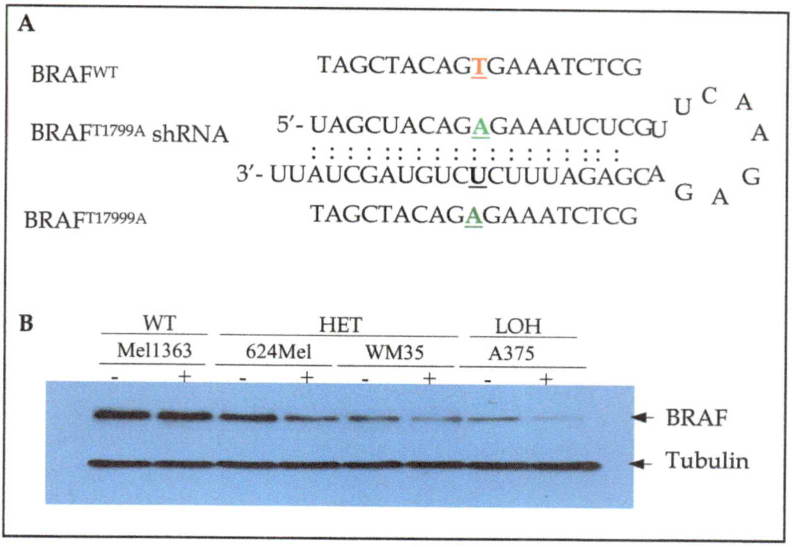

Fig. 3. T1799A mutant specific RNAi. Control and mut BRAF RNAi retroviruses are produced to infect melanoma cell lines. (A) The predicted BRAF^{T1796A} shRNA transcript encoded by pRS-BRAF^{T1799A}. Shown are sequences of the wt and T1799A mut alleles, and the predicted shRNA. (B) Western blot analysis of specific inhibition of mut BRAF by RNAi. Melanoma cells are stably infected with control (-) or pRS-BRAF^{T1799A}, a retrovirus expressing mut BRAF shRNA (+). Cell lysates are separated by sodium dodecyl sulfate polyacrylamide gel electrophoresis (SDS-PAGE), transferred to membrane, and probed with BRAF and tubulin antibodies. BRAF is not significantly affected in Mel1363 cells that have wt BRAF, but inhibited in 624Mel and WM35 cells that are heterozygous for mut BRAF (HET). Mut BRAF RNAi almost completely inhibited BRAF expression in A375 cells that are LOH of mut BRAF (Dong et al., 2003; Rotolo et al., 2005).

Other methods including real-time PCR, pyrosequencing, and allele-specific hybridization can be used to detect BRAF codon 600 mutations (e.g., reagents from Qiagen, Valencia, CA, USA; EntroGen, Tarzana, CA, USA; and Trimgen Sparks, Maryland, USA). Using various mutation assays, we and others reported high frequencies (approximately 70%) of BRAF mutations in benign melanocytic nevi (Dong et al., 2003; Pollock et al., 2003). This information is important in understanding BRAF mutation in tumor biology. Since nevi are much more common in the general population compared with the rare occurrence of melanoma, BRAF mutations alone are insufficient to cause malignant transformation in nevus cells. It has been shown that oncogenic BRAF cause proliferative senescence instead of unlimited proliferation in nevus cells (Michaloglou et al., 2005).

We designed mutant specific BRAF RNAi (siRNA and shRNA) to specifically target the T1799A mutant allele (Rotolo et al., 2005). Shown in Fig. 3 is the predicted mutant specific shRNA transcript, pRS-BRAF^{T1799A}, expressed from a retroviral vector pRETRO-SUPER-puro (pRS) (Brummelkamp et al., 2002). When a pRS-BRAF^{T1799A} construct is stably expressed in cultured melanoma cells using empty vector and a 19 bp firefly luciferase (luc) sequence as controls, BRAF expression is reduced in T1799A BRAF-positive but not in BRAF wild-type melanoma cells (Fig. 3B). Further, inhibition of BRAF expression is greatest in

A375 melanoma cells that show LOH at the BRAF locus and thus express only the T1799A mutant BRAF (Rotolo et al., 2005).

4. Loss of wild-type p16 and exogenous expression of INK4A in melanomas

Genetic and epigenetic lesions in the tumor suppressor gene INK4A are commonly found in cancer cells (Hanahan & Weinberg, 2000; Lowe & Sherr, 2003). Most melanomas, but not nevi, have lost the expression of wild-type INK4A either through DNA deletion/mutation or promoter hypermethylation (Castellano et al., 1997; Funk et al., 1998; von et al., 1999; Welch et al., 2001; Zhang et al., 2002). INK4A shares coding sequence with ARF in the CDKN2A locus (Fig. 4), but the proteins are translated in different reading frames (Sherr, 2001). ARF up-regulates p53 by interfering with the p53 negative regulator MDM2, while p16 binds to and inhibits cyclin-dependent kinases 4 and 6 (CDK4/6) promoting cell-cycle arrest via the RB tumor suppressor pathway (Chang et al., 2003; Lowe & Sherr, 2003). Although deletions and mutations may affect both INK4A and ARF genes, several studies have identified mutations in melanoma specimens affecting only INK4A without ARF involvement (Chin et al., 2006; Fargnoli et al., 1998). Consistent with a tumor suppressor role of INK4A in melanomas, a germ line Arg24Cys (R24C) mutation in CDK4 has been identified in familial melanoma patients (Wolfel et al., 1995; Zuo et al., 1996). This mutation abolishes CDK4 inhibition by p16 and thus is believed to be functionally equivalent to p16 loss. Cyclin D1 and D3 are over-expressed in melanomas, which is required for growth and survival of melanoma cells *in vitro* and *in vivo* (Bartkova et al., 1996; Florenes et al., 1996; Polsky & Cordon-Cardo, 2003). Mutational inactivation of RB tumor suppressor is rare in melanomas (Bartkova et al., 1996; Maelandsmo et al., 1996).

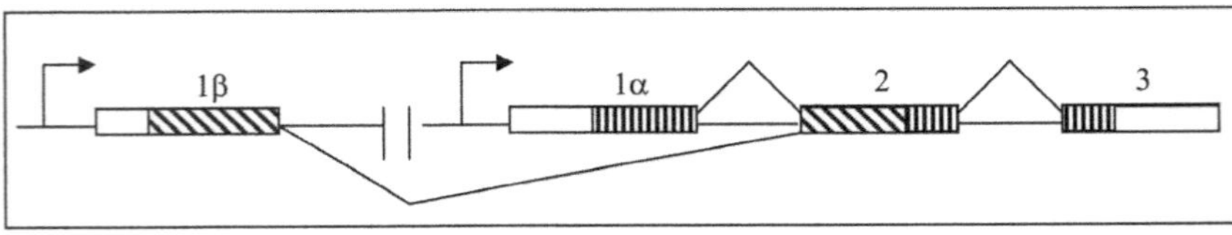

Fig. 4. Human CDKN2A locus. INK4A and ARF share sequences in the CDKN2A locus. The locus encodes two products, p16 and ARF (p14). Exons are shown as rectangles. Alternative first exons (1α and 1β) are transcribed from different promoters (arrows). The first exons are spliced to the same splicing acceptor site in exon 2 but are translated in alternative reading frames. INK4A coding sequences in exons 1α, 2, and 3 and ARF coding sequences in exons 1β and 2 are indicated by different shading patterns. Adopted from Sherr (Sherr, 2001).

We performed expression and mutation analyses of INK4A in melanoma cells. Immunohistochemical analysis shows that p16 is highly expressed in nevus cells (Fig. 5A), but expression descreases increasingly during tumor progression (Fig. 5B-D). Western blot analysis of cultured melanoma cells shows that p16 is barely detectable, if any, in melanoma cells (Fig. 5E). Mutation analysis of INK4A show that 624Mel cells have an 18 bp in-frame deletion of codons 32-37 (CTGGAGGCGGGGGCGCTG) in exon 1 α. The deleted sequence is located in the first ankyrin repeat and encodes an evolutionarily conserved 6 amino acids (LEAGAL) (Greenblatt et al., 2003). Deletions and mutations affecting these amino acid have been reported in melanomas and other cancers and significantly affect the CDK- and cell cycle-inhibitory activities of p16 (Harland et al., 1997; Muzeau et al., 1997; Ruas & Peters,

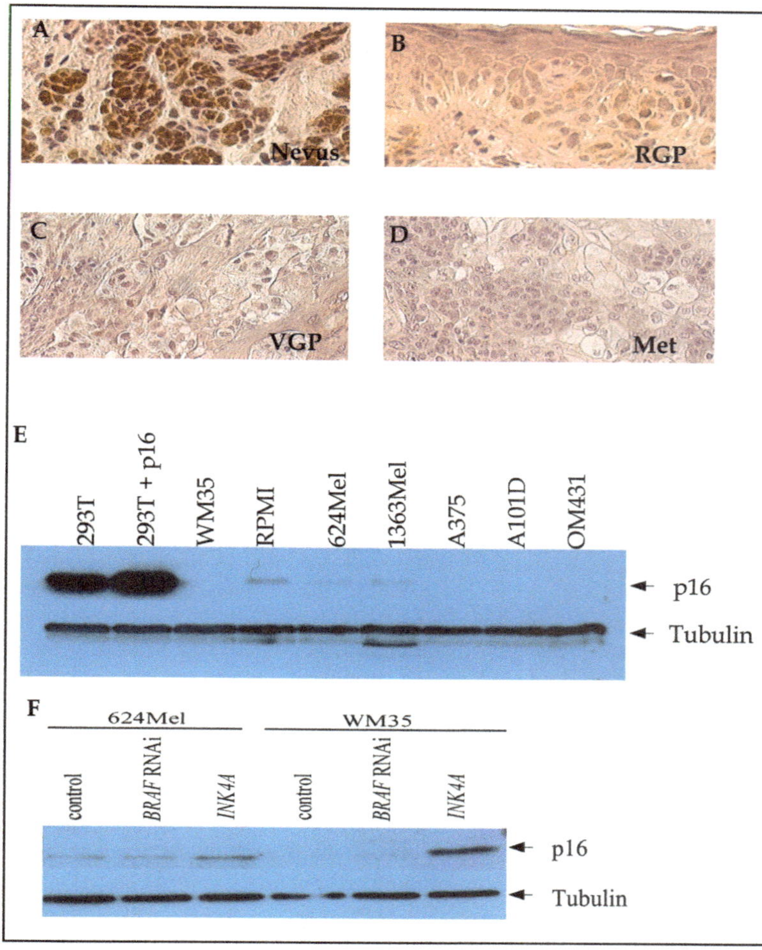

Fig. 5. Endogenous and exogenous expression of p16 in melanoma cells. (A-D) Immunohistochemical analysis of p16 expression in melanocytic lesions. Formalin-fixed and paraffin-embedded (FFPE) tissue sections of nevus (A), RGP (B), VGP (C), and metastatic (D) melanomas are stained with p16 antibody. All the samples are also positive for BRAF T1796A mutation (not shown). Note the strong expression of p16 in nevus but not in melanoma cells. Magnification x 100. (E) Western blot analysis of p16 expression in melanoma cell lines. 293T control (293T), 293T transfected with INK4A cDNA (293T + p16) are used as controls. WM35, RPMI, 624Mel, 1363Mel, A375, A101D, and OM431 melanoma cell lines are cultured in regular media. Cell lysates are separated by SDS-PAGE. Western blot was probed with p16 and tubulin antibodies (arrows). WM35, RPMI, 624Mel, A375, A101D, and OM431 also have BRAF T1796A mutation. (F) Exogenous expression of wt INK4A in melanoma cells. Immunoblotting of 624Mel and WM35 controls (-), and cells stably infected with retroviruses expressing mut BRAF RNAi (BRAF RNAi) or INK4A cDNA (INK4A). Western blot is probed with p16 and tubulin antibodies (arrows). Note mutant BRAF inhibition has no detectable effect on endogenous (624Mel) or exogenous (WM35) p16 expression.

1998). The deletion shows LOH (data not shown), suggesting that either the wild-type copy of the gene is deleted or this is a homozygous deletion. Sequence analysis also shows that INK4A is wild-type in RPMI and 1363Mel and deleted in WM35 melanoma cells (data not shown). Mutant p16 is expressed at relatively lower levels in 624Mel cells compared to wild-type p16 in RPMI and 1363Mel cells (Fig. 5E). The expression of wild-type INK4A can be restored in melanoma cells by exogenous expression of INK4A cDNA (Rotolo et al., 2005; Zhao et al., 2008). As shown in Fig. 5F, 624Mel and WM35 melanoma cells are infected with either vector control or pBabe-neo-INK4A retroviruses. After G418 selection of mass culture, immunoblotting showed that p16 is expressed at approximately 3-5 fold more than endogenous p16 in 624Mel cells and at a higher level in WM35 cells (Fig. 5F).

5. Functional interaction of BRAF and INK4A lesions in melanoma cells

Activating BRAF mutations and loss of wild-type INK4A expression both occur at high frequencies in melanomas. However, BRAF and INK4A lesions can have overlapping roles in the regulation of the RB pathway (Fig. 6). As shown in Fig. 6, oncogenic BRAF can upregulate cyclin D through ERK pathway resulting in activation of CDK4/6. In contrast, p16 binds to and inactivates these CDKs. Therefore, CDK4/6 may be activated either by mutant BRAF through upregulation of cyclin D via ERK signaling or by loss of p16 activity. Activated CDKs phosphorylate and inactivate RB proteins resulting in the liberation of E2F transcription factors and cell cycle progression, which may contribute to the observed hyperphosphorylation of RB proteins and activation of E2F transcription in advanced melanoma cells (Halaban, 1999). There is also indirect evidence suggesting the cooperation between lesions of BRAF and INK4A in tumor development. In normal fibroblasts, oncogenic RAS and RAF have been shown to cause permanent growth arrest and/or senescence, rather than unrestricted proliferation, through a mechanism involving induction of INK4A expression (Lin et al., 1998; Zhu et al., 1998). Deficiencies in INK4A abrogate RAS-induced senescence, leading to transformation of human fibroblast cells (Brookes et al., 2002; Drayton & Peters, 2002; Drayton et al., 2003; Huot et al., 2002). In mice, neither oncogenic Ras nor Ink4a loss is sufficient to induce the development of melanomas. However, they generate spontaneous melanomas in combination (Chin et al., 1997).

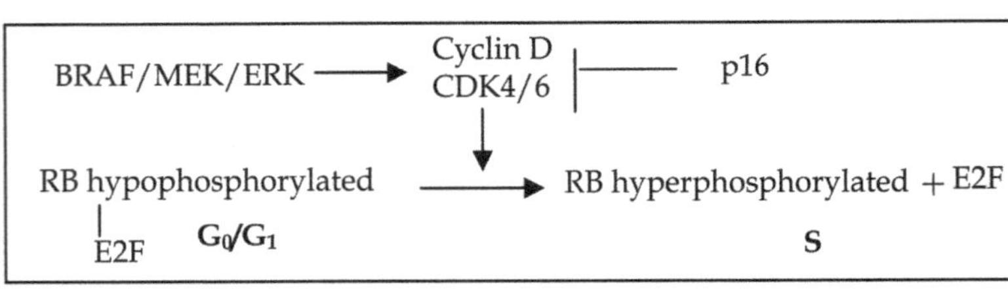

Fig. 6. The effects of BRAF and p16 can converge at the RB/E2F pathway through the opposite effects on cyclin-dependent kinases and cell cycle progression in the G_1/S phase.

6. Growth inhibition by either suppression of mutant BRAF or expression of wild-type INK4A

We performed experiments to examine the effects of inhibiting mut BRAF or expressing INK4A in melanoma cells. We found that 624Mel, A101D and WM35 cells that harbor both T1796A and INK4A mutations have intrinsic MEK activation (data not shown) that is

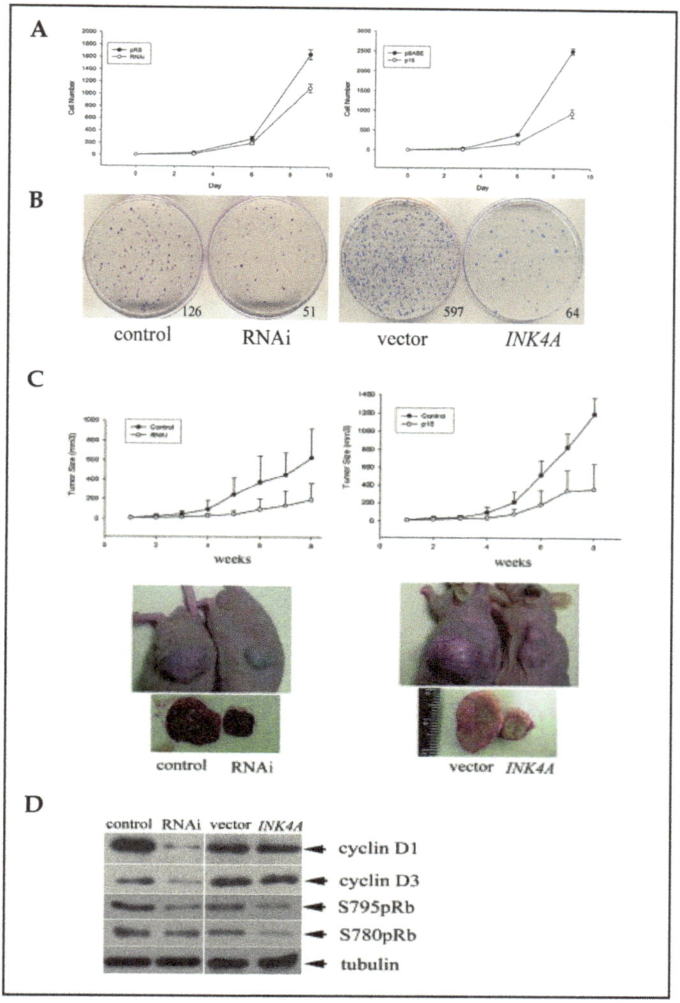

Fig. 7. Growth inhibition of melanoma cells by mutant BRAF RNAi or wild-type p16. Shown are *in vitro* and *in vivo* growth of 624Mel cells stably expressing either luc-RNAi (control) or mut BRAF RNAi (RNAi), vector control (vector) or wt INK4A (INK4A). (A) Cell counting. 5×10^4 624Mel cells are cultured and counted every 3 days using a hemocytometer ($P<0.05$, Student *t* test of day 9 cells). (B) Colony formation assay. 1×10^3 624Mel cells are plated in triplicate in 35 mm diameter plates and grown for 2 weeks. Colonies are fixed and stained. The colony numbers shown are the average colony counts from three plates ($P<0.001$, Two Poisson Parameters test). (C) Mouse xenograft assay. 5×10^5 624Mel cells are injected subcutaneously into flanks of nude mice ($n = 6$). Tumor growth is monitored. Pictures are taken 8 weeks after cell inoculation. The average tumor volumes are calculated and plotted ($p<0.01$, *t* test). (D) Expression of cyclin D1/D3 and phospho-pRB. Western blotting is performed using cell lysates from 624Mel control cells and cells expressing mut BRAF RNAi or INK4A and probed with cyclin D1 and cyclin D3 or Ser795 and Ser780 phosphorylated pRB (Rotolo et al., 2005).

inhibited by mut BRAF RNAi (Rotolo et al., 2005), consistent with earlier reports (Hingorani et al., 2003; Karasarides et al., 2004; Sumimoto et al., 2004; Wellbrock et al., 2004). Both mutant BRAF RNAi and wild-type INK4A significantly inhibited the growth of 624Mel cells in tissue culture, as measured by cell count (Fig. 7A) and colony formation assay (Fig. 7B). Population doubling times of mut BRAF RNAi and wild-type INK4A expressing 624Mel cells are on average 36 hr and 50 hr, respectively, compared to controls of approximately 24 hr (Rotolo et al., 2005). The effect on tumorigenesis is examined in a nude mice xenograft assay. Tumor growth is significantly inhibited by both mut BRAF shRNA and wild-type INK4A in 624Mel (Fig. 7C) and A101D and WM35 cells (not shown). Consistent with the observed growth inhibitory effects and with an overlapping role of BRAF and INK4A lesions in RB protein and cell cycle regulation (Fig. 6), cyclin D1 and D3 are downregulated in cells expressing mut BRAF RNAi, and phosphorylation of S780 and S795 of pRB, known cyclin D1/CDK4 targets are suppressed by both BRAF RNAi and INK4A (Fig. 7D).

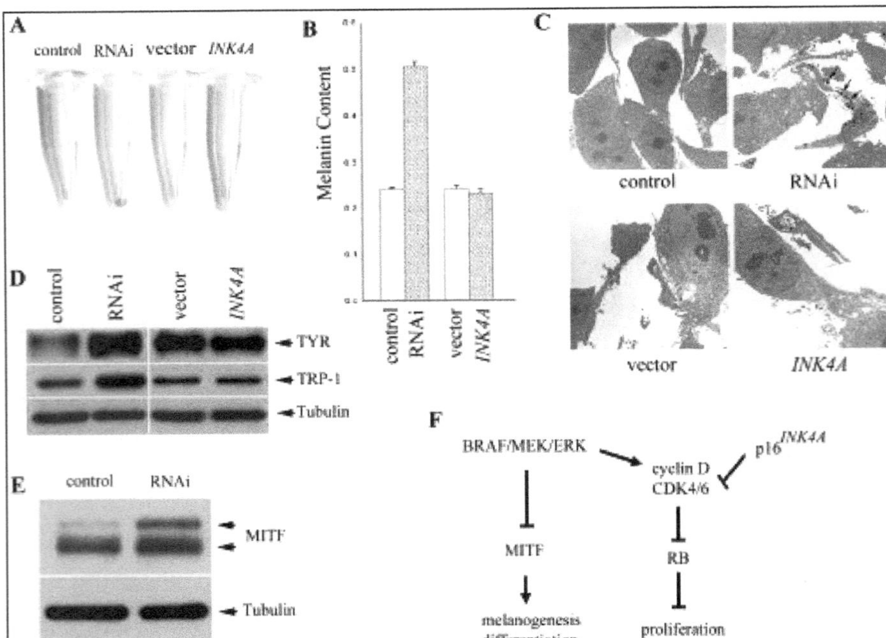

Fig. 8. Effect on melanogenesis. (A) Color of cell pellets. 5 × 10^6 624Mel controls and cells expressing mut BRAF RNAi or INK4A are pelleted. RNAi pellet shows a visible darker color. (B) Melanin contents; 5 × 10^6 cells are measured for melanin cotent. Data are means ± SE from 3 experiments performed in triplicate ($p < 0.001$, *t* test). (C) Representative electron micrographs of cultured 624Mel controls and cells expressing mut BRAF RNAi or INK4A. Note the increased numbers of mature melanosomes in RNAi-expressing cells (arrows). Magnification ×2,000. Similar changes are obtained using dissected xenograft tumors. (D) Western blot analysis of the expression of tyrosinase (TYR) and TRP-1 proteins. Western blot is probed with TYR, TRP-1 and α-tubulin antibodies. (E) Increased MITF in cells expressing ^{T1796A}BRAF RNAi, shown by Western blotting. (F) Model of separate regulation of proliferation and differentiation by mutant BRAF and p16 in melanoma cells.

Melanogenesis, a sign of melanocyte differentiation, is often changed in melanomas (Halaban, 2002). During normal development, differentiation stimuli trigger the activation of microphthalamia-associated transcription factor (MITF) to promote cell-cycle arrest and initiate the melanogenesis process (Fang & Setaluri, 1999; Setaluri, 2003; Widlund & Fisher, 2003). Melanogenesis is a multi-step biochemical process resulting in the formation of melanin in pigment cells. Melanogenic factors, tyrosinase (TYR), and tyrosinase-related protein-1 (TRP1) participate in the melanogenic pathway and are important melanocyte differentiation markers (Fang & Setaluri, 1999; Setaluri, 2003). Eberle et al (Eberle et al., 1995) compared the expression of TYR and TRP1 in cultured normal human melanocytes and melanoma cell lines by Northern blotting and reverse transcriptase-PCR (RT-PCR). They found that TYR and TRP1 genes are expressed in normal human melanocytes, but the expression is repressed in nearly all of the 14 melanoma cell lines examined and is completely absent in 4 of the 14 lines (Eberle et al., 1995). Hofbauer et al (Hofbauer et al., 1998) also found that tyrosinase expression level correlates inversely with clinical stage. These data suggest that the normal melanogenesis program is inhibited in melanoma cells. It is believed that differentiation and malignancy are inversely correlated and cancer is a disease of cell differentiation (Harris, 2004). Although unlimited proliferation and defects in cellular differentiation are characteristic of cancer growth, how the abnormal proliferation and pigmentation/differentiation are interconnected in the development of melanoma and other cancers is largely unknown (Coffman & Studzinski, 1999; Halaban, 2000).

Suppression of mutant BRAF inhibited ERK signaling, which may be attributed to the observed melanogenic effects. However, both activation and inhibition of ERK signaling can cause increased pigmentation. For example, although melanogenesis in melanocytes is suppressed both *in vitro* and *in vivo* by exogenous expression of Ras oncogene (Dotto et al., 1989; Tsukamoto et al., 1992; Wilson et al., 1989), transgenic mice expressing Ras under a mouse tyrosinase promoter demonstrated hyperpigmentation and melanocytic hyperplasia (Powell et al., 1995). Activation of ERK signaling by the c-Kit receptor plays a crucial role in the differentiation of pigment cells during development (Lassam & Bickford, 1992), whereas constitutive ERK signaling in melanoma cells is inhibitory to melanogenesis and inhibition of intrinsic ERK signaling in melanoma cells causes induction of melanogenesis and cellular differentiation (Englaro et al., 1998; Kim et al., 2004). Although our results demonstrate a melanogenic effect by inhibiting mutant BRAF, it is worth noting that activating BRAF mutations have been found in 70–80% of benign nevi that are mostly dark in color, and some malignant melanomas that are highly pigmented may have BRAF mutation. Thus, although BRAF mutation is important in blocking the melanogenic process in melanoma cells, it is not sufficient by itself to cause depigmentation. It is clear that the roles of BRAF mutation and ERK signaling in melanogenesis and melanocytic differentiation depend on the cellular context. Precisely what role is played by BRAF mutation and how it interacts with other signaling pathways in the determination of pigmentation phenotype needs to be further studied.

Since restoring p16 expression does not increase pigmentation, though cell proliferation is also suppressed, the differentiation effect of BRAF inhibition is not merely the result of general growth suppression. Rather, mutant BRAF actively participates in the differentiation program while simultaneously inducing proliferation. It is well known that malignant cells, including those of melanomas, maintain their differentiation program and sensitivity to differentiation modulators (Leszczyniecka et al., 2001). Therefore, understanding mutant BRAF in the regulation of the differentiation process may provide strategies by targeting mutant BRAF to reverse melanoma cells to a more mature and less malignant state. Melanogenesis is induced by inhibition of mutant BRAF but not by expression of wild-type p16, suggesting the existence of different mechanisms and nonoverlapping roles of the two most common genetic lesions in the malignant transformation of melanoma.

7. Growth inhibition and apoptosis by simultaneous inhibition of mutant BRAF and expression of INK4A in melanoma cells

Aberrant BRAF and INK4A often co-exist in melanoma and the regulatory relationship between BRAF and INK4A is unclear. It is possible that the co-occurrence is a result of genetic changes necessary for melanoma development without functional significance in melanoma cells. For example, in benign nevi, mutant BRAF turns on the expression of p16 resulting in proliferative senescence to counteract BRAF's proliferative drive (Bennett, 2008). Thus, loss of wild-type p16 is permissive to BRAF initiated melanoma development (Bennett, 2008). If mutant BRAF is still capable of turning on INK4A in melanoma (as in benign nevi), suppression of mutant BRAF, which has been actively explored to treat melanoma, may actually reduce the expression of any remaining functional p16 in melanoma cells and counteract the inhibitory effect of the treatment. On the other hand, the non-overlapping roles in melanogenesis suggest non-epistatic and additive/synergistic activities by the co-existing lesions. We hypothesize that simultaneous inhibition of BRAF-MEK and INK4A-CDK4 pathways is more effective than either alone in melanoma treatment. To test this hypothesis we performed experiments to co-express mut BRAF RNAi and INK4A in melanoma cells. Our initial studies revealed a sequence dependent difference when mut BRAF shRNA and wt INK4A are stably expressed in melanoma cells; the orders of introducing mut BRAF shRNA and wt INK4A generate different outcomes (Table 1, Table 2). 624Mel and WM35 cells stably expressing mut BRAF RNAi followed by wt INK4A expression (Set 1 in Table 1) are lethal although control 1363Mel cells are viable (Set 1 in Table 2). Whereas 624Mel and WM35 viable lines are eventually generated after weeks of tissue culture in experiments performed in the reverse order (Set 2 in Table 1 and Table 2). These results indicate that suppression of mut BRAF followed by restoration of wt INK4A generates more inhibitory effect than experiment performed in the reverse order in cells that harbor BRAF and INK4A lesions. We propose that inhibition of mut BRAF induces melanoma cells to a more differentiated state more susceptible to suppression by INK4A, whereas prior expression of INK4A interferes with differentiation program by mut BRAF inhibition. Therefore, the order of interventions could be important when targeting both BRAF and INK4A lesions in melanoma treatment.

Set 1*	Established line	pRS-puro	pRS-puro BRAF shRNA
	2nd control	pBabe-neo	pBabe-neo
	2nd Infection	pBabe-neo-INK4A	pBabe-neo-INK4A
Set 2*	Established line	pBabe-neo	pBabe-neo-INK4A
	2nd control	pRS-puro	pRS-puro
	2nd Infection	pRS-puro BRAF shRNA	pRS-puro BRAF shRNA

Table 1. Generation of melanoma cell lines expressing both mutant BRAF RNAi and INK4A

Cell line*	Set 1*		Set 2*	
624Mel	control	viable	control	viable
	BRAF shRNA + INK4A	**lethal**	INK4A + BRAF shRNA	viable
WM35	control	viable	control	viable
	BRAF shRNA + INK4A	**lethal**	INK4A + BRAF shRNA	viable
1363Mel	control	viable	control	viable
	BRAF shRNA + INK4A	viable	INK4A + BRAF shRNA	viable

*Set 1 and Set 2 experiments are performed in the reverse order. (Set 1) Cells infected and selected to stably expressing mut BRAF shRNA (pRS-puro BRAF RNAi) are subsequently infected with retrovirus pBabe-neo-INK4A. Cells are then under puro- and G418 double selection. (Set 2) Cells infected and selected to stably expressing pBabe-neo-INK4A are subsequently infected with retrovirus pRS-puro BRAF shRNA, and then double selected with puro- and G418. 624Mel and WM35 cells are positive for both BRAF and INK4A mutations, whereas 1363Mel is wt for both BRAF and INK4A.

Table 2. The sequence of expression of mut BRAF RNAi and wt INK4A affects cell survival

Melanoma cells under lengthy puro and G418 double selection seem to undergo various changes (e.g., change in ploidy as measured by flow cytometry, data not shown). We therefore choose to examine the more direct effect using transient transfection experiment. As described in Fig. 2 and Fig. 5, human melanoma cell line 624Mel is heterozygous for BRAF T1799A mutation (the ratio of T1799:A1799 alleles is about 1:1) and the cells have a six amino acid deletion in the exon 2 of INK4A although the smaller mutant protein is still detectable by Western blotting. Expression of BRAF RNAi and p16 cDNA each individually caused comparable levels of growth inhibition in melanoma cells through down-regulation of RB phosphorylation at the CDK4/6 sites (Fig. 7). 624Mel cells are transiently transfected with scrambled siRNA (5′--AAG UCC AUG GUG ACA GGA GAC-3′) and pBabe vector (control), BRAF siRNA (5′-AAG UGG CAU GGU GAU GUG GCA-3′) and pBabe vector (siRNA), scrambled siRNA and INK4A cDNA (INK4A), and BRAF siRNA and INK4A cDNA (siRNA-INK4A). The transfection efficiencies in 624Mel cells are approximately 30–50%, and the effects of transfection are assessed on unselected mass cultures. The RAS–RAF–MEK–ERK signaling pathway is viewed as upstream of the cyclin D-CDK4/6-p16-RB cascade; consistently, only melanomas with wild-type NRAS/BRAF have amplified CDK4 and cyclin D1 genes (Curtin et al., 2005). Therefore, expression of p16 may be epistatic to down-regulation of BRAF. If so, we would expect similar effects in cells expressing BRAF siRNA, INK4A cDNA, or BRAF siRNA plus INK4A cDNA. However, we found that simultaneous expression of BRAF siRNA and wild-type INK4A (siRNA-INK4A cells) inhibite cell growth more than either alone (siRNA or INK4A cells) as measured by cell counting (Fig. 9A, $p < 0.0001$, ANOVA; Tukey's Studentized range (HSD) test at 0.05 significance level) (Zhao et al., 2008) and colony formation (Fig. 9B).

Expression of BRAF siRNA and INK4A cDNA caused corresponding changes on levels of BRAF and p16 as detected by immunoblotting (Fig. 9D). BRAF levels are reduced in cells expressing BRAF siRNA (siRNA) and BRAF siRNA plus INK4A cDNA (siRNA–INK4A) but not in cells expressing INK4A cDNA (INK4A). The expression of p16 is increased in INK4A-transfected cells, and not in cells transfected with BRAF siRNA alone (Fig. 9D). Expression of BRAF siRNA caused reduction of MAPK signaling as indicated by ERK phosphorylation relative to ERK abundance (Fig. 9D), suggesting that the effects of BRAF inhibition are mediated by the BRAF–MEK–ERK signaling cascade. Since CDK4/6 kinases can be activated not only by RAF–MEK–ERK signaling, but also by other signaling pathways such as PI3K-AKT (Meier et al., 2007), exogenous p16 may generate broader inhibition of CDK4/6 activity not limited to that regulated by RAF-MEK-ERK. BRAF siRNA, on the other hand, may aid in p16 growth inhibition through reduced baseline activity of cyclin D-CDK4/6. Additionally, we found that levels of p27KIP1 are increased in siRNA, INK4A, and siRNA-INK4A cells (Fig. 9D). The changes of p27KIP1 are in line with the observed growth inhibition and with the well-established role of p27KIP1 in cell cycle regulation. p27KIP1, a negative regulator of cyclin E-CDK2, together with the reduced CDK4/6 activity as a result of BRAF siRNA and p16 expression, may block RB phosphorylation at both the CDK4/6 and CDK2 sites (note CDK2 level is not significantly altered, Fig. 9D), allowing RB to form complex with E2F and block cell cycle progression. p27KIP1 is regulated through different mechanisms (Bhatt et al., 2005), and further studies are required to understand the molecular mechanisms of the growth inhibition by BRAF siRNA and INK4A.

Induction of apoptosis by BRAF siRNA has been observed in some melanoma cells (Hingorani et al., 2003; Sumimoto et al., 2004), whereas p16 may act to block apoptosis (Maddika et al., 2007). To test whether expression of INK4A cDNA interferes with apoptosis induction by BRAF siRNA, we performed a TUNEL assay 72 h after transfection of 624Mel cells with BRAF siRNA and/or INK4A cDNA. Neither inhibition of BRAF siRNA nor expression of INK4A cDNA lead to significantly higher apoptosis than control (Fig. 10C, Tukey's Studentized range (HSD) test at 0.05 significance level does not detect statistically significant difference of apoptosis between siRNA, INK4A and control). However, coexpression of BRAF siRNA and INK4A cDNA triggered statistically significant difference of apoptosis (Fig. 9C, siRNA-INK4A in 624Mel cells generated significantly higher apoptosis than control or siRNA or INK4A, ANOVA $p = 0.0003$ and $p < 0.0001$, respectively; Tukey's Studentized range (HSD) test at 0.05 significance level). Note that there is no selection for transfected cells, so the maximum expected apoptosis is 50% (equivalent to the maximum transfection efficiency). The apoptotic effect, together with the enhanced growth inhibition (Fig. 9A and 9B), are consistent with the difficulty in generating stable cell lines expressing both BRAF short hairpin RNA and INK4A cDNA (Table 1 and Table 2). An anti-apoptotic effect of p16 has been previously reported that may be functionally equivalent to activation of RB since functional RB is known to suppress apoptosis (Harbour & Dean, 2000; Pucci et al., 2000). However, RB phosphorylation should be further inhibited in siRNA-INK4A expressing cells. The observed apoptosis may be mediated by other molecule(s) that over-ride or modify the anti-apoptotic effect of RB. Proteins in the BCL2 family are known to be critical regulators of apoptosis (Adams & Cory, 2007) which is in line with our observation that apoptosis is associated with the pro-apoptotic protein BIM (BCL2 interacting mediator of cell death (Collins et al., 2005), and BCL2, a critical prosurvival factor (Fig. 9D). The pro- and antiapoptotic counterparts of the BCL2 protein family can form heterodimers and neutralize each other's functions, suggesting that their relative concentrations play a pivotal role in the execution of programmed cell death. In BRAF siRNA cells, only an increase in BIM is detected, whereas in siRNA-INK4A cells, increased BIM occurs together with a decreased level of BCL2 (Fig. 9D). This could further offset the balance toward activation of apoptosis. The decrease in the levels of BCL2 protein is observed only in siRNA-INK4A cells but not in siRNA or INK4A cells suggesting a functional interaction between BRAF and p16 in the regulation of this pro-survival protein. Given the critical role of p53 in apoptosis, we performed sequencing analysis of p53 cDNA and found that 624Mel cells harbor a T1076G (Cys275Trp) mutation in the DNA binding domain that is likely to compromise the transcription and apoptosis function of p53 (Petitjean et al., 2007), suggesting that the observed apoptosis may not necessarily involve p53.

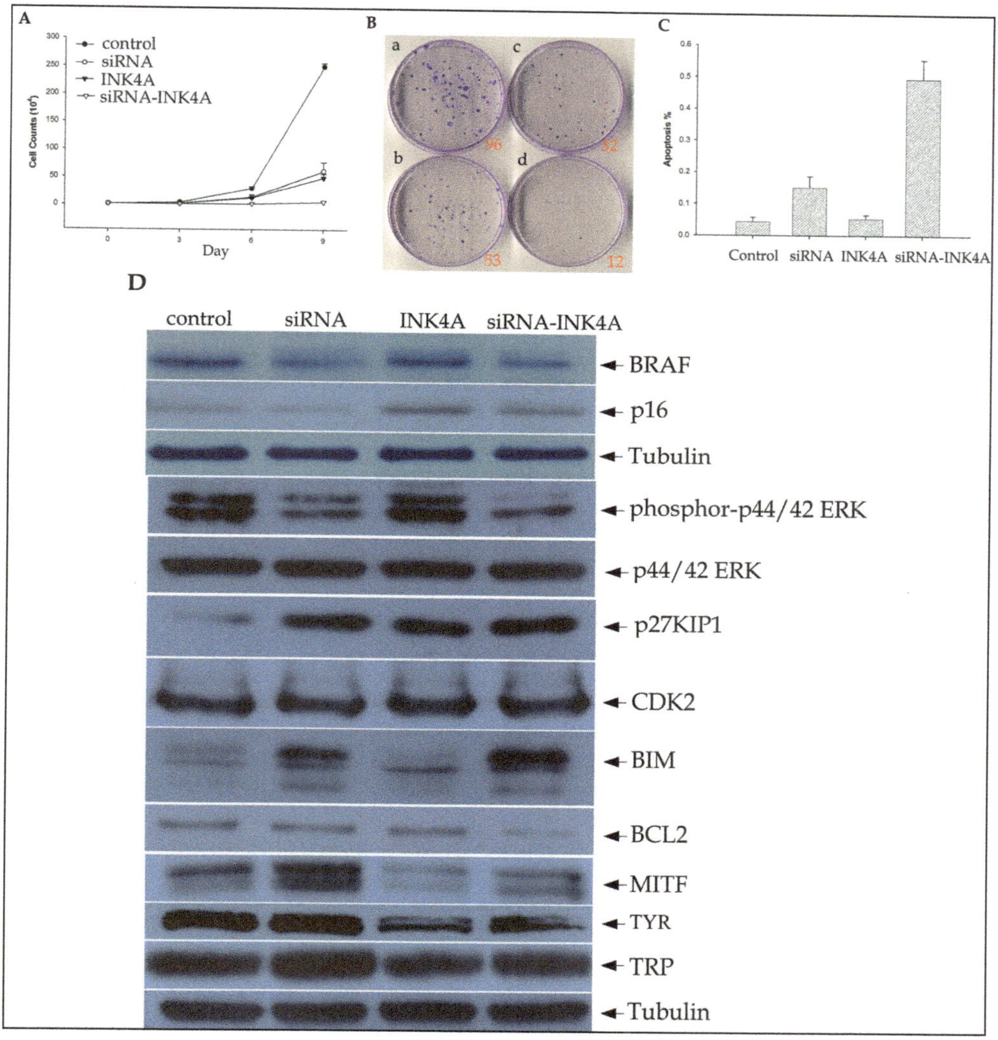

Fig. 9. Effects of simultaneous inhibition of BRAF by siRNA and expression of INK4A cDNA in 624Mel melanoma cells. 624Mel melanoma cells are transiently transfected with scrambled siRNA and pBabe vector (control), BRAF siRNA and pBabe vector (siRNA), scrambled siRNA and INK4A cDNA (INK4A), and BRAF siRNA and INK4A cDNA (siRNA-INK4A). (A) Growth inhibition measured by cell counting at day 3, 6, and 9 after transfection. (B) Growth inhibition measured by colony formation 2 weeks after transfection. (C) Apoptosis detected by TUNEL assay 72 h after transfection. (D) The expression of BRAF, p16 and several other proteins that are key regulators of proliferation (phosphor-p44/42 ERK, p27KIP1, CDK2), apoptosis (BIM, BCL2), and melanocytic differentiation (MITF, TYR, TRP1) are examined by Western blotting 48 hr after transfection. Tubulin is used as loading control (Zhao et al., 2008).

The mechanisms involved in the observed combinatory inhibition of proliferation and survival needs to be further explored. As the induced apoptosis is concomitant with growth arrest, it is possible that they are related. Alternatively, different cell populations, such as cells in different phases of the cell cycle, may respond differentially to BRAF siRNA and p16 under the same experimental condition. The observed growth inhibition and apoptosis may not simply be a quantitative/additive effect on CDK-RB since BRAF–MEK–ERK signaling has multiple targets that are not limited to CDK-RB regulation. Additionally, BRAF inhibition and p16 expression have different effects on melanogenesis (Fig. 8), suggesting that p16 may have qualitatively different activities not necessarily overlapping with BRAF, which may be the basis for the observed combinatory effects. In summary, our results show that simultaneous inhibition of mutant BRAF and expression of wild-type p16 cooperates in the inhibition of proliferation and enhances apoptosis, suggesting that BRAF and INK4A lesions - two of the most common genetic abnormalities in melanomas, interact functionally in melanoma cells and that strategies designed to correct both lesions could be effective for melanoma treatment.

8. Inhibition of MEK and CDK4 in melanoma cells

It has been shown that BRAF and INK4A may have activities independent of the corresponding canonical ERK and RB pathways, and the two pathways also mediate cellular signals independent of aberrant BRAF and INK4A. For example, RAF can act through apoptosis signal-regulating kinase-1 (ASK1)/c-Jun-NH2- kinase or mammalian sterile 20-like-kinase 2 (MST2) pathways (O'Neill et al., 2005); cyclin D:CDK4/6 can be activated by enhanced phosphatidylinositol 3-kinase (PI3K) and WNT signaling pathways in melanomas (Delmas et al., 2007; Schmitt et al., 2002). To examine whether the combinatorial effects of BRAF RNAi and INK4A cDNA in melanoma cells is specific to BRAF and INK4A or can be generalized to other components of the ERK and RB pathways, we tested PD98059 and 219476, commercially available inhibitors of MEK and CDK4, respectively, in human melanoma cells. Of note, deregulation of the RAS-RAF-MEK-ERK (ERK) and p16-cycylin D:CDK4/6-RB (RB) pathways are common in human malignancies and appears to be important for melanoma development. As shown in Fig. 1, chemotherapeutic agents targeting components of both pathways have been developed but clinical studies with monotherapy have been disappointing.

Human melanoma cell lines 624Mel, A101D, and A375 harbor heterozygous BRAF T1799A mutation and loss of wild-type p16 (Rotolo et al., 2005). The cells are treated, alone or in combination, with MEK inhibitor PD98059 (Waters et al., 1995) and CDK4 inhibitor 219476 (Zhu et al., 2003). As anticipated, ERK phosphorylation is reduced in cells treated with PD98059 and PD98059 plus 219476 (Fig. 10A). Levels of p27KIP1, a negative regulator of cyclin E:CDK2, are increased in cells treated with either PD98059 or 219476, and further increased in cells with combinatorial treatment (Fig. 10B). Phosphorylation of S780, S795, and S807/811 of RB, known cyclin D:CDK4 and cyclin E:CDK2 targets (Halaban, 2005), is decreased in cells treated with either PD98059 or 219476 (except S780 and S807/811 in OM431 cells), and further reduced in cells with combinatorial treatment (Fig. 10C). Of note, total RB is decreased under combinatorial treatment with PD98059 and 219476 in all three melanoma cells (Fig. 10C).

PD98059 and 219476 inhibit tumor cell growth in a dose dependent manner (Krasilnikov et al., 2003; Zhu et al., 2003). In order to make it possible to monitor the additional therapeutic

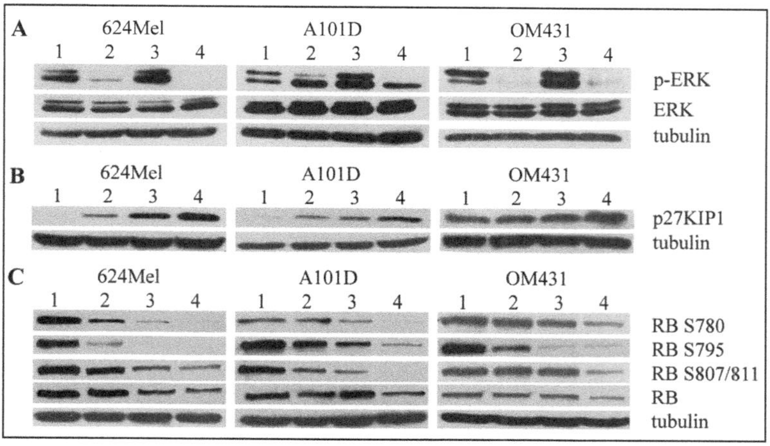

Fig. 10. Regulation of ERK phosphorylation, p27KIP1 expression, and RB phosphorylation by PD98059 and 219476, alone and in combination. Human melanoma cell lines 624Mel, A101D, and OM431 are treated with either vehicle solvent (1), PD98059 (2), 219476 (3), or PD98059 plus 219476 (4) (Li et al., 2010a). Western blot is performed using 20 μg total cell lysates. Tubulin is used as the loading control.

effects of the combinatorial treatment, both chemicals are used at dosages lower than that which would lead to maximal effect by either agent. The cytotoxicity of PD98059 and 219476 is measured using the MTS assay that measures the dehydrogenase enzyme activity found in metabolically active cells. In all the three cell lines, a significant difference in MTS counts exists for the control, PD98059, 219476, and PD98059 plus 219476 groups ($p < 0.0001$, R-Square 0.981444, 0.956956, and 0.991102 in 624Mel, A101D, and OM431, respectively, ANOVA). Further analysis showS that simultaneous treatment with PD98059 and 219476 results in significantly reduced numbers of cell survival than control or mono-treatment as measured by MTS in all the three cell lines (Fig. 11A, Tukey's Studentized Range (HSD) Test at 0.05 significance level). TUNEL DNA fragmentation assay is used to identify loss of viability due to programmed cell death. As shown in Fig. 11B, at the drug concentrations used, significantly different levels of apoptosis exist among control for PD98059, 219476, and combinatorial treatment groups ($p < 0.0001$, R-Square 0.973862, 0.990697, and 0.987900 in 624Mel, A101D, and OM431, respectively, ANOVA). Treatment with PD98059 alone results in no difference in apoptosis over controls in all three cell lines; 219476 enhances apoptosis in OM431 but not in the other two cell lines. However, combined treatment dramatically increases apoptosis over that seen for the control and mono-treatments (Fig. 11B, Tukey's Studentized Range (HSD) Test at 0.05 significance level).

We examined the expression of several pro- and anti-apoptotic proteins. Mono-treatment with PD98059 or 219476 causes a decreased or no change in the expression of anti-apoptotic proteins BCL2, BCL2L1, and BIRC5. While there are variations in the patterns of expression of BCL2, BCL2L1, and BIRC5 among the different cell lines, combinatorial treatment causes a comprehensive down-regulation of the proteins in all three cell lines (Fig. 12). In addition apoptosis facilitator BIM-EL is increased following treatment with PD98059 and PD98059 plus 219476 in all three cell lines. It is also increased in OM431 cells following treatment with 219476 (Fig. 12). Consistent with increased apoptosis, caspase 3 is activated by simultaneous treatment with PD98059 plus 219476 in all three cell lines, as shown by decreased pro-caspase 3, increased levels of the active form of caspase 3 (cleaved caspase 3), and degradation of PARP, a direct substrate of active caspase 3 (Fig. 12).

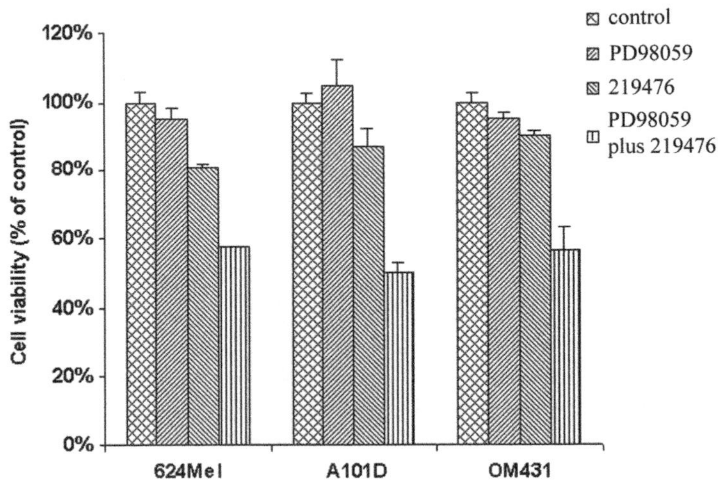

(A)

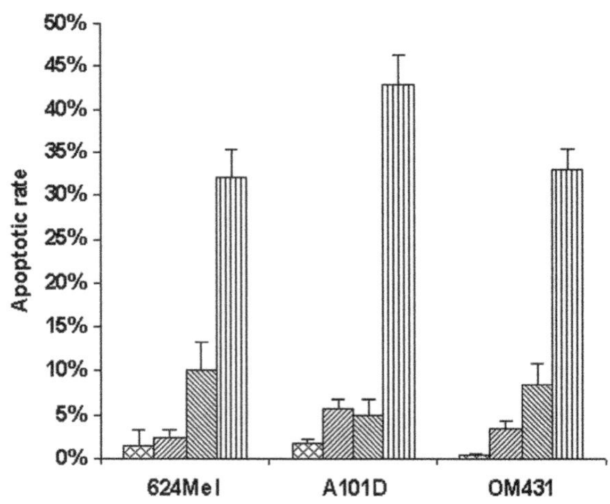

(B)

Fig. 11. Cytotoxicity by MEK inhibitor PD98059, CDK4 inhibitor 219476, and combinatorial treatment. (A) MTS cytotoxicity assay is performed in 624Mel, A101D and OM431 cells after 48h treatment in medium supplemented with 0.5% FBS. The results are given as means ± SD from three independent tests. (B) MEK and CDK4 inhibitors induce apoptosis of melanoma cells. TUNEL assay is performed in 624Mel, A101D and OM431 cells after 48h treatment with vehicle solvent, PD98059, 219476, or PD98059 plus 219476 in medium with 0.5% FBS. The results are given as means ± SD from three independent assays.

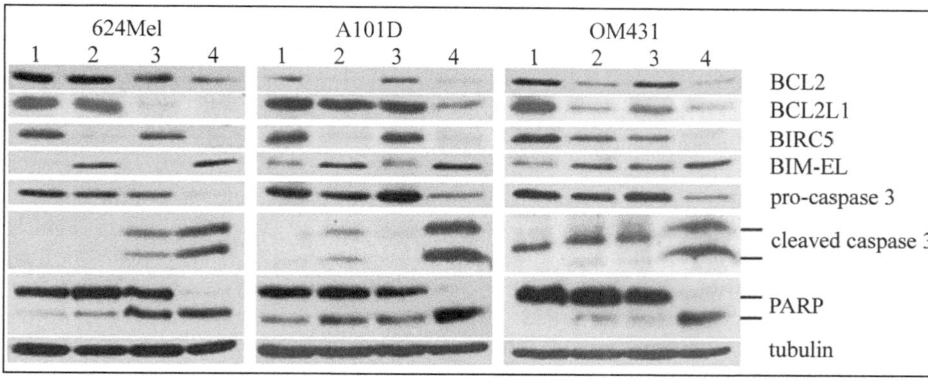

Fig. 12. Western blot analysis of changes in the expression of pro-survival and pro-apoptotic proteins. Cells are treated with solvent vehicle control (1), PD98059 (2), 219476 (3), and PD98059 plus 219476 (4) for 48 h in medium containing 5% FBS. 20 μg total cell extracts from 624Mel, A101D and OM431 cells are separated by SDS-PAGE and blotted using BCL2, BCL2L1, BIRC5, BIM, caspase-3, and PARP antibodies. Tubulin is used as loading control.

It has been well-established that constitutive activation of the ERK signaling induces the expression of cyclin D (Michaloglou et al., 2008; Rotolo et al., 2005), which binds to and activates CDK4 leading to the phosphorylation of RB protein facilitating cell cycle entry (Halaban, 2005). Consistent with an epistatic regulation between ERK pathway and cyclin D:CDK4, amplification of cyclin D1 and CDK4 genes have been identified mainly in melanomas that harbor wild-type NRAS and BRAF (Curtin et al., 2005; Smalley et al., 2008). Additionally, cyclin D:CDK4 can mediate resistance to inhibitors of the ERK signaling pathway (Smalley et al., 2008). Therefore, the enhanced apoptosis and decreased proliferation by simultaneously inhibiting ERK and RB pathways could result from the double hitting of ERK-cyclin D:CDK4-RB that regulate cell cycle progression and cell survival. Alternatively, in support of our previous results that BRAF and INK4A have a non-linear functional interaction (Rotolo et al., 2005; Zhao et al., 2008), additional cellular processes could be affected when cells are exposed to both PD98059 and 219476. ERK pathway has pleiopotent activities that regulate cell proliferation, survival, and differentiation through both cyclin D:CDK4 dependent and independent routes (Fecher et al., 2008; Panka et al., 2006a; Sekulic et al., 2008). Likewise, cyclin D:CDK4 can be regulated and converges multiple cellular signals. For example, while PI3K signaling can activate CDK4 through down-regulation of INK4A and up-regulation of cyclin D (Schmidt et al., 2002), WNT signaling can turn on CDK4 through suppression of INK4A transcription (Delmas et al., 2007). It is conceivable that inhibition of MEK and CDK4 not only affects ERK and RB pathways, but also PI3K, WNT, and other ERK signaling activities not mediated through the RB pathway. Therefore, simultaneous targeting of both ERK and RB pathways can generate enhanced effects by targeting both linear and non-overlapping activities.

Our results show that simultaneous inhibition of MEK and CDK4 using pharmacological inhibitors PD98059 and 219476 leads to significantly increased apoptosis compared to control and single agent treatment (Figs. 11, 12). This effect is consistent with results observed after simultaneous knockdown of mutant BRAF using siRNA and expression of INK4A cDNA in melanoma cells (Fig. 9). The apoptotic effect is associated with changes of apoptosis related proteins (Figs. 9 and 12). BCL2L1 and BIRC5 are highly expressed in melanoma cells, and increased expression correlates with tumor progression (Piras et al., 2007; Zhuang et al., 2007). A straightforward explanation for the observed apoptosis is that changes in the pro- and anti-apoptotic factors offset the balance and lead to apoptosis (Adams & Cory, 2007). Sequencing analysis of TP53 cDNA (Zhao et al., 2008) showed that 624Mel and OM431cells harbor a T1076G (Cys275Trp) and a G1048A (Gly266Glu) mutations, respectively, in the DNA binding domain that is likely to compromise the transcriptional and apoptotic function of p53 (Petitjean et al., 2007). No TP53 mutation has been detected in A101D cells. Although apoptosis is enhanced in all three cell lines, it is somewhat more pronounced in A101D than 624Mel and OM431 cells treated with PD98059 and 219476 (Fig. 11), suggesting that TP53 status may influence the magnitude of apoptosis. Combinatorial treated cells have further inhibited phosphorylation of ERK and RB, reduced total RB, and increased expression of p27KIP1 (Figs. 9 and 12). Yu et al. demonstrated that loss of Rb causes apoptosis without effecting cellular proliferation (Yu et al., 2003) and Wang et al. found that over-expression of p27KIP1 leads to apoptosis in melanoma cells (Wang et al., 1997). The mechanisms of these changes in relationship to each other and to the observed cooperative effects need to be further investigated.

Apoptosis resistance is a critical factor for therapy failure in melanoma patients. Encouragingly, our results demonstrate that an increase in apoptosis can be achieved through combinatorial targeting of BRAF-MEK-ERK and p16-CDK4-RB pathways. Deregulation of the RAS-RAF-MEK-ERK and p16-cycylin D:CDK4/6-RB pathways are common in human malignancies and appears to be important for melanoma development. There has been significant effort to target components of these pathways in cancer treatment. Pharmacologic agents targeting components of the ERK and RB pathways have been developed. However, clinical studies using monotherapy show that the clinical responses have failed expectations and maximum tolerated doses are often reached before reaching clinical efficacy (Burdette-Radoux et al., 2004; Fecher et al., 2008; Panka et al., 2006b; Sekulic et al., 2008). Our study suggests that combination targeting of ERK and RB pathways is a promising strategy for melanoma treatment and should encourage further in-depth investigations.

9. HERV-K expression correlates with MEK and CDK4 activation

The K type human endogenous retroviral sequence (HERV-K) is expressed in melanoma cells but not in melanocytes (Muster et al., 2003). Through millions of years of evolution and natural selection, HERVs have become indispensible parts of the human genome. For example, syncytin-1 and syncytin-2, encoded by the envelope (ENV) genes of HERV-W and HERV-FRD, respectively, mediate intercellular fusion of trophoblast cells to form syncytiotrophoblast as well as prevent maternal immune attack against the developing embryo, thereby facilitating implantation of the embryo (Krone & Grange, 2010; Rote et al., 2004). It is estimated that 8% of the human genome consists of retroviral elements (Singh et al., 2009). A complete HERV sequence is composed of GAG, POL, and ENV genes flanked by two long terminal repeats (LTRs), similar to exogenous retroviruses such as human immunodeficiency virus (HIV) (Ahn & Kim, 2009). HERVs can be classified into over 20 families based on tRNA specificity of the primer binding site used to initiate reverse transcription; thus, HERV-K would use lysine and HERV-W tryptophan if they were replicating viruses. Increased HERV expression has been found under pathological conditions, particularly in cancer and inflammatory disease (Voisset et al., 2008). Unlike most HERVs that harbor defective mutations, the HML-2 group of HERV-Ks has open reading frames that code for functional viral proteins, which may form noninfectious particles (Beimforde et al., 2008; Turner et al., 2001). We have demonstrated recently that expression of HERV-K correlates with ERK activation and p16 loss in human melanoma specimens, and that inhibition of MEK and CDK4, especially in combination, suppresses HERV-K expression (Li et al., 2010b), which suggests that HERV-K may mediate BRAF-MEK-ERK and p16-CDK4-RB signaling pathways in melanoma cells.

It is interesting to note that the growth characteristics of melanoma cells that can be modified by HERV-K activation (e.g., changes in cell shape, loss of melanin, anchorage-independent growth) (Serafino et al., 2009) overlap with those that can be blocked by suppression of the BRAF-MEK-ERK signaling pathway, especially with simultaneous restoration of p16 or inhibition of CDK4 (Li et al., 2010a; Rotolo et al., 2005; Zhao et al., 2008). This observation, together with the knowledge that aberrations in BRAF-MEK-ERK and p16-CDK4 pathways are early events and often co-exist during melanomagenesis, and the evidence that the RAF-MEK-ERK signaling pathway is required for the completion of HIV-1 reverse transcription (Mettling et al., 2008), prompted us to hypothesize that HERV-K is regulated by BRAF-MEK-ERK and p16-CDK4 pathways. We examined the expression of HERV-K GAG and ENV proteins, the active form of ERK (phospho-ERK, p-ERK), and p16 in a panel of human melanocytic specimens including 38 benign nevi and 34 melanomas. As summarized in Table 3, both HERV-K GAG and ENV proteins are largely cytoplasmic with occasional nuclear staining observed, whereas p-ERK is typically co-expressed in the nucleus and cytoplasm. Wild-type INK4A is expressed in both nucleus and cytoplasm, whereas mutant p16, if expressed, is either nuclear or cytoplasmic (Ghiorzo et al., 2004). HERV-K GAG cytoplasmic staining is over 10-fold more frequent in melanoma than in nevi (38% of melanomas vs. 3% of nevi, $p < 0.001$) (Table 3). Similarly, HERV-K ENV immunoreactivity is detected in the cytoplasm in 44% of melanomas and 11% of neval specimens (a 4-fold difference, $p = 0.003$). The nuclear staining of GAG and ENV are infrequently detected in both nevi and melanomas, and the differences do not reach statistical significance (Table 3). p-ERK staining is 5-fold more often positive in melanomas than in nevi (68% and 13%, respectively, $p < 0.001$). p16 staining, both in the cytoplasm and

Antigen	Positivity (%)		*p* value
	Nevi [n=38]	Melanoma [n=34]	
HERV-K GAG, cytoplasmic	3	38	$p < 0.001$**
HERV-K GAG, nuclear	0	6	$p = 0.493$
HERV-K ENV, cytoplasmic	11	44	$p = 0.003$**
HERV-K ENV, nuclear	8	12	$p = 0.7$
p-ERK, cytoplasmic and nuclear	13	68	$p < 0.001$**
p16, cytoplasmic	79	50	$p = 0.014$*
p16, nuclear	79	15	$p < 0.001$**

Protein immunoreactivity, cytoplasmic or nuclear, is dichotomized as negative/decreased (<30% of cells staining positively) or positive ($\geq$30% of cells staining positively).
** Difference is significant at the ≤0.01 level (2-tailed).
* Difference is significant at the ≤.05 level (2-tailed).

Table 3. Expression of HERV-K GAG and ENV, p-ERK and p16 in neval and melanoma specimens nucleus, is more frequently observed in nevi than in melanomas (cytoplasmic, 79% vs. 50%, $p = 0.014$; nuclear, 79% vs. 15%, $p < 0.001$) (Table 3). Figure 13 demonstrates representative staining patterns of HERV-K GAG, HERV-K ENV, p-ERK, and p16 in melanoma and neval specimens. Further analysis shows that the expression of HERV-K GAG in the cytoplasm of melanoma is positively correlated with p-ERK ($p = 0.005$) and negatively correlated with p16 cytoplasmic expression ($p = 0.012$) (Table 4). The expression of HERV-K ENV in the cytoplasm of melanomas is positively correlated with p-ERK ($p < 0.001$) and negatively correlated with p16 nuclear expression ($p = 0.046$) (Table 4).

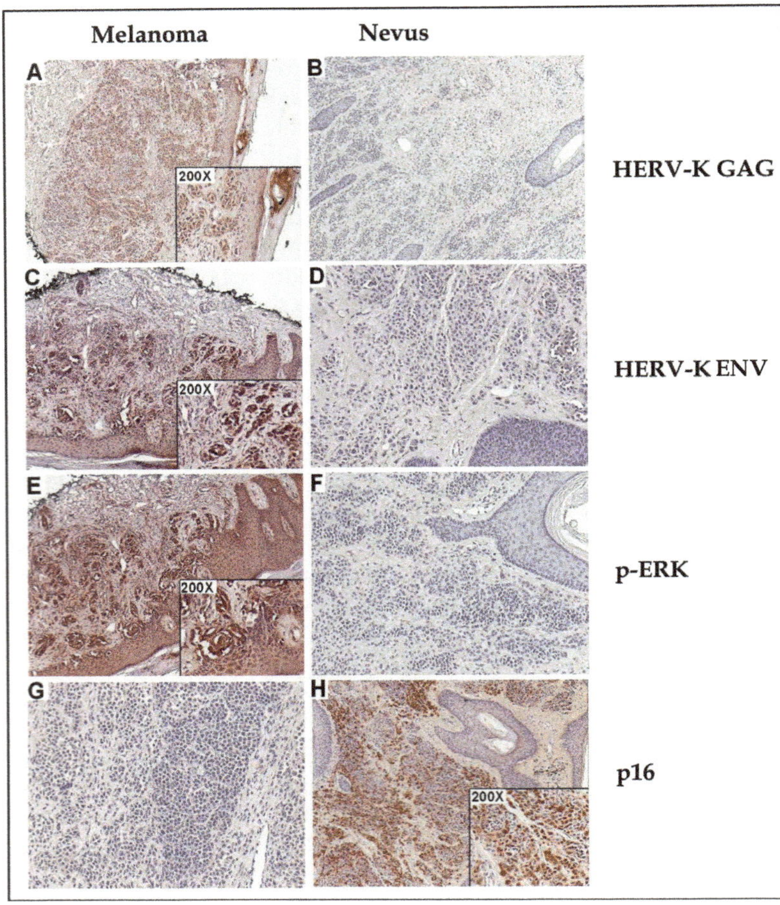

Fig. 13. Expression of HERV-K GAG and ENV, p-ERK and p16 in neval and melanoma specimens. Formalin-fixed and paraffin-embedded microscopic sections of melanoma (A, C, E, G) and nevus (B, D, F, H) are analyzed by immunohischemical staining using HERV-K GAG (A, B), ENV(C, D), p-ERK (E, F), and p16 (G, H) specific antibodies. Shown is a representative staining pattern. HERV-K GAG and ENV are mostly detected in melanoma cells (A and C), but rarely expressed in neval cells (B and D). p-ERK is mainly detected in melanoma cells (E) but rarely found in neval cells (F). p16 is not as prominently expressed in melanoma (G) as in neval cells (H). Magnification: ×100 and ×200 (insets).

	HERV-K GAG cytoplasmic	HERV-K GAG nuclear	HERV-K ENV cytoplasmic	HERV-K ENV nuclear
p-ERK, cytoplasmic and nuclear	$p = 0.005$**	$p = 0.093$	$p < 0.001$**	$p = 0.2$
p16, cytoplasmic	$p = 0.012$*	$p = 0.058$	$p = 0.114$	$p = 0.608$
p16, nuclear	$p = 0.123$	$p = 0.378$	$p = 0.046$*	$p = 0.251$

Note: ** Correlation is significant at the 0.01 level (2-tailed).
* Correlation is significant at the 0.05 level (2-tailed).

Table 4. Associations of the expression of p-ERK, p16, and HERV-K GAG and HERV-K ENV

The expression of HERV-K has been reported in several melanoma cell lines (Buscher et al., 2006; Buscher et al., 2005; Muster et al., 2003; Serafino et al., 2009). We examined HERV-K in four melanoma cell lines (624Mel, A375, A101D, and OM431) that have constitutive activation of p-ERK and loss of wild-type p16 with corresponding hyper-phosphorylation of RB protein (Li et al., 2010a; Rotolo et al., 2005; Zhao et al., 2008). HERV-K expression is detected using a specific HERV-K ENV antibody, as described (Muster et al., 2003; Serafino et al., 2009), that recognizes a 37 Kd spliced transmembrane domain of ENV protein (Buscher et al., 2006; Buscher et al., 2005; Muster et al., 2003). HERV-K ENV protein is prominently expressed in 624Mel and A375 cells, weakly positive in A101D cells, but barely detectable in OM431 cells (Fig. 14A). We extracted total cellular RNA from all the four cell lines and performed conventional RT-PCR using specific HERV-K POL and ENV primers as described (Serafino et al., 2009). Gel electrophoresis of RT-PCR end-products shows similar levels of POL and ENV RNAs in the four cell lines, in contrast to the dramatic differences in the case of ENV protein (data not shown). Direct sequencing of RT-PCR amplicons and NCBI BLAST analysis show that expressed sequences share 96%-98% overall homology with Group N HERV-K (Romano et al., 2006) (data not shown), as reported in other melanoma cells (Hirschl et al., 2007).
Multiple endogenous and exogenous factors have been linked to the activation of HERVs including hormones, cytokines, and cytotoxic chemicals (Taruscio & Mantovani, 2004). To our knowledge, a direct association between ERK and p16-CDK4 pathways and HERV expression has not been reported previously. It has been shown that HERV-K sequences, as other host genes, are regulated by DNA methylation in the promoter/enhancer sequences located in the 5′-LTR regions (Lavie et al., 2005). Since RB protein, a downstream mediator of BRAF-MEK-ERK and p16-CDK4 signaling pathways, is a key regulator of DNA methylation (Montoya-Durango et al., 2009), it is conceivable that the observed association between HERV-K, p-ERK, and p16-CDK4 may act through RB, a notion that will surely prompt further investigation. It is worth noting that the four melanoma cell lines examined, 624Mel, A375, A101D, and OM431, all have BRAF T1799A mutation, constitutive activation of ERK, loss of wild-type p16, over-expression of phospho-RB protein (Rotolo et al., 2005), and have comparable levels of HERV-K RNA transcripts (not shown). However, only 624Mel and A375 cells express high levels of HERV-K ENV protein (Fig. 14A), suggesting that HERV-K ENV protein is regulated by mechanisms in addition to ERK and p16-CDK4 pathways. Alternatively, A101D and OM431 cells may harbor mutant HERV-Ks affecting EVE expression, a notion that needs to be further investigated.
We examined whether HERV-K ENV expression is suppressed by MEK and CDK4 inhibitors using established experimental conditions (including time course and dose-

response curve) for PD98059 and 219476, specific inhibitors of MEK and CDK4, respectively (Li et al., 2010a). As expected, treatment with PD98059 inhibited ERK phosphorylation in both 624Mel and A375 cells (Fig. 14B, lane 2). Phosphorylation of serine 780, a CDK4 target in the RB protein, is reduced by PD98059 and 219476, especially in combination, in both cell lines (Fig. 14B). Similarly, HERV-K ENV expression is inhibited by either PD98059 or 219476, especially when used in combination (Fig. 14B). The results are consistent with findings of the association between HERV-K expression and p-ERK and p16 in melanocytic specimens (Table 4).

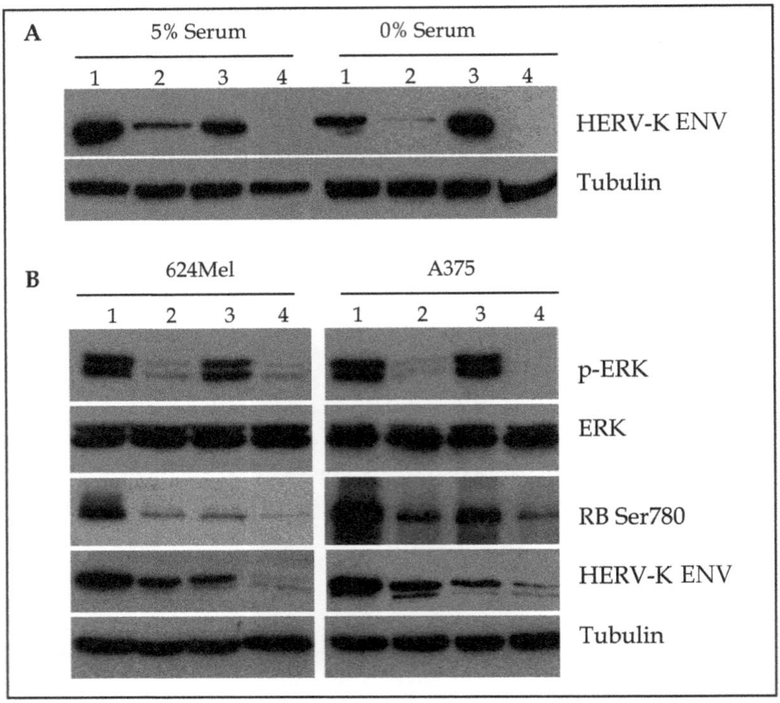

Fig. 14. MEK and CDK4 inhibitors suppress HERV-K ENV protein expression. (A) 624Mel (1), A101D (2), A375 (3), and OM431 (4) melanoma cells are cultured in DMEM with 5% serum or serum starved overnight, and cell lysates collected for Western blotting. (B) 624Mel and A375 melanoma cells are treated with solvent vehicle control (1), 25 μg MEK inhibitor PD98059 (2), 1 μg CDK4 inhibitor 219476 (3), and 25 μg PD98059 plus 1 μg 219476 (4) for 48 h under serum starvation, and cell lysates collected for Western blotting. Western blotting is performed using 50 μg total cell extracts and commercially available HERV-K ENV antibody that recognizes a 37 Kd spliced transmembrane domain of ENV protein. Tubulin is used as loading control.

HERVs have been implicated in the etiology of various diseases including cancer and chronic inflammation (Voisset et al., 2008), and emerging data support a role of HERV-K in melanomagenesis. For example, HERV-K is expressed in melanomas but not in normal melanocytes (Buscher et al., 2005; Muster et al., 2003), and specific inhibition of HERV-K by

RNAi suppresses melanoma cells *in vitro* and *in vivo* (Mangeney et al., 2005; Oricchio et al., 2007; Pothlichet et al., 2006; Serafino et al., 2009). There are several potential mechanisms to explain the role of HERV-Ks in melanomagenesis. First, HERV-K sequences may jump around by retro-transposition leading to mutagenesis and chromosomal abnormalities (Pothlichet et al., 2006; Tchenio & Heidmann, 1991) which may drive the evolution of aggressive clones. Second, HERV-K ENV, which is homologous to syncytin, may have fusogenic activity to mediate melanoma-melanoma and melanoma-target cell intercellular fusions and, therefore, can be the molecular link in the melanoma-normal cell fusion theory of metastasis (Carter, 2008; Pawelek & Chakraborty, 2008). Third, HERV-K proteins can be immunosuppressive (Mangeney et al., 2005) and may facilitate tumor progression by providing a critical survival/escape mechanism for tumor invasion and metastasis (Singh et al., 2009; Voisset et al., 2008), especially in the blood/lymph stream where circulating tumor cells are under attack by the host immune system.

HERV-K may prove to be a key mediator of BRAF-MEK-ERK and p16-CDK4-RB pathways during melanoma pathogenesis. Activation of BRAF/ERK is recently shown to drive chromosome abnormality and aneuploidy in melanocytes (Cui et al., 2010). It is conceivable that the effect may be mediated, at least partly, through HERV-K sequences that are capable of jumping around by retro-transposition leading to mutagenesis and chromosomal abnormalities (Pothlichet et al., 2006; Tchenio & Heidmann, 1991). It is possible that the observed growth promotion and anti-apoptotic effects of activated ERK and CDK4 (Li et al., 2010a; Zhao et al., 2008) can be mediated, at least in part, by HERV-K since HERV-K has been shown to directly affect melanoma cell proliferation, differentiation, and anchorage related survival (Oricchio et al., 2007; Serafino et al., 2009). Importantly, if HERV-K drives melanomagenesis downstream of the BRAF-MEK-ERK and p16/CDK4 pathways, when HERV-K is already turned on, cells may escape the inhibitory effects of therapies targeting BRAF-MEK-ERK and p16-CDK4. Triple therapies, such as simultaneous targeting of HERV-K, BRAF/MEK, and CDK4, may be necessary to produce more effective and long-lasting therapeutic effects than single or, as we have proposed previously, double inhibition of MEK-ERK and CDK4 (Li et al., 2010a; Zhao et al., 2008). This strategy is analogous to HIV "cocktail" therapy that disrupts HIV at different steps of replication and brought many AIDS patients from death to fairly normal and productive lives (Henkel, 1999).

10. Conclusion

Melanoma is the most lethal skin malignancy notorious for aggressive growth and therapeutic resistance. Multiple genetic and environmental factors have been linked to the development of melanoma. Approximately 60% of melanomas harbor mutations in v-raf murine sarcoma viral oncogene homolog B1 (BRAF) that lead to constitutive activation of the mitogen activated protein kinase/ERK kinase (MEK)-extracellular signal regulated kinase (ERK) signaling pathway. Results of the recent clinical trials with PLX4032, a specific inhibitor of mutant BRAF, have generated great excitement because approximately 80% of BRAF mutant metastatic melanomas regressed in response to PLX4032 treatment. Though this trial is considered a victory in the fight against melanomas, attention has been drawn to the fact that regressed tumors may resurge more aggressively within 8 months after the start of therapy indicating more research is needed to conquer melanoma. Most melanoma cells, but not nevi, have lost the expression of p16 inhibitor of CDK4 (INK4A), either through DNA mutation or promoter hypermethylation, resulting in a deregulated cyclin dependent kinase 4 (CDK4)-retinoblastoma (RB) pathway. We found that simultaneous inhibition of mutant BRAF and expression of wild-type INK4A or combinatorial application of MEK and CDK4 inhibitors in melanoma cells significantly inhibits growth and enhances apoptosis. Our results support the hypothesis that simultaneous targeting of BRAF-MEK-ERK and p16-CDK4 pathways may be a promising strategy for melanoma treatment. Additionally, we found that HERV-K activation in melanoma cells is associated with BRAF-MEK-ERK and p16INK4A-CDK4 pathways. Our results should help the better understanding of BRAF-MEK-ERK and p16INK4A–CDK4 pathways, as well as HERV-K involvement in melanomagenesis and facilitate the design of novel management strategies. Further studies are warranted to examine the molecular mechanisms and biological consequences of these associations.

11. References

Adams, J.M. & Cory, S. (2007). The Bcl-2 apoptotic switch in cancer development and therapy. *Oncogene*, 26, 1324-37.

Ahn, K. & Kim, H.S. (2009). Structural and quantitative expression analyses of HERV gene family in human tissues. *Mol Cells*, 28, 99-103.

Bartkova, J., Lukas, J., Guldberg, P., Alsner, J., Kirkin, A.F., Zeuthen, J. & Bartek, J. (1996). The p16-cyclin D/Cdk4-pRb pathway as a functional unit frequently altered in melanoma pathogenesis. *Cancer Res*, 56, 5475-83.

Beimforde, N., Hanke, K., Ammar, I., Kurth, R. & Bannert, N. (2008). Molecular cloning and functional characterization of the human endogenous retrovirus K113. *Virology*, 371, 216-25.

Bennett, D.C. (2008). How to make a melanoma: what do we know of the primary clonal events? *Pigment Cell Melanoma Res*, 21, 27-38.

Bhatt, K.V., Spofford, L.S., Aram, G., McMullen, M., Pumiglia, K. & Aplin, A.E. (2005). Adhesion control of cyclin D1 and p27Kip1 levels is deregulated in melanoma cells through BRAF-MEK-ERK signaling. *Oncogene*, 24, 3459-71.

Bollag, G., Hirth, P., Tsai, J., Zhang, J., Ibrahim, P.N., Cho, H., Spevak, W., Zhang, C., Zhang, Y., Habets, G., Burton, E.A., Wong, B., Tsang, G., West, B.L., Powell, B., Shellooe, R., Marimuthu, A., Nguyen, H., Zhang, K.Y., Artis, D.R., Schlessinger, J., Su, F., Higgins, B., Iyer, R., D'Andrea, K., Koehler, A., Stumm, M., Lin, P.S., Lee, R.J., Grippo, J., Puzanov, I., Kim, K.B., Ribas, A., McArthur, G.A., Sosman, J.A., Chapman, P.B., Flaherty, K.T., Xu, X., Nathanson, K.L. & Nolop, K. (2010). Clinical efficacy of a RAF inhibitor needs broad target blockade in BRAF-mutant melanoma. *Nature*.

Brookes, S., Rowe, J., Ruas, M., Llanos, S., Clark, P.A., Lomax, M., James, M.C., Vatcheva, R., Bates, S., Vousden, K.H., Parry, D., Gruis, N., Smit, N., Bergman, W. & Peters, G. (2002). INK4a-deficient human diploid fibroblasts are resistant to RAS-induced senescence. *Embo J*, 21, 2936-45.

Brummelkamp, T.R., Bernards, R. & Agami, R. (2002). Stable suppression of tumorigenicity by virus-mediated RNA interference. *Cancer Cell*, 243-7.

Burdette-Radoux, S., Tozer, R.G., Lohmann, R.C., Quirt, I., Ernst, D.S., Walsh, W., Wainman, N., Colevas, A.D. & Eisenhauer, E.A. (2004). Phase II trial of flavopiridol, a cyclin dependent kinase inhibitor, in untreated metastatic malignant melanoma. *Invest New Drugs*, 22, 315-22.

Buscher, K., Hahn, S., Hofmann, M., Trefzer, U., Ozel, M., Sterry, W., Lower, J., Lower, R., Kurth, R. & Denner, J. (2006). Expression of the human endogenous retrovirus-K transmembrane envelope, Rec and Np9 proteins in melanomas and melanoma cell lines. *Melanoma Res*, 16, 223-34.

Buscher, K., Trefzer, U., Hofmann, M., Sterry, W., Kurth, R. & Denner, J. (2005). Expression of human endogenous retrovirus K in melanomas and melanoma cell lines. *Cancer Res*, 65, 4172-80.

Carter, A. (2008). Cell fusion theory: can it explain what triggers metastasis? *J Natl Cancer Inst*, 100, 1279-81.

Castellano, M., Pollock, P.M., Walters, M.K., Sparrow, L.E., Down, L.M., Gabrielli, B.G., Parsons, P.G. & Hayward, N.K. (1997). CDKN2A/p16 is inactivated in most melanoma cell lines. *Cancer Res*, 57, 4868-75.

Chang, F., Steelman, L.S., Shelton, J.G., Lee, J.T., Navolanic, P.M., Blalock, W.L., Franklin, R. & McCubrey, J.A. (2003). Regulation of cell cycle progression and apoptosis by the Ras/Raf/MEK/ERK pathway (Review). *Int J Oncol*, 22, 469-80.

Chin, L., Garraway, L.A. & Fisher, D.E. (2006). Malignant melanoma: genetics and therapeutics in the genomic era. *Genes Dev*, 20, 2149-82.

Chin, L., Pomerantz, J., Polsky, D., Jacobson, M., Cohen, C., Cordon-Cardo, C., Horner, J.W., 2nd & DePinho, R.A. (1997). Cooperative effects of INK4a and ras in melanoma susceptibility in vivo. *Genes Dev*, 11, 2822-34.

Clark, W.H., Jr. & Tucker, M.A. (1998). Problems with lesions related to the development of malignant melanoma: common nevi, dysplastic nevi, malignant melanoma in situ, and radial growth phase malignant melanoma. *Hum Pathol*, 29, 8-14.

Coffman, F.D. & Studzinski, G.P. (1999). Differentiation-related mechanisms which suppress DNA replication. *Exp Cell Res*, 248, 58-73.

Collins, N.L., Reginato, M.J., Paulus, J.K., Sgroi, D.C., Labaer, J. & Brugge, J.S. (2005). G1/S cell cycle arrest provides anoikis resistance through Erk-mediated Bim suppression. *Mol Cell Biol*, 25, 5282-91.

Cui, Y., Borysova, M.K., Johnson, J.O. & Guadagno, T.M. (2010). Oncogenic B-Raf(V600E) induces spindle abnormalities, supernumerary centrosomes, and aneuploidy in human melanocytic cells. *Cancer Res*, 70, 675-84.

Curtin, J.A., Fridlyand, J., Kageshita, T., Patel, H.N., Busam, K.J., Kutzner, H., Cho, K.H., Aiba, S., Brocker, E.B., LeBoit, P.E., Pinkel, D. & Bastian, B.C. (2005). Distinct sets of genetic alterations in melanoma. *N Engl J Med*, 353, 2135-47.

Davies, H., Bignell, G.R., Cox, C., Stephens, P., Edkins, S., Clegg, S., Teague, J., Woffendin, H., Garnett, M.J., Bottomley, W., Davis, N., Dicks, E., Ewing, R., Floyd, Y., Gray, K., Hall, S., Hawes, R., Hughes, J., Kosmidou, V., Menzies, A., Mould, C., Parker, A., Stevens, C., Watt, S., Hooper, S., Wilson, R., Jayatilake, H., Gusterson, B.A., Cooper, C., Shipley, J., Hargrave, D., Pritchard-Jones, K., Maitland, N., Chenevix-Trench, G., Riggins, G.J., Bigner, D.D., Palmieri, G., Cossu, A., Flanagan, A., Nicholson, A., Ho, J.W., Leung, S.Y., Yuen, S.T., Weber, B.L., Seigler, H.F., Darrow, T.L., Paterson, H., Marais, R., Marshall, C.J., Wooster, R., Stratton, M.R. & Futreal, P.A. (2002). Mutations of the BRAF gene in human cancer. *Nature*, 417, 949-54.

Delmas, V., Beermann, F., Martinozzi, S., Carreira, S., Ackermann, J., Kumasaka, M., Denat, L., Goodall, J., Luciani, F., Viros, A., Demirkan, N., Bastian, B.C., Goding, C.R. & Larue, L. (2007). Beta-catenin induces immortalization of melanocytes by suppressing p16INK4a expression and cooperates with N-Ras in melanoma development. *Genes Dev*, 21, 2923-35.

Dong, J., Phelps, R.G., Qiao, R., Yao, S., Benard, O., Ronai, Z. & Aaronson, S.A. (2003). BRAF oncogenic mutations correlate with progression rather than initiation of human melanoma. *Cancer Res*, 63, 3883-5.

Dotto, G.P., Moellmann, G., Ghosh, S., Edwards, M. & Halaban, R. (1989). Transformation of murine melanocytes by basic fibroblast growth factor cDNA and oncogenes and selective suppression of the transformed phenotype in a reconstituted cutaneous environment. *J Cell Biol*, 109, 3115-28.

Drayton, S. & Peters, G. (2002). Immortalisation and transformation revisited. *Curr Opin Genet Dev*, 12, 98-104.

Drayton, S., Rowe, J., Jones, R., Vatcheva, R., Cuthbert-Heavens, D., Marshall, J., Fried, M. & Peters, G. (2003). Tumor suppressor p16INK4a determines sensitivity of human cells to transformation by cooperating cellular oncogenes. *Cancer Cell*, 4, 301-10.

Eberle, J., Garbe, C., Wang, N. & Orfanos, C.E. (1995). Incomplete expression of the tyrosinase gene family (tyrosinase, TRP-1, and TRP-2) in human malignant melanoma cells in vitro. *Pigment Cell Res*, 8, 307-13.

Elder, D. (1999). Tumor progression, early diagnosis and prognosis of melanoma. *Acta Oncol*, 38, 535-47.

Englaro, W., Bertolotto, C., Busca, R., Brunet, A., Pages, G., Ortonne, J.P. & Ballotti, R. (1998). Inhibition of the mitogen-activated protein kinase pathway triggers B16 melanoma cell differentiation. *J Biol Chem*, 273, 9966-70.

Fang, D. & Setaluri, V. (1999). Role of microphthalmia transcription factor in regulation of melanocyte differentiation marker TRP-1. *Biochem Biophys Res Commun*, 256, 657-63.

Fargnoli, M.C., Chimenti, S., Keller, G., Soyer, H.P., Dal Pozzo, V., Hofler, H. & Peris, K. (1998). CDKN2a/p16INK4a mutations and lack of p19ARF involvement in familial melanoma kindreds. *J Invest Dermatol*, 111, 1202-6.

Fecher, L.A., Amaravadi, R.K. & Flaherty, K.T. (2008). The MAPK pathway in melanoma. *Curr Opin Oncol*, 20, 183-9.

Flaherty, K.T., Puzanov, I., Kim, K.B., Ribas, A., McArthur, G.A., Sosman, J.A., O'Dwyer, P.J., Lee, R.J., Grippo, J.F., Nolop, K. & Chapman, P.B. (2010). Inhibition of mutated, activated BRAF in metastatic melanoma. *N Engl J Med*, 363, 809-19.

Florenes, V.A., Bhattacharya, N., Bani, M.R., Ben-David, Y., Kerbel, R.S. & Slingerland, J.M. (1996). TGF-beta mediated G1 arrest in a human melanoma cell line lacking p15INK4B: evidence for cooperation between p21Cip1/WAF1 and p27Kip1. *Oncogene*, 13, 2447-57.

Funk, J.O., Schiller, P.I., Barrett, M.T., Wong, D.J., Kind, P. & Sander, C.A. (1998). p16INK4a expression is frequently decreased and associated with 9p21 loss of heterozygosity in sporadic melanoma. *J Cutan Pathol*, 25, 291-6.

Ghiorzo, P., Villaggio, B., Sementa, A.R., Hansson, J., Platz, A., Nicolo, G., Spina, B., Canepa, M., Palmer, J.M., Hayward, N.K. & Bianchi-Scarra, G. (2004). Expression and localization of mutant p16 proteins in melanocytic lesions from familial melanoma patients. *Hum Pathol*, 35, 25-33.

Greenblatt, M.S., Beaudet, J.G., Gump, J.R., Godin, K.S., Trombley, L., Koh, J. & Bond, J.P. (2003). Detailed computational study of p53 and p16: using evolutionary sequence

analysis and disease-associated mutations to predict the functional consequences of allelic variants. *Oncogene*, 22, 1150-63.
Halaban, R. (1999). Melanoma cell autonomous growth: the Rb/E2F pathway. *Cancer Metastasis Rev*, 18, 333-43.
Halaban, R. (2000). The regulation of normal melanocyte proliferation. *Pigment Cell Res*, 13, 4-14.
Halaban, R. (2002). Pigmentation in melanomas: changes manifesting underlying oncogenic and metabolic activities. *Oncol Res*, 13, 3-8.
Halaban, R. (2005). Rb/E2F: a two-edged sword in the melanocytic system. *Cancer Metastasis Rev*, 24, 339-56.
Hanahan, D. & Weinberg, R.A. (2000). The hallmarks of cancer. *Cell*, 100, 57-70.
Harbour, J.W. & Dean, D.C. (2000). Rb function in cell-cycle regulation and apoptosis. *Nat Cell Biol*, 2, E65-7.
Harland, M., Meloni, R., Gruis, N., Pinney, E., Brookes, S., Spurr, N.K., Frischauf, A.M., Bataille, V., Peters, G., Cuzick, J., Selby, P., Bishop, D.T. & Bishop, J.N. (1997). Germline mutations of the CDKN2 gene in UK melanoma families. *Hum Mol Genet*, 6, 2061-7.
Harris, H. (2004). Putting on the brakes. *Nature*, 427, 201.
Henkel, J. (1999). Attacking AIDS with a 'cocktail' therapy? *FDA Consum*, 33, 12-7.
Hingorani, S.R., Jacobetz, M.A., Robertson, G.P., Herlyn, M. & Tuveson, D.A. (2003). Suppression of BRAF(V599E) in human melanoma abrogates transformation. *Cancer Res*, 63, 5198-202.
Hirschl, S., Schanab, O., Seppele, H., Waltenberger, A., Humer, J., Wolff, K., Pehamberger, H. & Muster, T. (2007). Sequence variability of retroviral particles derived from human melanoma cells melanoma-associated retrovirus. *Virus Res*, 123, 211-5.
Hofbauer, G.F., Kamarashev, J., Geertsen, R., Boni, R. & Dummer, R. (1998). Tyrosinase immunoreactivity in formalin-fixed, paraffin-embedded primary and metastatic melanoma: frequency and distribution. *J Cutan Pathol*, 25, 204-9.
Huot, T.J., Rowe, J., Harland, M., Drayton, S., Brookes, S., Gooptu, C., Purkis, P., Fried, M., Bataille, V., Hara, E., Newton-Bishop, J. & Peters, G. (2002). Biallelic mutations in p16(INK4a) confer resistance to Ras- and Ets-induced senescence in human diploid fibroblasts. *Mol Cell Biol*, 22, 8135-43.
Karasarides, M., Chiloeches, A., Hayward, R., Niculescu-Duvaz, D., Scanlon, I., Friedlos, F., Ogilvie, L., Hedley, D., Martin, J., Marshall, C.J., Springer, C.J. & Marais, R. (2004). B-RAF is a therapeutic target in melanoma. *Oncogene*.
Kim, D.S., Park, S.H. & Park, K.C. (2004). Transforming growth factor-beta1 decreases melanin synthesis via delayed extracellular signal-regulated kinase activation. *Int J Biochem Cell Biol*, 36, 1482-91.
Kolch, W. (2000). Meaningful relationships: the regulation of the Ras/Raf/MEK/ERK pathway by protein interactions. *Biochem J*, 351 Pt 2, 289-305.
Krasilnikov, M., Ivanov, V.N., Dong, J. & Ronai, Z. (2003). ERK and PI3K negatively regulate STAT-transcriptional activities in human melanoma cells: implications towards sensitization to apoptosis. *Oncogene*, 22, 4092-101.
Krone, B. & Grange, J.M. (2010). Melanoma, Darwinian medicine and the inner world. *J Cancer Res Clin Oncol*.

Lassam, N. & Bickford, S. (1992). Loss of c-kit expression in cultured melanoma cells. *Oncogene*, 7, 51-6.

Lavie, L., Kitova, M., Maldener, E., Meese, E. & Mayer, J. (2005). CpG methylation directly regulates transcriptional activity of the human endogenous retrovirus family HERV-K(HML-2). *J Virol*, 79, 876-83.

Leszczyniecka, M., Roberts, T., Dent, P., Grant, S. & Fisher, P.B. (2001). Differentiation therapy of human cancer: basic science and clinical applications. *Pharmacol Ther*, 90, 105-56.

Li, J., Xu, M., Yang, Z., Li, A. & Dong, J. (2010a). Simultaneous inhibition of MEK and CDK4 leads to potent apoptosis in human melanoma cells. *Cancer Invest*, 28, 350-6.

Li, Z., Sheng, T., Wan, X., Liu, T., Wu, H. & Dong, J. (2010b). Expression of HERV-K Correlates With Status of MEK-ERK and p16INK4A-CDK4 Pathways in Melanoma Cells. *Cancer Invest*.

Lin, A.W., Barradas, M., Stone, J.C., van, A.L., Serrano, M. & Lowe, S.W. (1998). Premature senescence involving p53 and p16 is activated in response to constitutive MEK/MAPK mitogenic signaling. *Genes Dev*, 12, 3008-19.

Lowe, S.W. & Sherr, C.J. (2003). Tumor suppression by Ink4a-Arf: progress and puzzles. *Curr Opin Genet Dev*, 13, 77-83.

Maddika, S., Ande, S.R., Panigrahi, S., Paranjothy, T., Weglarczyk, K., Zuse, A., Eshraghi, M., Manda, K.D., Wiechec, E. & Los, M. (2007). Cell survival, cell death and cell cycle pathways are interconnected: implications for cancer therapy. *Drug Resist Updat*, 10, 13-29.

Maelandsmo, G.M., Florenes, V.A., Hovig, E., Oyjord, T., Engebraaten, O., Holm, R., Borresen, A.L. & Fodstad, O. (1996). Involvement of the pRb/p16/cdk4/cyclin D1 pathway in the tumorigenesis of sporadic malignant melanomas. *Br J Cancer*, 73, 909-16.

Mangeney, M., Pothlichet, J., Renard, M., Ducos, B. & Heidmann, T. (2005). Endogenous retrovirus expression is required for murine melanoma tumor growth in vivo. *Cancer Res*, 65, 2588-91.

Meier, F., Busch, S., Lasithiotakis, K., Kulms, D., Garbe, C., Maczey, E., Herlyn, M. & Schittek, B. (2007). Combined targeting of MAPK and AKT signalling pathways is a promising strategy for melanoma treatment. *Br J Dermatol*, 156, 1204-13.

Mercer, K.E. & Pritchard, C.A. (2003). Raf proteins and cancer: B-Raf is identified as a mutational target. *Biochim Biophys Acta*, 1653, 25-40.

Mettling, C., Desmetz, C., Fiser, A.L., Reant, B., Corbeau, P. & Lin, Y.L. (2008). Galphai protein-dependant extracellular signal-regulated kinase-1/2 activation is required for HIV-1 reverse transcription. *Aids*, 22, 1569-76.

Michaloglou, C., Vredeveld, L.C., Mooi, W.J. & Peeper, D.S. (2008). BRAF(E600) in benign and malignant human tumours. *Oncogene*, 27, 877-95.

Michaloglou, C., Vredeveld, L.C., Soengas, M.S., Denoyelle, C., Kuilman, T., van der Horst, C.M., Majoor, D.M., Shay, J.W., Mooi, W.J. & Peeper, D.S. (2005). BRAFE600-associated senescence-like cell cycle arrest of human naevi. *Nature*, 436, 720-4.

Montoya-Durango, D.E., Liu, Y., Teneng, I., Kalbfleisch, T., Lacy, M.E., Steffen, M.C. & Ramos, K.S. (2009). Epigenetic control of mammalian LINE-1 retrotransposon by retinoblastoma proteins. *Mutat Res*, 665, 20-8.

Muster, T., Waltenberger, A., Grassauer, A., Hirschl, S., Caucig, P., Romirer, I., Fodinger, D., Seppele, H., Schanab, O., Magin-Lachmann, C., Lower, R., Jansen, B., Pehamberger, H. & Wolff, K. (2003). An endogenous retrovirus derived from human melanoma cells. *Cancer Res*, 63, 8735-41.

Muzeau, F., Flejou, J.F., Thomas, G. & Hamelin, R. (1997). Loss of heterozygosity on chromosome 9 and p16 (MTS1, CDKN2) gene mutations in esophageal cancers. *Int J Cancer*, 72, 27-30.

O'Neill, E.E., Matallanas, D. & Kolch, W. (2005). Mammalian sterile 20-like kinases in tumor suppression: an emerging pathway. *Cancer Res*, 65, 5485-7.

Oricchio, E., Sciamanna, I., Beraldi, R., Tolstonog, G.V., Schumann, G.G. & Spadafora, C. (2007). Distinct roles for LINE-1 and HERV-K retroelements in cell proliferation, differentiation and tumor progression. *Oncogene*, 26, 4226-33.

Panka, D.J., Atkins, M.B. & Mier, J.W. (2006a). Targeting the mitogen-activated protein kinase pathway in the treatment of malignant melanoma. *Clin Cancer Res*, 12, 2371s-2375s.

Panka, D.J., Wang, W., Atkins, M.B. & Mier, J.W. (2006b). The Raf inhibitor BAY 43-9006 (Sorafenib) induces caspase-independent apoptosis in melanoma cells. *Cancer Res*, 66, 1611-9.

Pawelek, J.M. & Chakraborty, A.K. (2008). Fusion of tumour cells with bone marrow-derived cells: a unifying explanation for metastasis. *Nat Rev Cancer*, 8, 377-86.

Pearson, G., Robinson, F., Beers, G.T., Xu, B.E., Karandikar, M., Berman, K. & Cobb, M.H. (2001). Mitogen-activated protein (MAP) kinase pathways: regulation and physiological functions. *Endocr Rev*, 22, 153-83.

Petitjean, A., Mathe, E., Kato, S., Ishioka, C., Tavtigian, S.V., Hainaut, P. & Olivier, M. (2007). Impact of mutant p53 functional properties on TP53 mutation patterns and tumor phenotype: lessons from recent developments in the IARC TP53 database. *Hum Mutat*, 28, 622-9.

Piras, F., Murtas, D., Minerba, L., Ugalde, J., Floris, C., Maxia, C., Colombari, R., Perra, M.T. & Sirigu, P. (2007). Nuclear survivin is associated with disease recurrence and poor survival in patients with cutaneous malignant melanoma. *Histopathology*, 50, 835-42.

Pollock, P.M., Harper, U.L., Hansen, K.S., Yudt, L.M., Stark, M., Robbins, C.M., Moses, T.Y., Hostetter, G., Wagner, U., Kakareka, J., Salem, G., Pohida, T., Heenan, P., Duray, P., Kallioniemi, O., Hayward, N.K., Trent, J.M. & Meltzer, P.S. (2003). High frequency of BRAF mutations in nevi. *Nat Genet*, 33, 19-20.

Polsky, D. & Cordon-Cardo, C. (2003). Oncogenes in melanoma. *Oncogene*, 22, 3087-91.

Pothlichet, J., Mangeney, M. & Heidmann, T. (2006). Mobility and integration sites of a murine C57BL/6 melanoma endogenous retrovirus involved in tumor progression in vivo. *Int J Cancer*, 119, 1869-77.

Poulikakos, P.I. & Rosen, N. (2011). Mutant BRAF melanomas--dependence and resistance. *Cancer Cell*, 19, 11-5.

Powell, M.B., Hyman, P., Bell, O.D., Balmain, A., Brown, K., Alberts, D. & Bowden, G.T. (1995). Hyperpigmentation and melanocytic hyperplasia in transgenic mice expressing the human T24 Ha-ras gene regulated by a mouse tyrosinase promoter. *Mol Carcinog*, 12, 82-90.

Pucci, B., Kasten, M. & Giordano, A. (2000). Cell cycle and apoptosis. *Neoplasia*, 2, 291-9.

Romano, C.M., Ramalho, R.F. & Zanotto, P.M. (2006). Tempo and mode of ERV-K evolution in human and chimpanzee genomes. *Arch Virol*, 151, 2215-28.

Rote, N.S., Chakrabarti, S. & Stetzer, B.P. (2004). The role of human endogenous retroviruses in trophoblast differentiation and placental development. *Placenta*, 25, 673-83.

Rotolo, S., Diotti, R., Gordon, R.E., Qiao, R.F., Yao, Z., Phelps, R.G. & Dong, J. (2005). Effects on proliferation and melanogenesis by inhibition of mutant BRAF and expression of wild-type INK4A in melanoma cells. *Int J Cancer*, 115, 164-9.

Ruas, M. & Peters, G. (1998). The p16INK4a/CDKN2A tumor suppressor and its relatives. *Biochim Biophys Acta*, 1378, F115-77.

Rubinstein, J.C., Sznol, M., Pavlick, A.C., Ariyan, S., Cheng, E., Bacchiocchi, A., Kluger, H.M., Narayan, D. & Halaban, R. (2010). Incidence of the V600K mutation among melanoma patients with BRAF mutations, and potential therapeutic response to the specific BRAF inhibitor PLX4032. *J Transl Med*, 8, 67.

Satyamoorthy, K., Li, G., Gerrero, M.R., Brose, M.S., Volpe, P., Weber, B.L., Van Belle, P., Elder, D.E. & Herlyn, M. (2003). Constitutive mitogen-activated protein kinase activation in melanoma is mediated by both BRAF mutations and autocrine growth factor stimulation. *Cancer Res*, 63, 756-9.

Schmidt, M., Fernandez de Mattos, S., van der Horst, A., Klompmaker, R., Kops, G.J., Lam, E.W., Burgering, B.M. & Medema, R.H. (2002). Cell cycle inhibition by FoxO forkhead transcription factors involves downregulation of cyclin D. *Mol Cell Biol*, 22, 7842-52.

Schmitt, C.A., Fridman, J.S., Yang, M., Lee, S., Baranov, E., Hoffman, R.M. & Lowe, S.W. (2002). A senescence program controlled by p53 and p16INK4a contributes to the outcome of cancer therapy. *Cell*, 109, 335-46.

Sekulic, A., Haluska, P., Jr., Miller, A.J., Genebriera De Lamo, J., Ejadi, S., Pulido, J.S., Salomao, D.R., Thorland, E.C., Vile, R.G., Swanson, D.L., Pockaj, B.A., Laman, S.D., Pittelkow, M.R. & Markovic, S.N. (2008). Malignant melanoma in the 21st century: the emerging molecular landscape. *Mayo Clin Proc*, 83, 825-46.

Serafino, A., Balestrieri, E., Pierimarchi, P., Matteucci, C., Moroni, G., Oricchio, E., Rasi, G., Mastino, A., Spadafora, C., Garaci, E. & Vallebona, P.S. (2009). The activation of human endogenous retrovirus K (HERV-K) is implicated in melanoma cell malignant transformation. *Exp Cell Res*, 315, 849-62.

Setaluri, V. (2003). The melanosome: dark pigment granule shines bright light on vesicle biogenesis and more. *J Invest Dermatol*, 121, 650-60.

Sherr, C.J. (2001). The INK4a/ARF network in tumour suppression. *Nat Rev Mol Cell Biol*, 2, 731-7.

Singh, S., Kaye, S., Gore, M.E., McClure, M.O. & Bunker, C.B. (2009). The role of human endogenous retroviruses in melanoma. *Br J Dermatol*.

Smalley, K.S., Lioni, M., Dalla Palma, M., Xiao, M., Desai, B., Egyhazi, S., Hansson, J., Wu, H., King, A.J., Van Belle, P., Elder, D.E., Flaherty, K.T., Herlyn, M. & Nathanson, K.L. (2008). Increased cyclin D1 expression can mediate BRAF inhibitor resistance in BRAF V600E-mutated melanomas. *Mol Cancer Ther*, 7, 2876-83.

Solit, D.B. & Rosen, N. (2011). Resistance to BRAF inhibition in melanomas. *N Engl J Med*, 364, 772-4.

Sosman, J.A., Moon, J., Tuthill, R.J., Warneke, J.A., Vetto, J.T., Redman, B.G., Liu, P.Y., Unger, J.M., Flaherty, L.E. & Sondak, V.K. (2011). A phase 2 trial of complete resection for stage IV melanoma: Results of Southwest Oncology Group Clinical Trial S9430. *Cancer*.

Sumimoto, H., Miyagishi, M., Miyoshi, H., Yamagata, S., Shimizu, A., Taira, K. & Kawakami, Y. (2004). Inhibition of growth and invasive ability of melanoma by inactivation of mutated BRAF with lentivirus-mediated RNA interference. *Oncogene*.

Taruscio, D. & Mantovani, A. (2004). Factors regulating endogenous retroviral sequences in human and mouse. *Cytogenet Genome Res*, 105, 351-62.

Tawbi, H.A. & Buch, S.C. (2010). Chemotherapy resistance abrogation in metastatic melanoma. *Clin Adv Hematol Oncol*, 8, 259-66.

Tchenio, T. & Heidmann, T. (1991). Defective retroviruses can disperse in the human genome by intracellular transposition. *J Virol*, 65, 2113-8.

Tsukamoto, K., Ueda, M. & Hearing, V.J. (1992). Melanogenesis in murine melanocytes is suppressed by infection with the v-rasHa oncogene. *Pigment Cell Res*, Suppl 2, 181-4.

Turner, G., Barbulescu, M., Su, M., Jensen-Seaman, M.I., Kidd, K.K. & Lenz, J. (2001). Insertional polymorphisms of full-length endogenous retroviruses in humans. *Curr Biol*, 11, 1531-5.

Voisset, C., Weiss, R.A. & Griffiths, D.J. (2008). Human RNA "rumor" viruses: the search for novel human retroviruses in chronic disease. *Microbiol Mol Biol Rev*, 72, 157-96, table of contents.

von, E.F., Werner, G., Theuer, C., Riese, U., Dahse, R., Fiedler, W., Schimmel, B., Ernst, G., Karte, K., Claussen, U. & Wollina, U. (1999). Analysis of the tumor suppressor gene p16(INK4A) in microdissected melanoma metastases by sequencing, and microsatellite and methylation screening. *Arch Dermatol Res*, 291, 474-7.

Wang, X., Gorospe, M., Huang, Y. & Holbrook, N.J. (1997). p27Kip1 overexpression causes apoptotic death of mammalian cells. *Oncogene*, 15, 2991-7.

Waters, S.B., Holt, K.H., Ross, S.E., Syu, L.J., Guan, K.L., Saltiel, A.R., Koretzky, G.A. & Pessin, J.E. (1995). Desensitization of Ras activation by a feedback disassociation of the SOS-Grb2 complex. *J Biol Chem*, 270, 20883-6.

Weber, J. (2011). Immunotherapy for melanoma. *Curr Opin Oncol*, 23, 163-9.

Welch, J., Millar, D., Goldman, A., Heenan, P., Stark, M., Eldon, M., Clark, S., Martin, N.G. & Hayward, N.K. (2001). Lack of genetic and epigenetic changes in CDKN2A in melanocytic nevi. *J Invest Dermatol*, 117, 383-4.

Wellbrock, C., Ogilvie, L., Hedley, D., Karasarides, M., Martin, J., Niculescu-Duvaz, D., Springer, C.J. & Marais, R. (2004). V599EB-RAF is an oncogene in melanocytes. *Cancer Res*, 64, 2338-42.

Widlund, H.R. & Fisher, D.E. (2003). Microphthalamia-associated transcription factor: a critical regulator of pigment cell development and survival. *Oncogene*, 22, 3035-41.

Wilson, R.E., Dooley, T.P. & Hart, I.R. (1989). Induction of tumorigenicity and lack of in vitro growth requirement for 12-O-tetradecanoylphorbol-13-acetate by transfection of murine melanocytes with v-Ha-ras. *Cancer Res*, 49, 711-6.

Wolfel, T., Hauer, M., Schneider, J., Serrano, M., Wolfel, C., Klehmann-Hieb, E., De, P.E., Hankeln, T., Meyer, z.B.K.H. & Beach, D. (1995). A p16INK4a-insensitive CDK4 mutant targeted by cytolytic T lymphocytes in a human melanoma. *Science*, 269, 1281-4.

Yu, B.D., Becker-Hapak, M., Snyder, E.L., Vooijs, M., Denicourt, C. & Dowdy, S.F. (2003). Distinct and nonoverlapping roles for pRB and cyclin D:cyclin-dependent kinases 4/6 activity in melanocyte survival. *Proc Natl Acad Sci U S A*, 100, 14881-6.

Zhang, H., Schneider, J. & Rosdahl, I. (2002). Expression of p16, p27, p53, p73 and Nup88 proteins in matched primary and metastatic melanoma cells. *Int J Oncol*, 21, 43-8.

Zhao, Y., Zhang, Y., Yang, Z., Li, A. & Dong, J. (2008). Simultaneous knockdown of BRAF and expression of INK4A in melanoma cells leads to potent growth inhibition and apoptosis. *Biochem Biophys Res Commun*, 370, 509-13.

Zhu, G., Conner, S.E., Zhou, X., Shih, C., Li, T., Anderson, B.D., Brooks, H.B., Campbell, R.M., Considine, E., Dempsey, J.A., Faul, M.M., Ogg, C., Patel, B., Schultz, R.M., Spencer, C.D., Teicher, B. & Watkins, S.A. (2003). Synthesis, structure-activity relationship, and biological studies of indolocarbazoles as potent cyclin D1-CDK4 inhibitors. *J Med Chem*, 46, 2027-30.

Zhu, J., Woods, D., McMahon, M. & Bishop, J.M. (1998). Senescence of human fibroblasts induced by oncogenic Raf. *Genes Dev*, 12, 2997-3007.

Zhuang, L., Lee, C.S., Scolyer, R.A., McCarthy, S.W., Zhang, X.D., Thompson, J.F. & Hersey, P. (2007). Mcl-1, Bcl-XL and Stat3 expression are associated with progression of melanoma whereas Bcl-2, AP-2 and MITF levels decrease during progression of melanoma. *Mod Pathol*, 20, 416-26.

Zuo, L., Weger, J., Yang, Q., Goldstein, A.M., Tucker, M.A., Walker, G.J., Hayward, N. & Dracopoli, N.C. (1996). Germline mutations in the p16INK4a binding domain of CDK4 in familial melanoma. *Nat Genet*, 12, 97-9.

8

Melanoma Immunomodulation: A War of Attrition

Bently P. Doonan, Jessica D. Hathaway and Azizul Haque
Medical University of South Carolina
United States of America

1. Introduction

Melanoma is an aggressive skin cancer that has an occurrence rate of about 1 in every 50 Americans (Giblin & Thomas, 2007). It is the 6th most common cancer, with a lifetime risk of 2.04% for men and 1.38% for women (Jemal et al., 2008; Jilaveanu et al., 2009). According to the American Cancer Society, in 2009 the number of new cases of melanoma rose to 68,720 with 8,650 new deaths attributed to the disease (ACS, 2010). There are many known factors that contribute to the formation of melanoma. One major factor influencing the increase in melanoma cases is increased exposure to ultra-violet radiation (UVR). Other risk factors include skin type, hair/eye color, the presence of dysplastic nevi and/or increased nevi, and a family history of melanoma (Jilaveanu et al., 2009). Also, mutations in BRAF, CDKN2A, and CDK4 genes have all been attributed to melanoma development. BRAF mutations have been found in 70% of all melanomas and greater than 90% of these mutations carry a single missense (single nucleotide change) mutation (Meyle & Guldberg, 2009). CDKN2A is involved in melanoma pathogenesis and is a germline mutation found in younger patients (Liu et al., 2007). CDK4 is involved in cell-cycle arrest and has been identified in 10% of melanomas (Bennett, 2008). These mutations are mostly detected in non-chronic sun-induced damage melanomas, while chronic sun-induced damage melanomas are more commonly observed.

When melanoma arises, early diagnosis is crucial to survival. With early diagnosis, more than 80% of cases can be treated successfully through surgery (Zhu et al., 2009). This surgery includes excision of the tumor and surrounding tissue; lymph nodes near the tumor may also be removed if evidence of metastasis is present. Other treatments for melanoma include radiation and chemotherapy, used particularly in cases of highly aggressive and metastatic disease (ACS, 2010). Side-effects from these treatments include fatigue, malaise, and an increased susceptibility to non-melanoma cancers (Kamposioras et al., 2010). Also, these therapies are severely toxic to the patients, suggesting a need for improved, less toxic treatment options that specifically target melanoma tumors, like immunotherapy. The multiple ways that melanoma alters the immune system locally, at the site of the tumor, and systemically makes the disease difficult to treat but ideal for the study of immunomodulation (Berinstein, 2009). Immunomodulation, the alteration of the immune system or its function, is exploited in multiple forms by melanoma tumors from changes in the cellular and sub-cellular makeup of the tumor to changes in the tumor microenvironment that suppress localized and systemic attempts at disease reduction.

At the cellular level, melanoma tumors differentially express cytokines, chemokines, and soluble molecules responsible for immunosuppression and tumor proliferation which will be discussed further in this chapter, particularly those with potential for targeting or with therapeutic benefits (Lazar-Molnar et al., 2000). Melanoma cells are also less efficient in antigen (Ag) presentation to CD4+ T cells, reducing immune detection of melanoma tumors and the effectiveness of some immunotherapy strategies (Norton & Haque, 2009). Multiple defects along the HLA class II pathway are present in melanoma cells, the alteration of which could prove useful in novel tumor targeting and immunotherapeutic vaccination strategies. These defects and the potential to overcome them will be further explained in this chapter. Costimulatory molecules are also altered in melanoma cells, reducing positive cellular interaction with T cells and professional antigen presenting cells (APCs), while promoting immunosuppressive interactions through CD28, CTLA-4, and the B7 family of immune inhibitors (Pardee et al., 2009; Wolchok & Saenger, 2008). Study focused on enhancing these secondary stimulation signals would promote complete T cell stimulation and activation of anti-tumor CD8+ T cells, a current goal of most immunotherapy strategies. Melanoma cells are also capable of modulating the surrounding immune cells including: suppression of tumor infiltrating lymphocytes (TILs), enhancement of CD4+CD25+FoxP3+ T regulatory cells (Tregs), increased immature myeloid suppressor cells, increased pro-tumorigenic m2 macrophages, and generation of melanoma-associated fibroblasts (Oble et al., 2009; Camisaschi et al., 2010; Balsamo et al., 2009; Ilkovitch & Lopez, 2008). These topics will be further dissected throughout the chapter as they relate to both immune suppression and multimodal treatment strategies. The course of tumor progression not only adds more problems to immune regulation of the disease, but also more potential targets for therapeutic intervention. Melanoma angiogenesis and metastasis aggravate immune suppression in distinct and specific ways increasing the morbidity and mortality of the disease, while reducing the effectiveness of current treatment options (Schadendorf et al., 2009; Zbytek et al., 2008; Mahabeleshwar & Byzova, 2007). Both of these topics will be further examined with specific emphasis on the relationship between Interleukin (IL)-8, vascular endothelial growth factor (VEGF), the matrix metalloproteinases (MMPs), and the distinct problems faced when tumors metastasize, particularly to lymph nodes, the lungs, liver, and brain (Sloan et al., 2009; Vahrmeijer et al., 2008; Huang et al., 2008; Yang et al., 2009).

Melanoma also represents one of the most widely studied tumors in terms of immunotherapy design, clinical evaluation, and therapeutic application (Jandus et al., 2009). This chapter will discuss the successes and failures of melanoma immunotherapy strategies like IL-2 therapy, melanoma vaccines like canvaxin, and adoptive cell transfer in terms of immunomodulation and its effect on treatment (Atkins, 2006; Goldman & DeFrancesco, 2009). This chapter will also discuss current strategies being developed and potential new directions in treatment that address the immunomodulatory nature of melanoma. These include combined chemoimmunotherapy, melanoma monoclonal antibodies, and multimodal therapy strategies (Kudo-Saito et al., 2005; Ascierto et al., 2010; Flaherty, 2006). The goal of this chapter is to summarize the multiple roadblocks in melanoma treatment associated with the immunomodulation instigated by melanoma tumors. By understanding these issues, novel targets for melanoma therapy can be developed and the shortcomings of current treatment modalities can be enhanced leading to improved patient care and patient outcomes. The fight against melanoma in many ways is a war of attrition: gradual gains can and must be made by making treatment more effective through improved knowledge of the immunomodulatory mechanisms that melanoma tumors employ.

2. The tumor microenvironment

When discussing the ability of melanoma tumors to induce both local and systemic immunomodulation, it is important to first understand the tumor microenvironment itself, and how the alterations at this level affect both tumor progression and limit the effectiveness of some treatment strategies. Melanoma arises through a complex process of cellular mutation and a loss of keratinocyte control over melanocyte growth and differentiation (Hsu et al., 2002; Shirakata, 2010). This imbalance leads to the formation of early stage nevi, appearing localized near the basement membrane of the skin. As malignant melanoma progresses, it develops through interaction between dysfunctional melanocytes and the tumor microenvironment. The progression from nevocellular nevi to dysplastic nevi is accompanied with changes in both keratinocytes and local adhesion molecules allowing for increased melanocyte-melanocyte interaction and the formation of nevocyte nests at the dermal-epidermal junction (Danen et al., 1996; Hsu et al., 2002). Following this development, melanocytes fail to respond to keratinocyte or epidermal cell signaling, they no longer form dendrites, and start to modulate the immune environment through the release of cytokines and immune activation factors which will be described in this chapter (Ilkovitch & Lopez, 2008). Tumors next proceed through two distinct growth phases, radial and vertical growth, accompanied by increased inflammation, immune modulation, and healthy cell destruction. In this sense, the abuse of the immune system drives the progression of disease to a more aggressive phenotype, again through shed factors which will be further explained in this chapter. Finally, following vertical growth through the basement membrane of the dermis following periods of high angiogenesis, melanoma cells are now free to metastasize to local and distant sites resulting in poor disease prognosis (Ria et al., 2010). This section will also focus on the distinct ways melanoma cells respond to the tumor microenvironment during the course of melanoma progression, and how these alterations could be exploited in developing novel melanoma therapies.

2.1 Shed molecules and immunosuppression

At the cellular level, melanoma tumors differentially express cytokines, chemokines, and soluble molecules responsible for immunosuppression and tumor proliferation. Initially, these molecules can have regulatory roles in the tumor microenvironment through growth inhibition, but these functions are lost as tumors slowly progress to a state of localized immune suppression (Lu & Kerbel, 1993). Table 1 is a brief summary of some of the cytokines and growth factors associated with melanoma progression and immunosuppression. A more thorough examination of these factors is expertly presented in a review by Ilkovitch et al (Ilkovitch & Lopez, 2008).

Some cytokines appear to have dual roles within the tumor microenvironment depending on the stage and advancement of disease. During initial tumor formation the inflammatory cytokine IL-6 shed by localized keratinocytes, epithelial, and immune cells inhibits tumor proliferation. IL-6-induced growth inhibitor during early stages of melanoma garnered some attention as an immunological target, but clinical application failed to show any benefit (Lu & Kerbel, 1993). During late stages of disease, IL-6's control of over-growth is lost and autocrine usage of IL-6 produced by melanoma cells actively enhances tumor progression through the STAT3 pathway, which can be further enhanced through interactions with IL-17 (Wang et al., 2004; Hodge et al., 2005; Wang et al., 2009). Elevated STAT3 activity regulates tumor oncogenic factors, cell survival, and cell proliferation

Molecule	Role
IL-1(α and β)	Melanoma derived IL-1α and IL-1β induce fibroblast and endothelial growth factors as well as surface adhesion molecules allowing for the growth and metastasis of melanoma cells, also can stimulate IL-6 production.
IL-6	Initial tumor suppression, then stimulates tumor growth through autocrine regulation by activating Stat3, IL-17 can also be induced in this system further stimulating Stat3.
IL-8	Highly involved in angiogenesis through chemoattraction of infiltrating lymphocytes and cell adhesion regulation.
IL-10	Anti-inflammatory, induces T cell and DC suppression, can be excreted by tumors and by tolerized or regulatory T cells.
IDO	Inhibits T lymphocyte mediated antigen-specific immune responses through suppression of tryptophan, also promotes immune tolerance.
FasL	Melanoma cells lack functional FasL, which prevent FasL interaction with Fas receptor on lymphocytes, and modulate apoptosis induction.
TGF-β	Multiple roles in immunosuppression, can be secreted by melanoma tumors acting in both autocrine and paracrine manner, converts immune cells to suppressive regulatory phenotype.
PGE2	Released from melanoma associated fibroblasts, inhibits NK T cell activity and adds to immunosuppression.

Table 1. Immunomodulatory Molecules Influencing Melanoma Growth

molecules resulting in angiogenesis, tumor growth, and in some cases (i.e. brain) metastasis (Xie et al., 2006). Similarly to IL-6, TGF-β also displays growth inhibitor paracrine function during early stages of disease, and autocrine tumor growth in later stages of progression (Ma et al., 2009; Pardali & Moustakas, 2007).

Anti-inflammatory cytokines and immunomodulatory molecules are often exploited by melanoma cells, most notably IL-10. Melanoma cells, melanoma recruited myeloid suppressor cells, and Tregs actively secrete IL-10 to induce tolerized T cells and dendritic cells (DC) (Huang et al., 1999; Polak et al., 2007). The chemokine IL-8 also plays a major role in melanoma progression, particularly in angiogenesis. Autocrine produced IL-8 can stimulate melanoma growth and induce expression of cellular adhesion molecules allowing for tumor cell migration. The chemoattractant nature of IL-8 also allows for the recruitment of monocytes and macrophages to the tumor site which release growth factors modulating vascular permeability contributing to cell migration. The tumorigenic properties of IL-8 are well summarized by Waugh and Williams (Waugh & Wilson, 2008). Based on these characteristics, targeting IL-8 could reduce the angiogenic nature of melanoma cells allowing for improved clearance of tumors, an area that should be further studied for its therapeutic potential. Additionally, two shed molecules indoleamine-2,3-deoxyginase (IDO) and prostaglandin E2 (PGE2) also contribute to melanoma induced immunosuppression and represent interesting potential targets in immunotherapy design. IDO is produced primarily by suppressive lymphocytes and immature myeloid/dendritic cells. IDO also acts as a tryptophan sink in the tumor microenvironment, severely inhibiting T cell activation (Polak et al., 2007; Honig et al., 2004). Recent study suggests that PGE2 is produced by melanoma-associated fibroblasts and immature myeloid cells and aids in the recruitment of a specific lineage of migratory DC with low cytokine expression profiles (Luft et al., 2002). PGE2 also inhibits NK T cell anti-tumor activity contributing to immunosuppression in the tumor microenvironment (Balsamo et al., 2009). Taken together, these molecules represent hurdles to most immunotherapy strategies employed, which rely on the state of the immune system at the time of treatment to overcome the tumor burden. Steps should be taken to inhibit PGE2 and IDO, as well as the suppressive cytokines mentioned prior to immunotherapy, allowing for a more robust immune response. These cytokines are not solely responsible for the deficiency in current treatment strategies; the cellular makeup of TILs and the melanoma-associated neighboring cells may play major roles in immune subversion.

2.2 Immune cells

As seen in the description of shed molecules, there is dynamic crosstalk between tumors and surrounding tissues and infiltrating immune cells that result in both tumor challenge and in tumor progression. Often, autocrine and paracrine signaling pathways between melanoma cells and surrounding cells contribute to tumor progression and metastasis as reviewed by Lazar-Molnar et al (Lazar-Molnar et al., 2000). The shift from tumor suppression to tumor progression and metastasis results, in part, from the alteration in the type and characteristics of TILs. These changes include the enhancement of $CD4^{+}CD25^{+}FoxP3^{+}$ Tregs, increased immature myeloid suppressor cells, increased pro-tumorigenic m2 macrophages, and the generation of melanoma-associated fibroblasts (Kalluri & Zeisberg, 2006; Mantovani et al., 2002; Almand et al., 2001; Bronte et al., 2001). From a treatment perspective, understanding the alterations in immune cells localized to the tumor site provides both the reason for the failures of some immunotherapy and some novel ways to treat the disease. As stated previously, the progression from healthy melanocyte to melanoma occurs through both mutations within the tumor and through alterations of the cellular environment around the melanoma. In the skin, tissue homeostasis is critical in cellular regulation as well as immune control, and melanoma tumors disrupt this regulation through multiple processes.

Melanoma cells release high levels of basic fibroblast growth factor (bFGF) which results in the generation and localization of melanoma-associated fibroblasts to the tumor microenvironment (Meier et al., 2000). These cells are unlike normal skin fibroblasts in that they proliferate rapidly and eventually outnumber most other cell types within the tumor microenvironment (Li et al., 2003; Lee et al., 2005). They also release molecules that support the growth and movement of melanoma tumors in the extracellular matrix (ECM) of surrounding tissue and affect the function of NK T cells, aiding in immune inhibition (Balsamo et al., 2009). Melanoma tumors also recruit immune suppressor cells such as immature dendritic cells, myeloid derived suppressor/immature myeloid cells, and M2 macrophages (Kusmartsev & Gabrilovich, 2006; Bronte et al., 2001; Hanson et al., 2009). These cells work together releasing immunosuppressive molecules like TGF-β, IL-1α, IDO, IL-10, PGE2, and reactive oxygen species (ROS) (Kusmartsev & Gabrilovich, 2003; Almand et al., 2001; Valenti et al., 2006). Functionally, these cells are deficient in melanoma tumor antigen presentation, resulting in indirect tumor tolerance through interaction with CD8+ T cells (Almand et al., 2001). These factors work against the anti-tumor infiltrating lymphocytes creating a network of immune suppression surrounding the tumor, and through localized inflammation and dysregulation of cell adhesion molecules, they aid in tumor growth, movement, and angiogenesis (Brigati et al., 2002). Thus, targeting these cells in combination with melanoma tumors should improve the efficacy of immunotherapy strategies, such as targeting shared signaling pathways between tumors and surrounding tissue like STAT3 and BRAF/MAPK (Sumimoto et al., 2006; Inamdar et al., 2010).

Figure 1 illustrates the cells melanoma tumors induce for their benefit and the effect that they have on anti-tumor immunity. When discussing melanoma immunosuppression, one cannot leave out the role that T cells play in the tumor microenvironment, in particular the detrimental role of FoxP3+ Tregs, reviewed by Oble et al (Oble et al., 2009). Tregs are normally involved in regulating immune responses to avoid autoimmunity and in reigning in the cytolytic effects of effector CD8+ T cells. They represent the suppressive arm of CD4+ T cells, and are best identified by their high expression of CD25 and FoxP3 (Camisaschi et al., 2010; Vence et al., 2007). In melanoma, particularly in advanced disease states, Tregs are the primary infiltrating lymphocyte where they directly inhibit any cytotoxic antitumor activity through direct contact inhibition, and the release of high levels of IL-10 (Baumgartner et al., 2007). Study suggests that high serum concentrations of Tregs are associated with poor prognosis, poor treatment responses, and an increased risk of recurrence (Vence et al., 2007).

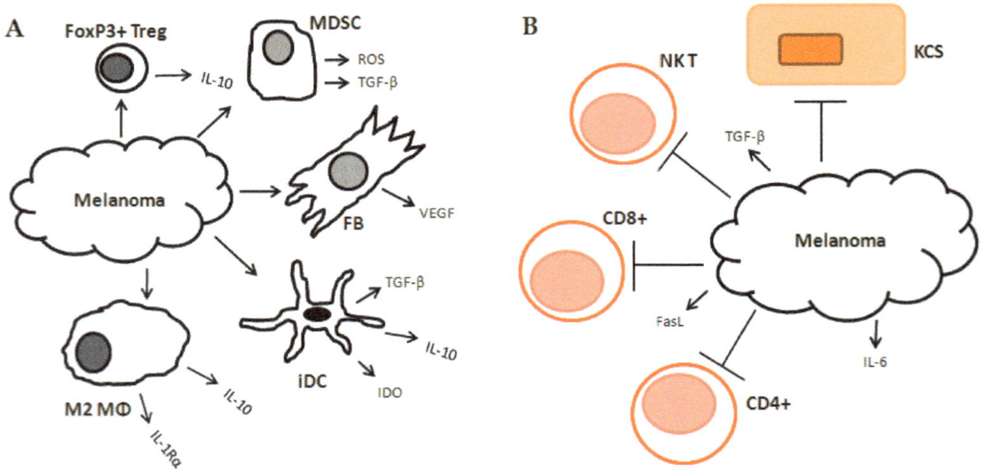

Fig. 1. Microenvironment and immune cell dysfunction. A. Melanoma cells recruit melanoma-associated epithelial and immune cells. These include fibroblasts (FB), immature dendritic cells (iDC), myeloid derived suppressor cells (MDSC), M2 macrophages (M2 MΦ). And CD4+CD25highFoxP3+ T cells (FoxP3+Treg) which release molecules like IL-10, IL-1Rα, IDO, TGF-β, VEGF, and ROS that can inhibit antitumor activity and promote tumor growth. B. Melanoma cells directly interfere with limiting endothelial and immune cells like keratinocytes (KCS), NK T cells (NK T), cytotoxic lymphocytes (CD8+), and CD+ effector cells (CD4+) through the expression of TGF-β, shed and surface FasL, and IL-6.

Tregs are also found in high numbers in sentinel lymph nodes and peripheral blood in cases of metastatic melanoma where they interfere with the expansion of CD8+ and CD4+ effector cells trough IL-2 suppression (Viguier et al., 2004). Study in mice revealed that Treg depletion resulted in the expansion of highly reactive CD8+ T cells resulting in tumor clearance, and in human studies, depleting lymphocytes prior to adoptive cell transfer (ACT) improved the effectiveness of treatment (Mahnke et al., 2007; Matsushita et al., 2008). These results could be associated with the deletion of the large pool of Tregs in the tumor microenvironment and represent an important immunotherapeutic option going forward.

The multiple ways of targeting these immunosuppressive cells in therapy design will be highlighted later in this chapter.

3. Melanoma antigen processing and presentation

In conjunction with these observed deficiencies in the tumor microenvironment leading to immune dysfunction, it is important to understand the direct interplay between melanoma tumors and the immune cells attempting to regulate and destroy tumors. Much focus has been paid to the suppressive nature of Tregs, yet melanoma cells have their own mechanisms of directly inhibiting CD8+ cytotoxic and CD4+ effector T cells (Viguier et al., 2004; Lampen & van Hall, 2011; Norton & Haque, 2009). CD8+ and CD4+ T cells interact with melanoma tumors through contact with HLA class I and HLA class II molecules on their cell surface, respectively. Multiple defects exist in melanoma cells ranging from complete loss of class I and II expression to subversive Ag generation attributed to defects in endosomal/lysosomal machinery. These issues and how they represent novel mechanisms for disease treatment and immunotherapy design will be discussed in this section.

3.1 Antigen processing and presentation

The general consensus when describing immunological strategies against melanoma is in the induction of a cytotoxic immune response mainly generated by the activation of anti-tumor CD8+ T cells. Though CD8+ T cells perform the bulk of the tumor destruction, by focusing solely on activating these cells and not CD4+ T cells, melanoma tumors are capable of devising strategies to avoid CD8+ T cell detection and activation. Clinical evidence supports this notion, as even in patients with advanced disease there are detectable CD8+ T cells specific for melanoma tumor Ag, yet the tumor remains unchallenged (Harlin et al., 2006). This occurs through multiple mechanisms from the immunosuppression described in the previous sections of this chapter, and also through flaws in melanoma Ag processing, presentation, and costimulation. Melanoma tumors have also been shown to downregulate HLA class I surface expression, preventing any T cell activation and tumor clearance (Lopez-Nevot et al., 1988; Cabrera et al., 2007). Tumors also differentially express costimulatory molecules required for complete T cell activation, which will be discussed further in the next section of this chapter. An additional reason for the inability of CD8+ T cells to clear a tumor completely is that there are few to no support signals driving the anti-tumor immune response further following the initial activation and a complete lack of potent antitumor immunological memory. The support signals needed are supposed to come from activated CD4+ effector T cells, differentiated from Tregs by their low CD25 expression and the lack of FoxP3 (Lizee et al., 2006). CD4+ T cells release immune stimulatory cytokines and can directly cross present Ag to professional antigen presenting cells (APCs), driving a complete immune response that can lead to the development of immunological memory. CD4+ T are also crucial as they interact with HLA class II on melanoma tumors which present self tumor Ags (Figure 2). However, melanoma cells are severely hindered in their ability to present endogenous tumor Ags (Goldstein et al., 2008). Although melanoma cells can reduce their HLA class II, studies have shown that detectable levels of surface class II are still present that could be exploited in immunotherapeutic vaccine design.

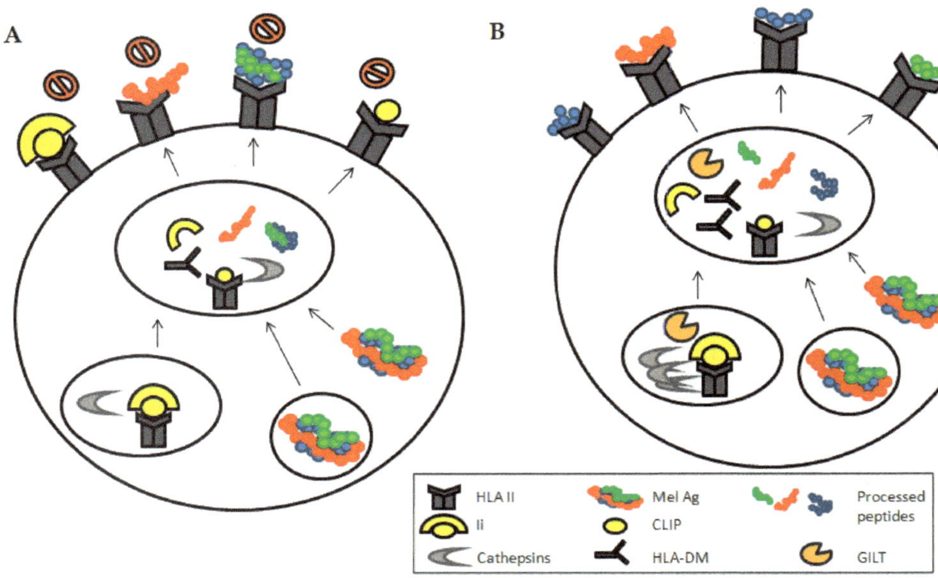

Fig. 2. Defects in HLA class II Ag Processing in Melanoma cells. A. Melanoma cells differentially process endogenous and exogenous Ags in endolysosomal compartments through deficiencies in Ii, HLA-DM, acidic cathepsin activity, and the failure to reduce oxidized peptides. This results in the presentation of a peptide milieu which fails to stimulate interacting CD4+ T cells, limiting the effects of CD8+ antitumor responses. B. The presence of GILT in endolysosomal compartments facilitates increase in both acidic cathepsin processing of tumor Ag and HLA class II components, and the functional processing of cysteinylated or oxidized peptides for improved CD4+ T cell activation.

Melanoma cells also differentially express acidic cathepsins which catalytically process endogenous and exogenous Ags in endolysosomal compartments. The lack of these enzymes or their limited activity results in poor Ag processing and the generation of nonfunctional antigenic determinant(s), that when presented are incapable of stimulating T cells (Goldstein et al., 2008). They also express low levels of HLA-DM, a nonclassical class II molecule responsible for peptide loading onto HLA class II molecules and the removal of the class II-associated invariant chain (Ii) peptide (CLIP) (Norton & Haque, 2009). Without active HLA-DM function, low affinity peptides are loaded onto class II proteins and in some cases CLIP is not removed, the result of which is again poor immune activation (Weber et al., 1996). Melanoma cells also lack an important enzyme, Gamma Interferon-inducible Lysosomal Thiol Reductase (GILT), which is required for the functional reduction of cysteinylated or oxidized proteins and peptides (Haque et al., 2002). Spontaneous cysteinylation of peptides and Ags occurs through the formation of disulfide bonds between cysteine residues or when cysteine residues bind to free floating cysteine in biological fluid (Haque et al., 2002). These peptides display high binding affinity for the HLA class II binding groove, yet they are nonfunctional at CD4+ T cell activation. Figure 2 illustrates some of the defects in HLA class II processing and presentation utilized by melanoma tumors and the ability for GILT induction to improve or reverse some of these deficiencies.

GILT is a lysosomal reductase that is highly expressed in professional APCs, but is absent or expressed at low levels in melanoma (Phan et al., 2002). GILT can be induced in melanoma cells and in other tumor cells when treated with interferon-gamma (IFN-γ) (Goldstein et al., 2008). The expression of GILT in melanoma cells upregulates active forms of cysteinyl and aspartyl cathepsins such as cathepsins S, B, and D; and GILT expression also upregulates the non-classical class II molecule DM (Goldstein et al., 2008). GILT also breaks disulfide bonds within Ags/peptides providing further access for loading and processing by cathepsins (Goldstein et al., 2008). Melanoma cells expressing GILT may be able to efficiently process and present peptides to CD4+ T cells for immunological recognition and elimination of tumors. Unfortunately, the numerous defects illustrated here do not form the complete picture of melanoma immunomodulation in terms of Ag processing. Once functional peptides are loaded into either HLA class I or class II compartments and CD8+ and CD4+ T cells recognize these molecules, a second signal received from costimulatory molecules on the surface of the tumor is needed to activate these immune cells.

3.2 Costimulatory molecules

Surprisingly, melanoma tumors represent immunogenic cancers with various activation of antitumor immunity, yet the natural immune responses are incapable of eradicating the tumor, the reason for which is not fully understood (Pandolfi et al., 2008). A contributing factor to this is the previously mentioned immunosuppressive microenvironment and the altered Ag processing and presentation in melanoma that can stimulate T cells, but not in the same way as APCs which would drive a strong immune response against the tumor. A second factor influencing this inhibition is the lack of, or inhibition of, costimulatory signals required for optimum T cell activation. Following Ag processing and the loading of tumor derived peptides into the HLA class II groove, this complex is translocated to the cell surface for presentation to T cells. CD4+ T cells recognize functional class II complexes with antigenic peptides and tight junction binding occurs between the T cell receptor (TcR) and the class II/Ag complex (Cochran et al., 2000). CD4 molecules on T cells then bind to a different site on the HLA class II molecule and T cells receive their first stimulation signal (Chambers, 2001). A second signal is then required for activation/regulation of the T cell. If the T cells receive a stimulatory signal from the tumor in the form of CD80/CD86 (B7-1/2) binding to T cell expressed CD28, then T cells become activated and mount an antitumor response (Figure 3). However, costimulatory molecules are often modified on melanoma tumor cells inhibiting T cell activation. Melanoma tumors have been shown to express high levels of CTLA-4, a cell surface receptor that also interacts with CD28 but in a regulatory role, inhibiting T cell activation (Weber, 2008). Naturally, this function may inhibit autoimmune conditions, but tumors exploit this process, functionally silencing CD4+ T cell activation and shifting the environment to a T-regulatory setting.

These issues are further compounded by the presence of death receptor ligands on the surface of melanoma tumors (Pilon-Thomas et al., 2010). T cells naturally express programmed death receptors (PD-1) on their cell surface as a limiting factor during T cell activation, sparing healthy "self" cells that may activate these T cells. TIL's have been specifically shown to express higher levels of PD-1 than circulating T cells, a paradigm that is not completely understood (Ahmadzadeh et al., 2009). Study shows that melanoma tumors express high levels of the ligand for PD-1, PD-L, which during TcR-HLA interaction sends a death signal to both CD4+ and CD8+ T cells causing them to undergo apoptosis

(Pilon-Thomas et al., 2010). Melanoma specific-myeloid suppressor cells also express PD-L, further accelerating immunosuppression. Thus, these molecules represent ideal targets in developing improved melanoma immunotherapy strategies which will be discussed further in the following sections, particularly the use of anti-CTLA-4 monoclonal Ab (mAb).

An additional signal worth mentioning is the much debated role of tumor FasL (CD95) (Hallermalm et al., 2004). FasL is a transmembrane protein belonging to the TNF superfamily, which when bound to its receptor induces apoptosis (Hallermalm et al., 2004). Multiple studies have shown melanoma tumors express detectable surface FasL expression both in vivo and in vitro and that this ligand may act as a first line immunosuppressor through inhibiting CTL activity (Shukuwa et al., 2002; Andreola et al., 2002). High surface FasL expression also correlates with poor disease prognosis, but whether this is due to enhanced immune impairment or through an autocrine tolerization against FasL-FasR binding remains unknown (Hallermalm et al., 2004).

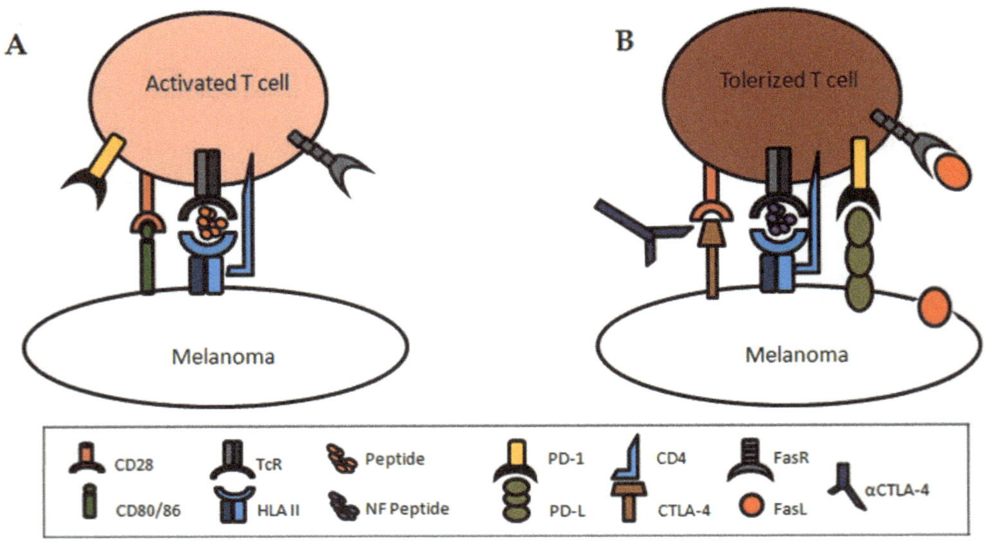

Fig. 3. Costimulatory Signals in Melanoma. A. Complete T cell activation requires binding between HLA class II-Ag complexes with T cell receptors on CD4+ T cells. A second signal between B7-1/2(CD80/86) molecules on melanoma tumors with CD28 on T cells activates CD4+ T cells initiating a robust immune response B. Melanoma cells differentially present oxidized peptides to the TcR which can inhibit T cell activation. They also express high levels of CTLA-4 which preferentially binds CD28 and suppresses T cell function. Blockade of CTLA-4 using mAb can restore immune recognition. Melanoma cells also express programmed death ligands (PD-L) which bind PD-1 on T cells inducing T cell tolerance. In addition, tumors also express surface and secretory FasL which bind FasR on T cells favoring apoptosis.

Study in uveal melanoma has also shown the potential for shed FasL encapsulated in a microvesicle that degranulates in the microenvironment and binds to FasR expression on lymphocytes (Andreola et al., 2002). More research is needed to fully develop this concept, but the targeting of surface FasL on melanoma tumor may improve the immune environment allowing immunotherapy strategies to be more effective. More effective targeting of these factors is also paramount in limiting disease progression before tumors undergo angiogenesis and eventually metastasize, which pose their own issues in targeting the disease.

4. Issues with advanced disease

The previous sections have discussed the immunological concerns with melanoma in the tumor microenvironment and the interplay between the tumor and the immune system. However, the course of tumor progression further complicates this picture as tumors develop microvasculature, migrate to the blood stream, and metastasize to distant sites. Angiogenesis is tightly linked with the vertical growth phase of melanoma; a process which restructures the surrounding environment allowing tumor cells to migrate to the blood stream. This process is accompanied by a shift in the immune environment as infiltrating monocytes and macrophages converge at the site of angiogenesis and are misused by tumor cells to further proliferate. Following angiogenesis, melanoma tumors often metastasize to distant and local sites contributing to the great number of melanoma associated mortality. Once melanoma tumors invade the vasculature and colonize distant sites, new immunologic dysfunction is enacted at the site, further complicating and reducing the efficacy of therapeutic strategies, particularly in the lymph nodes and the brain. This section will further examine the immunological issues presented during angiogenesis and metastasis, and stress the need for new techniques at targeting these processes and how it will require specialized immunotherapy strategies.

4.1 Angiogenesis

As melanoma tumors progress, there is a distinct shift from the radial growth phase to the vertical growth phase which is accompanied by many changes to the cellular and immune environment. This change is also closely linked with angiogenesis. Angiogenesis is the formation of new blood vessels, and is abused and unregulated in advanced melanoma (Mahabeleshwar & Byzova, 2007). Figure 4A shows some of the molecules involved in angiogenesis, and in the switch from radial growth to vertical growth in melanoma tumors. With the formation of new blood vessels and the vertical growth of tumors, an influx of immune cells occurs as a result of shed molecules like IL-8 (Waugh & Wilson, 2008).

As previously discussed, IL-8 as well as IL-6 can act as circulating tumor cell attractants, which can accelerate tumor growth, angiogenesis, and recruitment of other chemo-attractants (Kim et al., 2009). IL-8 signaling has also been shown to increase the transcription of nuclear factor-κB in melanoma, which may be increased through protein kinase C (PKC) activity (Wang & Richmond, 2001). Along with NF-κB, STAT3, and β-catenin, IL-8 indirectly upregulates the activity of AP-1 and mTOR, which are both implicated in cell proliferation, invasion, and cell survival (Karst et al., 2009). VEGF is also linked with IL-8 signaling through its activation by the GPCR of the IL-8 receptor. VEGF is the primary molecule responsible for angiogenesis in both natural and melanoma settings (Srivastava et al., 2003). Melanoma cells have also been shown to utilize VEGF in an autocrine fashion to fuel progression and growth. Tumor-derived molecules like basic fibroblast growth factor (bFGF), placental growth factor (PGF), and platelet derived growth factor (PDGF) aid in melanoma angiogenesis, and may represent potential targets in immunotherapy design (Figure 4). Other angiogenic factors involved in melanoma are the matrix metalloproteinases

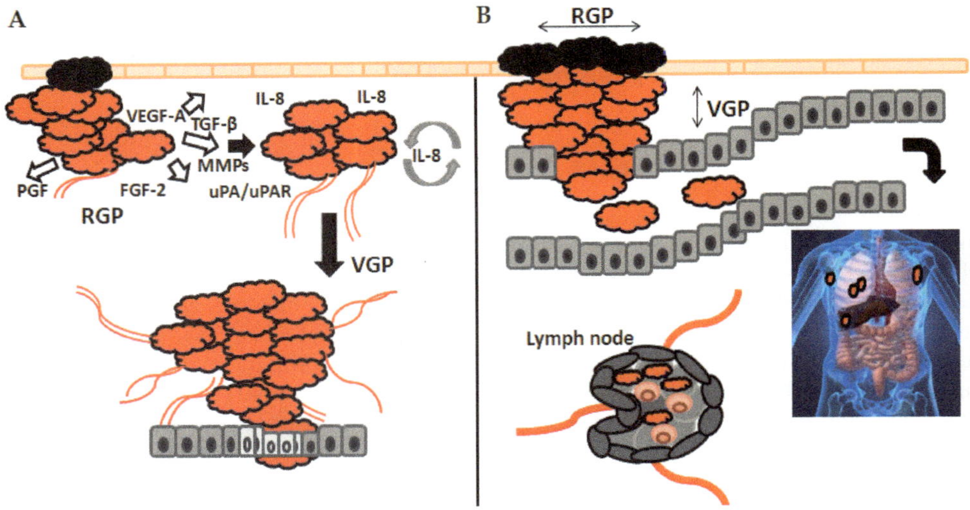

Fig. 4. Angiogenesis and Metastasis in Melanoma. A. Extracellular restructuring molecules are shed by both metastatic tumors and infiltrating bystander cells. These molecules (VEGF, PGF, FGF-2, and MMPs) lead to increased cell-cell contact, movement, and vascularization. The transition into vertical growth phase is then accompanied by increased autocrine IL-8 signaling which supports angiogenesis through recruitment of tissue destabilizing molecules and immune cells. Urokinase plasminogen activator and its receptor (uPA/uPAR) further angiogenesis by promoting cell movement and reorganization of endothelial cells into tube-like structure allowing tumors to reach the blood stream. B. Following RGP and VGP tumors metastasize to colonize distant sites such as sentinel lymph nodes, the lungs, liver and brain by entering the blood stream or through the lymphatic network. Within lymph nodes further immune suppression is induced through high levels of T regs, IL-10, and immature DC.

(MMPs). MMPs are a large group of secreted proteases that are involved in normal physiological and pathologic processes such as embryogenesis, wound healing, angiogenesis, tissue remodeling, tumor invasion, and metastasis (Kondratiev et al., 2008). Within this family of proteins, MMP-2, MMP-9, MMP-13, and MMP-14 have been found in melanoma, and are used as biomarkers for staging (Bosserhoff, 2006; Beshir et al., 2010). MMP-2 and MMP-9 degrade connective tissue and basement membrane collagen, and are believed to play an important role in skin and uveal melanoma progression (Kondratiev et al., 2008; Seftor et al., 2001). During the utilization of these molecules and others, there is localized inflammation occurring with the influx of lymphocytes, monocytes and macrophages. These cells are then activated and secrete TNF-α and IL-1 α in response to the shed VEGF and IL-8, which tumor cells then use in furthering their proliferation (Moldovan, 2002; Moldovan & Moldovan, 2005). In this system, the inhibition of macrophage/monocytes activation could aid in limiting tumor progression and angiogenesis. In an expert review of angiogenesis in melanoma, Ria et al describe the complete angiogenic process, the molecules involved, and the strategies designed to target these factors (Ria et al., 2010). The targeting of these molecules and the inhibition of the pro-tumorigenic influx of immune cells should aid in improving melanoma immunotherapy strategies.

4.2 Metastasis

Following melanoma angiogenesis and the vertical growth of melanoma into localized blood vessels, tumors metastasize to multiple distant sites including lymph nodes, the liver, lungs and brain (Streit & Detmar, 2003; Zbytek et al., 2008). This process has often occurred by the time melanoma is detected clinically, further complicating the treatment of the disease (Murakami et al., 2004). The first site of tumor metastasis is often the sentinel lymph node, which also serves as an important prognostic marker of melanoma progression (Takeuchi et al., 2004; Streit & Detmar, 2003). This progression to sentinel lymph nodes is closely related with angiogenesis, as these sites in metastatic melanoma patients have high expression of VEGF molecules (VEGF-C and VEGF-D) providing the link from tumor progression to metastasis. This process is also further driven by chemoattractive activity of tumor associated lymphatic endothelial cells which may act to draw melanoma cells to the lymph node (Kakinuma & Hwang, 2006; Streit & Detmar, 2003). This activity is a natural means of attracting mature dendritic cells to sentinel lymph nodes, but some melanoma tumors express the same surface receptor (CCR7) as dendritic cells, and are mistakenly drawn to the lymph nodes (Murakami et al., 2004). This is interesting, as targeting this surface receptor may aid in the prevention of melanoma metastasis.

The deregulated immune environment is also responsible for the spread of melanoma tumors from tissue to lymph nodes. The highly immunogenic nature of melanoma and the manipulation of immune cells by tumors, particularly in the development of Tregs, could contribute to the movement to sentinel lymph nodes. Within these lymph nodes, melanoma tumors further suppress the influx of anti-tumor immune cells through the tolerization of DC and the large number of Treg cells accompanying the tumor (Figure 4B) (Shu et al., 2006). As described in the immune cell section of this chapter, these Treg cells in the lymph are now capable of more widespread suppression allowing for the colonization of distant sites by travelling through the lymphoid network as veritable "body guards" surrounding the tumor. Tumors are also capable of traveling through the vascular network to colonize distant sites, which requires surviving the vascular environment, adhering to the desired organ, and invading the desired tissues. These processes are accomplished through upregulation of adhesion molecules on melanoma tumors like integrins allowing for adhesion and passage into distant tissue (Yoshimura et al., 2009).

Melanoma tumors now metastasize to distant sites including the liver, lungs, and brain. Single solitary tumors are effectively cleared through surgery, but multiple metastatic lesions limit surgeries effectiveness. The involvement of major organs represents a sharp decrease in the efficacy of treatment options, and with respect to brain metastasis, accounts for the overwhelming majority of melanoma deaths (Zbytek et al., 2008). Liver metastasis is often seen in cases of uveal melanoma and is treated through chemotherapy and surgery (Vahrmeijer et al., 2008). Unfortunately, unlike other cancers that metastasize to the liver, melanoma metastasis often cannot be resected due to the gross number of tumors and the location of the tumor (Vahrmeijer et al., 2008). Melanoma tumors which metastasize to the lungs often pose the same problems that liver metastases do, in which surgical resection is often impossible, and, to compound problems, brain metastases are often concurrent with lung metastasis, though the lungs are probably colonized first (Fidler et al., 1999). In these unique cases immunotherapy may be considered in place of or in conjunction with chemotherapy. A recent in vitro study on preferential liver metastasis of melanoma showed a correlation between the presence of high integrin 2α on invading tumor cells versus those that did not metastasize to the liver (Yoshimura et al., 2009). Targeting this surface molecule through the use of a monoclonal antibody could then prove useful in inhibiting disease before it progresses to the liver. Lung cancer can pose additional concerns; airway passage epithelial cells, like those found in the lungs, can possess TLR2 surface expression, which in vitro study has shown to be upregulated in metastatic melanoma cell lines (Yang et al., 2009). TLR2 activation can promote an influx of lymphocytes and cytokine production through STAT3 regulated pathways, which we have already mentioned, are deregulated in cases of melanoma. This same study showed that inhibiting TLR2 through the use of an anti-TLR2 antibody inhibited the extent of pulmonary melanoma metastasis, a concept which could prove useful in devising novel immunotherapy strategies (Yang et al., 2009). Despite brain metastasis resulting in the majority of melanoma deaths, relatively little is known about the processes involved in brain metastasis (Sloan et al., 2009). Patients with multiple melanoma brain lesions have few treatment options. When 1-3 brain metastases are present, surgery and stereotactic radiosurgery are routinely performed, but when more metastases are present surgery loses efficacy and response rates to chemotherapy remain low (Sloan et al., 2009; Aboody et al., 2006). Unfortunately, the presence of brain metastasis was often used as an exclusion criterion for immunotherapy trials of metastatic melanoma. Some studies using both biological response modifiers like IL-2/IFNα and cellular immunotherapy employing MART-reactive TIL's have shown some success (Sloan et al., 2009). Given the ability for some immune passage through the blood brain barrier, immunotherapy should be on the forefront of treatment for melanoma brain metastases, yet clinical manifestations of successful immunotherapy remain limited (Sloan et al., 2009).

5. Issues with immunotherapy

In many ways, melanoma represents the gold standard in immunotherapy design and clinical application. Melanoma is a highly immunogenic tumor, and clinical evidence has shown spontaneous regression of primary lesions in a significant number of tumors (Komenaka et al., 2004). This should not be confused with the outlined immunomodulation and immune deficiencies outlined in this chapter, melanoma tumors still evade immune clearance and detection, particularly in advanced metastatic disease. The study of melanoma immunotherapy has existed in some form for the last 30 years, with some major breakthroughs to show for all this hard work (Weber, 2011). In general, immunotherapy refers to any therapeutic intervention designed to stimulate, inhibit, support, or alter the immune system as a means of inducing tumor destruction. Immunotherapy strategies include the use of immunostimulatory cytokine administration like IL-2 and IFNα, adoptive cell transfer (ACT), multiple cancer vaccination strategies, and the use of monoclonal antibodies which target tumor Ag or suppress melanoma derived inhibitory signals (Weber, 2011). Some of the strategies used in a clinical setting are highlighted in Table 2. Surprisingly, with all of this work done, only recently has an immunotherapy shown a survival advantage in patients with advanced disease (Hodi et al., 2010). This section will briefly highlight some of the successes and issues with current immunotherapy, and try to determine how these deficiencies may be overcome. A more complete review of melanoma immunotherapy strategies can also be found from Sivendran et al (Sivendran et al., 2010).

The first immunotherapy strategies to show clinical promise were the immune stimulating cytokines IFNα and IL-2, both receiving FDA approval for the treatment of melanoma in the 1990's, IFNα in the treatment of stage III melanoma with Decarbazine and IL-2 in stage IV

Name	Action	Approval status	Clinical results	Issues
IFN-α (IFN-α2β, PEG-IFN)	Activates and stimulates DC and T cells, while cytotoxic to melanoma through STAT1 activation and STAT3 downregulation.	1995, As adjuvant with surgery or cytotoxic chemotherapy, most notably dacarbazine.	10-15% response rate, useful in cases of limited disease.	As single agent, high toxicity profile, adjuvant therapy has been linked with psychiatric issues like depression and mania.
IL-2 (Proleukin)	Expands and activates T cells, administered in bollus high dose.	1998, Stage IV melanoma.	15% response rate, some patients having durable responses to treatment, when in high dosage treatment regimen.	High toxicity profile. Best results only seen in a small inclusion group with limited disease progression and minimal organ involvement.
Canvaxin (onamelatucel-L)	Antigen-rich, allogeneic whole-cell vaccine.	Phase III trials ended in 2005 due to inefficacy.	Initial clinical trials were promising showing increased overall survival gains of 19 %and 12% in stage III and IV melanoma respectively.	During phase III clinical trails an independent safety reviewed board reveled Canvaxin was no more effective than control arm.
Adoptive cell therapy (ACT-CTL or ACT-TIL therapy)	Patient PBMCs are pulsed in vitro with melanoma peptide/ Ag or stimulatory cytokines and CTL clones are isolated, expanded and injected.	Ongoing clinical trials using pretreatment of lymphodepletion through irradiation or chemotherapy prior to ACT injection.	Response rates have been reported as high as 50%, particularly in large bulk tumor cases when following lymphodepletion .	Lymphodepletion required for efficacy, but all patients can't tolerate.
Ontak (DAB/IL-2, Denileukin Diftitox)	Recombinant IL-2/ diptheria toxin conjugate binds to IL-2R expressing cells depleting these lymphocytes.	Currently in Phase II clinical trial as intervention.	Promising results from phase II trials where lymphodepletion was observed with the formation of anti-melanoma CD8+ T cells.	While it depletes detrimental T reg cells, CD8+ and CD4+ effector cells are also depleted limiting overall efficacy.

Table 2. Issues Associated with Various Melanoma Immunotherapy Strategies

disease (Fang et al., 2008). IL-2 therapy remains the only immunotherapy strategy for late stage melanoma but significant issues remain with its use. IL-2 therapy displays moderate to severe toxicity and relatively low efficacy in patients with non-cutaneous metastasis and metastatic organ involvement (Petrella et al., 2007). Thus, the key to improving IL-2's use in a clinical setting is in the selection of patients receiving treatment. Younger patients who are in good health, with little to no organ metastasis would see the most benefit from IL-2 therapy, and patients with stage II/III tumors may see even greater response to this treatment. Similarly, IFNα displays toxicity similar to cytotoxic drug therapy and this toxicity increases greatly when administered over longer periods of time. Some study also showed a correlation between IFNα and clinical manifestations of depression, mania, and suicidal tendencies (Greenberg et al., 2000). The cause behind these effects is poorly understood, but will remain a concern to monitor with IFNα therapy moving forward. However, the main concern with IFNα is the lack of improvement in overall survival, with only transient gains seen in relapse-free survival (RFS) (Kirkwood et al., 2004). Efforts to combine IFNα with a cancer vaccine strategy were disappointing, but seem to reflect issues in the design and selection of the melanoma vaccine (Kirkwood et al., 2004). The use of IFNα

to boost an antitumor response paired with an effective vaccine or with ACT could still prove beneficial and shouldn't be ruled out in therapeutic design.
Another very promising concept in immunotherapy design which has failed to aid in the clinical setting is melanoma cancer vaccines. These can come in the form of whole cell cancer vaccines, tumor cell lysates, protein/peptide vaccines, DC loaded vaccines, viral vectors, and DNA vaccines (Terando et al., 2007). To date, the largest phase III melanoma vaccine clinical trial involving late stage III and IV melanoma compared the use of CanVaxin with the nonspecific immune stimulator Bacillus Calmette-Guerin (BCG) or BCG alone (Morton et al., 2002). BCG is currently being evaluated in phase III clinical trial administered following surgery versus best standard medical care alone in patients with advanced metastatic disease. CanVaxin is an allogeneic whole cell cancer vaccine using three of the most widely studied melanoma cell lines which encompassed a vast pool of Ag targets and showed great promise during phase II clinical trials.
Unfortunately, an independent safety review board halted the phase III trial when evidence showed no detectable advantage in the treatment arm, virtually stopping CanVaxin in its tracks (Eggermont, 2009). A key issue with the design and application of CanVaxin could be the lack of host Ag presented in the vaccine, given differences between the tumor cell lines used versus the primary tumor. Studies utilizing host-derived irradiated tumor cells instead of cell lines, have shown immune reactivity and limited toxicity, but the time required for their generation remains a concern. These cancer vaccine strategies have been investigated in early clinical trials but the clinical manifestation of strong antitumor T cell activation remains elusive (Goldman & DeFrancesco, 2009). Some efforts to improve the design and application of these vaccines will be further discussed in the next section.
Currently, an immunotherapy strategy with the potential for success is adoptive cell therapy (ACT). As previously mentioned, the highly immunogenic nature of melanoma tumors generates large pools of melanoma reactive CD8+ T cells in vivo, which can be extracted and expanded in vitro. This expansion of patient lymphocytes can be done through stimulation with T cell growth factors like IL-2 or through stimulation with melanoma tumor Ags (Rosenberg et al., 2003). Following expansion, these T cells are then reinjected into patients to attack the tumor. This method has resulted in durable response rates, particularly in stage II/III patients; and in some cases, complete tumor reduction (Rosenberg et al., 2003). However, trials in late stage melanoma failed to show durable tumor clearance, most likely due to the high percentage of Treg cells and immunosuppressive cytokines in the microenvironment (Rosenberg et al., 2008). To combat this, the combination of lymphodepletion with chemotherapy or radiation prior to reinfusion of T cells can greatly improve the response to treatment (Dudley et al., 2008). Unfortunately, lymphodepletion in itself is hazardous to the patient as it destroys both the antitumor CD8+ and CD4+ effector cells along with the Treg cells, and leaves patients vulnerable to bacterial and viral infections (Dudley et al., 2008). Agents capable of specific Treg depletion would aid ACT therapy greatly, and a few molecules in clinical trials potentially fit this need. Ontak (Denileukin Diftitox), a recombinant fusion protein combining IL-2 with Diptheria toxin, binds to IL-2R expressing cells and induces apoptosis through toxin release. It has been shown to deplete Treg cells, resulting in a CD8+ antitumor response in phase II clinical trials (Mahnke et al., 2007). However, CD4+ effector cells were also depleted following Ontak administration, a potentially limiting factor in the long term durable anti-tumor response. The combination then of Ontak with ACT could improve the efficacy of immunotherapy in advanced disease patients, but an important aspect of immune stimulation remains absent from this

therapeutic design: the activation of CD4+ effector T cells. As mentioned previously, CD4+ T cells play an important role in anti-tumor immunity particularly in the presentation of tumor Ags to professional APCs and CD8+ T cells, and in the induction of long-lasting anti-tumor immunological memory (Hung et al., 1998). Therefore, future strategies should aim to activate both CD4+ and CD8+ T cells in ACT therapy design, an idea which will be further explored in the following section.

6. Potential new directions

As highlighted in the previous section, our lack of success in melanoma immunotherapy is not for a lack of effort. With the last thirty years of immunotherapy design and clinical trials we can now apply what we've learned to novel ways of addressing the complex problem of metastatic melanoma. This may include revisiting some previously attempted ideas, but applied within a new context, particularly with what we know about the localized immune inhibition in melanoma patients. This section will discuss current strategies being developed and potential new directions in treatment that address the immunomodulatory nature of melanoma. These include novel chemoimmunotherapy ideas and techniques, the further use of monoclonal antibodies against melanoma Ags and T cell inhibitory factors and finally, on how combining multiple approaches in multimodal immunotherapy design represents a fight on multiple fronts with the potential for increased tumor destruction and disease free survival.

6.1 Chemoimmunotherapy

Therapeutic approaches combining cytotoxic chemotherapy with immunotherapy is not a new concept by any means (LoRusso et al., 1990). In fact, both IFNα and IL-2 have been extensively tested in combination with chemotherapeutics like decarbazine (DTIC), temozolamide, and cisplatin (Schadendorf et al., 2009). Yet, only the pegylated (PEG)-IFNα + DTIC or PEG-IFNα + temozolomide showed enhanced response rates, and all other trials failed to show any significant survival rates (Schadendorf et al., 2009). Moreover, the combination of these molecules increased overall toxicity greater than individual treatment, another limiting factor in the use of combined chemoimmunotherapy (Schadendorf et al., 2009). However, these results only indicate that the combination of two highly cytotoxic agents with limited efficacy in their own right are incapable of enhancing patient survival in highly advanced stages of diseases. Similar approaches should be carefully studied and considered in patients with diminished risk who demonstrate high tolerability to treatment, like the concession currently made for those receiving high dose IL-2 therapy. In selecting the right patient for this therapy, considerable gains may still be made in the combination of these agents. A second approach may be to limit the toxicity of the chemotherapeutic and select a drug with immunostimulatory properties. These molecules may include the highly en vogue antioxidant molecules like green tea extracts, holistic mushroom extracts, and flavinoids, each displaying cytotoxicity in tumor models in vitro with limited toxicity to healthy cells (Baliga & Katiyar, 2006; Harhaji Trajkovic et al., 2009; Craig, 1999). More importantly, these molecules may work synergistically with immune stimulating molecules through enhanced immune activation (Banerjee et al., 2008). Extensive research needs to be performed to ensure similar results in vivo as displayed in vitro, but the combination of these more tolerable antitumor agents with immunostimulatory cytokines may generate increased tumor clearance while reducing the toxic burden to individuals. Similarly, altering the immune cytokine used could aid in the efficacy and reduced toxicity of chemoimmunotherapy.

Cytokines like IL-15, IL-7, and IL-21 could prove more beneficial in stimulating antitumor immune cells during chemotherapy, with reduced toxicity when compared to IL-2 or IFNα (Epardaud et al., 2008; Ribas, 2006). IL-21 has the added benefit of more selective T cell expansion versus IL-2, in which Tregs are not responsive to IL-21 stimulation (Sivendran et al., 2010). Currently IL-21 is being tested in phase I/II clinical trials displaying promising results (Sivendran et al., 2010). IL-15 shares similarity with IL-2 through a shared receptor subunit, but IL-15 has been shown to enhance both ACT and chemotherapy strategies in mouse models with almost no cytokine associated toxicity (Epardaud et al., 2008). Current research performed using IL-15 preconjugated with its receptor (IL-15α) increased both the half life and activity of the cytokine, and improved its ability to destroy advanced solid tumors (Epardaud et al., 2008). Though preliminary, this discovery could prove beneficial in the use of cytokine therapy as both single agent, and in combination with chemotherapeutics to more effectively destroy melanoma. An additional strategy for combined chemoimmunotherapy use is in cancer vaccination design and application. In this case, chemotherapy prior to or concurrent with peptide or DC loaded vaccine techniques could allow for improved efficacy of a single treatment alone. Unfortunately, clinical trials have yet to show significant advantages to combining cytotoxic therapy with vaccine strategies over chemotherapy alone (Lens, 2008). To address this issue, study should incorporate drugs which target progression or metastasis of melanoma in conjunction with immunotherapy as a means of limiting tumor movement and increasing the chances of immune induced tumor clearance. As previously mentioned, Ria et al describe multiple anti-angiogenic drug candidates which could halt the progression of tumors through inhibiting VEGF, VEGFR, tyrosine kinase receptors, integrins, and MMPs (Ria et al., 2010). Combining these inhibitors with immune vaccines to stimulate antitumor immunity or with ACT could allow the reduction of both localized and metastatic tumors.

Currently, the most beneficial chemoimmunotherapy strategy uses lymphodepleting chemotherapeutics (cyclophosphamide and fludarabine) prior to reinjection with expanded TILs and high dose IL-2. This strategy vastly improves the response rate and efficacy of ACT through depletion of Tregs allowing for greater TIL expansion in vivo following reinjection. Unfortunately, lymphodepletion leaves the patient susceptible to both bacterial and viral infection, and is not specific for Tregs; all supportive anti-melanoma CD8+ and CD4+ T cells are also destroyed in the process. Treg-specific reduction prior to ACT represents the gold standard of improved treatment, yet as described previously our best efforts using drugs like Ontak are still shy of clinical relevance (Mahnke et al., 2007). Increased effort needs to be placed on developing Treg specific lymphodepleting chemotherapy, allowing for the full effect of ACT to show clinical benefit. These improvements to chemoimmunotherapy design are not the only potential new directions in melanoma therapy; the most promising option in the near future appears to be the use of monoclonal antibodies in the fight against advanced disease.

6.2 Monoclonal antibodies

Monoclonal antibodies (mAb) have been the focus of much research in cancer since their discovery some thirty plus years ago (Oldham & Dillman, 2008). Though some mAb have been approved to treat other cancers, most notably Trastuzumab (Herceptin) in the treatment of breast cancer, there is only one FDA approved mAb for the treatment of advanced melanoma, ipilimumab (Dillman, 2011). Ipilimumab is one of a number of mAb designed to selectively block CTLA-4 activity in melanoma tumors allowing for the expansion and activation of CD8+ and CD4+ anti-melanoma T cells (Robert & Ghiringhelli, 2009). This chapter previously described the effect high CTLA-4 expression has on melanoma tumors by inhibiting the costimulatory signal needed for T cell activation, shifting the immune response from active to suppressive. Ipilimumab has been tested in clinical trials both as a single agent and in combination with chemotherapy and vaccine strategies (Wolchok et al., 2010; Weber et al., 2009). Recent phase III clinical trials of advanced disease showed, for the first time, a significant survival advantage of patients treated with ipilimumab versus a gp100 vaccine alone, representing a huge breakthrough in these advanced disease patients (Hodi et al., 2010). A larger phase III comparison study using DTIC ± ipilimumab involving more than 500 patients has been performed, the results of which led to the approval of Ipilimumab in the treatment of advanced melanoma on March 25, 2011. Ipilimumab, like any other treatment, is not without issue, as patients undergoing treatment have experienced immune-induced side effects including dermatitis, enterocolitis, hepatitis, and most significantly diarrhea (Sivendran et al., 2010). Some interesting treatment effects have also been observed in a number of patients treated with ipilimumab which will require close attention in determining the best treatment protocol. A number of patients receiving ipilimumab displayed delayed slow ongoing responses lasting a year or more, delayed responses taking up to 6-12 months, and surprisingly, tumor growth and progression followed by tumor regression (Weber, 2011). These interesting effects could lead to the withdrawal from treatment due to the appearance of tumor growth or the delayed response, but these patients need to remain in treatment as the patients who displayed these characteristics often had better disease prognosis than others (Weber, 2011). New immune criteria for the judgment of drug efficacy should be included in determining the best course of patient treatment to avoid issues like these, particularly as ipilimumab has great potential as a combined agent with vaccination and cytotoxic drug therapy, and most interestingly with ACT.

Ipilimumab is not the only mAb targeting advanced disease receiving clinical attention; anti-PD-1, anti-CD137, and anti-CD40 are all undergoing clinical investigation (Sivendran et al., 2010). Anti-PD-1 has shown promise in melanoma cell lines and small phase I/II clinical trials displayed immune activity without major drug associated toxicity, opening the door for its use in combination with other mAb and immunotherapeutic strategies (Brahmer et al., 2010). Clinical trials are ongoing, pairing anti-PD-1 with CTLA-4 blockade or with multiple melanoma peptide vaccine strategies (Curran et al., 2010). Anti-CD137 binds to 4-1BB expressed on activated immune cells sending a costimulatory signal promoting lymphocyte activation (Meseck et al., 2011). In trials using anti-CD137 with GM-CSF-secreting tumor cell immunotherapy induced complete rejection of tumor in a B16 mouse model, displaying proof of principal in melanoma immunotherapy use (Li et al., 2007). Results of a phase I clinical trial revealed antibody activity associated with minimal toxicity in patients with advanced solid-tumor malignancies (Sivendran et al., 2010).

Similarly, anti-CD40 binding with CD40 on the surface of immune cells results in the activation of T cells, and the upregulation of MHC class II complexes and costimulatory molecules, two characteristics we have previously described as being major roadblocks to immunotherapy of advanced melanoma (Law & Grewal, 2009). Anti-CD40 has been tested in advanced solid tumors, refractory Hodgkin lymphoma, and multiple myeloma (French et al., 1999). In melanoma, anti-CD40 seems ideal for combination with protein/peptide vaccine strategies as upregulation of MHC class II complexes and costimulatory molecules would increase the amount of tumor-vaccine interaction and presentation to T cells where increased costimulatory molecules would promote T cell activation instead of suppression or T cell anergy. Future efforts in melanoma mAb design should include the targeting of immunosuppressive cytokines and molecules like those outlined at the start of the chapter as a novel mechanism of enhanced immune activation. These molecules include, but are not limited to, IL-10, TGF-β, PGE2, IDO, and VEGF. Through the targeting and inhibition of these molecules a more immunosupportive tumor microenvironment could increase the efficacy of current and future immunotherapy strategies. Along with cytokine therapy, the use of mAbs in the treatment of metastatic melanoma appear to have the fastest course to clinical use, but the ideal immunotherapeutic strategy would combine these techniques with ACT or vaccination strategies, promoting long-term, sustained immunological anti-tumor responses.

6.3 Multimodal therapy strategies

As outlined in this chapter, melanoma tumors deploy multiple immune evasion techniques to subvert both natural and therapy induced anti-melanoma immune responses, despite the highly immunogenic nature of melanoma tumors. It should then make logical sense that targeting one of these pathways or suppressive mechanisms would incompletely abrogate the problem, as different mechanisms would take over the immunomodulatory duties of melanoma tumors inhibiting the treatments efficacy. Thus, strategies to target melanoma should target multiple suppressive pathways preventing tumors from avoiding single agent strategies. This is accomplished by the administration of multimodal therapy design, in which the combination of therapies enhances the effectiveness of each individual therapy increasing the durability and intensity of the anti-tumor response (Kudo-Saito et al., 2005). Multiple in vitro and melanoma mouse models support the notion of multimodal therapy as a way to completely ablate tumor burden and prevent its recurrence (Ascierto et al., 2010). Clinically, the combination of strategies is not a new method by any means, and even current immunotherapy techniques often combine chemotherapeutic agents with immune cytokines and mAbs for improved treatment (Bhatia et al., 2009). However, in moving forward in the design of improved melanoma therapy, combining multiple immunotherapy strategies like, ACT, gene therapy, DC or peptide vaccines, cytokine therapy, mAb therapy, and novel tumor molecule targeting could represent the future standard of advanced melanoma therapy. Before this ideal can be realized, there are some issues with each technique individually that need to be fixed prior to their combination. Some of these issues we have already mentioned: the inherent toxicity of immune stimulatory cytokine like IL-2 and IFNα, the failures of ACT to fully stimulate long-term anti-tumor immunity, the time required in generating an expanded pool of TIL for ACT therapy, and the inefficacy of vaccine strategies in vivo like those seen with CanVaxin (Berinstein, 2009). The first two issues we have already addressed; the use of less toxic cytokines like IL-7, IL-15/IL-15R, and IL-21 could alleviate toxicity concerns while promoting the expansion of activated immune cells, particularly those which promote immunological memory, and through lymphodepletion prior to ACT expanded lymphocytes are capable of repopulating the immune environment with anti-tumor CD8+ T cells leading to longer efficacy (Dudley et al., 2008). The last two issues are more difficult to solve, but there is hope on the horizon.

The effect that melanoma has on the immune system both hinders our ability to treat the disease, and also allows for treatment like ACT to effectively kill tumors due to the immunogenic nature of melanoma. Unfortunately, only about 50% of melanoma patients have TILs capable of being expanded in vitro for reinjection, a number still much higher than in other cancers where the feat is near impossible (Rosenberg et al., 2008). Further complicating things, the generation of expanded activated TILs takes a few weeks, during which, valuable treatment time is lost for those patients with advanced disease, and with lymphodepletion the chances of an infection increase greatly (Rosenberg et al., 2003). Thus, the ability to expand activated patient TILs from all patients and the rapid generation of anti-tumor lymphocytes would further the effectiveness and clinical application of ACT (Rosenberg, 2001). To achieve this, rapid selection of CD8+ T cells with characteristics predetermined beneficial for anti-tumor immunity can be separated in culture and expanded with administration of anti-CD3 and the presence of feeder cells to increase the activation and expansion rate. Results from this treatment manipulation have shown benefit over previous strategies (Rosenberg et al., 2008). To combat the inability of all patients to generate active TIL, strategies which clone TcRs from activated TIL population into peripheral blood mononuclear cells (PBMCs) of melanoma patients allows for the reinjection of primed anti-tumor lymphocytes without the need for expanded TILs (Weber, 2011). An additional benefit of cloning in these TcRs is that they can be manufactured to express theoretically any melanoma Ag capable of synthetic production, improving the chances of T cell stimulation in vivo through cross-presentation (Robbins et al., 2011). Study using this method has shown benefit in a number of cancers, even in the absence of prior lymphodepletion, further reducing treatment associated toxicity (Robbins et al., 2011).

An additional strategy which should be explored is the expansion of CD4+ effector TIL in the same fashion as CD8+ CTL for combined ACT capable of a more prolonged interaction resulting in increased tumor clearance. These CD4+ TIL can be expanded and raised against patient derived or synthetically generated melanoma Ag, allowing for direct cross-presentation with patient lymphocytes in vivo. This could then lead to the development and support of CD8+ memory T cells, as long as the synthetic Ag is highly immunogenic and replicates the immunodominant HLA matched tumor epitopes. This last point, the ability to present synthesized melanoma Ag capable of stimulating patient immune cells in vivo is also a major issue in vaccine development. As previously mentioned, melanoma vaccine strategies are as varied as they are disappointing in the clinical setting facing issues of inefficacy, inferiority to chemotherapy, and a failure to work in collaboration with other techniques (Berinstein, 2009). Two key issues face melanoma vaccine strategies, the selection of immunogenic tumor associated Ags and the reliance on only CD8+ CTL stimulation in vaccine design, and in many ways these two problems go hand in hand (Sondak et al., 2006). In this chapter, we have highlighted the importance of stimulating CD4+ effector T cells in developing a robust immune response through cross-presentation to CD8+ T cells and other APC, but also for their release of immunostimulatory cytokines like IFNγ (Corthay et al., 2005). Yet, until recently, vaccine strategies (protein/peptide, whole cell, or DC loaded vaccines) have solely used tumor Ags designed for CD8+ CTL activation (Terando et al., 2007). Though these T cells are responsible for the bulk of tumor destruction, time and time again they fail clinically to eradicate host tumors, often due to induced T cell tolerance against these Ags propagated by tumors (Terando et al., 2007). Only through the discovery and application of HLA class II specific anti-tumor melanoma Ags, effector CD4+ T cells may get the much needed stimulation required for a complete T cell response.

Excellent work has been done in the field of HLA class II specific melanoma Ags in recent years, specifically in the identification of an HLA-DR4 restricted Melan-A/Mart-1_{51-73} epitope (RNGYRALMDKSLHVGTQCALTRR) capable of stimulating CD4+ anti-tumor T cells in a number of DR matched patients (Zarour et al., 2000). The identification of Ags like these should be added to patient specific vaccine strategies matching both HLA class I and HLA class II allele specific immunogenic Ags in order to improve the efficacy of melanoma tumor vaccines. A second vaccine strategy which stimulates both CD8+ and CD4+ T cells utilized a natural process of HLA class II peptide presentation in a whole cell cancer vaccine design for enhanced Ag-T cell interaction (Bosch et al., 2010; Thompson et al., 2008). This class II vaccine uses tumor cells genetically modified to express surface class II and costimulatory molecules without expressing invariant chain (Ii). As previously described, Ii blocks the loading of antigenic peptides into the HLA class II peptide binding groove prior to presentation in the endolysosomal compartments (Thompson et al., 2008). By silencing Ii, numerous novel class II peptides are loaded onto the HLA binding groove which would have normally been blocked (Thompson et al., 2008). These peptides may or may not be functionally active, but they do represent peptides which T cells are not tolerant against, allowing for potential T cell activation. The presence of costimulatory molecules on the vaccine-cell surfaces furthers the chance of immune activation, as T cells receive the support signal needed for activation. A third way to generate novel immunogenic peptides for HLA class II presentation, which has been briefly stated, is the induction of GILT into whole cell vaccine strategies. GILT has been shown to increase HLA-DM expression, cysteinyl protease activity, and functionally reduces cysteinylated or oxidized Ags/peptides when transfected into melanoma cells (Goldstein et al., 2008; Rausch et al., 2010). In much the same fashion as the previously described vaccine design, GILT's presence could generate novel immunogenic tumor Ags capable of stimulating CD4+ T cells in vivo. Though early in discovery, techniques like these should be pursued in the improved design of melanoma cancer vaccines. The combination of these improved techniques, with those already described, in a multimodal immunotherapeutic design could then provide the most benefit in terms of long-term tumor free survival. A proposed outline of a multimodal immunotherapy regime is shown in Figure 5.

By first clearing the Tregs from the tumor microenvironment, any immunotherapy strategy will see improved efficacy, similar to those seen in ACT clinical trials (Dudley et al., 2008). ACT TIL therapy utilizing both CD4+ and CD8+ activated and expanded T cells or through the addition of TcR-Ag specific transfected PBMCs are then free to repopulate the immune environment. TIL responses against the tumor should then sustain for much longer than previously observed with the addition of activated CD4+ T cells using HLA class II specific tumor Ags and with concurrent stimulation with mAb against CTLA-4. The patient should then be monitored for response to treatment seen in tumor reduction and by extracting a sample of patient TILs checked for tumor reactivity. The addition of an improved DC loaded vaccine pulsed with processed tumor peptide-GM-CSF fusion protein, like those used in the successful prostate cancer therapeutic Sipuleucel-T (Provenge), could then act as a boost to the anti-tumor TILs present sustaining the development of immunological memory (Brower, 2010). Finally, using less toxic cytokine therapy through IL-15/IL-15R or with IL-7, IL-21 will support the continuation of CD8+ memory T cells and fuel the remaining anti-tumor lymphocytes into attacking the tumor. Though complex, the combination of these procedures would more effectively target the multiple

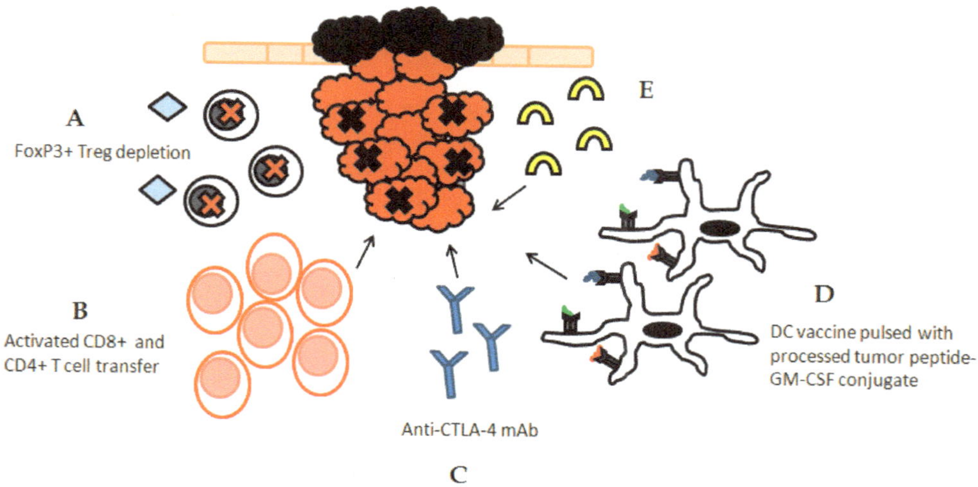

Fig. 5. Multimodal Therapy Design. A. Most of not all immunotherapy strategies should include a means of Treg depletion to prime antitumor immune responses. B. This may come in the form of an adoptive cell therapy (ACT) using autologous TIL's expanded in vitro and pulsed with tumor specific peptides targeting both CD8+ andCD4+ T cells. C. The addition of anti-CTLA-4 mAb could further support these TIL's life and prevent de novo generation of Treg cells D. Following a resting period to limit the chances of autoimmune reactions, concomitant challenge with a dendritic cell vaccine loaded processed tumor peptide and GM-CSF could then further expand the tumor specific immune response of the ACT. E. IL-15a therapy could also be administered during vaccination protocol to stimulate and expand T cell responsive with significantly less toxicity than through IL-2 addition.

immunomodulatory mechanism employed by tumors to evade the immune system. Much work will be needed to bring these theoretical ideals into clinical reality, but through improved understanding of melanoma tumors and their ability to modulate the immune environment, substantial gains can be made in both therapeutic design and patient care.

7. Conclusions

The future looks promising for melanoma immunotherapy, even with the multiple disadvantages that research scientists and clinicians face from the disease. This chapter attempted to summarize the multiple steps of immunomodulation that melanoma tumors employ to thwart even the most well thought out therapy strategies. By understanding both the mechanisms tumors employ to suppress and abuse the immune system and the ways that previous immunotherapy strategies have failed to meet our expectation, we can move forward in devising new strategies in improved immunotherapeutics and disease management. These improved concepts include combining chemotherapy and immunotherapy strategies in new ways to more effectively shift the balance of the tumor microenvironment from immunosuppressive to immunostimulatory prior to immunological intervention, and the targeting of protumorigenic pathways like the BRAF/MAPK and STAT3 pathways to aid in tumor destruction and promote immune responses. Improved understanding of the defective Ag processing and presentation pathways in melanoma presents novel targeting strategies through genetic manipulation of tumors by induction of GILT capable of generating novel immunogenic Ags/peptides. The importance of incorporating strategies to expand and activate both CD8+ and CD4+ T cells will also help in the design and efficacy of ACT, whole-cell, and protein/peptide based vaccine therapy with improved durable immune responses and the development of immunological memory. New cytokine adjuvants like IL-15 and IL-7 may also expand the efficacy of these techniques and aid in the reduction of toxicity seen in IL-2 or IFNα strategies. Monoclonal antibodies like ipilimumab also represent the very near future in melanoma therapy following its recent FDA approval. More strategies combining these molecules with ACT and vaccine strategies should be explored as a means of enhancing the expansion and activation of immune cells and in avoiding immunosuppression induced by melanoma cells. More collaborative efforts need to be made between basic scientists, clinical investigators, and physicians to devise the best way to take discoveries made on the bench into the clinic, particularly in the immunomodulation of melanoma tumors. It appears that for every step we take forward in targeting melanoma, the tumors develop a new suppressive mechanism to avoid our efforts. These deficits must be understood and overcome for immunotherapy to become a true therapeutic option for late stage melanoma patients. As always our best weapon in the fight against melanoma is knowledge, and the collective knowledge gained from understanding melanoma immunomodulation will lead to the next generation of techniques capable of alleviating this deadly disease.

8. Acknowledgements

The authors would like to thank our funding and support provided by the National Cancer Institute (CA129560 and CA129560-S1) to Dr. Azizul Haque. We would also like to thank Drs. Jason God and Laura Kasman for reviewing this chapter.

9. References

Aboody, K. S., J. Najbauer, N. O. Schmidt, W. Yang, J. K. Wu, Y. Zhuge, W. Przylecki, R. Carroll, P. M. Black, and G. Perides. 2006. Targeting of melanoma brain metastases using engineered neural stem/progenitor cells. *Neuro Oncol* 8 (2):119-26.

ACS, American Cancer Society. 2010. Cancer Facts & Figures 2010.4.

Ahmadzadeh, M., L. A. Johnson, B. Heemskerk, J. R. Wunderlich, M. E. Dudley, D. E. White, and S. A. Rosenberg. 2009. Tumor antigen-specific CD8 T cells infiltrating the tumor express high levels of PD-1 and are functionally impaired. *Blood* 114 (8):1537-44.

Almand, B., J. I. Clark, E. Nikitina, J. van Beynen, N. R. English, S. C. Knight, D. P. Carbone, and D. I. Gabrilovich. 2001. Increased production of immature myeloid cells in cancer patients: a mechanism of immunosuppression in cancer. *J Immunol* 166 (1):678-89.

Andreola, G., L. Rivoltini, C. Castelli, V. Huber, P. Perego, P. Deho, P. Squarcina, P. Accornero, F. Lozupone, L. Lugini, A. Stringaro, A. Molinari, G. Arancia, M. Gentile, G. Parmiani, and S. Fais. 2002. Induction of lymphocyte apoptosis by tumor cell secretion of FasL-bearing microvesicles. *J Exp Med* 195 (10):1303-16.

Ascierto, P. A., H. Z. Streicher, and M. Sznol. 2010. Melanoma: a model for testing new agents in combination therapies. *J Transl Med* 8:38.

Atkins, M. B. 2006. Cytokine-based therapy and biochemotherapy for advanced melanoma. *Clin Cancer Res* 12 (7 Pt 2):2353s-2358s.

Baliga, M. S., and S. K. Katiyar. 2006. Chemoprevention of photocarcinogenesis by selected dietary botanicals. *Photochem Photobiol Sci* 5 (2):243-53.

Balsamo, M., F. Scordamaglia, G. Pietra, C. Manzini, C. Cantoni, M. Boitano, P. Queirolo, W. Vermi, F. Facchetti, A. Moretta, L. Moretta, M. C. Mingari, and M. Vitale. 2009. Melanoma-associated fibroblasts modulate NK cell phenotype and antitumor cytotoxicity. *Proc Natl Acad Sci U S A* 106 (49):20847-52.

Banerjee, T., J. B. Duhadaway, P. Gaspari, E. Sutanto-Ward, D. H. Munn, A. L. Mellor, W. P. Malachowski, G. C. Prendergast, and A. J. Muller. 2008. A key in vivo antitumor mechanism of action of natural product-based brassinins is inhibition of indoleamine 2,3-dioxygenase. *Oncogene* 27 (20):2851-7.

Baumgartner, J., C. Wilson, B. Palmer, D. Richter, A. Banerjee, and M. McCarter. 2007. Melanoma induces immunosuppression by up-regulating FOXP3(+) regulatory T cells. *J Surg Res* 141 (1):72-7.

Bennett, D. C. 2008. How to make a melanoma: what do we know of the primary clonal events? *Pigment Cell Melanoma Res* 21 (1):27-38.

Berinstein, N. L. 2009. Strategies to enhance the therapeutic activity of cancer vaccines: using melanoma as a model. *Ann N Y Acad Sci* 1174:107-17.

Beshir, A. B., G. Ren, A. N. Magpusao, L. M. Barone, K. C. Yeung, and G. Fenteany. 2010. Raf kinase inhibitor protein suppresses nuclear factor-kappaB-dependent cancer cell invasion through negative regulation of matrix metalloproteinase expression. *Cancer Lett.*

Bhatia, S., S. S. Tykodi, and J. A. Thompson. 2009. Treatment of metastatic melanoma: an overview. *Oncology (Williston Park)* 23 (6):488-96.

Bosch, J. J., U. K. Iheagwara, S. Reid, M. K. Srivastava, J. Wolf, M. Lotem, B. R. Ksander, and S. Ostrand-Rosenberg. 2010. Uveal melanoma cell-based vaccines express MHC II molecules that traffic via the endocytic and secretory pathways and activate CD8(+) cytotoxic, tumor-specific T cells. *Cancer Immunol Immunother* 59 (1):103-12.

Bosserhoff, A. K. 2006. Novel biomarkers in malignant melanoma. *Clin Chim Acta* 367 (1-2):28-35.

Brahmer, J. R., C. G. Drake, I. Wollner, J. D. Powderly, J. Picus, W. H. Sharfman, E. Stankevich, A. Pons, T. M. Salay, T. L. McMiller, M. M. Gilson, C. Wang, M. Selby, J. M. Taube, R. Anders, L. Chen, A. J. Korman, D. M. Pardoll, I. Lowy, and S. L. Topalian. 2010. Phase I study of single-agent anti-programmed death-1 (MDX-1106) in refractory solid tumors: safety, clinical activity, pharmacodynamics, and immunologic correlates. *J Clin Oncol* 28 (19):3167-75.

Brigati, C., D. M. Noonan, A. Albini, and R. Benelli. 2002. Tumors and inflammatory infiltrates: friends or foes? *Clin Exp Metastasis* 19 (3):247-58.

Bronte, V., P. Serafini, E. Apolloni, and P. Zanovello. 2001. Tumor-induced immune dysfunctions caused by myeloid suppressor cells. *J Immunother* 24 (6):431-46.

Brower, V. 2010. Approval of provenge seen as first step for cancer treatment vaccines. *J Natl Cancer Inst* 102 (15):1108-10.

Cabrera, T., E. Lara, J. M. Romero, I. Maleno, L. M. Real, F. Ruiz-Cabello, P. Valero, F. M. Camacho, and F. Garrido. 2007. HLA class I expression in metastatic melanoma correlates with tumor development during autologous vaccination. *Cancer Immunol Immunother* 56 (5):709-17.

Camisaschi, C., C. Casati, F. Rini, M. Perego, A. De Filippo, F. Triebel, G. Parmiani, F. Belli, L. Rivoltini, and C. Castelli. 2010. LAG-3 expression defines a subset of CD4(+)CD25(high)Foxp3(+) regulatory T cells that are expanded at tumor sites. *J Immunol* 184 (11):6545-51.

Chambers, C. A. 2001. The expanding world of co-stimulation: the two-signal model revisited. *Trends Immunol* 22 (4):217-23.

Cochran, J. R., T. O. Cameron, and L. J. Stern. 2000. The relationship of MHC-peptide binding and T cell activation probed using chemically defined MHC class II oligomers. *Immunity* 12 (3):241-50.

Corthay, A., D. K. Skovseth, K. U. Lundin, E. Rosjo, H. Omholt, P. O. Hofgaard, G. Haraldsen, and B. Bogen. 2005. Primary antitumor immune response mediated by CD4+ T cells. *Immunity* 22 (3):371-83.

Craig, W. J. 1999. Health-promoting properties of common herbs. *Am J Clin Nutr* 70 (3 Suppl):491S-499S.

Curran, M. A., W. Montalvo, H. Yagita, and J. P. Allison. 2010. PD-1 and CTLA-4 combination blockade expands infiltrating T cells and reduces regulatory T and myeloid cells within B16 melanoma tumors. *Proc Natl Acad Sci U S A* 107 (9):4275-80.

Danen, E. H., T. J. de Vries, R. Morandini, G. G. Ghanem, D. J. Ruiter, and G. N. van Muijen. 1996. E-cadherin expression in human melanoma. *Melanoma Res* 6 (2):127-31.

Dillman, R. O. 2011. Cancer immunotherapy. *Cancer Biother Radiopharm* 26 (1):1-64.

Dudley, M. E., J. C. Yang, R. Sherry, M. S. Hughes, R. Royal, U. Kammula, P. F. Robbins, J. Huang, D. E. Citrin, S. F. Leitman, J. Wunderlich, N. P. Restifo, A. Thomasian, S. G. Downey, F. O. Smith, J. Klapper, K. Morton, C. Laurencot, D. E. White, and S. A. Rosenberg. 2008. Adoptive cell therapy for patients with metastatic melanoma: evaluation of intensive myeloablative chemoradiation preparative regimens. *J Clin Oncol* 26 (32):5233-9.

Eggermont, A. M. 2009. Immunostimulation versus immunosuppression after multiple vaccinations: the woes of therapeutic vaccine development. *Clin Cancer Res* 15 (22):6745-7.

Epardaud, M., K. G. Elpek, M. P. Rubinstein, A. R. Yonekura, A. Bellemare-Pelletier, R. Bronson, J. A. Hamerman, A. W. Goldrath, and S. J. Turley. 2008. Interleukin-15/interleukin-15R alpha complexes promote destruction of established tumors by reviving tumor-resident CD8+ T cells. *Cancer Res* 68 (8):2972-83.

Fang, L., A. S. Lonsdorf, and S. T. Hwang. 2008. Immunotherapy for advanced melanoma. *J Invest Dermatol* 128 (11):2596-605.

Fidler, I. J., G. Schackert, R. D. Zhang, R. Radinsky, and T. Fujimaki. 1999. The biology of melanoma brain metastasis. *Cancer Metastasis Rev* 18 (3):387-400.

Flaherty, K. T. 2006. Chemotherapy and targeted therapy combinations in advanced melanoma. *Clin Cancer Res* 12 (7 Pt 2):2366s-2370s.

French, R. R., H. T. Chan, A. L. Tutt, and M. J. Glennie. 1999. CD40 antibody evokes a cytotoxic T-cell response that eradicates lymphoma and bypasses T-cell help. *Nat Med* 5 (5):548-53.

Giblin, A. V., and J. M. Thomas. 2007. Incidence, mortality and survival in cutaneous melanoma. *J Plast Reconstr Aesthet Surg* 60 (1):32-40.

Goldman, B., and L. DeFrancesco. 2009. The cancer vaccine roller coaster. *Nat Biotechnol* 27 (2):129-39.

Goldstein, O. G., L. M. Hajiaghamohseni, S. Amria, K. Sundaram, S. V. Reddy, and A. Haque. 2008. Gamma-IFN-inducible-lysosomal thiol reductase modulates acidic proteases and HLA class II antigen processing in melanoma. *Cancer Immunol Immunother* 57 (10):1461-70.

Greenberg, D. B., E. Jonasch, M. A. Gadd, B. F. Ryan, J. R. Everett, A. J. Sober, M. A. Mihm, K. K. Tanabe, M. Ott, and F. G. Haluska. 2000. Adjuvant therapy of melanoma with interferon-alpha-2b is associated with mania and bipolar syndromes. *Cancer* 89 (2):356-62.

Hallermalm, K., A. De Geer, R. Kiessling, V. Levitsky, and J. Levitskaya. 2004. Autocrine secretion of Fas ligand shields tumor cells from Fas-mediated killing by cytotoxic lymphocytes. *Cancer Res* 64 (18):6775-82.

Hanson, E. M., V. K. Clements, P. Sinha, D. Ilkovitch, and S. Ostrand-Rosenberg. 2009. Myeloid-derived suppressor cells down-regulate L-selectin expression on CD4+ and CD8+ T cells. *J Immunol* 183 (2):937-44.

Haque, M. A., P. Li, S. K. Jackson, H. M. Zarour, J. W. Hawes, U. T. Phan, M. Maric, P. Cresswell, and J. S. Blum. 2002. Absence of gamma-interferon-inducible lysosomal thiol reductase in melanomas disrupts T cell recognition of select immunodominant epitopes. *J Exp Med* 195 (10):1267-77.

Harhaji Trajkovic, L. M., S. A. Mijatovic, D. D. Maksimovic-Ivanic, I. D. Stojanovic, M. B. Momcilovic, S. J. Tufegdzic, V. M. Maksimovic, Z. S. Marjanovic, and S. D. Stosic-Grujicic. 2009. Anticancer properties of Ganoderma lucidum methanol extracts in vitro and in vivo. *Nutr Cancer* 61 (5):696-707.

Harlin, H., T. V. Kuna, A. C. Peterson, Y. Meng, and T. F. Gajewski. 2006. Tumor progression despite massive influx of activated CD8(+) T cells in a patient with malignant melanoma ascites. *Cancer Immunol Immunother* 55 (10):1185-97.

Hodge, D. R., E. M. Hurt, and W. L. Farrar. 2005. The role of IL-6 and STAT3 in inflammation and cancer. *Eur J Cancer* 41 (16):2502-12.

Hodi, F. S., S. J. O'Day, D. F. McDermott, R. W. Weber, J. A. Sosman, J. B. Haanen, R. Gonzalez, C. Robert, D. Schadendorf, J. C. Hassel, W. Akerley, A. J. van den Eertwegh, J. Lutzky, P. Lorigan, J. M. Vaubel, G. P. Linette, D. Hogg, C. H. Ottensmeier, C. Lebbe, C. Peschel, I. Quirt, J. I. Clark, J. D. Wolchok, J. S. Weber, J. Tian, M. J. Yellin, G. M. Nichol, A. Hoos, and W. J. Urba. 2010. Improved Survival with Ipilimumab in Patients with Metastatic Melanoma. *N Engl J Med.*

Honig, A., L. Rieger, M. Kapp, M. Sutterlin, J. Dietl, and U. Kammerer. 2004. Indoleamine 2,3-dioxygenase (IDO) expression in invasive extravillous trophoblast supports role of the enzyme for materno-fetal tolerance. *J Reprod Immunol* 61 (2):79-86.

Hsu, M. Y., F. Meier, and M. Herlyn. 2002. Melanoma development and progression: a conspiracy between tumor and host. *Differentiation* 70 (9-10):522-36.

Huang, F. J., P. S. Steeg, J. E. Price, W. T. Chiu, P. C. Chou, K. Xie, R. Sawaya, and S. Huang. 2008. Molecular basis for the critical role of suppressor of cytokine signaling-1 in melanoma brain metastasis. *Cancer Res* 68 (23):9634-42.

Huang, S., S. E. Ullrich, and M. Bar-Eli. 1999. Regulation of tumor growth and metastasis by interleukin-10: the melanoma experience. *J Interferon Cytokine Res* 19 (7):697-703.

Hung, K., R. Hayashi, A. Lafond-Walker, C. Lowenstein, D. Pardoll, and H. Levitsky. 1998. The central role of CD4(+) T cells in the antitumor immune response. *J Exp Med* 188 (12):2357-68.

Ilkovitch, D., and D. M. Lopez. 2008. Immune modulation by melanoma-derived factors. *Exp Dermatol* 17 (12):977-85.

Inamdar, G. S., S. V. Madhunapantula, and G. P. Robertson. 2010. Targeting the MAPK pathway in melanoma: why some approaches succeed and other fail. *Biochem Pharmacol* 80 (5):624-37.

Jandus, C., D. Speiser, and P. Romero. 2009. Recent advances and hurdles in melanoma immunotherapy. *Pigment Cell Melanoma Res* 22 (6):711-23.

Jemal, A., R. Siegel, E. Ward, Y. Hao, J. Xu, T. Murray, and M. J. Thun. 2008. Cancer statistics, 2008. *CA Cancer J Clin* 58 (2):71-96.

Jilaveanu, L. B., S. A. Aziz, and H. M. Kluger. 2009. Chemotherapy and biologic therapies for melanoma: do they work? *Clin Dermatol* 27 (6):614-25.

Kakinuma, T., and S. T. Hwang. 2006. Chemokines, chemokine receptors, and cancer metastasis. *J Leukoc Biol* 79 (4):639-51.

Kalluri, R., and M. Zeisberg. 2006. Fibroblasts in cancer. *Nat Rev Cancer* 6 (5):392-401.

Kamposioras, K., G. Pentheroudakis, D. Pectasides, and N. Pavlidis. 2010. Malignant melanoma of unknown primary site. To make the long story short. A systematic review of the literature. *Crit Rev Oncol Hematol*.

Karst, A. M., K. Gao, C. C. Nelson, and G. Li. 2009. Nuclear factor kappa B subunit p50 promotes melanoma angiogenesis by upregulating interleukin-6 expression. *Int J Cancer* 124 (2):494-501.

Kim, S. H., D. H. Kim, P. Lavender, J. H. Seo, Y. S. Kim, J. S. Park, S. J. Kwak, and Y. K. Jee. 2009. Repression of TNF-alpha-induced IL-8 expression by the glucocorticoid receptor-beta involves inhibition of histone H4 acetylation. *Exp Mol Med* 41 (5):297-306.

Kirkwood, J. M., J. Manola, J. Ibrahim, V. Sondak, M. S. Ernstoff, and U. Rao. 2004. A pooled analysis of eastern cooperative oncology group and intergroup trials of adjuvant high-dose interferon for melanoma. *Clin Cancer Res* 10 (5):1670-7.

Komenaka, I., H. Hoerig, and H. L. Kaufman. 2004. Immunotherapy for melanoma. *Clin Dermatol* 22 (3):251-65.

Kondratiev, S., D. R. Gnepp, E. Yakirevich, E. Sabo, D. J. Annino, E. Rebeiz, and N. V. Laver. 2008. Expression and prognostic role of MMP2, MMP9, MMP13, and MMP14 matrix metalloproteinases in sinonasal and oral malignant melanomas. *Hum Pathol* 39 (3):337-43.

Kudo-Saito, C., J. Schlom, K. Camphausen, C. N. Coleman, and J. W. Hodge. 2005. The requirement of multimodal therapy (vaccine, local tumor radiation, and reduction of suppressor cells) to eliminate established tumors. *Clin Cancer Res* 11 (12):4533-44.

Kusmartsev, S., and D. I. Gabrilovich. 2003. Inhibition of myeloid cell differentiation in cancer: the role of reactive oxygen species. *J Leukoc Biol* 74 (2):186-96.

Kusmartsev, S., and D. I. Gabrilovich. 2006. Role of immature myeloid cells in mechanisms of immune evasion in cancer. *Cancer Immunol Immunother* 55 (3):237-45.

Lampen, M. H., and T. van Hall. 2011. Strategies to counteract MHC-I defects in tumors. *Curr Opin Immunol.*

Law, C. L., and I. S. Grewal. 2009. Therapeutic interventions targeting CD40L (CD154) and CD40: the opportunities and challenges. *Adv Exp Med Biol* 647:8-36.

Lazar-Molnar, E., H. Hegyesi, S. Toth, and A. Falus. 2000. Autocrine and paracrine regulation by cytokines and growth factors in melanoma. *Cytokine* 12 (6):547-54.

Lee, J., M. Fassnacht, S. Nair, D. Boczkowski, and E. Gilboa. 2005. Tumor immunotherapy targeting fibroblast activation protein, a product expressed in tumor-associated fibroblasts. *Cancer Res* 65 (23):11156-63.

Lens, M. 2008. The role of vaccine therapy in the treatment of melanoma. *Expert Opin Biol Ther* 8 (3):315-23.

Li, B., J. Lin, M. Vanroey, M. Jure-Kunkel, and K. Jooss. 2007. Established B16 tumors are rejected following treatment with GM-CSF-secreting tumor cell immunotherapy in combination with anti-4-1BB mAb. *Clin Immunol* 125 (1):76-87.

Li, G., K. Satyamoorthy, F. Meier, C. Berking, T. Bogenrieder, and M. Herlyn. 2003. Function and regulation of melanoma-stromal fibroblast interactions: when seeds meet soil. *Oncogene* 22 (20):3162-71.

Liu, J., K. G. Suresh Kumar, D. Yu, S. A. Molton, M. McMahon, M. Herlyn, A. Thomas-Tikhonenko, and S. Y. Fuchs. 2007. Oncogenic BRAF regulates beta-Trcp expression and NF-kappaB activity in human melanoma cells. *Oncogene* 26 (13):1954-8.

Lizee, G., L. G. Radvanyi, W. W. Overwijk, and P. Hwu. 2006. Improving antitumor immune responses by circumventing immunoregulatory cells and mechanisms. *Clin Cancer Res* 12 (16):4794-803.

Lopez-Nevot, M. A., E. Garcia, C. Romero, M. R. Oliva, S. Serrano, and F. Garrido. 1988. Phenotypic and genetic analysis of HLA class I and HLA-DR antigen expression on human melanomas. *Exp Clin Immunogenet* 5 (4):203-12.

LoRusso, P. M., S. L. Aukerman, L. Polin, B. G. Redman, M. Valdivieso, L. Biernat, and T. H. Corbett. 1990. Antitumor efficacy of interleukin-2 alone and in combination with adriamycin and dacarbazine in murine solid tumor systems. *Cancer Res* 50 (18):5876-82.

Lu, C., and R. S. Kerbel. 1993. Interleukin-6 undergoes transition from paracrine growth inhibitor to autocrine stimulator during human melanoma progression. *J Cell Biol* 120 (5):1281-8.

Luft, T., M. Jefford, P. Luetjens, T. Toy, H. Hochrein, K. A. Masterman, C. Maliszewski, K. Shortman, J. Cebon, and E. Maraskovsky. 2002. Functionally distinct dendritic cell (DC) populations induced by physiologic stimuli: prostaglandin E(2) regulates the migratory capacity of specific DC subsets. *Blood* 100 (4):1362-72.

Ma, Y. M., T. Sun, Y. X. Liu, N. Zhao, Q. Gu, D. F. Zhang, S. Qie, C. S. Ni, Y. Liu, and B. C. Sun. 2009. A pilot study on acute inflammation and cancer: a new balance between IFN-gamma and TGF-beta in melanoma. *J Exp Clin Cancer Res* 28:23.

Mahabeleshwar, G. H., and T. V. Byzova. 2007. Angiogenesis in melanoma. *Semin Oncol* 34 (6):555-65.

Mahnke, K., K. Schonfeld, S. Fondel, S. Ring, S. Karakhanova, K. Wiedemeyer, T. Bedke, T. S. Johnson, V. Storn, S. Schallenberg, and A. H. Enk. 2007. Depletion of CD4+CD25+ human regulatory T cells in vivo: kinetics of Treg depletion and alterations in immune functions in vivo and in vitro. *Int J Cancer* 120 (12):2723-33.

Mantovani, A., S. Sozzani, M. Locati, P. Allavena, and A. Sica. 2002. Macrophage polarization: tumor-associated macrophages as a paradigm for polarized M2 mononuclear phagocytes. *Trends Immunol* 23 (11):549-55.

Matsushita, N., S. A. Pilon-Thomas, L. M. Martin, and A. I. Riker. 2008. Comparative methodologies of regulatory T cell depletion in a murine melanoma model. *J Immunol Methods* 333 (1-2):167-79.

Meier, F., M. Nesbit, M. Y. Hsu, B. Martin, P. Van Belle, D. E. Elder, G. Schaumburg-Lever, C. Garbe, T. M. Walz, P. Donatien, T. M. Crombleholme, and M. Herlyn. 2000. Human melanoma progression in skin reconstructs : biological significance of bFGF. *Am J Pathol* 156 (1):193-200.

Meseck, M., T. Huang, G. Ma, G. Wang, S. H. Chen, and S. L. Woo. 2011. A functional recombinant human 4-1BB ligand for immune costimulatory therapy of cancer. *J Immunother* 34 (2):175-82.

Meyle, K. D., and P. Guldberg. 2009. Genetic risk factors for melanoma. *Hum Genet* 126 (4):499-510.

Moldovan, L., and N. I. Moldovan. 2005. Role of monocytes and macrophages in angiogenesis. *EXS* (94):127-46.

Moldovan, N. I. 2002. Role of monocytes and macrophages in adult angiogenesis: a light at the tunnel's end. *J Hematother Stem Cell Res* 11 (2):179-94.

Morton, D. L., E. C. Hsueh, R. Essner, L. J. Foshag, S. J. O'Day, A. Bilchik, R. K. Gupta, D. S. Hoon, M. Ravindranath, J. A. Nizze, G. Gammon, L. A. Wanek, H. J. Wang, and R. M. Elashoff. 2002. Prolonged survival of patients receiving active immunotherapy with Canvaxin therapeutic polyvalent vaccine after complete resection of melanoma metastatic to regional lymph nodes. *Ann Surg* 236 (4):438-48; discussion 448-9.

Murakami, T., A. R. Cardones, and S. T. Hwang. 2004. Chemokine receptors and melanoma metastasis. *J Dermatol Sci* 36 (2):71-8.

Norton, D. L., and A. Haque. 2009. Insights into the Role of GILT in HLA Class II Antigen Processing and Presentation by Melanoma. *J Oncol* 2009:142959.

Oble, D. A., R. Loewe, P. Yu, and M. C. Mihm, Jr. 2009. Focus on TILs: prognostic significance of tumor infiltrating lymphocytes in human melanoma. *Cancer Immun* 9:3.

Oldham, R. K., and R. O. Dillman. 2008. Monoclonal antibodies in cancer therapy: 25 years of progress. *J Clin Oncol* 26 (11):1774-7.

Pandolfi, F., R. Cianci, S. Lolli, I. S. Dunn, E. E. Newton, T. J. Haggerty, L. A. Boyle, and J. T. Kurnick. 2008. Strategies to overcome obstacles to successful immunotherapy of melanoma. *Int J Immunopathol Pharmacol* 21 (3):493-500.

Pardali, K., and A. Moustakas. 2007. Actions of TGF-beta as tumor suppressor and pro-metastatic factor in human cancer. *Biochim Biophys Acta* 1775 (1):21-62.

Pardee, A. D., A. K. Wesa, and W. J. Storkus. 2009. Integrating costimulatory agonists to optimize immune-based cancer therapies. *Immunotherapy* 1 (2):249-64.

Petrella, T., I. Quirt, S. Verma, A. E. Haynes, M. Charette, and K. Bak. 2007. Single-agent interleukin-2 in the treatment of metastatic melanoma. *Curr Oncol* 14 (1):21-6.

Phan, U. T., R. L. Lackman, and P. Cresswell. 2002. Role of the C-terminal propeptide in the activity and maturation of gamma -interferon-inducible lysosomal thiol reductase (GILT). *Proc Natl Acad Sci U S A* 99 (19):12298-303.

Pilon-Thomas, S., A. Mackay, N. Vohra, and J. J. Mule. 2010. Blockade of programmed death ligand 1 enhances the therapeutic efficacy of combination immunotherapy against melanoma. *J Immunol* 184 (7):3442-9.

Polak, M. E., N. J. Borthwick, F. G. Gabriel, P. Johnson, B. Higgins, J. Hurren, D. McCormick, M. J. Jager, and I. A. Cree. 2007. Mechanisms of local immunosuppression in cutaneous melanoma. *Br J Cancer* 96 (12):1879-87.

Rausch, M. P., K. R. Irvine, P. A. Antony, N. P. Restifo, P. Cresswell, and K. T. Hastings. 2010. GILT accelerates autoimmunity to the melanoma antigen tyrosinase-related protein 1. *J Immunol* 185 (5):2828-35.

Ria, R., A. Reale, A. Castrovilli, G. Mangialardi, F. Dammacco, D. Ribatti, and A. Vacca. 2010. Angiogenesis and progression in human melanoma. *Dermatol Res Pract* 2010:185687.

Ribas, A. 2006. Update on immunotherapy for melanoma. *J Natl Compr Canc Netw* 4 (7):687-94.

Robbins, P. F., R. A. Morgan, S. A. Feldman, J. C. Yang, R. M. Sherry, M. E. Dudley, J. R. Wunderlich, A. V. Nahvi, L. J. Helman, C. L. Mackall, U. S. Kammula, M. S. Hughes, N. P. Restifo, M. Raffeld, C. C. Lee, C. L. Levy, Y. F. Li, M. El-Gamil, S. L. Schwarz, C. Laurencot, and S. A. Rosenberg. 2011. Tumor Regression in Patients With Metastatic Synovial Cell Sarcoma and Melanoma Using Genetically Engineered Lymphocytes Reactive With NY-ESO-1. *J Clin Oncol* 29 (7):917-24.

Robert, C., and F. Ghiringhelli. 2009. What is the role of cytotoxic T lymphocyte-associated antigen 4 blockade in patients with metastatic melanoma? *Oncologist* 14 (8):848-61.

Rosenberg, S. A. 2001. Progress in the development of immunotherapy for the treatment of patients with cancer. *J Intern Med* 250 (6):462-75.

Rosenberg, S. A., N. P. Restifo, J. C. Yang, R. A. Morgan, and M. E. Dudley. 2008. Adoptive cell transfer: a clinical path to effective cancer immunotherapy. *Nat Rev Cancer* 8 (4):299-308.

Rosenberg, S. A., J. C. Yang, P. F. Robbins, J. R. Wunderlich, P. Hwu, R. M. Sherry, D. J. Schwartzentruber, S. L. Topalian, N. P. Restifo, A. Filie, R. Chang, and M. E. Dudley. 2003. Cell transfer therapy for cancer: lessons from sequential treatments of a patient with metastatic melanoma. *J Immunother* 26 (5):385-93.

Schadendorf, D., S. M. Algarra, L. Bastholt, G. Cinat, B. Dreno, A. M. Eggermont, E. Espinosa, J. Guo, A. Hauschild, T. Petrella, J. Schachter, and P. Hersey. 2009. Immunotherapy of distant metastatic disease. *Ann Oncol* 20 Suppl 6:vi41-50.

Seftor, R. E., E. A. Seftor, N. Koshikawa, P. S. Meltzer, L. M. Gardner, M. Bilban, W. G. Stetler-Stevenson, V. Quaranta, and M. J. Hendrix. 2001. Cooperative interactions of laminin 5 gamma2 chain, matrix metalloproteinase-2, and membrane type-1-

matrix/metalloproteinase are required for mimicry of embryonic vasculogenesis by aggressive melanoma. *Cancer Res* 61 (17):6322-7.

Shirakata, Y. 2010. Regulation of epidermal keratinocytes by growth factors. *J Dermatol Sci*.

Shu, S., A. J. Cochran, R. R. Huang, D. L. Morton, and H. T. Maecker. 2006. Immune responses in the draining lymph nodes against cancer: implications for immunotherapy. *Cancer Metastasis Rev* 25 (2):233-42.

Shukuwa, T., I. Katayama, and T. Koji. 2002. Fas-mediated apoptosis of melanoma cells and infiltrating lymphocytes in human malignant melanomas. *Mod Pathol* 15 (4):387-96.

Sivendran, S., B. Glodny, M. Pan, M. Merad, and Y. Saenger. 2010. Melanoma immunotherapy. *Mt Sinai J Med* 77 (6):620-42.

Sloan, A. E., C. J. Nock, and D. B. Einstein. 2009. Diagnosis and treatment of melanoma brain metastasis: a literature review. *Cancer Control* 16 (3):248-55.

Sondak, V. K., M. S. Sabel, and J. J. Mule. 2006. Allogeneic and autologous melanoma vaccines: where have we been and where are we going? *Clin Cancer Res* 12 (7 Pt 2):2337s-2341s.

Srivastava, A., R. Ralhan, and J. Kaur. 2003. Angiogenesis in cutaneous melanoma: pathogenesis and clinical implications. *Microsc Res Tech* 60 (2):208-24.

Streit, M., and M. Detmar. 2003. Angiogenesis, lymphangiogenesis, and melanoma metastasis. *Oncogene* 22 (20):3172-9.

Sumimoto, H., F. Imabayashi, T. Iwata, and Y. Kawakami. 2006. The BRAF-MAPK signaling pathway is essential for cancer-immune evasion in human melanoma cells. *J Exp Med* 203 (7):1651-6.

Takeuchi, H., D. L. Morton, C. Kuo, R. R. Turner, D. Elashoff, R. Elashoff, B. Taback, A. Fujimoto, and D. S. Hoon. 2004. Prognostic significance of molecular upstaging of paraffin-embedded sentinel lymph nodes in melanoma patients. *J Clin Oncol* 22 (13):2671-80.

Terando, A. M., M. B. Faries, and D. L. Morton. 2007. Vaccine therapy for melanoma: current status and future directions. *Vaccine* 25 Suppl 2:B4-16.

Thompson, J. A., M. K. Srivastava, J. J. Bosch, V. K. Clements, B. R. Ksander, and S. Ostrand-Rosenberg. 2008. The absence of invariant chain in MHC II cancer vaccines enhances the activation of tumor-reactive type 1 CD4+ T lymphocytes. *Cancer Immunol Immunother* 57 (3):389-98.

Vahrmeijer, A. L., C. J. van de Velde, H. H. Hartgrink, and R. A. Tollenaar. 2008. Treatment of melanoma metastases confined to the liver and future perspectives. *Dig Surg* 25 (6):467-72.

Valenti, R., V. Huber, P. Filipazzi, L. Pilla, G. Sovena, A. Villa, A. Corbelli, S. Fais, G. Parmiani, and L. Rivoltini. 2006. Human tumor-released microvesicles promote the differentiation of myeloid cells with transforming growth factor-beta-mediated suppressive activity on T lymphocytes. *Cancer Res* 66 (18):9290-8.

Vence, L., A. K. Palucka, J. W. Fay, T. Ito, Y. J. Liu, J. Banchereau, and H. Ueno. 2007. Circulating tumor antigen-specific regulatory T cells in patients with metastatic melanoma. *Proc Natl Acad Sci U S A* 104 (52):20884-9.

Viguier, M., F. Lemaitre, O. Verola, M. S. Cho, G. Gorochov, L. Dubertret, H. Bachelez, P. Kourilsky, and L. Ferradini. 2004. Foxp3 expressing CD4+CD25(high) regulatory T

cells are overrepresented in human metastatic melanoma lymph nodes and inhibit the function of infiltrating T cells. *J Immunol* 173 (2):1444-53.
Wang, D., and A. Richmond. 2001. Nuclear factor-kappa B activation by the CXC chemokine melanoma growth-stimulatory activity/growth-regulated protein involves the MEKK1/p38 mitogen-activated protein kinase pathway. *J Biol Chem* 276 (5):3650-9.
Wang, L., T. Yi, M. Kortylewski, D. M. Pardoll, D. Zeng, and H. Yu. 2009. IL-17 can promote tumor growth through an IL-6-Stat3 signaling pathway. *J Exp Med* 206 (7):1457-64.
Wang, T., G. Niu, M. Kortylewski, L. Burdelya, K. Shain, S. Zhang, R. Bhattacharya, D. Gabrilovich, R. Heller, D. Coppola, W. Dalton, R. Jove, D. Pardoll, and H. Yu. 2004. Regulation of the innate and adaptive immune responses by Stat-3 signaling in tumor cells. *Nat Med* 10 (1):48-54.
Waugh, D. J., and C. Wilson. 2008. The interleukin-8 pathway in cancer. *Clin Cancer Res* 14 (21):6735-41.
Weber, D. A., B. D. Evavold, and P. E. Jensen. 1996. Enhanced dissociation of HLA-DR-bound peptides in the presence of HLA-DM. *Science* 274 (5287):618-20.
Weber, J. 2011. Immunotherapy for melanoma. *Curr Opin Oncol* 23 (2):163-9.
Weber, J. S. 2008. Tumor evasion may occur via expression of regulatory molecules: a case for CTLA-4 in melanoma. *J Invest Dermatol* 128 (12):2750-2.
Weber, J., J. A. Thompson, O. Hamid, D. Minor, A. Amin, I. Ron, R. Ridolfi, H. Assi, A. Maraveyas, D. Berman, J. Siegel, and S. J. O'Day. 2009. A randomized, double-blind, placebo-controlled, phase II study comparing the tolerability and efficacy of ipilimumab administered with or without prophylactic budesonide in patients with unresectable stage III or IV melanoma. *Clin Cancer Res* 15 (17):5591-8.
Wolchok, J. D., B. Neyns, G. Linette, S. Negrier, J. Lutzky, L. Thomas, W. Waterfield, D. Schadendorf, M. Smylie, T. Guthrie, Jr., J. J. Grob, J. Chesney, K. Chin, K. Chen, A. Hoos, S. J. O'Day, and C. Lebbe. 2010. Ipilimumab monotherapy in patients with pretreated advanced melanoma: a randomised, double-blind, multicentre, phase 2, dose-ranging study. *Lancet Oncol* 11 (2):155-64.
Wolchok, J. D., and Y. Saenger. 2008. The mechanism of anti-CTLA-4 activity and the negative regulation of T-cell activation. *Oncologist* 13 Suppl 4:2-9.
Xie, T. X., F. J. Huang, K. D. Aldape, S. H. Kang, M. Liu, J. E. Gershenwald, K. Xie, R. Sawaya, and S. Huang. 2006. Activation of stat3 in human melanoma promotes brain metastasis. *Cancer Res* 66 (6):3188-96.
Yang, H. Z., B. Cui, H. Z. Liu, S. Mi, J. Yan, H. M. Yan, F. Hua, H. Lin, W. F. Cai, W. J. Xie, X. X. Lv, X. X. Wang, B. M. Xin, Q. M. Zhan, and Z. W. Hu. 2009. Blocking TLR2 activity attenuates pulmonary metastases of tumor. *PLoS One* 4 (8):e6520.
Yoshimura, K., K. F. Meckel, L. S. Laird, C. Y. Chia, J. J. Park, K. L. Olino, R. Tsunedomi, T. Harada, N. Iizuka, S. Hazama, Y. Kato, J. W. Keller, J. M. Thompson, F. Chang, L. H. Romer, A. Jain, C. Iacobuzio-Donahue, M. Oka, D. M. Pardoll, and R. D. Schulick. 2009. Integrin alpha2 mediates selective metastasis to the liver. *Cancer Res* 69 (18):7320-8.
Zarour, H. M., J. M. Kirkwood, L. S. Kierstead, W. Herr, V. Brusic, C. L. Slingluff, Jr., J. Sidney, A. Sette, and W. J. Storkus. 2000. Melan-A/MART-1(51-73) represents an immunogenic HLA-DR4-restricted epitope recognized by melanoma-reactive CD4(+) T cells. *Proc Natl Acad Sci U S A* 97 (1):400-5.

Zbytek, B., J. A. Carlson, J. Granese, J. Ross, M. C. Mihm, and A. Slominski. 2008. Current concepts of metastasis in melanoma. *Expert Rev Dermatol* 3 (5):569-585.

Zhu, S., H. Wurdak, Y. Wang, A. Galkin, H. Tao, J. Li, C. A. Lyssiotis, F. Yan, B. P. Tu, L. Miraglia, J. Walker, F. Sun, A. Orth, P. G. Schultz, and X. Wu. 2009. A genomic screen identifies TYRO3 as a MITF regulator in melanoma. *Proc Natl Acad Sci U S A* 106 (40):17025-30.

9

Promising Experimental Therapies for Metastatic Melanoma

Bao Lam, Patrick A. Ott and Anna C. Pavlick
New York University School of Medicine
USA

1. Introduction

Advanced melanoma has the highest per-death loss of years of potential life expectancy second only to adult leukemia. The incidence of melanoma continues to rise worldwide at approximately 3% per year, and in 2009 there were an estimated 68,720 new cases in the United States and 8650 deaths (Balch et al. 2009). According to Surveillance Epidemiology and End Results (SEER) data, roughly 4% of melanomas are metastatic at time of diagnosis. Locally advanced or recurrent unresectable, and disseminated melanoma is notoriously unresponsive to standard treatment, and is associated with a dismal prognosis. Patients with metastatic melanoma have a median survival of 8 months and 2-year survival rates of 10% to 15%. (Tsao et al. 2004). Until March of 2011, only 2 drugs were approved by the Food and Drug Administration (FDA) in the United States (US) for metastatic melanoma: interleukin 2 (IL-2) and dacarbazine (ipilimumab was approved in March of 2011 and will be discussed in this chapter). Dacarbazine is an alkalyting agent that in 1975 became the first chemotherapeutic drug approved by the US FDA for metastatic melanoma. Response rates for this regimen were 20% in a 30-year overview (Serrone et al. 2000), whereas more recent studies showed response rates in the 10-14% range (Bedikian et al. 2006; Chapman et al. 1999; Middleton et al. 2000). Temozolomide, an orally available congener of dacarbazine, was shown to be non-inferior in efficacy in comparison to dacarbazine in a randomized phase III trial (Middleton et al. 2000). Temozolomide had a similar objective response rate and overall survival compared to dacarbazine, and a significantly longer disease free survival. IL-2 was approved by the US FDA in 1998 for the treatment of metastatic melanoma. Single agent IL-2, when given in high dose intravenous boluses, leads to objective responses in 16% of patients, with complete responses in 6% and partial responses in 10%. Many patients maintained a complete response even after 7 years follow-up (Atkins et al. 2000). The toxicities of high dose IL-2 are substantial, including constitutional symptoms (fevers, chills, fatigue), hypotension, renal insufficiency, emesis, diarrhea and thrombocytopenia, and up to 2% of mortality is directly related to the treatment (Atkins et al. 2000). A systemic review of 41 randomized clinical trials including patients receiving various treatment schedules including biochemotherapy did not show improved progression-free survival (PFS) or overall survival (OS) (Eigentler et al. 2003). More recently, another meta-analysis of 18 trials involving nearly 2,500 patients with metastatic melanoma suggested an increase in response rate to biochemotherapy, but overall survival was not improved (Ives et al. 2007). Until today, biochemotherapy and combination chemotherapy built upon IL-2 and dacarbazine or temozolomide has not shown statistically significant improvement in overall survival and cannot be regarded as standard therapeutic options for metastatic melanoma. Thus, more effective treatment modalities are urgently needed.

2. Agents targeting the immune system

2.1 CTLA-4

Increasing knowledge of T-cell regulation has uncovered potential immunologic targets for the treatment of melanoma. The interaction between antigen-presenting cells (APC) and T lymphocytes is crucial for inducing melanoma-specific T-cell responses. In addition to the antigen specific interaction between the HLA peptide complex on the APC and the T-cell receptor (TCR), several different co-stimulatory and co-inhibitory molecules modulate the T cell response. For instance, the T-cell surface molecule CD28 interacts with the B7 receptor on the APC to mediate a co-stimulatory signal (which is necessary in addition to the HLA-peptide-TCR interaction for efficient priming of the T cell), whereas the T-cell cytotoxic T-lymphocyte antigen (CTLA)-4 interacts with B7 to downregulate T-cell activation, acting as a natural "checkpoint" on the T-cell mediated immunologic response. Blocking interaction between CTLA-4 and B7 can overcome this checkpoint and enhance T-cell-mediated antitumor activity. This can be achieved by an anti-CTLA-4 monoclonal antibody (mAb). To date, two fully human anti-CTLA-4 mAb's have been developed for metastatic melanoma: tremelimumab (CP-675,206; Pfizer Inc., New York) and ipilimumab (MDX-010; Bristol-Myers, New Jersey).

In the initial phase I study, tremelimumab was relatively well tolerated and demonstrated encouraging clinical activity including several complete responses. However, in a randomized phase III study comparing single-agent tremelimumab with either dacarbazine or temozolomide in patients with advanced melanoma, tremelimumab failed to demonstrate a significant improvement in OS in comparison to standard chemotherapy (Ribas 2008). On the other hand, ipilimumab, in a randomized phase III clinical trial comparing ipilimumab alone versus gp100 vaccine alone to the combination of ipilimumab and gp100 vaccine, resulted in improved OS of nearly four months (median survival duration of 10.1 and 10.0 months in the ipilimumab arm and the combined arm, respectively, in comparison to 6.4 months in the vaccination alone (HR 0.66; 95% CI = 0.51-0.87; $p = .033$ and HR 0.68; 95% CI = 0.55-0.85; $p < .001$, respectively). A total of 676 HLA-A*0201-positive patients with unresectable stage III or IV melanoma, whose disease had progressed after one or more of the following therapeutic regimens: dacarbazine, temozolomide, fotemustine, carboplatin, or interleukin-2, were included in this study. This was the first randomized clinical trial that showed a statistically significant improvement in OS for metastatic melanoma (Hodi et al. 2010). This agent has now received FDA approval for use in metastatic melanoma.

The activity and side-effect profile of anti-CTLA-4 antibodies have several characteristics that reflect their immune-mediated mechanism of action. Objective responses observed in patients with metastatic melanoma with either tremelimumab or ipilimumab were seen in approximately 7-10% of patients. Remarkably, as much as 70% of responses were durable (Hodi et al. 2010; Ribas 2008). The unique pattern of response to CTLA-4 mAbs such as initial apparent progression of disease, even with emergence of new lesions, followed by regression and responses over the course of several months to years, has been seen with these agents (Hamid 2007). The recognition of this unusual kinetics of response has led to a

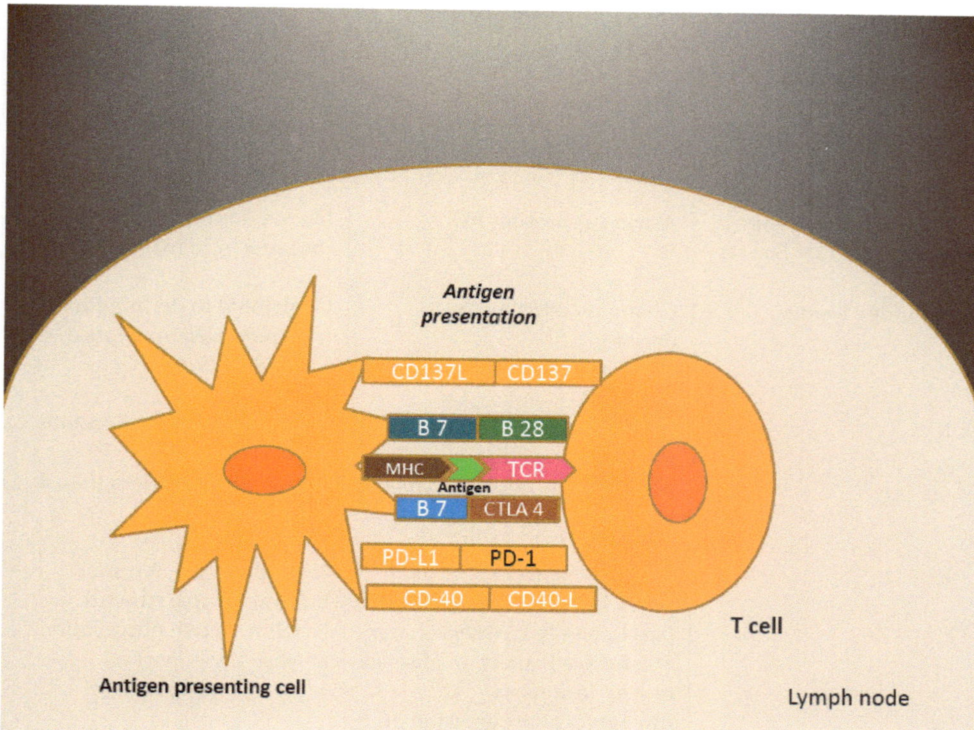

Fig. 1. T-cell response in melanoma: co-stimulatory and co-inhibitory signals. B7 proteins on antigen-presenting cells serve as ligands for both CD28 receptors and CTLA-4 inhibitory molecules on T cells. Upon T-cell receptor binding to antigen presented on MHCs, B7 proteins expressed on APCs can bind to CD28 or CTLA-4 receptors on T cells depending upon the precise expression patterns of the receptors and ligands and on the state of activation of the respective cells. Ligation of B7 to the CTLA-4 receptor results in inhibitory signals for T-cell activation and proliferation. Conversely, ligation of CD28 provides stimulatory signals to T cells leading to their activation. Interaction between PD-1 and PD-L1 results in inhibitory signals, whereas interaction between CD40 and CD40-L leads to T cell activation. Ag: antigen; CTLA-4: cytotoxic T-lymphocyte antigen 4; PD-1: programmed death 1; TCR: T-cell receptor.

proposal of immune-related response criteria (irRC) when evaluating treatment responses to anti-CTLA-4 mAb's (Wolchok JD 2009) (table 1). Immune related response criteria should replace currently accepted Response Evaluation Criteria in Solid Tumors (RECIST) for the evaluation of melanoma patients treated with immunotherapy. Indeed, it is possible that clinical efficacy of tremelimumab may have been missed in the phase III clinical trial owing to the failure to recognize that immune response criteria are needed for adequate response assessment.

The growing clinical experience with anti-CTLA-4 mAbs also identifies a constellation of autoimmune side effects, which have been designated "immune-related adverse events" or irAEs (Di Giacomo et al. 2010). These irAEs, including rash, autoimmune colitis, hepatitis,

	RECIST	irRC
New, measurable lesions (i.e., ≥5 × 5 mm)	Always represent PD	Incorporated into tumor burden
New, nonmeasurable lesions (i.e., <5 × 5 mm)	Always represent PD	Do not define progression (but preclude irCR)
Non-index lesions	Changes contribute to defining BOR of CR, PR, SD, and PD	Contribute to defining irCR (complete disappearance required)
CR	Disappearance of all lesions in two consecutive observations not less than 4 wk apart	Disappearance of all lesions in two consecutive observations not less than 4 wk apart
PR	≥50% decrease in SPD of all index lesions compared with baseline in two observations at least 4 wk apart, in absence of new lesions or unequivocal progression of non-index lesions	≥50% decrease in tumor burden compared with baseline in two observations at least 4 wk apart
SD	50% decrease in SPD compared with baseline cannot be established nor 25% increase compared with nadir, in absence of new lesions or unequivocal progression of non-index lesions	50% decrease in tumor burden compared with baseline cannot be established nor 25% increase compared with nadir
PD	At least 25% increase in SPD compared with nadir and/or unequivocal progression of non-index lesions and/or appearance of new lesions (at any single time point)	At least 25% increase in tumor burden compared with nadir (at any single time point) in two consecutive observations at least 4 wk apart

Table 1. Comparison between RECIST criteria and the irRC. BOR: best overall response; irCR: immune-related complete response; PD: progressive disease; PR: partial response; SD: stable disease; SPD: sum of the products of the two largest perpendicular diameters.

and less frequently hypophysitis and uveitis tend to be not harmful provided the clinician is aware of these unusual side effects, monitors the symptoms adequately, and knows when to intervene. IrAEs are thought to be a result of non-specific or cross-reactive tissue damage caused by activated T-cells. The most commonly reported rash is a macular and papular exanthema affecting trunk and extremities, which has been reported in 47–68 % of patients (O'Day et al. 2010; Weber et al. 2009; Wolchok et al. 2010). These dermatologic irAEs are generally mild and symptomatic relief is provided by antihistamines, while grade 3/4 autoimmune dermatitis is successfully treated with slowly tapered corticosteroids. At our institution, we reported the unique occurrence of hair depigmentation following therapy with CTLA-4 monoclonal antibody that correlated with durable clinical responses (figure 2). Six of 43 patients developed sudden hair depigmentation starting with the eyebrows, and continued to have either complete depigmentation of all body hair or the development of diffuse vitiligo. The median time to depigmentation was 10 months. All of these patients achieved partial response or complete response that sustained during the follow-up period of 24-36 months (Pavlick 2010).

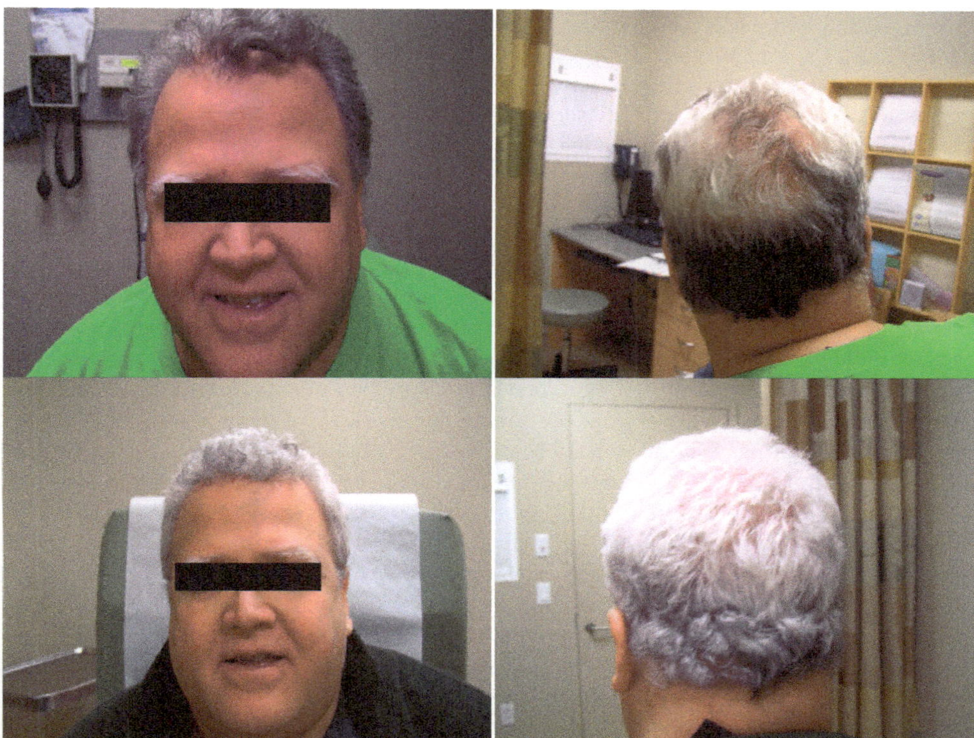

Fig. 2. Progressive hair depigmentation due to ipilimumab over 3-month period. These photographs are published with patient's permission.

Diarrhea due to immune-mediated colitis is the most frequent gastrointestinal irAE; if untreated, it may lead to serious complications such as intestinal perforation (<1%) (Beck et al. 2006). Although grade 3–4 diarrhea is generally reversible with standard anti-inflammatory therapies, experience suggests that patients with colitis treated with high-dose corticosteroids combined with mesalamine, and with seeming resolution of the adverse effects, can have an early recrudescence of the symptoms requiring either prolonged corticosteroid administration, tumor necrosis factor (TNF) blockade with infliximab, or prolonged bowel rest with total parenteral hyperalimentation (Yang et al. 2007). Other irAEs such as hepatitis, iridocyclitis and endocrinopathies including hypophyisitis, hypothyroidism and adrenal insufficiency are uncommon but worth mentioning. Hepatitis generally presents as asymptomatic rise in the levels of alanine aminotransferase (*ALT*) and aspartate aminotransferase (AST). In most cases, a delayed schedule of anti-CTLA 4 mAb leads to normalization of these levels. However, unlike other irAEs, hypophysitis, which occurs in 1.5% of patients treated with ipilimumab (Hodi et al. 2010) often does not improve with high-dose corticosteroids, and permanent hormone replacement therapy is required. Similarly the frequency of hypothyroidism and adrenal insufficiency is 1.5% each (Hodi et al. 2010). Interestingly, development and increasing severity of irAEs generally associate with tumor regression and with a prolonged time to relapse; nevertheless, this association is not absolute and patients without evidence of irAEs have also experienced significant clinical responses (Downey et al. 2007; Kahler and Hauschild 2010).

Melanoma is notorious for its propensity to metastasize to the brain. Up to 75% of patients develop this complication in autopsy series (de la Monte et al. 1983; Patel et al. 1978), and at least one third to one half of patients in clinical practice are found to have one or more brain metastases during the clinical course of their metastatic disease (Amer et al. 1978; Sampson et al. 1998). Brain metastasis portends a grave prognosis. The currently available treatment options for brain metastasis from melanoma include surgical and radiation therapies which may improve the outcome of selected patients with brain metastasis. The most favorable outcomes have been reported in patients who are candidates for stereotactic radiosurgery (Fife et al. 2004). Even though systemic treatment using cytotoxic agents, such as temozolomide in the US, often is employed in the setting of brain metastasis by virtue of the ability of temozolomide to cross the blood-brain barrier, its impact on overall survival remains unproven (Agarwala et al. 2004; Antonadou et al. 2002; Hwu et al. 2005). Up to date, no single treatment modality has been systematically tested in a randomized clinical trial to demonstrate an impact on disease-specific survival. Encouragingly, treatment with CTLA-4 mAb has resulted in durable control of brain metastases (Hodi et al. 2008b; Margolin et al. 2010; Schartz et al. 2010). While the phase III trials with ipilimumab excluded patients with prior or current brain metastasis, a parallel expanded access trial of ipilimumab enrolled patients who were later found to have small brain metastases that had not been treated with radiation. Among those patients, several were noted to have tumor regression in the brain. This unexpected observation led to a clinical trial initiated by the Cytokine Working Group specifically designed for melanoma patients with one or more brain metastases that did not require immediate surgery or radiotherapy. In this trial, patients were candidates for ipilimumab therapy if they had no systemic disease, untreated disease, or were no longer responding to a prior regimen for systemic disease. Brain metastases and extracranial disease were assessed separately, using standard criteria for tumor assessment based on the World Health Organization system and a composite global response status. The results of this trial, reported at the 2010 ASCO meeting, were encouraging. At week 12, for brain alone, the disease control rate was 21.5% (5 of 51 patients achieved partial response, and 6 of 51 patients achieved stable disease); the duration of brain disease control ranged from 3 to 15 months (Lawrence 2010).

2.2 PD-1

The programmed death 1 (PD-1) receptor is a negative regulator of antigen-activated T cells (Fourcade et al. 2009). It bears homology to CTLA-4 but provides distinct co-inhibitory signals. The cytoplasmic domain of PD-1 contains 2 tyrosine signaling motifs that can attenuate the TCR/CD28 signal (Parry et al. 2005). There are two known ligands for PD1: B7-H1/PD-L1 (hereafter PD-L1), the predominant mediator of PD-1-dependent immunosuppression, and B7-DC/PD-L2. PD-L1 is expressed by many tumors including melanoma, and its interaction with PD-1 resulted in tumor escape in experimental models (Iwai et al. 2002). Blockade of the PD-1: PD-L1 pathway in combination with prolonged antigen stimulation with melanoma cells augments the number of cytokine-producing, proliferating, and total NY-ESO-1-specific CD8 +T cells. In murine tumor models, the inhibition of PD-1: PD-L1 interactions was shown to reverse the generation of functional anergy and exhaustion in CD 8+ T cells (Chikuma et al. 2009), and to restore a considerable proportion of the effector activity of CD8+ T cells (Blank et al. 2004), which can reinstate their antitumor effects (Blank et al. 2004; Iwai et al. 2002; Strome et al. 2003). Current data indicate that there is a correlation between the degree of PD-L1 expression and the vertical growth of primary tumors in melanoma (Hino et al. 2010). Multivariate analysis demonstrated that PD-L1 expression is an independent prognostic factor for melanoma (Hino et al. 2010). Therefore, blockade of PD-1: PD-L1 interaction represents a rational strategy for cancer immunotherapy.

MDX-1106 (BMS-936558/ONO-4538) is a fully human immunoglobulin G4 (IgG4) mAb specific for PD-1. The drug binds PD-1 with high affinity and blocks its interaction with both PD-L1 and PD-L2. A phase I study of single agent MDX-1106 in refractory solid tumors was conducted in 39 patients with advanced metastatic non-small cell lung carcinoma (NSCLC), melanoma, castrate-resistant prostate cancer, renal cell carcinoma (RCC), or colorectal carcinoma (CRC). Although efficacy was not the primary endpoint of this phase I study, of the 39 treated patients, 1 durable complete response (CRC) and 2 partial responses (melanoma, RCC) were seen. Two additional patients (melanoma, NSCLC) had significant lesional tumor regressions, which did not meet criteria for PR. This study suggested a more benign immune-related toxicity profile for anti-PD-1 mAb than one seen associated with anti-CTLA-4 mAb. Only 1 patient with metastatic ocular melanoma developed grade 3 inflammatory colitis following five doses (1 mg/kg) administered over 8 months, which responded to steroids and infliximab, while grade 2 immune related adverse events occurred in 3 patients presenting with polyarticular arthropathies requiring oral steroids and hypothyroidism requiring hormone replacement. (Brahmer et al. 2010). Another phase I trial was conducted on 16 patients with metastatic disease including melanoma. Objective responses were documented in 37.5% of patients lasting 3-13+ months; half of the patients had melanoma and there were few irAEs (Sznol 2010).

2.3 Adoptive cell therapy

The transfer of tumor specific T cells has emerged as a promising therapeutic strategy for melanoma. Adoptive cell therapy (ACT) was pioneered at the Surgery Branch of the National Cancer Institute (NCI; Bethesda, MD), and to date, has shown some of the most impressive response rates (up to 72%) in patients with metastatic melanoma. The most developed approach is based on the *ex vivo* selection of highly reactive, tumor-infiltrating lymphocytes (TIL), their activation and numerical expansion before reinfusion to the autologous tumor-bearing host (Dudley et al. 2005). Adoptive transfer after a nonmyeloablative conditioning regimen was shown to result in the persistent clonal repopulation of T-cells in patients with metastatic melanoma, with the transferred cells proliferating *in vivo*, displaying functional activity, and trafficking to tumor sites (Dudley et al. 2002).

By eliminating competition for endogenous serum cytokines, lymphodepletion may affect survival and proliferation of the adoptively transferred TIL. Data from animal models suggested that increased levels of lymphodepletion could improve ACT efficacy. In murine models, lymphodepletion seemed to enhance the antitumor effects of transferred T cells *in vivo* by several mechanisms including the elimination of suppressive CD4+, CD25+ T-regulatory lymphocytes, the elimination of cellular "sinks" for homeostatic cytokines such as IL-7 and IL-15, and the engagement of toll-like receptors on antigen-presenting cells after damage to the integrity of the gut epithelial lining (Antony et al. 2005; Gattinoni et al. 2005; Paulos et al. 2007). Cyclophosphamide and fludarabine have been employed for nonmyeloablative lymphodepletion. In a series of 35 patients, Dudley et al. showed that adoptive transfer of autologous TIL after nonmyeloablative but lymphodepleting chemotherapy with cyclophosphamide and fludarabine followed by high dose IL-2 resulted in objective responses in 51% of heavily pretreated patients with metastatic melanoma (Dudley et al. 2005). Further increasing intensity of host preparative lymphodepletion by adding total-body irradiation (TBI) of either 2 or 12 Gy prior to cell transfer in cyclophosphamide and fludarabine lymphodeleted patients was shown to generate response rates up to 52% and 72%, respectively. Of the 25 patients studied in the 12 Gy TBI arm, there were 4 complete responders and at least 2 substantial partial responders (Dudley et al. 2008).

The caveat of adoptive cell therapy is its complexity of several critical preparative steps that are both labor intensive and costly which may be the major obstacle to the widespread application of this approach. Up to 4 to 6 weeks of cell culture are required to obtain adequate numbers of reactive lymphocytes for adoptive transfer. Additionally, much akin to the limitation of high dose IL-2, only patients with an excellent functional status are be able to withstand the intensity of adoptive cell therapy which may also involve TBI in addition to IL-2. On the other hand, as the data from the NCI suggest, such potent therapy in highly selected patients does have the potential to induce durable responses and a potential cure. To date, however, only small phase II clinical trials have been completed and no phase III study has been initiated. Meanwhile, further innovations beyond current TIL technology are underway. Current strategies seek to improve the yield of TIL cultures, to use vaccines to stimulate the transferred T cells *in vivo*, and to employ gene therapy using genetically engineered lymphocytes that express highly reactive T-cell receptors (TCRs) with specific anti-melanoma differentiation antigen activity (gp-100 or MART-1), produce IL-2 or other molecules promoting an effective immune response. The gene therapy approach is of particular interest because the anti-tumor effector T cells could be rapidly expanded for adoptive transfer. Furthermore, it could be of tremendous benefit to patients who do not have autologous reactive TIL available and would otherwise be ineligible for adoptive immunotherapy (Johnson et al. 2009; Yang et al. 2010). The objective response rates in trials employing gene therapy have been reported to be 20% to 45%, and durable tumor regression at all disease sites including the brain has also been observed (Johnson et al. 2009; Morgan et al. 2006; Robbins et al. 2011).

3. Agents targeting oncogenic signaling pathways

The MAPK pathway (figure 3) has been of keen interest in melanoma in particular since Davies et al. first reported that 66% of melanomas harbor activating somatic missense mutations in the BRAF gene (V600E), leading to constitutive activation of this pathway (Davies et al. 2002; Meier et al. 2005). The RAF/MEK/ERK pathway is an important regulator of growth, survival and migration and it is constitutively activated in many human cancers (Fecher et al. 2008). Physiologically, the RAF/MEK/ERK signaling pathway is activated upon binding of extracellular ligands to growth factor receptors with intrinsic tyrosine kinase activity such as epidermal growth factor receptor (EGFR), c-Kit, platelet-derived growth factor receptor (PDGFR), vascular endothelial growth factor receptor

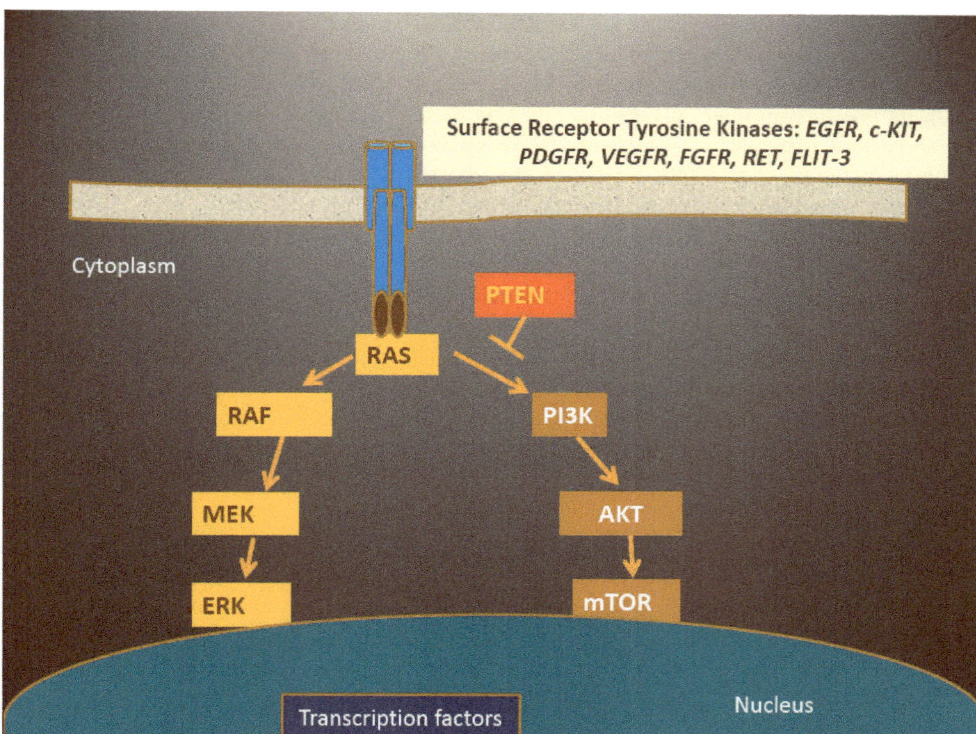

Fig. 3. Molecular targets in melanoma: the MAPK and PI3K pathways. Binding of growth factors to cell surface receptors induces their dimerization and activation of the MAPK tyrosine kinase cascade, which includes RAS RAF, MEK and ERK. Activated (phosphorylated) ERK translocates into the nucleus, and phosphorylates transcription factors for genes involved in cell growth and proliferation. This pathway is constitutively activated in many human melanomas. An alternate pathway via PI3K, AKT, and mTOR is also activated in some melanomas.

(VEGFR), and fibroblast growth factor receptor (FGFR). Signaling through the RAF/MEK/ERK pathway eventually leads to the transcription of hundreds if not thousands of genes related to cellular proliferation, survival, apoptosis, tumor invasion, and motility (Fecher et al. 2008; Shields et al. 2007). Another kinase signaling pathway involves PI3K/AKT activating mTOR which promotes signaling to the nucleus and activates genes involved in cell growth and proliferation (Stahl et al. 2004). Studies have shown that a high proportion of melanomas carry alterations in the PI3K/AKT pathway (PTEN deletion or AKT amplification) independent of the $BRAF^{V600E}$ mutation (Haluska et al. 2007; Vivanco and Sawyers 2002). These findings reveal a complex, interlinked network of cellular signaling pathways that contain several potentially synergistic therapeutic targets for metastatic melanoma.

3.1 RAF

Sorafenib (Bay 43-9006) was the first RAF inhibitor to enter early clinical trials. It is a small-molecule, multi-targeted tyrosine kinase inhibitor that blocks EGFR, c-Kit, Flt-3, PDGF and VEGF in addition to BRAF (Adnane et al. 2006; Wilhelm et al. 2004). Although Sorafenib does not have meaningful activity in melanoma as a single agent (Eisen et al. 2006; Ott et al. 2010), its use in combination with dacarbazine or temozolomide led to superior objective responses and progression –free survival compared to historical response rates to these agents (Amaravadi et al. 2009). However, in a phase III randomized trial (E2603) comparing carboplatin, paclitaxel and sorafenib versus carboplatin, paclitaxel and placebo in chemotherapy-naïve patients, the futility analysis demonstrated no benefit of the three drug combination compared to the two drug chemotherapy combination. In the PRISM study, the addition of Sorafenib to the combination of carboplatin and paclitaxel as second-line treatment after chemotherapy with dacarbazine or temozolomide failed to improve progression-free survival, response rate and time-to-disease progression in metastatic melanoma patients (Hauschild et al. 2009).

Since then, second generation selective RAF inhibitors have been developed and are actively tested in various clinical trials. RG7204 (Roche Pharmaceuticals, formerly PLX4032, Plexxikon) is an oral, highly selective inhibitor of the oncogenic V600E mutant BRAF kinase, which showed promising results in early clinical studies. In a dose-finding phase I trial, 11/16 (68%) of patients with mutant BRAF metastatic melanoma achieved PR and four patients had minor responses leading to a PFS of 8-9 months (Flaherty 2009). A dose extension phase I trial with 32 patients demonstrated an objective response rate of 81% (2 CRs, 24 PRs) (Flaherty et al. 2010). The median PFS among these patients was more than 7 months. RG7204 is generally well tolerated with rash, photosensitivity, arthralgia and nausea. Of note, 31% of patients developed grade 3 squamous cell carcinoma (SCC), keratoacanthoma (KA) type. The median time to the appearance of a cutaneous squamous cell carcinoma was 8 weeks with no reported involvement of other organs. Treatment with RG7204 was not interrupted by the appearance of these skin lesions and the majority of them were resected (Flaherty et al. 2010). On the basis of these promising results, a phase II trial (BRIM 2) is now fully accrued and a phase III trial (BRIM 3) met its primary end points with RG7204 improving both PFS and OS (Chapman, PB, N Engl J Med. 2011 Jun 30;364(26):2507-16. Epub 2011 Jun 5) comparing RG7204 to dacarbazine in untreated patients with BRAF V600E mutant metastatic melanoma.

GSK 2118436 is another oral, highly potent and selective inhibitor of the V600E/K/D mutant BRAF. In a phase I/II study, treatment with GSK 2118436 led to a decrease in FDG-PET metabolic uptake with 11/14 (79%) of melanoma patients showing a decrease from baseline (range -5 to -100%), and 18/ 30 (60%) patients demonstrated a > 20% tumor decrease by RECIST at first restaging (8-9 wks). GSK 2118436 showed good tolerability and low grade nausea, vomiting, fatigue, headaches and skin changes (including low grade SCC) were the main adverse effects (Kefford 2010). A phase II study of GSK2118436 as salvage therapy (NCT01153763), and a phase III study of GSK2118436 versus dacarbazine (NCT01227889) as front line therapy for mutant BRAF metastatic melanoma patients are underway.

Judging from the data available to date and the experience in our center, selective RAF inhibitors are relatively well tolerated, high grade adverse events are uncommon. Unique side effects associated with these novel drugs are the emergence of KA and SCC. These lesions can appear as early as 2 weeks after the initiation of therapy and are reported in 15-30% of the patients (Arnault et al. 2009; Flaherty et al. 2010). Histologically, KA is almost indistinguishable from a well differentiated SCC. In contrast to KA, SCC is a malignant lesion that does not regress spontaneously and has the potential for metastasis. The biologic mechanism and natural history of these lesions in the context of RAF inhibitors, in comparison to their spontaneous counterparts, are currently unknown (Arnault et al. 2009; Robert et al. 2010).

3.2 MEK

The serine/threonine tyrosine kinase MEK acts downstream from RAF in the RAF/MEK/ERK pathway; its inhibition is an attractive anticancer strategy as it has the potential to block upregulated signal transduction through this pathway, regardless of the upstream position of the oncogenic aberration. AZD6244 (ARRY-142886, Array BioPharma, AstraZeneca) is a selective MEK1/2 inhibitor that has shown preclinical activity (Yeh et al. 2007) and demonstrated clinical activity in a phase I study with a relatively benign toxicity profile (Adjei et al. 2008). These results led to a randomized phase II trial comparing AZD6244 versus temozolomide in chemotherapy naïve advanced melanoma patients (Dummer 2008). A total of 200 patients were enrolled with 104 and 96 patients randomized to AZD6244 and temozolomide, respectively; those who progressed on temozolomide could crossover to AZD6244. Results showed a trend toward OS in patients with BRAF mutations in the AZD6244 arm (Dummer 2008). At the 2010 ASCO annual meeting, the early results of a phase I study with AZD6244 in combination with docetaxel, dacarbazine or temsirolimus suggests the presence of BRAF mutation was significantly associated with clinical responses and increased time to progression. (Patel 2010). Several phase II studies of AZD6244 are underway for advanced melanoma patients with BRAF mutations as front line therapy: for treatment-naïve patients versus temozolomide (NCT00338130), in combination with dacarbazine versus dacarbazine alone (NCT00936221), as well as salvage therapy (NCT00866177). GSK1120212 is another potent and selective inhibitor of the MEK1/2 enzymes with promising anti-tumor activity in a phase I clinical trial, resulting in response rate > 70% in advanced melanoma patients with known BRAF mutations, including one patient who was previously treated with PLX4032 (Infante 2010). This drug is currently investigated in phase II and III clinical trials for advanced BRAF mutant melanoma patients who were either previously treated with a BRAF inhibitor or not. (NCT01245062, NCT01037127).

Although targeting the MAPK pathway is a promising new therapeutic approach for the treatment of melanoma, and treatment with selective BRAF and MEK inhibitors can induce high response rates, the limited duration of these responses in most patients, most likely because of emerging resistance to these inhibitors represents a significant clinical challenge. Molecular redundancy, in part due to the existence of RAF isoforms and signaling through alternative oncogenic pathways, such as PI3K/AKT/mTOR pathway (Jiang et al. 2011; Paraiso et al. 2010), receptor tyrosine kinase (PDGFRβ)-dependent pathway (Nazarian et al. 2010) and COT (MAP3K8) (Johannessen et al. 2010), may provide the melanoma cells' escape mechanisms to specific pathway inhibitors and underscore their ability to adapt to pharmacological challenges (Jiang et al. 2011; Paraiso et al. 2010). In preclinical models, it has been reported that acquired resistance of melanoma cells to the BRAF inhibitors was associated with rebound activation of the RAF/MEK/ERK pathway (Paraiso et al. 2010). In line with this finding, activating signals to downstream MEK/ERK has been shown to switch to ARAF (Villanueva et al. 2010) or CRAF (Montagut et al. 2008; Villanueva et al. 2010) via N-RAS upregulation (Nazarian et al. 2010) to overcome the effect of BRAF inhibition. Moreover, the majority of melanoma cells harboring the BRAF V600E mutation retained the wild-type BRAF allele which could be rescued from the effects of BRAF knock-down by extracellular growth factors such as basic fibroblast growth factor, hepatocyte growth factor or endothelin-1 (Christensen and Guldberg 2005).

3.3 C-Kit

Imatinib is a selective tyrosine kinase inhibitor with multiple targets, including c-Kit and PDGR receptors, and has shown to be highly efficacious in chronic myelogenous leukemia and GIST tumors (Heinrich et al. 2000). Initial phase II trials with this agent in melanoma were disappointing with no objective responses (Ugurel et al. 2005; Wyman et al. 2006). However, gain of function mutations, gene amplifications and over-expression of c-kit were subsequently reported in 30-40% of mucosal, acral and cutaneous melanomas with chronic sun damage (Curtin et al. 2006). Impressive tumor regression was documented in a patient with mucosal melanoma who carried a mutation in the juxtamembranous domain of c-Kit (exon 11) in response to single agent imatinib (Hodi et al. 2008a). Moreover, preclinical studies showed sensitivity of c-Kit mutant mucosal melanoma, providing a rationale for the use of imatinib in this melanoma type. Preliminary results of a phase II trial evaluating the effect of imatinib in patients with metastatic melanoma with c-kit aberrations were presented at ASCO 2009. Over 30% of patients achieved a response (complete and partial response), whereas 50% had disease stability (Carvajal 2009). Another phase I/II study to define safety and efficacy of imatinib in combination with temozolomide in patients with unresectable, stage III/IV melanoma is currently underway. After the data on c-kit alterations became available when the trial was already in progress, patients with mucosal, acral and chronic sun damage melanomas were preferentially enrolled in the phase II part of the study. Early results of the trial were presented at ASCO 2008 (Fecher 2008). Of the 23 patients treated, 16 had been enrolled in phase I and 7 in phase II. The combination was well tolerated and demonstrated anti-tumor activity in melanoma. Of the 7 patients treated in the phase II trial, 1 patient had a CR and 6 had PRs (Fecher 2008). Phase II studies with a second generation c-kit inhibitor (nilotinib) in first or second line therapies for advanced melanoma with c-Kit mutation or amplification are ongoing (NCT01168050, NCT01099514). In addition, the multi-targeted receptor tyrosine kinase inhibitor sunitinib has shown potential efficacy in patients with c-kit mutated melanoma in an early phase clinical trial (Minor 2010).

3.4 MTOR

Resistance of mutant BRAF melanoma cells to RAF/MEK inhibition may also be due to activation of other survival signaling pathways such as the PI3K/AKT/mTOR pathway (figure 3) resulting in melanoma development and progression (Shao and Aplin 2010; Stahl et al. 2004; Villanueva et al. 2010). Recent reports suggested a significant correlation of increased PI3K-AKT activity with resistance to RAF/MEK inhibitors in melanoma (Gopal et al. 2010; Villanueva et al. 2010) and that inhibition of the PI3K/AKT/mTOR pathway could suppress MEK inhibitor-induced activation of AKT and resulted in synergistic cell killing with a MEK inhibitor (AZD6244) (Gopal et al. 2010). This provides a rationale for combinatorial therapy leading to dual inhibition of both RAF/MEK/ERK and PI3K/AKT/mTOR pathways. A phase II trial of the mTOR inhibitor temsirolimus (CCI-779) combined with the MEK inhibitor AZD6244 is currently recruiting treatment-naïve patients with BRAF mutant advanced melanoma (NCT01166126). In addition, inhibition of the PI3K/AKT/mTOR signaling pathway was found to sensitize melanoma cells to chemotherapeutic agents such as cisplatin and temozolomide *in vitro* as evidenced by enhanced apoptosis and suppressed invasive tumor growth (Sinnberg et al. 2009). A Phase II study of the mTOR inhibitor everolimus in combination with paclitaxel and carboplatin in patients with metastatic melanoma is in progress (NCT01014351).

4. Other targeted drugs currently in clinical development

4.1 PARP Inhibitors

Poly-ADP ribose polymerase (PARP) is a key enzyme in DNA repair. ADP- ribosylation is involved in DNA excision repair and inhibition of the enzyme enhances the cytotoxicity of DNA damaging agents (Durkacz et al. 1980). PARP inhibition in BRCA-deficient breast cancers has shown a favorable therapeutic index. In a phase II trial, olaparib, a novel poly-ADP ribose polymerase (PARP) inhibitor, achieved an objective response rate of 41% in women with BRCA1 or BRCA2 mutations and advanced breast cancer (Tutt et al. 2010). In melanoma, PARP-1 expression has been shown to correlate with tumor thickness (Staibano et al. 2005), a poor prognostic factor for melanoma, and over-expression of PARP-1 is correlated with recurrence and/or progression of the disease (Csete et al. 2009), suggesting that it potentially is as a promising new therapeutic target. AG014699 is the first PARP inhibitor to enter a clinical trial and was studied in combination with temozolomide in a phase II study with 40 chemotherapy-naïve metastatic melanoma patients. Of the 20 evaluable patients, there were 4 confirmed PRs and 4 SDs (Plummer 2006).

4.2 Antibody-drug conjugate

Glycoprotein NMB (GPNMB) is over-expressed in a variety of cancers including melanoma. CR011-vcMMAE is an antibody-drug conjugate comprised of a fully-human monoclonal antibody directed at the extracellular domain of GPNMB linked to a potent tubulin destabilizing agent, monomethyl auristatin E (MMAE). The enzyme-sensitive linker is designed to be stable in the bloodstream and to release MMAE inside tumor cells, resulting in cancer cell death. A phase I/II study of CR011-vcMMAE in patients with advanced, pretreated melanoma has completed accrual (NCT00412828). At the ASCO annual meeting in 2010, CR-vcMMAE at 1.88mg/kg, when given every three weeks, was reported to produce an objective response rate of 15% (Hamid 2010).

4.3 Antibodies against integrins

Integrins of the α_v family, such as $\alpha_v\beta3$ and $\alpha_v\beta5$, are implicated in tumor-induced angiogenesis and are thought to play a role in tumor growth. CNTO 95 is a fully human monoclonal antibody directed against α_v Integrins, which has demonstrated anti-tumor and anti-angiogenic activities in animal models (Trikha et al. 2004). Results of a phase I study to assess safety and pharmacokinetics of CNTO 95 in patients with advanced refractory solid tumors demonstrated good tolerability (Jayson 2004). A phase I/II multicenter, randomized and double-blind study to assess the safety and efficacy of CNTO 95, alone and in combination with dacarbazine, in stage IV melanoma patients has been completed and result pending publication (NCT00246012). Another phase I trial of CNTO 95 in patients with metastatic melanoma and angiosarcoma recently demonstrated a manageable toxicity profile, and encouragingly, 2 of 18 patients with melanoma, who had failed several therapeutic regimens, sustained stable disease 5 and 7 months, respectively (O'Day et al. 2011).

5. Conclusion

Understanding the molecular biology of melanoma and unraveling of several signaling pathways over the last few years, as well as advances in immunology have led to the development of a number of promising novel therapeutic treatment options for metastatic melanoma. Immune-checkpoint blockade with ipilimumab has demonstrated increased overall survival in a randomized phase III clinical study (Hodi et al. 2010). Other immune-related approaches, such as anti-PD1/PD-L1 and adoptive cell therapy, are on the horizon. The identification of the BRAF V600E mutation led to the development of new agents that specifically block the MAPK pathway. Improved PFS and OS as a result of treatment with the V600E mutant BRAF kinase inhibitor RG7204 in BRIM 3 have been reported. Encouraging response rates with imatinib therapy in patients with mucosal, acral, and sun-damaged skin melanomas that harbor mutations or amplification in the c-kit gene have also been documented. These results herald the era of individualized therapies based on specific tumor genotypes, of which scientifically thoughtful combinations will usher in a new standard of care for metastatic melanoma in the near future.

6. References

Adjei, A. A., Cohen, R. B., Franklin, W., Morris, C., Wilson, D., Molina, J. R., Hanson, L. J., Gore, L., Chow, L., Leong, S., Maloney, L., Gordon, G., Simmons, H., Marlow, A., Litwiler, K., Brown, S., Poch, G., Kane, K., Haney, J., and Eckhardt, S. G. (2008). Phase I pharmacokinetic and pharmacodynamic study of the oral, small-molecule mitogen-activated protein kinase kinase 1/2 inhibitor AZD6244 (ARRY-142886) in patients with advanced cancers. *J Clin Oncol*, 26(13), 2139-2146

Adnane, L., Trail, P. A., Taylor, I., and Wilhelm, S. M. (2006). Sorafenib (BAY 43-9006, Nexavar), a dual-action inhibitor that targets RAF/MEK/ERK pathway in tumor cells and tyrosine kinases VEGFR/PDGFR in tumor vasculature. *Methods Enzymol*, 407, 597-612

Agarwala, S. S., Kirkwood, J. M., Gore, M., Dreno, B., Thatcher, N., Czarnetski, B., Atkins, M., Buzaid, A., Skarlos, D., and Rankin, E. M. (2004). Temozolomide for the treatment of brain metastases associated with metastatic melanoma: a phase II study. *J Clin Oncol*, 22(11), 2101-2107

Amaravadi, R. K., Schuchter, L. M., McDermott, D. F., Kramer, A., Giles, L., Gramlich, K., Carberry, M., Troxel, A. B., Letrero, R., Nathanson, K. L., Atkins, M. B., O'Dwyer, P. J., and Flaherty, K. T. (2009). Phase II Trial of Temozolomide and Sorafenib in Advanced Melanoma Patients with or without Brain Metastases. *Clin Cancer Res*, 15(24), 7711-7718

Amer, M. H., Al-Sarraf, M., Baker, L. H., and Vaitkevicius, V. K. (1978). Malignant melanoma and central nervous system metastases: incidence, diagnosis, treatment and survival. *Cancer*, 42(2), 660-668

Antonadou, D., Paraskevaidis, M., Sarris, G., Coliarakis, N., Economou, I., Karageorgis, P., and Throuvalas, N. (2002). Phase II randomized trial of temozolomide and concurrent radiotherapy in patients with brain metastases. *J Clin Oncol*, 20(17), 3644-3650

Antony, P. A., Piccirillo, C. A., Akpinarli, A., Finkelstein, S. E., Speiss, P. J., Surman, D. R., Palmer, D. C., Chan, C. C., Klebanoff, C. A., Overwijk, W. W., Rosenberg, S. A., and Restifo, N. P. (2005). CD8+ T cell immunity against a tumor/self-antigen is augmented by CD4+ T helper cells and hindered by naturally occurring T regulatory cells. *J Immunol*, 174(5), 2591-2601

Arnault, J. P., Wechsler, J., Escudier, B., Spatz, A., Tomasic, G., Sibaud, V., Aractingi, S., Grange, J. D., Poirier-Colame, V., Malka, D., Soria, J. C., Mateus, C., and Robert, C. (2009). Keratoacanthomas and squamous cell carcinomas in patients receiving sorafenib. *J Clin Oncol*, 27(23), 59-61

Atkins, M. B., Kunkel, L., Sznol, M., and Rosenberg, S. A. (2000). High-dose recombinant interleukin-2 therapy in patients with metastatic melanoma: long-term survival update. *Cancer J Sci Am*, 6 Suppl 1, 11-14

Balch, C. M., Gershenwald, J. E., Soong, S. J., Thompson, J. F., Atkins, M. B., Byrd, D. R., Buzaid, A. C., Cochran, A. J., Coit, D. G., Ding, S., Eggermont, A. M., Flaherty, K. T., Gimotty, P. A., Kirkwood, J. M., McMasters, K. M., Mihm, M. C., Jr., Morton, D. L., Ross, M. I., Sober, A. J., and Sondak, V. K. (2009). Final version of 2009 AJCC melanoma staging and classification. *J Clin Oncol*, 27(36), 6199-6206

Beck, K. E., Blansfield, J. A., Tran, K. Q., Feldman, A. L., Hughes, M. S., Royal, R. E., Kammula, U. S., Topalian, S. L., Sherry, R. M., Kleiner, D., Quezado, M., Lowy, I., Yellin, M., Rosenberg, S. A., and Yang, J. C. (2006). Enterocolitis in patients with cancer after antibody blockade of cytotoxic T-lymphocyte-associated antigen 4. *J Clin Oncol*, 24(15), 2283-2289

Bedikian, A. Y., Millward, M., Pehamberger, H., Conry, R., Gore, M., Trefzer, U., Pavlick, A. C., DeConti, R., Hersh, E. M., Hersey, P., Kirkwood, J. M., and Haluska, F. G. (2006). Bcl-2 antisense (oblimersen sodium) plus dacarbazine in patients with advanced melanoma: the Oblimersen Melanoma Study Group. *J Clin Oncol*, 24(29), 4738-4745

Blank, C., Brown, I., Peterson, A. C., Spiotto, M., Iwai, Y., Honjo, T., and Gajewski, T. F. (2004). PD-L1/B7H-1 inhibits the effector phase of tumor rejection by T cell receptor (TCR) transgenic CD8+ T cells. *Cancer Res*, 64(3), 1140-1145

Brahmer, J. R., Drake, C. G., Wollner, I., Powderly, J. D., Picus, J., Sharfman, W. H., Stankevich, E., Pons, A., Salay, T. M., McMiller, T. L., Gilson, M. M., Wang, C., Selby, M., Taube, J. M., Anders, R., Chen, L., Korman, A. J., Pardoll, D. M., Lowy, I., and Topalian, S. L. (2010). Phase I study of single-agent anti-programmed death-1 (MDX-1106) in refractory solid tumors: safety, clinical activity, pharmacodynamics, and immunologic correlates. *J Clin Oncol*, 28(19), 3167-3175

Carvajal, R. D., Chapman, P.B, Wolchok, J.D., Cane, L., Teitcher, J.B., Lutzky, J., Pavlick, A.C., Bastian, B.C., Antonescu, C.R., Schwartz, G.K. (2009). A phase II study of imatinib mesylate (IM) for patients with advanced melanoma harboring somatic alterations of KIT. *J Clin Oncol*, 27, ASCO Annual Meeting, Abstr 9001

Chapman, P. B., Einhorn, L. H., Meyers, M. L., Saxman, S., Destro, A. N., Panageas, K. S., Begg, C. B., Agarwala, S. S., Schuchter, L. M., Ernstoff, M. S., Houghton, A. N., and Kirkwood, J. M. (1999). Phase III multicenter randomized trial of the Dartmouth regimen versus dacarbazine in patients with metastatic melanoma. *J Clin Oncol*, 17(9), 2745-2751

Chikuma, S., Terawaki, S., Hayashi, T., Nabeshima, R., Yoshida, T., Shibayama, S., Okazaki, T., and Honjo, T. (2009). PD-1-mediated suppression of IL-2 production induces CD8+ T cell anergy in vivo. *J Immunol*, 182(11), 6682-6689

Christensen, C., and Guldberg, P. (2005). Growth factors rescue cutaneous melanoma cells from apoptosis induced by knockdown of mutated (V 600 E) B-RAF. *Oncogene*, 24(41), 6292-6302

Csete, B., Lengyel, Z., Kadar, Z., and Battyani, Z. (2009). Poly(adenosine diphosphate-ribose) polymerase-1 expression in cutaneous malignant melanomas as a new molecular marker of aggressive tumor. *Pathol Oncol Res*, 15(1), 47-53

Curtin, J. A., Busam, K., Pinkel, D., and Bastian, B. C. (2006). Somatic activation of KIT in distinct subtypes of melanoma. *J Clin Oncol*, 24(26), 4340-4346

Davies, H., Bignell, G. R., Cox, C., Stephens, P., Edkins, S., Clegg, S., Teague, J., Woffendin, H., Garnett, M. J., Bottomley, W., Davis, N., Dicks, E., Ewing, R., Floyd, Y., Gray, K., Hall, S., Hawes, R., Hughes, J., Kosmidou, V., Menzies, A., Mould, C., Parker, A., Stevens, C., Watt, S., Hooper, S., Wilson, R., Jayatilake, H., Gusterson, B. A., Cooper, C., Shipley, J., Hargrave, D., Pritchard-Jones, K., Maitland, N., Chenevix-Trench, G., Riggins, G. J., Bigner, D. D., Palmieri, G., Cossu, A., Flanagan, A., Nicholson, A., Ho, J. W., Leung, S. Y., Yuen, S. T., Weber, B. L., Seigler, H. F., Darrow, T. L., Paterson, H., Marais, R., Marshall, C. J., Wooster, R., Stratton, M. R., and Futreal, P. A. (2002). Mutations of the BRAF gene in human cancer. *Nature*, 417(6892), 949-954

de la Monte, S. M., Moore, G. W., and Hutchins, G. M. (1983). Patterned distribution of metastases from malignant melanoma in humans. *Cancer Res*, 43(7), 3427-3433

Di Giacomo, A. M., Biagioli, M., and Maio, M. (2010). The emerging toxicity profiles of anti-CTLA-4 antibodies across clinical indications. *Semin Oncol*, 37(5), 499-507

Downey, S. G., Klapper, J. A., Smith, F. O., Yang, J. C., Sherry, R. M., Royal, R. E., Kammula, U. S., Hughes, M. S., Allen, T. E., Levy, C. L., Yellin, M., Nichol, G., White, D. E., Steinberg, S. M., and Rosenberg, S. A. (2007). Prognostic factors related to clinical response in patients with metastatic melanoma treated by CTL-associated antigen-4 blockade. *Clin Cancer Res*, 13(22 Pt 1), 6681-6688

Dudley, M. E., Wunderlich, J. R., Robbins, P. F., Yang, J. C., Hwu, P., Schwartzentruber, D. J., Topalian, S. L., Sherry, R., Restifo, N. P., Hubicki, A. M., Robinson, M. R., Raffeld, M., Duray, P., Seipp, C. A., Rogers-Freezer, L., Morton, K. E., Mavroukakis, S. A., White, D. E., and Rosenberg, S. A. (2002). Cancer regression and autoimmunity in patients after clonal repopulation with antitumor lymphocytes. *Science*, 298(5594), 850-854

Dudley, M. E., Wunderlich, J. R., Yang, J. C., Sherry, R. M., Topalian, S. L., Restifo, N. P., Royal, R. E., Kammula, U., White, D. E., Mavroukakis, S. A., Rogers, L. J., Gracia, G. J., Jones, S. A., Mangiameli, D. P., Pelletier, M. M., Gea-Banacloche, J., Robinson, M. R., Berman, D. M., Filie, A. C., Abati, A., and Rosenberg, S. A. (2005). Adoptive cell transfer therapy following non-myeloablative but lymphodepleting chemotherapy for the treatment of patients with refractory metastatic melanoma. *J Clin Oncol*, 23(10), 2346-2357

Dudley, M. E., Yang, J. C., Sherry, R., Hughes, M. S., Royal, R., Kammula, U., Robbins, P. F., Huang, J., Citrin, D. E., Leitman, S. F., Wunderlich, J., Restifo, N. P., Thomasian, A., Downey, S. G., Smith, F. O., Klapper, J., Morton, K., Laurencot, C., White, D. E., and Rosenberg, S. A. (2008). Adoptive cell therapy for patients with metastatic melanoma: evaluation of intensive myeloablative chemoradiation preparative regimens. *J Clin Oncol*, 26(32), 5233-9

Dummer, R., Robert, C., Chapman, P. B. , Sosman, J. A., Middleton, M., Bastholt, L. , Kemsley, K. , Cantarini, M. V. , Morris, C. , Kirkwood, J. M. . (2008). AZD6244 (ARRY-142886) vs temozolomide (TMZ) in patients (pts) with advanced melanoma: An open-label, randomized, multicenter, phase II study. *J Clin Oncol*, 26(May 20 suppl), ASCO annual meeting abstract 9033

Durkacz, B. W., Omidiji, O., Gray, D. A., and Shall, S. (1980). (ADP-ribose)n participates in DNA excision repair. *Nature*, 283(5747), 593-596

Eigentler, T. K., Caroli, U. M., Radny, P., and Garbe, C. (2003). Palliative therapy of disseminated malignant melanoma: a systematic review of 41 randomised clinical trials. *Lancet Oncol*, 4(12), 748-759

Eisen, T., Ahmad, T., Flaherty, K. T., Gore, M., Kaye, S., Marais, R., Gibbens, I., Hackett, S., James, M., Schuchter, L. M., Nathanson, K. L., Xia, C., Simantov, R., Schwartz, B., Poulin-Costello, M., O'Dwyer, P. J., and Ratain, M. J. (2006). Sorafenib in advanced melanoma: a Phase II randomised discontinuation trial analysis. *Br J Cancer*, 95(5), 581-586

Fecher, L. A., Amaravadi, R. K. & Flaherty, K. T. (2008). The MAPK pathway in melanoma. *Curr Opin Oncol*, 20(2), 183-9

Fecher, L. A., Nathanson, K. , Flaherty, K. T. , Amaravadi, R. , Giles, L. , McGettigan, S. , Carberry, M. , Elder, D. , Schuchter, L. . (2008). Phase I/II trial of imatinib and temozolomide in advanced unresectable melanoma. *J Clin Oncol*, 26(ASCO 2008 Meeting Abstract 9059)

Fife, K. M., Colman, M. H., Stevens, G. N., Firth, I. C., Moon, D., Shannon, K. F., Harman, R., Petersen-Schaefer, K., Zacest, A. C., Besser, M., Milton, G. W., McCarthy, W. H., and Thompson, J. F. (2004). Determinants of outcome in melanoma patients with cerebral metastases. *J Clin Oncol*, 22(7), 1293-1300

Flaherty, K., Puzanov, I., Sosman, J., Kim, K., Ribas, A., McArthur, G., Lee, R.J., Grippo, J.F., Nolop, K., Chapman, P. (2009). Phase I study of PLX4032: Proof of concept for V600E BRAF mutation as a therapeutic target in human cancer. *J Clin Oncol*, 27(15s), ASCO Annual Meeting Abstract (suppl; abstr 9000)

Flaherty, K. T., Puzanov, I., Kim, K. B., Ribas, A., McArthur, G. A., Sosman, J. A., O'Dwyer, P. J., Lee, R. J., Grippo, J. F., Nolop, K., and Chapman, P. B. (2010). Inhibition of mutated, activated BRAF in metastatic melanoma. *N Engl J Med*, 363(9), 809-819

Fourcade, J., Kudela, P., Sun, Z., Shen, H., Land, S. R., Lenzner, D., Guillaume, P., Luescher, I. F., Sander, C., Ferrone, S., Kirkwood, J. M., and Zarour, H. M. (2009). PD-1 is a regulator of NY-ESO-1-specific CD8+ T cell expansion in melanoma patients. *J Immunol*, 182(9), 5240-5249

Gattinoni, L., Finkelstein, S. E., Klebanoff, C. A., Antony, P. A., Palmer, D. C., Spiess, P. J., Hwang, L. N., Yu, Z., Wrzesinski, C., Heimann, D. M., Surh, C. D., Rosenberg, S. A., and Restifo, N. P. (2005). Removal of homeostatic cytokine sinks by lymphodepletion enhances the efficacy of adoptively transferred tumor-specific CD8+ T cells. *J Exp Med*, 202(7), 907-912

Gopal, Y. N., Deng, W., Woodman, S. E., Komurov, K., Ram, P., Smith, P. D., and Davies, M. A. (2010). Basal and treatment-induced activation of AKT mediates resistance to cell death by AZD6244 (ARRY-142886) in Braf-mutant human cutaneous melanoma cells. *Cancer Res*, 70(21), 8736-8747

Haluska, F., Pemberton, T., Ibrahim, N., and Kalinsky, K. (2007). The RTK/RAS/BRAF/PI3K pathways in melanoma: biology, small molecule inhibitors, and potential applications. *Semin Oncol*, 34(6), 546-554

Hamid, O., Sznol, M. , Pavlick, A. C. , Kluger, H. M., Kim, K. B. , Boasberg, P. D. , Simantov, R. , Davis, T. A. , Crowley, E., Hwu, P. . (2010). Frequent dosing and GPNMB expression with CDX-011 (CR011-vcMMAE), an antibody-drug conjugate (ADC), in patients with advanced melanoma. *J Clin Oncol*, 28(15s), ASCO Annual Meeting Abstract 8525

Hamid, O., Urba, W. J. , Yellin, M., Nichol, G. M. , Weber, J., Hersh, E. M. , Tchekmedyian, S. , Hodi, F. S., Weber R. , O'Day, S. . (2007). Kinetics of response to ipilimumab (MDX-010) in patients with stage III/IV melanoma. *J Clin Oncol*, 25 (18S (June 20 Supplement)), Abstract 8525

Hauschild, A., Agarwala, S. S., Trefzer, U., Hogg, D., Robert, C., Hersey, P., Eggermont, A., Grabbe, S., Gonzalez, R., Gille, J., Peschel, C., Schadendorf, D., Garbe, C., O'Day, S., Daud, A., White, J. M., Xia, C., Patel, K., Kirkwood, J. M., and Keilholz, U. (2009). Results of a phase III, randomized, placebo-controlled study of sorafenib in combination with carboplatin and paclitaxel as second-line treatment in patients with unresectable stage III or stage IV melanoma. *J Clin Oncol*, 27(17), 2823-2830

Heinrich, M. C., Griffith, D. J., Druker, B. J., Wait, C. L., Ott, K. A., and Zigler, A. J. (2000). Inhibition of c-kit receptor tyrosine kinase activity by STI 571, a selective tyrosine kinase inhibitor. *Blood*, 96(3), 925-932

Hino, R., Kabashima, K., Kato, Y., Yagi, H., Nakamura, M., Honjo, T., Okazaki, T., and Tokura, Y. (2010). Tumor cell expression of programmed cell death-1 ligand 1 is a prognostic factor for malignant melanoma. *Cancer*, 116(7), 1757-1766

Hodi, F. S., Friedlander, P., Corless, C. L., Heinrich, M. C., Mac Rae, S., Kruse, A., Jagannathan, J., Van den Abbeele, A. D., Velazquez, E. F., Demetri, G. D., and Fisher, D. E. (2008a). Major response to imatinib mesylate in KIT-mutated melanoma. *J Clin Oncol*, 26(12), 2046-2051

Hodi, F. S., O'Day, S. J., McDermott, D. F., Weber, R. W., Sosman, J. A., Haanen, J. B., Gonzalez, R., Robert, C., Schadendorf, D., Hassel, J. C., Akerley, W., van den

Eertwegh, A. J., Lutzky, J., Lorigan, P., Vaubel, J. M., Linette, G. P., Hogg, D., Ottensmeier, C. H., Lebbe, C., Peschel, C., Quirt, I., Clark, J. I., Wolchok, J. D., Weber, J. S., Tian, J., Yellin, M. J., Nichol, G. M., Hoos, A., and Urba, W. J. (2010). Improved survival with ipilimumab in patients with metastatic melanoma. *N Engl J Med*, 363(8), 711-723

Hodi, F. S., Oble, D. A., Drappatz, J., Velazquez, E. F., Ramaiya, N., Ramakrishna, N., Day, A. L., Kruse, A., Mac Rae, S., Hoos, A., and Mihm, M. (2008b). CTLA-4 blockade with ipilimumab induces significant clinical benefit in a female with melanoma metastases to the CNS. *Nat Clin Pract Oncol*, 5(9), 557-561

Hwu, W. J., Lis, E., Menell, J. H., Panageas, K. S., Lamb, L. A., Merrell, J., Williams, L. J., Krown, S. E., Chapman, P. B., Livingston, P. O., Wolchok, J. D., and Houghton, A. N. (2005). Temozolomide plus thalidomide in patients with brain metastases from melanoma: a phase II study. *Cancer*, 103(12), 2590-2597

Infante, J. R., Fecher, L. A. , Nallapareddy, S., Gordon, M. S., Flaherty, K. T., Cox, D. S., DeMarini, D. J. , Morris, S. R., Burris, H. A., Messersmith, W. A. (2010). Safety and efficacy results from the first-in-human study of the oral MEK 1/2 inhibitor GSK1120212. *J Clin Oncol*, 28(15s), ASCO annual meeting abstract 2503

Ives, N. J., Stowe, R. L., Lorigan, P., and Wheatley, K. (2007). Chemotherapy compared with biochemotherapy for the treatment of metastatic melanoma: a meta-analysis of 18 trials involving 2,621 patients. *J Clin Oncol*, 25(34), 5426-5434

Iwai, Y., Ishida, M., Tanaka, Y., Okazaki, T., Honjo, T., and Minato, N. (2002). Involvement of PD-L1 on tumor cells in the escape from host immune system and tumor immunotherapy by PD-L1 blockade. *Proc Natl Acad Sci U S A*, 99(19), 12293-12297

Jayson, G. C., Mullamitha, S. , Ton, C. , Valle, J. , Saunders, M., Munteanu, M. C. , Jang, H., Trikha, M., Davis, H. M. , Beckman, R. A. . (2004). Phase I study of CNTO 95, a fully human monoclonal antibody (mAb) to αv integrins, in patients with solid tumors. *J Clin Oncol*, 22(14s), ASCO Meeting, Abstract 3119

Jiang, C. C., Lai, F., Thorne, R. F., Yang, F., Liu, H., Hersey, P., and Zhang, X. D. (2011). MEK-Independent Survival of B-RAFV600E Melanoma Cells Selected for Resistance to Apoptosis Induced by the RAF Inhibitor PLX4720. *Clin Cancer Res*, 19(4), 721-730

Johannessen, C. M., Boehm, J. S., Kim, S. Y., Thomas, S. R., Wardwell, L., Johnson, L. A., Emery, C. M., Stransky, N., Cogdill, A. P., Barretina, J., Caponigro, G., Hieronymus, H., Murray, R. R., Salehi-Ashtiani, K., Hill, D. E., Vidal, M., Zhao, J. J., Yang, X., Alkan, O., Kim, S., Harris, J. L., Wilson, C. J., Myer, V. E., Finan, P. M., Root, D. E., Roberts, T. M., Golub, T., Flaherty, K. T., Dummer, R., Weber, B. L., Sellers, W. R., Schlegel, R., Wargo, J. A., Hahn, W. C., and Garraway, L. A. (2010). COT drives resistance to RAF inhibition through MAP kinase pathway reactivation. *Nature*, 468(7326), 968-672

Johnson, L. A., Morgan, R. A., Dudley, M. E., Cassard, L., Yang, J. C., Hughes, M. S., Kammula, U. S., Royal, R. E., Sherry, R. M., Wunderlich, J. R., Lee, C. C., Restifo, N. P., Schwarz, S. L., Cogdill, A. P., Bishop, R. J., Kim, H., Brewer, C. C., Rudy, S. F., VanWaes, C., Davis, J. L., Mathur, A., Ripley, R. T., Nathan, D. A., Laurencot, C. M., and Rosenberg, S. A. (2009). Gene therapy with human and mouse T-cell receptors mediates cancer regression and targets normal tissues expressing cognate antigen. *Blood*, 114(3), 535-546

Kahler, K. C., and Hauschild, A. (2010). Treatment and side effect management of CTLA-4 antibody therapy in metastatic melanoma. *J Dtsch Dermatol Ges*, 9(4), 277-286

Kefford, R., Arkenau, H. , Brown, M. P. , Millward, M. , Infante, J. R. , Long, G. V. , Ouellet, D., Curtis, M. , Lebowitz, P. F. , Falchook, G. S. (2010). Phase I/II study of GSK2118436, a selective inhibitor of oncogenic mutant BRAF kinase, in patients with metastatic melanoma and other solid tumors. *J Clin Oncol*, 28(15s), ASCO Annual Meeting, Abstract 8503

Lawrence, D. P., Hamid, O., McDermott, D. F. , Puzanov, I. , Sznol, M. , Clark, J. , Logan, T. , Hodi, F. S. , Heller, K. N. , Margolin, K. A. . (2010). Phase II trial of ipilimumab monotherapy in melanoma patients with brain metastases. *J Clin Oncol*, 28(15s), (suppl; abstr 8523)

Margolin, K. A., Di Giacomo, A. M., and Maio, M. (2010). Brain metastasis in melanoma: clinical activity of CTLA-4 antibody therapy. *Semin Oncol*, 37(5), 468-472

Meier, F., Schittek, B., Busch, S., Garbe, C., Smalley, K., Satyamoorthy, K., Li, G., and Herlyn, M. (2005). The RAS/RAF/MEK/ERK and PI3K/AKT signaling pathways present molecular targets for the effective treatment of advanced melanoma. *Front Biosci*, 10, 2986-3001

Middleton, M. R., Grob, J. J., Aaronson, N., Fierlbeck, G., Tilgen, W., Seiter, S., Gore, M., Aamdal, S., Cebon, J., Coates, A., Dreno, B., Henz, M., Schadendorf, D., Kapp, A., Weiss, J., Fraass, U., Statkevich, P., Muller, M., and Thatcher, N. (2000). Randomized phase III study of temozolomide versus dacarbazine in the treatment of patients with advanced metastatic malignant melanoma. *J Clin Oncol*, 18(1), 158-166

Minor, D. R., O'Day, S. , Kashani-Sabet, M. , Daud, A. , Salman, Z. , Bastian, B. . (2010). Sunitinib therapy for metastatic melanomas with KIT aberrations. *J Clin Oncol*, 28, ASCO 2010 Meeting, Abstract 8545.

Montagut, C., Sharma, S. V., Shioda, T., McDermott, U., Ulman, M., Ulkus, L. E., Dias-Santagata, D., Stubbs, H., Lee, D. Y., Singh, A., Drew, L., Haber, D. A., and Settleman, J. (2008). Elevated CRAF as a potential mechanism of acquired resistance to BRAF inhibition in melanoma. *Cancer Res*, 68(12), 4853-4861

Morgan, R. A., Dudley, M. E., Wunderlich, J. R., Hughes, M. S., Yang, J. C., Sherry, R. M., Royal, R. E., Topalian, S. L., Kammula, U. S., Restifo, N. P., Zheng, Z., Nahvi, A., de Vries, C. R., Rogers-Freezer, L. J., Mavroukakis, S. A., and Rosenberg, S. A. (2006). Cancer regression in patients after transfer of genetically engineered lymphocytes. *Science*, 314(5796), 126-129

Nazarian, R., Shi, H., Wang, Q., Kong, X., Koya, R. C., Lee, H., Chen, Z., Lee, M. K., Attar, N., Sazegar, H., Chodon, T., Nelson, S. F., McArthur, G., Sosman, J. A., Ribas, A., and Lo, R. S. (2010). Melanomas acquire resistance to B-RAF(V600E) inhibition by RTK or N-RAS upregulation. *Nature*, 468(7326), 973-977

O'Day, S. J., Maio, M., Chiarion-Sileni, V., Gajewski, T. F., Pehamberger, H., Bondarenko, I. N., Queirolo, P., Lundgren, L., Mikhailov, S., Roman, L., Verschraegen, C., Humphrey, R., Ibrahim, R., de Pril, V., Hoos, A., and Wolchok, J. D. (2010). Efficacy and safety of ipilimumab monotherapy in patients with pretreated advanced melanoma: a multicenter single-arm phase II study. *Ann Oncol*, 21(8), 1712-1717

O'Day, S. J., Pavlick, A. C., Albertini, M. R., Hamid, O., Schalch, H., Lang, Z., Ling, J., Mata, M., Reddy, M., and Foster, B. (2011). Clinical and pharmacologic evaluation of two dose levels of intetumumab (CNTO 95) in patients with melanoma or angiosarcoma. *Invest New Drugs*, 2011 Feb 18.[Epub ahead of print]

Ott, P. A., Hamilton, A., Min, C., Safarzadeh-Amiri, S., Goldberg, L., Yoon, J., Yee, H., Buckley, M., Christos, P. J., Wright, J. J., Polsky, D., Osman, I., Liebes, L., and Pavlick, A. C. (2010). A phase II trial of sorafenib in metastatic melanoma with tissue correlates. *PLoS One*, 5(12), e15588

Paraiso, K. H., Fedorenko, I. V., Cantini, L. P., Munko, A. C., Hall, M., Sondak, V. K., Messina, J. L., Flaherty, K. T., and Smalley, K. S. (2010). Recovery of phospho-ERK activity allows melanoma cells to escape from BRAF inhibitor therapy. *Br J Cancer*, 102(12), 1724-1730

Parry, R. V., Chemnitz, J. M., Frauwirth, K. A., Lanfranco, A. R., Braunstein, I., Kobayashi, S. V., Linsley, P. S., Thompson, C. B., and Riley, J. L. (2005). CTLA-4 and PD-1 receptors inhibit T-cell activation by distinct mechanisms. *Mol Cell Biol*, 25(21), 9543-9553

Patel, J. K., Didolkar, M. S., Pickren, J. W., and Moore, R. H. (1978). Metastatic pattern of malignant melanoma. A study of 216 autopsy cases. *Am J Surg*, 135(6), 807-810

Patel, S. P., Lazar, A. J. , Mahoney, S. , Vaughn, C. , Gonzalez, N. , Papadopoulos, N. E. , Liu, P. , Infante, J. R., LoRusso, P., Kim, K. B. (2010). Clinical responses to AZD6244 (ARRY-142886)-based combination therapy stratified by gene mutations in patients with metastatic melanoma. *J Clin Oncol*, 28(15s)

Paulos, C. M., Kaiser, A., Wrzesinski, C., Hinrichs, C. S., Cassard, L., Boni, A., Muranski, P., Sanchez-Perez, L., Palmer, D. C., Yu, Z., Antony, P. A., Gattinoni, L., Rosenberg, S. A., and Restifo, N. P. (2007). Toll-like receptors in tumor immunotherapy. *Clin Cancer Res*, 13(18 Pt 1), 5280-5289

Pavlick, A. C., Ott, P. A. , Kannan, R. , Madden, K. M., Sorlie, C. , Escano, C. , Escalon, J. , Hernando-Monge, E. , Osman, I. , Bhardwaj, N. (2010). Hair depigmentation as an indicator of a durable response to CTLA-4 therapy. *J Clin Oncol*, 28 suppl(15s), ASCO Annual Meeting, abstract 8571

Plummer, R., Lorigan, P., Evans, J., Steven, N., Middleton, M., Wilson, R., Snow, K., Dewji, R., Calvert, H. . (2006). First and final report of a phase II study of the poly(ADP-ribose) polymerase (PARP) inhibitor, AG014699, in combination with temozolomide (TMZ) in patients with metastatic malignant melanoma (MM). *J Clin Oncol*, 24(18s), ASCO Meeting, Abstract 8013

Ribas, A., Hauschild, A., Kefford, R. , Punt, C. J. , Haanen, J. B. , Marmol, M. , Garbe, C. , Gomez-Navarro, J. , Pavlov D. , Marshall, M. . (2008). Phase III, open-label, randomized, comparative study of tremelimumab (CP-675,206) and chemotherapy (temozolomide [TMZ] or dacarbazine [DTIC]) in patients with advanced melanoma. *J Clin Oncol*, 26(15S (May 20 Supplement)), Abstract 9011

Robbins, P. F., Morgan, R. A., Feldman, S. A., Yang, J. C., Sherry, R. M., Dudley, M. E., Wunderlich, J. R., Nahvi, A. V., Helman, L. J., Mackall, C. L., Kammula, U. S., Hughes, M. S., Restifo, N. P., Raffeld, M., Lee, C. C., Levy, C. L., Li, Y. F., El-Gamil, M., Schwarz, S. L., Laurencot, C., and Rosenberg, S. A. (2011). Tumor Regression in Patients With Metastatic Synovial Cell Sarcoma and Melanoma Using Genetically Engineered Lymphocytes Reactive With NY-ESO-1. *J Clin Oncol*, 29(7), 917-924

Robert, C., Arnault, J. P., and Mateus, C. (2010). "RAF inhibition and induction of cutaneous squamous cell carcinoma." *Curr Opin Oncol*, 23(2), 177-182

Sampson, J. H., Carter, J. H., Jr., Friedman, A. H., and Seigler, H. F. (1998). Demographics, prognosis, and therapy in 702 patients with brain metastases from malignant melanoma. *J Neurosurg*, 88(1), 11-20

Schartz, N. E., Farges, C., Madelaine, I., Bruzzoni, H., Calvo, F., Hoos, A., and Lebbe, C. (2010). Complete regression of a previously untreated melanoma brain metastasis with ipilimumab. *Melanoma Res*, 20(3), 247-50

Serrone, L., Zeuli, M., Sega, F. M., and Cognetti, F. (2000). Dacarbazine-based chemotherapy for metastatic melanoma: thirty-year experience overview. *J Exp Clin Cancer Res*, 19(1), 21-34

Shao, Y., and Aplin, A. E. (2010). Akt3-mediated resistance to apoptosis in B-RAF-targeted melanoma cells. *Cancer Res*, 70(16), 6670-6681

Shields, J. M., Thomas, N. E., Cregger, M., Berger, A. J., Leslie, M., Torrice, C., Hao, H., Penland, S., Arbiser, J., Scott, G., Zhou, T., Bar-Eli, M., Bear, J. E., Der, C. J., Kaufmann, W. K., Rimm, D. L., and Sharpless, N. E. (2007). Lack of extracellular signal-regulated kinase mitogen-activated protein kinase signaling shows a new type of melanoma. *Cancer Res*, 67(4), 1502-1512

Sinnberg, T., Lasithiotakis, K., Niessner, H., Schittek, B., Flaherty, K. T., Kulms, D., Maczey, E., Campos, M., Gogel, J., Garbe, C., and Meier, F. (2009). Inhibition of PI3K-AKT-mTOR signaling sensitizes melanoma cells to cisplatin and temozolomide. *J Invest Dermatol*, 129(6), 1500-1515

Stahl, J. M., Sharma, A., Cheung, M., Zimmerman, M., Cheng, J. Q., Bosenberg, M. W., Kester, M., Sandirasegarane, L., and Robertson, G. P. (2004). Deregulated Akt3 activity promotes development of malignant melanoma. *Cancer Res*, 64(19), 7002-7010

Staibano, S., Pepe, S., Lo Muzio, L., Somma, P., Mascolo, M., Argenziano, G., Scalvenzi, M., Salvatore, G., Fabbrocini, G., Molea, G., Bianco, A. R., Carlomagno, C., and De Rosa, G. (2005). Poly(adenosine diphosphate-ribose) polymerase 1 expression in malignant melanomas from photoexposed areas of the head and neck region. *Hum Pathol*, 36(7), 724-731

Strome, S. E., Dong, H., Tamura, H., Voss, S. G., Flies, D. B., Tamada, K., Salomao, D., Cheville, J., Hirano, F., Lin, W., Kasperbauer, J. L., Ballman, K. V., and Chen, L. (2003). B7-H1 blockade augments adoptive T-cell immunotherapy for squamous cell carcinoma. *Cancer Res*, 63(19), 6501-6505

Sznol, M., Powderly, J.D. , Smith, D.C , Brahmer, J.R. , Drake, C.G. , McDermott, D.F. , Lawrence, P.D. , Wolchok, J.D. , Topalian, S.L. , Lowy, I. (2010). Safety and antitumor activity of biweekly MDX-1106 (Anti-PD-1, BMS-936558/ONO-4538) in patients with advanced refractory malignancies. *J Clin Oncol 28:15s, 2010 (suppl; abstr 2506)*

Trikha, M., Zhou, Z., Nemeth, J. A., Chen, Q., Sharp, C., Emmell, E., Giles-Komar, J., and Nakada, M. T. (2004). CNTO 95, a fully human monoclonal antibody that inhibits alphav integrins, has antitumor and antiangiogenic activity in vivo. *Int J Cancer*, 110(3), 326-335

Tsao, H., Atkins, M. B. & Sober, A. J. (2004). Management of cutaneous melanoma. *N Engl J Med*, 351(10), 998-1012

Tutt, A., Robson, M., Garber, J. E., Domchek, S. M., Audeh, M. W., Weitzel, J. N., Friedlander, M., Arun, B., Loman, N., Schmutzler, R. K., Wardley, A., Mitchell, G.,

Earl, H., Wickens, M., and Carmichael, J. (2010). Oral poly(ADP-ribose) polymerase inhibitor olaparib in patients with BRCA1 or BRCA2 mutations and advanced breast cancer: a proof-of-concept trial. *Lancet*, 376(9737), 235-244

Ugurel, S., Hildenbrand, R., Zimpfer, A., La Rosee, P., Paschka, P., Sucker, A., Keikavoussi, P., Becker, J. C., Rittgen, W., Hochhaus, A., and Schadendorf, D. (2005). Lack of clinical efficacy of imatinib in metastatic melanoma. *Br J Cancer*, 92(8), 1398-1405

Villanueva, J., Vultur, A., Lee, J. T., Somasundaram, R., Fukunaga-Kalabis, M., Cipolla, A. K., Wubbenhorst, B., Xu, X., Gimotty, P. A., Kee, D., Santiago-Walker, A. E., Letrero, R., D'Andrea, K., Pushparajan, A., Hayden, J. E., Brown, K. D., Laquerre, S., McArthur, G. A., Sosman, J. A., Nathanson, K. L., and Herlyn, M. (2010). Acquired resistance to BRAF inhibitors mediated by a RAF kinase switch in melanoma can be overcome by cotargeting MEK and IGF-1R/PI3K. *Cancer Cell*, 18(6), 683-695

Vivanco, I., and Sawyers, C. L. (2002). The phosphatidylinositol 3-Kinase AKT pathway in human cancer. *Nat Rev Cancer*, 2(7), 489-501

Weber, J., Thompson, J. A., Hamid, O., Minor, D., Amin, A., Ron, I., Ridolfi, R., Assi, H., Maraveyas, A., Berman, D., Siegel, J., and O'Day, S. J. (2009). A randomized, double-blind, placebo-controlled, phase II study comparing the tolerability and efficacy of ipilimumab administered with or without prophylactic budesonide in patients with unresectable stage III or IV melanoma. *Clin Cancer Res*, 15(17), 5591-5598

Wilhelm, S. M., Carter, C., Tang, L., Wilkie, D., McNabola, A., Rong, H., Chen, C., Zhang, X., Vincent, P., McHugh, M., Cao, Y., Shujath, J., Gawlak, S., Eveleigh, D., Rowley, B., Liu, L., Adnane, L., Lynch, M., Auclair, D., Taylor, I., Gedrich, R., Voznesensky, A., Riedl, B., Post, L. E., Bollag, G., and Trail, P. A. (2004). BAY 43-9006 exhibits broad spectrum oral antitumor activity and targets the RAF/MEK/ERK pathway and receptor tyrosine kinases involved in tumor progression and angiogenesis. *Cancer Res*, 64(19), 7099-7109

Wolchok JD, H. A., O'Day S, Weber JS, Hamid O, Lebbé C, Maio M, Binder M, Bohnsack O, Nichol G, Humphrey R, Hodi FS. (2009). Guidelines for the Evaluation of Immune Therapy Activity in Solid Tumors: Immune-Related Response Criteria. *Clin Cancer Res*, 15(23), 7412-7420

Wolchok, J. D., Neyns, B., Linette, G., Negrier, S., Lutzky, J., Thomas, L., Waterfield, W., Schadendorf, D., Smylie, M., Guthrie, T., Jr., Grob, J. J., Chesney, J., Chin, K., Chen, K., Hoos, A., O'Day, S. J., and Lebbe, C. (2010). Ipilimumab monotherapy in patients with pretreated advanced melanoma: a randomised, double-blind, multicentre, phase 2, dose-ranging study. *Lancet Oncol*, 11(2), 155-164

Wyman, K., Atkins, M. B., Prieto, V., Eton, O., McDermott, D. F., Hubbard, F., Byrnes, C., Sanders, K., and Sosman, J. A. (2006). Multicenter Phase II trial of high-dose imatinib mesylate in metastatic melanoma: significant toxicity with no clinical efficacy. *Cancer*, 106(9), 2005-2011

Yang, J. C., Hughes, M., Kammula, U., Royal, R., Sherry, R. M., Topalian, S. L., Suri, K. B., Levy, C., Allen, T., Mavroukakis, S., Lowy, I., White, D. E., and Rosenberg, S. A. (2007). Ipilimumab (anti-CTLA4 antibody) causes regression of metastatic renal cell cancer associated with enteritis and hypophysitis. *J Immunother*, 30(8), 825-830

Yang, S., Dudley, M. E., Rosenberg, S. A., and Morgan, R. A. (2010). A simplified method for the clinical-scale generation of central memory-like CD8+ T cells after transduction with lentiviral vectors encoding antitumor antigen T-cell receptors. *J Immunother*, 33(6), 648-658

Yeh, T. C., Marsh, V., Bernat, B. A., Ballard, J., Colwell, H., Evans, R. J., Parry, J., Smith, D., Brandhuber, B. J., Gross, S., Marlow, A., Hurley, B., Lyssikatos, J., Lee, P. A., Winkler, J. D., Koch, K., and Wallace, E. (2007). Biological characterization of ARRY-142886 (AZD6244), a potent, highly selective mitogen-activated protein kinase kinase 1/2 inhibitor. *Clin Cancer Res*, 13(5), 1576-1583

Part 4

Electrochemotherapy

10

Pulse Power Ablation of Melanoma with Nanosecond Pulsed Electric Fields

Stephen J. Beebe, Wentia E. Ford, Wei Ren and Xinhua Chen
Old Dominion University / Frank Reidy Research Center for Bioelectrics
Norfolk, Virginia,
USA

1. Introduction

Melanocytes are cells that originate in the neural crest. In the dermis, their well characterized role is to produce melanin and through interactions with keratinocytes transfer this pigment to determine skin color and protect the largest organ in the body, the skin, from ultraviolet light. As an effective free radical scavenger, melanin protects against reactive oxygen species that would otherwise damage DNA [Rózanowska et al., 1999]. Melanocytes may also have other roles such as immune, neuroendocrine, and signaling functions through interactions with cells other than keratinocytes, such as lymphocytes, mast cells and endothelial cells [see Tsatmali et al., 2002 for review]. However, keratinocytes regulate melanocyte number, differentiation and melanin production in response to UV radiation. It may be that the resilience of melanocytes to protect the skin, their extraordinary regenerative capacity and their origin as neural crest migratory cells makes them one of the most deadly forms of metastatic skin cancers when they undergo tumorogenesis. It is known that there is a great deal of common cellular and genetic events among embryonic development, tissue regeneration and cancer. Further, typical self-renewal and migration capacity of cancer are shared with embryonic and regenerative cells [White and Zon, 2008]. The recapitulation of embryonic genetic programs is facilitated by overexposure to extreme sunlight (UVA and UVB) or tanning bed light (mostly UVA). The American Cancer Society estimated that in the US in 2009, 68,720 new cases of melanoma (188 new cases / day) will be diagnosed and 8,650 people will die from the disease (24 melanoma deaths / day). The continued increase in melanoma is a significant cause of morbidity and mortality in the Western world. Thus, metastatic melanoma remains a persistent therapeutic challenge. There are limited successes in preventing this often fatal disease and there are even fewer successes in developing a cure.

2. Standard melanoma therapies

Presently available treatment strategies have had limited impact on progression and overall survival of patients with melanoma. In addition to surgery, currently approved treatments for metastatic melanoma include chemotherapy, radiation and/or immunotherapy. Chemotherapy is mostly limited to dacarbazine, cisplatin, carmustine and vinblastin. The addition of systemic immunotherapy with IL-2 and/or INFα to these chemotherapeutic agents resulted in major toxicities. INFά is approved for use but is not included as a standard of care due to minimal impact on overall survival and significant toxicities [Amaravadi et al., 2007; Gogas et al., 2007; Tarhini et al., 2006]. Unfortunately, metastatic melanoma is one of the most resistant cancers to a wide range of treatment modalities including single-agents and combination chemotherapy, immunotherapy, chemoimmunotherapy and a host of immune stimulators [Riker et al., 2007].

3. Targeted melanoma therapies

One of the major problems that cancer therapeutics face today is coping with a diversity of cancer diseases and melanoma is no exception. However, Hanahan and Weinberg [2000, 2011] reasoned that since all mammalian cells express the same molecular mechanisms for proliferation, differentiation and death, most if not all cancers should share a limited number of common molecular, biochemical and cellular traits that govern their behavior. This is insightful since cancers exhibit hundreds of genotypes and subtypes of tumors can be found in specific organs. In addition, different mutations can be found within the same tumor.
In order to promote the development of cancer research into a more logical science, to provide more focused characterization of cancer and to manage this array of diseases, Hanahan and Weinberg [2000,2011] initially defined six major hallmarks of cancer that exhibit physiological anomalies that control cell homeostasis and proliferation. These include self-sufficiency in growth signals, insensitivity to growth-inhibitory (antigrowth) signals, evasion of apoptosis, limitless replicative potential, sustained angiogenesis, and tissue invasion and metastasis. They later included reprogramming of energy metabolism and evasion of immune detection as cancer hallmarks [2011]. Kroemer and Pouyssegur [2007] included evasion of immune surveillance as a seventh hallmark. Luo et al. [7] expanded these classic hallmarks to include stress phenotypes of tumorigenesis and defined a large class of non-oncogenes that are essential for cancer cell survival. Treatment strategies to develop targeted, mutation-specific small molecule drugs or monoclonal antibodies to treat melanomas is an outcome of an evolving understanding of the molecular mechanisms of melanoma in the perspective of these defined cancer hallmarks.
A number of new agents for advanced melanoma are being tested in clinical trials. Considering the hallmarks of cancer, the most recent new drugs for treating melanoma have found some successes in the inhibition of self sufficiency of growth signals, immune surveillance evasion, sustained angiogenesis and evasion of apoptosis. These agents are directed towards proteins that are involved in cell signaling pathways that are responsible for cell division and proliferation, immune responses, blood vessel formation and programmed cell death. Several considerations are appropriate when taking targeted drugs into account. First, targeted therapies are generally effective for individuals identified with a specific mutation, so patients can be screened before treatment to determine if they have the specific mutation for which the drug is designed to affect. This exemplifies the impact of personalized medicine on oncology and if successful will become a common procedure. This can be achieved by relatively simple and inexpensive procedures. The second concern is issues of heterogeneity within a patient's melanoma. While a specific mutation may be determined in a biopsy sample, the targeted mutation may not be present in all of the patient's melanoma cells. This provides a potential means for resistance and recurrences. A third issue is the continued "pressure" exerted or relieved by a targeted agent on cell signaling in the affected cancer cells. Such events modify signaling dynamics with responses

that attempt to "escape" the modification, which may also lead to resistance and recurrences. These issues may complicate uses of targeted medicine in melanoma treatments.

Although other causes of cancer are known, mutations that often lead to malignant growth and metastasis frequently occur in protein kinases [Blume-Jensen and Hunter, 2001; Chenga and Force, 2010]. Protein tyrosine kinases transduce extracellular signals into intracellular functions that regulate a wide array of cellular activity. Tumorigenesis is often driven by constitutively active protein kinases that modulate cell cycle, angiogenesis or apoptosis. Two general classes of protein kinase inhibitors include monoclonal antibodies or small molecular weight inhibitors that are directed against specific protein tyrosine kinase receptors or their ligands. A common site for protein kinase inhibitor drug design is the ATP binding site because transfer of phosphate to substrates cannot occur without the gamma-phosphate from ATP. However, the binding sites are so highly conserved among kinases that kinase genes can be identified without phosphotransferase activity by the presence of specific sequences that define ATP binding. Two major concerns in designing these drugs are issues of specificity and potency. Specificity is one issue because of the ATP binding site conservation among all protein kinases. Given the broad range of kinase functions, it becomes important to inhibit kinases involved in tumorigenesis without affecting other kinases. Potency is the other concern because ATP is at relative high concentrations in the cell (milliMolar) and an orally active small molecular weight drug must have a high affinity to be an effective inhibitor. Kinase inhibitors are divided into three major classes based on binding to their ATP site [Chenga and Force, 2010]. Type I inhibitors have high affinity for the ATP binding pocket. Therefore type I kinase inhibitors generally have broad kinase specificity. Type II kinase inhibitor (e.g., imatinib) are more selective because they not only have specificity for the ATP binding site but also sites adjacent the ATP binding site. In addition, unlike type I inhibitors, type II inhibitors can bind to kinases in their inactive conformation. Type III kinase inhibitors (e.g., families of mitogen-activated protein/extracellular signal-regulated kinase kinase inhibitors) are more selective but more difficult to design because they bind to sites distant from the ATP binding pocket.

A number of monoclonal antibodies and targeted small molecular weight protein tyrosine kinase inhibitors are in clinical trials for the treatment of melanoma. Regarding the hallmarks of cancer, these agents are directed to prevent limitless replicative potential and/or self-sufficiency in growth signals, evasion of immune surveillance, sustained angiogenesis, and evasion of apoptosis. Because protein tyrosine kinases are involved in many of these hallmarks, many of these agents are multi-protein tyrosine kinase inhibitors that are directed towards more than one of these hallmarks and kinases so have overlapping targets. For example, Sunitinib, Sorafenib and Imatinib target VEGFRs and/or PDGFRs and can act as anti-angiogenesis agents. In addition, these drugs can also act on either c-Kit and/or Raf-1/B-Raf and are directed towards limitless replicative potential and/or self-sufficiency in growth signals. Current data indicate that melanomas with activating c-KIT mutations and possibly also with KIT gene amplifications respond to therapy with tyrosine kinase inhibitors blocking c-KIT. It was suggested that subgroups of patients with metastatic melanoma prone to *KIT* mutations, such as primary mucosal and acrolentiginous melanomas, should be analyzed for their *KIT* status [Satzger et al., 2010].

A significant number of melanomas are mutated at V600E in BRAF (~60%), an oncogene that is a signal transduction enzyme near the origin or proximal end of a cascade of phosphorylation events that promotes proliferation through the Raf/Mek/Erk pathway and survival of cells through the PI3K/Akt/mTor pathway. PLX4032, a B-raf kinase inhibitor has been shown to induce programmed cell death by inhibiting proliferation, growth and survival. It is also known to be involved in overcoming apoptosis evasion. In a recent multi-phase phase I dose-escalation trial among 16 patients with melanoma exhibiting the V600E BRAF mutation, 62% (10 patients) had a partial response and 1 had a complete response when given PLX4032 (240mg or more twice daily). Among 32 patients in the extension cohort receiving as much as 960mg twice daily, 75% (24 patients) had a partial response and 2 patients had a complete response. The estimated median progression-free survival among all patients was more than 7 months [Flaherty et al., 2010]. This represents an important new therapeutic development in the treatment of melanoma. For those who experienced relapses, second mutation(s) continue to drive tumorigenesis. Two mechanism of resistance to PLX4032 (covering 40% of cases) have been discovered. In one of these the cancer cells begin to overexpress a cell surface Beta-type protein platelet derived growth factor receptor creating an alternate survival pathway. In a second mechanism of resistance, the oncogene *N-Ras* mutates, reactivating the normal BRAF survival pathway [Nazarian et al., 2010].

Several new agents have been evaluated for targeting the immune system. Several agonist monoclonal antibodies have shown promise including those directed against members of the tumor necrosis factor receptor superfamily such as 4-1BB (CD137), Ox40 (CD134), and CD40. Two human antagonists monoclonal antibodies have been investigated in melanoma patients that bind to CTLA-4 (cytotoxic T lymphocyte-associated antigen 4), which is a molecule on helper T-cells that appears to play an important role in regulating natural immune responses. These include Ipilimumab and Tremelimumab. Ipilimumab was recently evaluated alone and in combination with gp100 as compared with gp100 alone. In this phase III trial, it showed improved overall survival in patients with previously treated metastatic melanoma. Although there were some severe adverse reactions associated with this therapy they were reversible with appropriate treatment [Hodi et al., 2010; Peggs and Quezada, 2010]. Tremelimumab has been shown to induce durable tumor responses in patients with metastatic melanoma in Phase I and Phase II clinical studies [Reubens et al., 2006] and more recently has shown promise in treatment of patients with metastatic melanoma, in a completed randomized, double-blind phase III trial [Callahan et al., 2010].

While most of the potential therapeutic agents are given orally, other delivery methods have begun to be used for more localized treatments and include the utilization of electric fields. One of these approaches is to maintain cell survival using conventional electroporation to deliver plasmids that express genes for therapeutic effects [Neumann et al., 2002]. This method is referred to as electrogene therapy. This is an outgrowth of electrochemotherapy that uses conventional electroporation to deliver impermeable chemotherapeutic drugs such as bleomycin to tumors [Heller et al., 1996; Mir et al., 1991]. The delivery of IL-12 to melanoma lesions to activate the immune system against melanoma by electrogene therapy has demonstrated safety and efficacy in phase I clinical trials. Results demonstrated a bystander effect where lesions surrounding electrogene-treated lesions showed tumor regression [Daud et al., 2008]. The use of electrogene therapy to deliver plasmids for gene expression in pre-clinical and clinical trials is reviewed elsewhere [Beebe et al., 2010].

Two other therapies are based on uses of electric fields that extend conventional electroporation (EP). The first is irreversible electroporation (IRE), which extends EP by increasing the electric field to produce cell necrosis through irreversible plasma cell membrane defects [Al-Sakere et al., 2007; Davalos et al., 2005; Onik et al., 2007;], although some evidence suggests that ablation zones may also exhibit apoptotic cells [Guo et al., 2010;

Lee et al., 2010], a possibility that requires further investigation. IRE is also reported to affect only cell membranes and limits effects to cells within the ablation zone, sparing blood vessels, bile ducts and extracellular matrix structures [Maor et al., 2007; Phillips et al., 2010]. However, a major drawback is muscle contractions induced by microsecond pulses that are absent or significantly reduced with nanosecond pulses in a porcine model [Long et al., 2011]. While IRE could be considered a blunt tool that forces cell death by necrosis (or apoptosis), it exhibits precision for applications because it can clearly define the intended treatment zone and spares larger vessels and ducts [Ivorra et al., 2009; Granot et al., 2009].
Another extension of conventional electroporation uses pulse power technology with nanosecond pulse electric fields (nsPEFs), which continues to be explored for tumor ablation. While there are some comparisons with conventional electroporation, pulse power is distinct in several regards. Compared to conventional electroporation, pulse power ablation (PPA) with nsPEFs uses exceptionally short pulse durations (ns vs. micro-second or milli-second) with exceptionally fast rise times (2-4ns vs. ~100ns). It is hypothesized that fast rise times with short pulse durations have advantages for intracellular effects [Schoenbach et al., 2001]. The electric fields used in these applications of pulse power are higher than conventional electroporation (10-350 kV/cm vs. about 1 kV/cm). Further, the power deposited in cells or tissues is much higher (~180MW vs. ~500W) and energy is lower (mJ/cc vs. J/cc); they are non-thermal. The combination of these conditions causes cell membrane supra-electroporation in *all* cellular membranes resulting in high density "nanopores" (nm diameter) [Gowrishankar et al., 2006; Stewart et al., 2004,].

4. Applications of ultra-high pulse power ablation for the treatment of melanoma

Pulsed power is a technology designed to store energy and release it very quickly to produce immediate high power. It was initially developed during World War II for use in radar, which requires short high power pulses. Since then pulse power technology has been used in particle accelerators, ultra-strong magnetic fields, electromagnetics, fusion research and high power pulsed lasers. An example of how pulse power works is to compare the storage of one joule of energy released in one second versus releasing the same energy in one microsecond or one nanosecond [Wikipedia]. If the stored joule of energy is released all at once to a suspension of cells or tumor tissue in one second, the peak power delivered would only be 1 watt. If all of the stored energy were released within one microsecond, the power would be one megawatt, a million times greater and if release in one nanosecond the peak power would be one gigawatt, a billion times greater. Within the last ten years, applications of ultra-high pulse power have been extended to biology and medicine [Beebe et al., 2002, 2003a, 2004; Beebe and Schoenbach, 2005; Schoenbach et al., 2001, 2004; Vernier et al., 2003a,b], including the treatment of melanoma [Chen, 2009, 2010; Ford et al., 2010; Nuccitelli et al., 2006, 2009, 2010]. In applications of pulse power ablation for treatment of melanoma, as much as 6 kV of potential energy were release in multiple 300ns bursts at 60kV/cm into murine B16f10 melanoma cells or tumors. In addition, the pulses included an extremely fast rise and fall time of about 4-5ns so the 300ns pulses were at maximum power for about 97% of each pulse. It is hypothesized, but not yet proven, that this rapid rise time is important for targeting intracellular organelles and may be an important aspect for therapeutic efficacy.
Another factor that results from nsPEF conditions is the absence of significant temperature increases during treatment. Both *in vitro* and *in vivo* nsPEF studies have shown non-thermal

effects [Chen et al., 2009; Nuccitelli et al., 2006; Pakhomov et al., 2004;]. However, the presence or absence of thermal effects depends on the pulse repetition rate and heat dissipation rates of *in vitro* and *in vivo* systems. Higher frequency applications are more prone to thermal effects. While initial strategies for biological and medical applications were to achieve non-thermal effects, there may be advantages of synergistic effects between electric fields and heating.

A combination of an ultrashort pulses and rapid rise times (shorter than the charging and relaxation time of plasma membranes), created conditions that were hypothesized and shown to have effects on permeabilization of intracellular granules in calcein-loaded human eosinophils without calcein release through the plasma membrane [Schoenbach et al., 2001]. Selective permeabilization of intracellular vesicles was also shown using a mixed population of phospholipid vesicles as well as in endosomal membrane vacuoles in COS-7 cells [Tekle et al., 2005]. Several other studies demonstrated effects that suggested selective permeabilization of intracellular calcium storage sites [Beebe et al., 2003b, 2004; Buescher and Schoenbach, 2003; Vernier et al., 2003a; White et al., 2004] and effects on plasma membranes that were unique compared to conventional electroporation pulses [Beebe et al., 2003a; Deng et al., 2004; Ibey et al., 2010]. However, it was shown later that apparent absences of plasma membrane effects were likely due to formation of plasma membrane pores that were smaller than the reporter molecules, such as propidium iodide or ethidium homodimer [Bowman et al., 2010; Pakhomov et al., 2007a, b]. While these nsPEF applications are known to have effects on all cell membranes, differences among cell types and their sensitivities to pulse power conditions have been reported and will be discussed here.

NsPEF effects have been observed on plasma membranes and intracellular membranes of the cytoskeletal structure, endoplasmic reticulum, mitochondria and nucleus. Many of these effects are hypothesized to be caused by the formation of "nanopores", which occur during supra-electroporation [Gowrishankar et al., 2006; Stewart et al., 2004]. As stated earlier, this effect includes small pores on a large proportion of all cell membranes as opposed to larger pores on a small proportion of the cells membranes during conventional electroporation. However, this may need to be re-considered since more recent modeling approaches suggest that electroporation pulses generate fields inside cells that are high enough to permeabilize intracellular membranes and vesicles [Esser et al., 2010]. This paper predicts for EP that these membrane pores expand and become larger than nanopores arising from nsPEF. It will be important to experimentally test this in cells and tissues to discern real differences between conventional electroporation and nsPEFs concerning intracellular effects and therapeutic relevance. Nevertheless, nanopores allow small ion transport especially ions like sodium, calcium and potassium that can affect cell excitability. Conventional electroporation pores occur primarily in plasma membranes and allow transport of ions and larger molecules such as impermeable chemotherapeutic drugs and plasmids that express therapeutic genes. Like all dose related biological effects, the induction of nanopores has a threshold related to the pulse characteristics including duration, electric field and number. Thus, as pulse conditions increase to longer pulse durations, nanopores will begin to expand and assume characteristics of conventional electroporation. Thus, as pulse durations increase from very short durations to longer duration, there is a continuum from the presence of nanopores on all cell membranes to larger pores primarily on plasma membranes. Further, each cell type has different thresholds presumably based on cell membrane characteristics.

In addition to pulse duration alone, other pulse conditions such as pulse amplitude and pulse number can also influence cell behavior. Modeling results using molecular dynamics [Hu et al., 2006; Tieleman et al., 2003; Vernier et al., 2006] and continuum models [Joshi et al., 2001; 2002; Kotnic and Miklavcic, 2006; Smith et al., 2006] have provided insight into the mechanism of permeabilization of membranes with a single pulse. From an experimental point, Jurkat cells treated with 10ns and 60ns single pulses at various electric fields demonstrated an enhanced uptake of ethidium homodimer, a marker for membrane integrity, and an enhanced binding of Annexin V, a marker for phosphatidylserine externalization, both indicative of membrane permeabilization [Beebe et al., 2004]. In studies using Jurkat and U937 cells [Pakhomov et al., 2004] or GH3 and CHO cells [Ibey et al., 2009] under a variety of conditions, viability scaled with the absorbed dose as defined as the electrical energy density. Another study evaluating cell viability of murine B16f10 melanoma cells with trypan blue using 0.8ns pulses seemed to confirm this [Schoenbach et al., 2008]. However these studies used different cell types and different pulse condition variables but did not include conditions of variable pulse durations, amplitudes and numbers together. When all three variables were included, the results scales with the product of the pulse duration (τ), pulse amplitude (E) and the square root of the pulse number ($n^{0.5}$). This square root dependence on the pulse number indicates a statistical motion of cells between pulses with respect to the applied electric field, and can be explained using an extension of the random walk statistical results to random rotations of cells in solution [Schoenbach et al., 2009]. These studies can be of significant value to determine the underling interaction mechanism(s) between pulsed electric fields and cells and tissues. Collectively, these data suggest that there are multiple mechanisms of action of nsPEFs on biological systems.

When effects of nsPEFs on cells are considered, it remains to be determined which effects are due to direct actions of electric fields on cell structure and function and which are due to secondary downstream cellular or biological effects that include responses from the cytoskeleton, endoplasmic reticulum, mitochondria, nucleus and DNA damage. Given conventional electroporation effects on cell membranes and now reports of nsPEF effects on all cell membranes including intracellular structures, it becomes difficult to determine which effects are direct and which are indirect. It seems clear that nanopore formation is a direct electric field effect, but it remains to be seen whether these nanopores are primarily responsible for initiation of all observed nsPEF effects, from specific structural effects to broadly based effects such as cell survival and cell death. It is possible that effects other than nanopore formation are present that may be unrelated to membrane charging events. However, there are presently no available published data to address this issue. While nanopores must have significant effects on cells, other downstream biological effects are still under investigation. Given that pulse power applications for the purposes of this review are for melanoma tumor ablation, we can ask how nanopores or other consequences of electric fields result in effects that we observe as melanoma cells die and melanoma tumors regress. Here we review literature that has led to understanding these effects from a number of cell types and then to recall some literature examples and present some data using nsPEFs on B16f10 melanoma cells and tumors. Given that pulse power using nanosecond pulsed electric fields can eliminate B16f10 tumors and prevent their return, we will focus on nsPEF effects that bear on hallmarks of cancer including reversing evasion of apoptosis and opposing sustained angiogenesis in tumors *in vivo*. However, both of these effects are related to a number of actions on cell membrane and organelles that lead to cell demise.

5. Effects of ultra-high pulse power on cell plasma membranes

Although pulse power influences both plasma membranes and intracellular membranes, responses from the plasma membrane are relatively easy to analyze. It was initially hypothesized that pulse power fields could pass through the plasma membrane with significant effects. Using propidium iodide and ethidium homodimer as conventional probes for membrane permeability, initial studies suggested that our prediction was correct [Beebe et al., 2003; Schoenbach et al., 2001; Vernier et al., 2003]. However by using smaller fluorescent probes and more sensitive analytical methods, it has become clear that nsPEFs produce unique pores or aqueous channels that are distinct from conventional electroporation pores in that they are much smaller and are thus called nanopores. Pakhomov and coworkers have provided significant detail to the behavior of nanopores induced by nsPEFs [Bowman et al., 2010; Pakhomov et al., 2007a, b, 2009] but have only begun to fully characterize them. Pulses with durations of 60ns and electric fields of 12 kV/cm showed long-lasting (minutes) reduction of the cell membrane resistance and a corresponding loss of the plasma membrane potential. The formation of nanopores was demonstrated by patch clamp analysis and verified by non-electrophysiological methods using Tl+-sensitive fluorophore and using Tl+ uptake as a marker for nanoporation. These nanopores are voltage sensitive, exhibit an inwardly rectifying current that resembles those of nonselective cation ion channels but do not appear to exhibit outward currents. These pore properties are distinct from conventional electro-pores, disappear when they become larger propidium permeable pores and are not blocked by broad-spectrum K+ channel inhibitors or Ca2+ chelators. Tl+ uptake was observed at electric field intensities far below the threshold for propidium iodide uptake and they remained stable for as long as ten minutes. Overall, nsPEF applications to cells *in vitro* provide evidence from models and experimental observations that they open lipid nanopores that create unique aqueous channels for cation-selective transport into cells from the extracellular environment. These plasma membrane nanopores are likely to be responsible, at least in part, for many nsPEF-induced biological effects. Given that there is evidence for effects on intracellular membranes, it is highly likely that pulse power-induced nanopores are present in intracellular membranes and are responsible for at least some of the biological response from cells as will be discussed later.

The plasma membrane separates cells from the external environment, but is much more than an external covering to contain intracellular organelles. This lipid bilayer includes a wide variety of integral membrane proteins that allow both passive and active transport of ions into and out of cells. In addition, the plasma membrane exhibits symmetry in lipid constituents on the inner and outer leaf of the membrane. Normally, phosphatidylserine is on the inner leaflet and phosphatidyl-ethanolamine is on the outer leaflet. During apoptosis, phosphatidylserine is externalized, signaling to other cells in the micro-environment that these cells are undergoing cell death by apoptosis. Under these conditions macrophages will engulf the dying cells by phagocytosis before cells lose their integrity through membrane permeabilization preventing inflammatory responses. However, since nsPEF conditions that lead to cell death will induce nanopore formation, cells may become permeable to membrane integrity markers such as propidium iodide or ethidium homodimer. Whether cell plasma membranes become permeable depends on EP conditions as discussed earlier. In addition, the cell type is also an important consideration as indicated in some of the following examples.

When ten 100ns pulses at 60kV/cm were applied to 3T3 pre-adipocytes and analyzed by flow cytometry, there was no increase in ethidium homodimer or propidium iodide uptake, indicating that the plasma membrane was impermeable to molecules on the order of about 1 nm or larger. Using Annexin-V-FITC as a phosphatidylserine externalization marker, there was a time-dependent increase in Annexin-V binding but no increase in ethidium homodimer uptake 30 minutes after treatment [Beebe et al., 2003a]. Eighteen to twenty-four hours later less than 10% of the cells survived. These cells also exhibited active caspases, suggesting caspase-associated apoptosis.

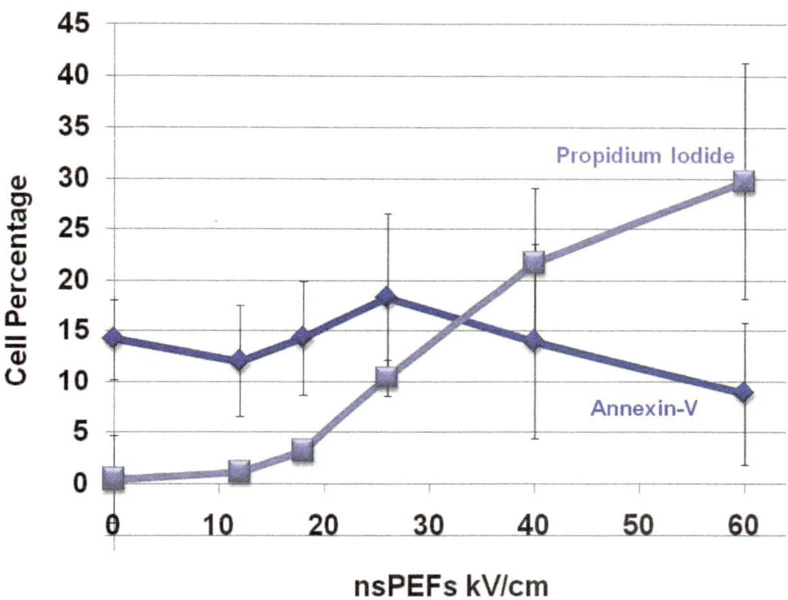

Fig. 1. Effect of nsPEFs on B16f10 melanoma cell permeability and phosphatidylserine orientation

As indicated in Figure 1, B16f10 cells were also exposed to ten 300ns pulses with electric fields as high as 60 kV/cm. In contrast to 3T3 pre-adipocytes under these same conditions, there was very little if any Annexin-V binding indicating no phosphatidylserine externalization. However about 20-40% of cells took up propidium iodide at 60 kV/cm, suggesting that a minority of cells exhibited nanopores larger than about a nanometer. B16f10 cells also exhibited caspase activity (Ford et al., 2010, see below). Thus, 3T3-L1 pre-adipocytes exhibited Annexin-V binding but no propidium iodide uptake while B16f10 cells exhibited no significant Annexin-V binding, but uptake of propidium iodide in a small population of cells. Both cell types showed increases in active caspases. When Jurkat cells were treated with nsPEFs, 300ns pulses at 60 kV/cm resulted in significant and immediate cell necrosis indicating that the plasma membranes of Jurkat cells were significantly more sensitive to pulse power than 3T3-L1 cells. Jurkat cells exposed to 60ns pulses at 60kV/cm exhibited Annexin-V binding but a delayed uptake of propidium [Beebe et al., 2003a]. The delayed permeability to propidium iodide was distinctly different than the immediate propidium uptake when cells were exposed to 10 microsecond pulses typical of conventional electroporation [Deng et al., 2004]. When HCT116 cells that were wild-type and null for p53 were treated with nsPEFs, addition of ethidium homodimer-1 and Annexin-V-FITC post-pulse demonstrated greater fluorescence in p53 null cells versus p53 wild-type cells, suggesting a p53-dependent biological effect on plasma membranes [Hall et al., 2005]. It is possible that relative levels of p53 may affect plasma membrane response to pulse power.

The comparisons among these cell types demonstrates that different cells have unique responses to the same nsPEF conditions and that some cells respond to lower pulse conditions than others. The conclusion that there are cell-type specific responses to pulse power is consistent with several other studies [Hair et al., 2003; Ibey et al., 2010; Stacey et al., 2003]. While these data indicate the possibility to selectively targeting specific cells in a mixed population, specificity for cancer versus normal cells has not been demonstrated. Nevertheless, it is highly likely that when electric fields are sufficiently high, pulse power is expected to eliminate all cell types, including slowly proliferating cancer stem cells, which are not readily affected by chemotherapeutic agents, and host cells that are collaborating with malignant cells.

While propidium iodide uptake is a well-characterized marker for cell viability and phosphatidylserine externalization is a well characterized marker for apoptosis, both of these indicators and their indications should be reconsidered when cells are exposed to nsPEFs or conventional electroporation. It is well known from conventional electroporation studies that cells can be transiently permeable to relative large molecules and remain viable. The primary aim of conventional electroporation is transient membrane permeability in cells that survive. Transient permeability has also been demonstrated using nanosecond pulsed electric fields in HCT116 cells [Hall et al., 2007b]. It was hypothesized from modeling analysis [Hu et a., 2005, 2006; Vernier et al., 2006a, b] and demonstrated experimentally [Vernier et al., 2006] that exposure to nsPEFs could externalize phosphatidylserine through nanopores that were created in the plasma membrane. These nanopores are distinct from pores created by EP in that they are too small to allow transport of large molecules but do allow transport of ions and externalization of PS. Conventional electroporation induces phospholipid rearrangements in plasma membranes [Haest et al., 1997; Schwarz et al., 1999]. Tekle et al. [2008] demonstrate that phosphatidylserine externalization induced by nsPEFs in the absence of caspase activity, resulted in phagocytic clearance of B cells by mouse macrophages in part by electric field-induced apoptosis mimicry. Thus, analysis of phosphatidylserine externalization as an apoptosis marker in response to nsPEFs should be carefully considered and as always demonstration of apoptosis should include several different markers.

It is also possible that nsPEFs have effects on other structures such as those with roles for transport across membranes or other biological effects. For example, ligand receptor interactions or the structure and function of membrane receptors could be affected by pulse power. Effects of pulse power have not been investigated on caveolae, which have been reported to play roles in endocytosis, lipid trafficking and signal transduction; and on lipid rafts, which have been implicated in cell signaling, membrane fluidity and protein and receptor trafficking [Brown and London, 1998]. Thus, while plasma membrane and putative intracellular membrane nanopores are likely important in biological responses to ultra-high pulse power effects on cells and tissues, other membrane structures and functions may also be modulated by pulse power.

6. Effect of nsPEFs on the endoplasmic reticulum

The endoplasmic reticulum is composed of intracellular membranes with a similar composition to the plasma membrane, forming an intracellular network of tubules and cisternae or "little nets" (from the Latin reticulum). It carries out several specialized functions including translation, folding and transport of proteins, sequestration of calcium, glycogen storage, and responses to stress. Given that nsPEFs were hypothesized to have intracellular effects and these effects were most likely due to membrane charging events, it was reasonable to consider that they would have effects on this extensive intracellular membrane array. Since the endoplasmic reticulum is a storage site for calcium, a number of studies demonstrated effects of nsPEFs on calcium mobilization in the presence and absence of extracellular calcium [Beebe et al., 2003b, 2004; Buescher and Schoenbach, 2003; Vernier et al., 2003; White et al., 2004]. In fact, of all the cellular responses that have been elicited with nsPEFs, calcium mobilization is the one of the most sensitive, occurring at shorter pulse durations and lower electric fields than other measured cell responses. In experiments with HL-60 and Jurkat cells [Beebe et al., 2004; White et al., 2004] using 60ns pulses, calcium release was observed from intracellular storage sites in the absence or presence of extracellular calcium chelators at electric fields as low as 2-4kV/cm. Based on studies that depleted calcium stores in the endoplasmic reticulum, it was determined that calcium was mobilized from this site in these cells. For phosphatidylserine externalization in these same cells, 60ns pulses required electric fields 10-20 times higher (40 kV/cm). Calcium mobilization was also observed in Jurkat cells with ten 30ns pulses at 25kV/cm under conditions that did not allow Na+ transport across the plasma membrane [Vernier et al., 2003]. NsPEFs also acted as an agonist to activate platelets to form platelet gels [Zhang et al., 2008]. This effect was electric field dependent and was postulated to result from an increase in calcium mobilization through nanopores in the plasma membranes as well as from intracellular calcium stores, most likely alpha-granules in platelets. A study evaluating calcium responses in chromaffin cells exposed to nanosecond electric pulses suggested a role for L-type calcium channels for calcium entry, but not from intracellular calcium [Vernier et al., 2008]. A more recent study exposing chromaffin cells in the presence and absence of a variety of channel inhibitors concluded that 5ns pulses opened multiple types of voltage-gated calcium channels involving sodium transport across plasma membranes by either non-selective cation channels and/or lipid nanopores [Craviso et al., 2010]. Another study analyzed fluorescent calcium sensitive probes in isolated rat ventricular myocytes exposed to pulses of 4ns and electric fields at 10-80 kV/cm [Wang et al., 2009]. This study demonstrated that these ultrashort pulses triggered action potentials through tetrodotoxin-insensitive, non-selective ion channels that were consistent with the presence of nanopores in the sarcolemmal.

NsPEFs also mobilized calcium in B16f10 melanoma cells [Ford et al., 2010]. Calcium is involved in most, if not all cell functions [Berridge et al., 2000]. Mitochondria have a huge capacity to accumulate calcium and the permeability transition pore (PTP) complex is activated by calcium. When calcium levels markedly increase, the PTP complex can enter an irreversible high conduction state which dissipates the mitochondria membrane potential ultimately leading to cytochrome c release and initiation of apoptosis. We were interested to see if caspase activation was calcium-dependent. Chelators of calcium (EGTA and BAPTA) were used to prevent calcium effects and caspase activation was analyzed using the cell permeable, irreversible pan-caspase inhibitor, z-VAD-fmk. Ionomycin increased Ca2+ 3.1-

fold and ten 300ns pulses at 60 kV/cm increased calcium nearly 2-fold using fluo-3 as a calcium indicator. Ionomycin, a calcium ionophore did not activate platelets above control levels. These same pulses increased the presence of active caspase by about two fold and increased the number of caspase positive cells from 20% in control cells to about 80% in nsPEF-treated cells. The presence of EGTA and BATA had no effect on the presence of active caspases.

In a more recent study with E4 squamous carcinoma cells roles for calcium were more specifically identified [Ren and Beebe, 2011]. When conditions were sufficient to kill about 95% of the E4 cell population (ten 300ns pulses at 60kV/cm), cytochrome *c* release and cleavage of the BH3 only protein Bid to t-Bid was only partially caspase-dependent. An analysis of effects of calcium on Bid cleavage using EGTA and BAPTA-AM to chelate extra- and intra-cellular calcium, respectively, determined that intracellular calcium as an intrinsic mechanism was responsible for about 30% of calcium-dependent Bid cleavage and extracellular calcium as an extrinsic mechanism was responsible for about 70% of calcium-dependent Bid cleavage. This study also observed that nsPEFs activated calpains in a calcium-dependent manner, but experiments did not rule out involvement of other proteases. The results indicated that multiple mechanisms were involved in Bid cleavage and cytochrome *c* was released and calcium was mobilized from intracellular and extracellular sources. A possible common mechanism could be formation of nanopores in these membranes.

There are other possible effects of nsPEFs on the endoplasmic reticulum. It is highly likely that other endoplasmic reticulum responses to pulse power will occur especially under conditions that are below the threshold or just above the threshold for cell death when a population of cells will not survive. This is especially relevant given roles for the endoplasmic reticulum in protein translation and folding. Cells respond to stress through changes in gene expression and the regulation of protein levels can be modulated by the endoplasmic reticulum. Regulation of eukaryotic initiation factor-2alpha by phosphorylation and internal ribosome initiation through the internal ribosome-entry site are two examples for direct roles of the endoplasmic reticulum in translation control in cellular stress responses and apoptosis [Holcik and Sonenberg, 2005]. Stress responses from the endoplasmic reticulum can also occur by crosstalk with the mitochondria to induce cytochrome *c* release or through caspase-12, which is transported to and/or located in the mitochondria and can act without cytochrome *c* release [Momoi, 2004; Szegezdi et al., 2003]. Under these conditions, the downstream responses of endoplasmic reticulum stress include a mitochondria-mediated response, often involving calcium mobilization or a mitochondria-independent response that involves the activation of caspase-12 and caspase-4. Both of these "pathways" lead to the activation of executioner caspases. Effects of nsPEFs in the stress response, control of translation and caspase activation through effects on the endoplasmic reticulum have not been investigated.

7. Effect of nsPEFs on mitochondria

Mitochondria are often referred to as the cell's "power plant" since they are responsible for production of ATP. However, another important function of mitochondria is in programmed cell death. A primary focus here will be on the role of mitochondria in pulse power-induced cell death, which will be discussed with specific references to effects on ATP levels, mitochondria membrane potential and release of pro-apoptotic factors. Analyses of nsPEF effects on mitochondria have only just begun by analysis in B16f10 melanoma [Ford et al., 2010] as well as E4 squamous cell carcinoma [Ren and Beebe, 2011]. Ford and co-workers [2010] recently demonstrated that nsPEFs induced a decrease in cellular ATP levels and decreased the mitochondria membrane potential in B16f10 melanoma cells. The loss of the mitochondria membrane potential is a common event during apoptosis. Figure 2 shows effects of nsPEFs on the mitochondria membrane potential in B16f10 melanoma cells.

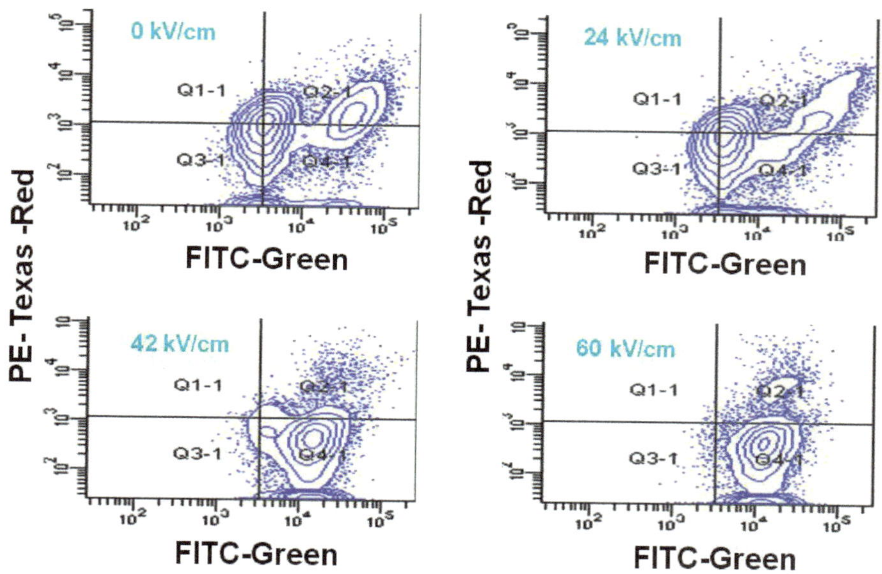

Fig. 2. NsPEFs decreases the mitochondria membrane potential in B16f10 cells.

In non-apoptotic cells, JC-1 (5,5′,6,6′-tetrachloro-1,1′,3,3′-tetraethylbenzimidazolylcarbocyanine iodide) exists as a monomer in the cytosol as a FITC fluorophore as shown through the green channel on the X-axis. It also accumulates as aggregates in the mitochondria which stain red as shown through the PE-Texas Red channel on the Y-axis. In apoptotic and necrotic cells, aggregated, red JC-1 decreases and monomeric, green JC-1 increases. The top left panel of Figure 2 shows control cells in two populations with different green monomeric JC-1 intensities. As nsPEFs are applied to the cells with increasing electric fields, red JC-1 aggregate intensities decrease (Y-axis) and green JC-1 monomer intensities increase (X-axis). The decrease in the mitochondria membrane potential occurred as quickly as it could be measure by flow cytometry (minutes). This transformation occurs in an electric field-dependent manner indicating that electric fields caused a decrease in the mitochondria membrane potential. As expected, the levels of ATP drop significantly in a similar manner [Ford et al., 2010]. Given that nsPEFs cause nanopore formation in the plasma membrane and also have effects on intracellular membranes it is possible that the electric fields cause nanopore formation in the inner mitochondria membrane resulting in a decrease in the potential across the membrane. Another possibility is that nanopore formation in the plasma membrane causes an increase in sodium in the cytosol, which causes the decrease in the mitochondria membrane potential. Further experimentation will be required to differentiate between these two possibilities.

Another common event during apoptosis is the release of pro-apoptotic factors from the mitochondria. Several methods are available to analyze cytochrome *c* release including immunoblots using mitochondrial-free cytosolic fractions [Beebe et al., 2003a]. Using this assay it is more difficult to quantify cytochrome *c* release and it is not possible to determine the number of cells in a population that release cytochrome *c*. Another approach is to use fluorescent antibody detection of cytochrome *c* by fluorescent microscopy and/or flow cytometry.

Cytochrome *c* release using immunoblot analysis was demonstrated in Jurkat cells exposed to nsPEFs [Beebe et al., 2003a]. Cytochrome *c* release occurred within 30-45 minutes after treatment and was coincident with caspase activation, which was determined with the cell permeable irreversible inhibitor z-VAD-fmk. NsPEFs also initiated cytochrome *c* release in HCT116 colon carcinoma cells, albeit it did not occur until the second hour, which was after active caspases were present. In B16f10 melanoma cells cytochrome *c* release was analyzed as well as release of the pro-apoptotic factors Smac/Diablo and apoptosis initiating factor (AIF). These results are shown in Figure 3 (below).

Unlike all other cells tested for cytochrome *c* release in response to nsPEFs, and in contrast to ethanol treated cells, B16f10 cells did not release cytochrome *c* while active caspases were detected using z-VAD-fmk [Ford et al., 2010]. Cells in experiments shown in Figure 3 were analyzed 3 hours after treatment. However, when analyzed between 1 and 7 hours after treatment, cytochrome *c* released was not detected. In data not shown, a second assay was used that was based on a loss of cytosolic cytochrome *c* from permeabilized cells before analysis with fluorescent antibodies (Innocyte assay, Cal Biochem) based on the procedure described by Waterhouse and Trapani [2003]. We were unable to detect cytochrome *c* release using this assay while about 50% of E4 squamous carcinoma cells released cytochrome c 1 hour after treatment with nsPEFs [Ren and Beebe, 2011]. However, as indicated in Figure 3, we did detect small increases in fluorescence with antibodies to Smac/Diablo and apoptosis initiating factor (AIF), albeit in small populations of cells (10-15%). Given that cytochrome *c* release was detected in Jurkat cells coincident with activation of caspases (Beebe et al., 2003a] as well as in HCT 116 cells [Hall et al., 2007a] and E4 squamous carcinoma cells [Ren and Beebe, 2011] after caspase activation, this suggests that nsPEFs have cell type-specific effects on mitochondria-mediated events associated with apoptosis-like mechanisms.

8. Effects of nsPEFs on nucleus / DNA

Possible effects of nsPEFs on the nucleus have been of specific interest since the technology was applied to cells and tissues. Given that these effects on cells and tissues are high in power and low in energy density, it would be expected that the energy deposited into cells from these electric fields would not be sufficient to break hydrogen bonds, especially those in DNA. However, some experimental data suggests that this might not be true in cells *in vitro* and tumor tissues *in vivo*. Fibrosarcoma tumors grown in mice and treated with nsPEFs *ex vivo* exhibited DNA damage using TUNEL analysis [Beebe et al., 2002, 2003b]. Stacey and colleagues [2003] evaluated possible genotoxic stress effects of ultra-high pulse power using nanosecond pulsed electric fields on 11 suspension and adherent cell lines. They evaluated cell survival assessed by clonogenic formation or live cell counts; DNA damage was determined by the comet assay and chromosome aberrations and cell cycle parameters by measuring the mitotic indices of exposed cells. Not all cell types were affected in the same

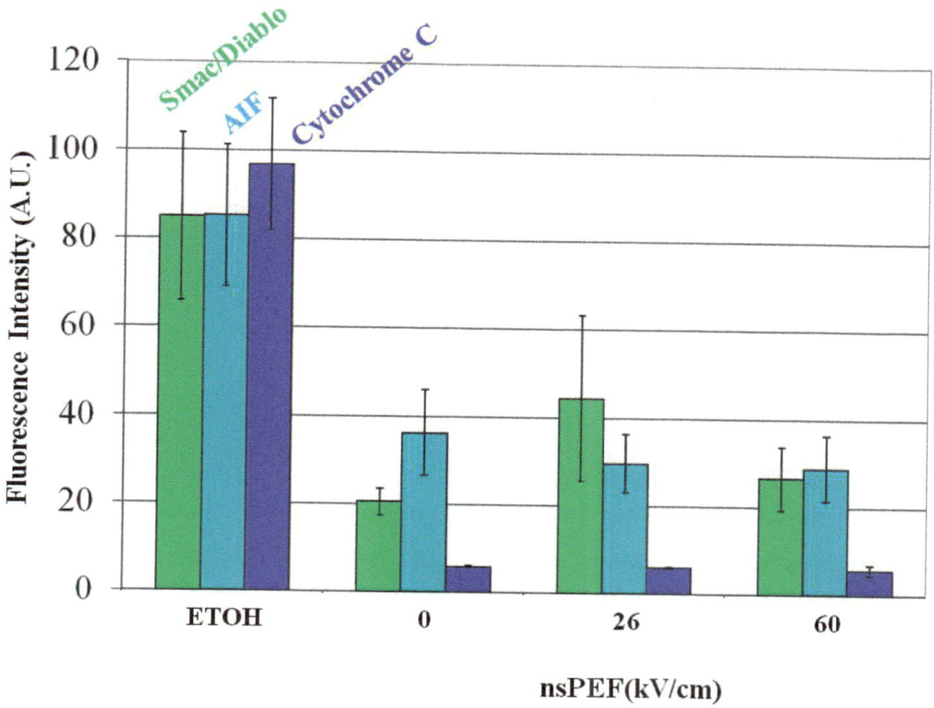

Fig. 3. NsPEFs have minimal effects on release of pro-apoptotic factors from mitochondria in B16f10 melanoma cells.

ways. After one 60 ns pulse with an electric field intensity of 60 kV/cm, non-adherent cultures exhibited a rapid decline in cell viability (90%), DNA damage, and a reduction in the number of cells reaching mitosis. Adherent cultures did not exhibit these effects under the same conditions with the exception of mouse 3T3 cells, which behaved as the suspended cells did. These results suggested that pulse-power-induced genotoxicity may be cell type-specific and therefore have possible applications in the selective removal of one cell type within a heterogeneous population of cells such as in diseased states. The comet assay also suggested possibilities for DNA damage in B16 cells *in vitro* when treated with nanosecond pulsed electric fields [Nuccitelli et al., 2009].

Another approach to identify effects on DNA was to use phosphorylation of Histone 2AX to identify possible DNA double strand breaks using fluorescent antibodies by flow cytometry or fluorescent microscopy. When DNA double strand breaks occur, Histone 2AX, a histone variant, is phosphorylated on Serine 139 and serves as a sensitive and early monitor to identify these events [Bonner et al., 2008; Rogakou et al., 1999]. When B16f10 cells were exposed to 300ns pulses at 60kV/cm, it was not possible to determine an increased Histone 2AX phosphorylation. While there were significant levels of phosphorylated Histone2AX, there were no significant differences between control and treated cells, even though >95% of treated cells were eliminated 24 hours later [Ford et al., 2010]. This suggests that DNA double strands breaks are not uncommon in control B16f10 cells. However, results were different in HCT116 cells.

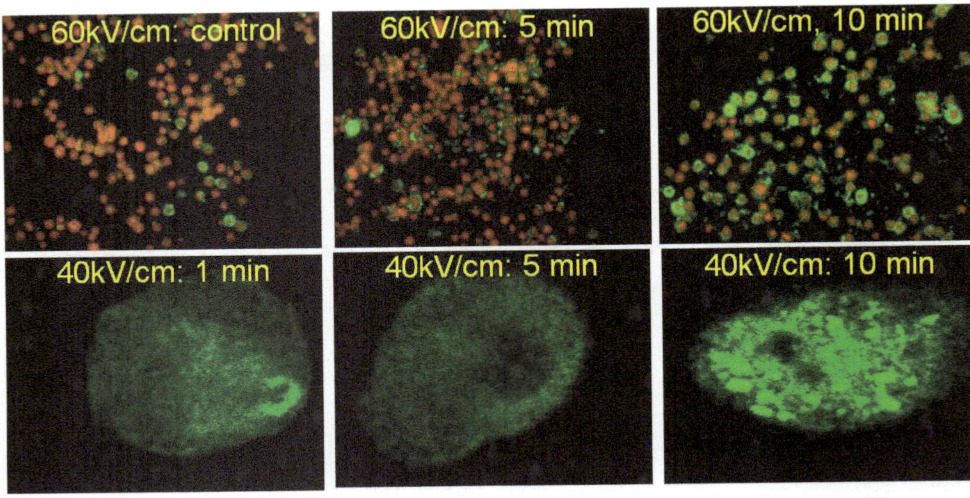

Fig. 4. NsPEFs induce DNA double strand breaks in HCT 116 colon carcinoma cells.

HCT116 colon carcinoma cells were exposed to ten 300ns pulses at various electric fields and analyzed for Histone 2AX phosphorylation with fluorescent antibodies specific for phosphorylation at the serine 139 site. Figure 4 (above) shows identification of phosphorylated Histone 2AX in HCT116 cells treated with ten 300ns pulses at 40 or 60 kV/cm. The top panels show 20x magnifications of cells treated with 60kV/cm, a condition that resulted in death of >95% of cells. Within 5-10 minutes HCT116 cells were positive for phosphorylation of Histone 2AX. The bottom panels shows 60x oil magnifications of representative HCT116 cell nuclei that were phosphorylated at Serine 139. The rapidity of phosphorylation was surprising if nsPEFs did not have direct effects on DNA. A common mechanism for DNA damage in response to ionizing radiation is the generation of reactive oxygen species. However, we were unable to detect reactive oxygen species in B16f10 cells treated in the same way [Ford et al. 2010]. These results were consistent with results of DNA damage using the comet assay, which identified rapid DNA damage [Stacey et al., 2004; Nuccitelli et al, 2009]. In experiments analyzing nsPEF effects on DNA double strand breaks in Jurkat cells that resulted in >95% cell death, Histone 2AX phosphorylation occurred several hours after treatment and was caspase-dependent, suggesting that this DNA damage was due to apoptosis [Ren and Beebe, unpublished results]. Taking all of this data together, it appears that nsPEF-induced DNA damage is cell type specific.

More general nsPEF effects on cell nuclei in HL-60 cells were determined in cells when non-lethal pulse power conditions caused the nucleus in acridine orange-stained HL-60 cells to become irregularly shaped as the fluorescence decreased [Chen et al., 2004]. When HCT116 cells were treated with non-lethal pulse power using nanosecond pulsed electric fields, reversible changes in nuclear size and morphology were observed indicating effects on nuclei even under conditions that resulted in cell survival [Hall et al., 2005]. In a different approach to analyze nsPEF effects on cell nuclei, Chen and co-workers [2007] used confocal microscopy and flow cytometry to observe Smith antigen antibody (Y12) binding to nuclear speckles, known as small nuclear ribonucleoprotein particles (snRNPs) or intrachromatin granule clusters (IGCs), in Jurkat cells following one or five non-lethal 10ns pulses at 150 kV/cm. These experiments indicated that nsPEFs disrupted pre-messenger RNA splicing mechanisms but did not allow propidium uptake, suggesting the nuclear effects occurred in the absence of plasma membrane pores larger than about a nanometer. Furthermore, these effects were cell cycle dependent. When cells were synchronized to the G2-M phase with nocodazole, exposing cells in the mitotic phase to five consecutive 10ns pulses immediately and significantly increased the number of nuclear speckled substructures, suggesting direct effects to inhibit RNA transcription mechanisms. While these pulse power conditions resulted in significant cell survival, the long term effects after these responses have not been analyzed.

NsPEF effects reviewed thus far have been with B16f10 cells and other cell types *in vitro*. Effects on DNA in B16f10 tumors in mice have been analyzed [Chen et al., 2010]. In these studies, hairless female SKH-1 mice were injected subcutaneously with $1x10^6$ B16-F10 cells. Tumors developed within 8-10 days. B16f10 tumors were treated *in vivo* with one hundred 300ns pulses at 40kV/cm and analyzed for phosphorylated Histone 2AX, 1, 3, 6 and 24 hours after treatment. The results indicated a time-dependent increase in γH2AX in melanoma, with significant differences occurring at 1 hour (15% of cells), reaching a peak at 3 hours (85% of cells) and decreasing to control levels thereafter. These transient peaks in Histone 2AX phosphorylation coincided with TUNEL positive cells and pyknotic nuclei. Quantitative differences were observed by calculating mean nuclear area (μm^2) between control and treated tumor nuclei during the first 24 hours after treatment with nsPEFs. Treated tumor nuclei were significantly smaller than control nuclei. The transient nature of histone 2AX phosphorylation and TUNEL positive cells suggested that DNA repair was initiated but not completed. When DNA was analyzed by agarose gel electrophoresis large DNA fragments, but not 180bp fragmentation ladders, were observed. The presence of active caspases peaked after peaks of histone 2AX phosphorylation and TUNEL positive cells. Taken together, these results suggested that the DNA damage occurred by a caspase-independent mechanisms and that apoptosis did not go to completion (see nsPEF effects on apoptosis mechanisms, below).

Most data for effects of pulse power-induced effects on DNA in cells and tissues suggests that at least some DNA damage may be caused by direct nsPEF effects. DNA damage in B16f10 melanoma cells and tumors does not appear to be a caspase-associated apoptosis marker. However, the mechanism(s) remain to be defined. Pulse power is not expected to generate sufficient energy to break hydrogen bonds and it may not be expected to generate reactive oxygen species through ionization of water. However, reactive oxygen species can be generated by effects on mitochondria, which are clearly present after pulse power treatment of B16f10 and other cells. Nevertheless, pulse-power induced reactive oxygen species in B16f10 cells [Ford et al., 2010] or E4 squamous carcinoma cells [Ren and Beebe, 2011] *in vitro* were not detected when CM-H_2DCFDA was used as a reactive oxygen species marker. Since ATM (ataxia telangiectasia mutated) kinase and/or ATR (ATM and Rad 3-related) kinase are activated with ionizing radiation and UV light, it would be of interest to carry out kinetic analysis of these kinases after cells are exposed to pulse power and correlate this with histone 2AX phosphorylation.

9. Effect of nsPEFs on actin cytoskeleton

The cytoskeleton forms a dynamic network of filamentous protein structures that crisscrosses the cytoplasm, providing shape, mechanical support, modes for intracellular transport of synthesized proteins and the capacity for motility. It is contiguous with the plasma membrane. Given that nsPEFs have effects on plasma membranes and intracellular structures and the cytoskeleton is an extension of the plasma membrane, it was likely that nanosecond pulsed electric fields would affect the cytoskeleton.

Effects of pulse power ablation on the actin cytoskeleton have been demonstrated [Hall et al., 2007a]. Human HCT 116 colon carcinoma cells were synchronized to S phase (95%) by thymidine block or analyzed unsynchronized (50% S phase). The actin cytoskeleton was labeled with rhodamine phalloidin and pulsed with three 60ns pulses at 60kV/cm and visualized by fluorescent microscopy. Both S-phase synchronized and unsynchronized control cells exhibited well-defined peripheral cytoskeletal structures around large nuclei. One hour after treatment, the cytoskeletal structure of unsynchronized cells exhibited a more random, less organized structure near the plasma membrane with blebbed-like structures. In contrast, the cytoskeletal structure of S phase cells exposed to the same pulses was not significantly perturbed. Five hours after treatment with these conditions, control and treated cell were indistinguishable with 90-95% survival [Hall et al., 2007a]. When these cells were pulsed with three 300ns pulses at 60kV/cm, which killed 90% of cells, S-phase cells and unsynchronized cells exhibited rearranged actin cytoskeletons.

These experiments demonstrated several new facts about nsPEF effects on actin and how actin functions in HCT 116 cells. First, nsPEFs have differential cytoskeletal effects on cells in S phase, but no differential effects on survival. A second aspect is the capacity of the actin cytoskeleton to resist effects of nsPEFs during DNA synthesis. This is contrary to the idea that proliferating cells, with potentially vulnerable DNA in the absence a nuclear membrane, would be more susceptible to nsPEFs. Third, when nsPEFs perturb the actin structure with low level pulse power (three 60kV/cm pulses at 60 or 300ns), there is a transient influence that allows recovery between 1 and 5 hours after treatment with cell survival. However, when pulse power conditions are sufficiently intense, cells cannot survive the exposure. In these studies, two nsPEF thresholds are demonstrated. One threshold is for pulse power intensity that supersedes the capacity of actin cytoskeleton to resist rearrangement during DNA synthesis in S-phase and a second threshold is pulse power intensity that surpasses the capability of cells to survive nsPEF ablation. This suggests that in some tumors this treatment could complement chemotherapeutic agents such as vincristine, vinblastine and other vinca alkaloids that bind to tubulin and prevent polymerization as well as paclitaxel and other taxanes that bind to tubulin and prevent depolymerization.

Effects of nsPEFs on B16f10 cell actin cytoskeletal structures using ten 300ns pulses at 60kV/cm, like that used in HCT 116 cells had unnoticeable effects on the cytoskeleton [JA Liu and SJ Beebe, unpublished]. This again suggests cell type-specific differences. This may not be too surprising since pulse power-induced plasma membrane effects were different between B16f10 and HCT116 cells as well as other cells. However, Ford et al. [2010] observed that when active caspases were expressed in B16f10 cells, the actin cytoskeleton was not readily observed 2-3 hours after pulse power treatment. Since actin is a caspase substrate, this suggested that the actin cytoskeleton is dismantled by active caspases after pulse power treatment.

10. Effect of pulse power on apoptosis-like cell death mechanisms

The landscape for defining cell death mechanisms has become more complex as our understanding of life and death advances. Since apoptosis initiation and progression are complex processes and are cell type-specific, apoptosis mechanisms and pathways are often simplified by classifying pathways as intrinsic and extrinsic. The extrinsic pathways is further classified as type I cells that do not use mitochondria cytochrome *c* release and type II cells that do [Fulda and Debatin, 2006; Lavrik, 2010]. The fate of cells depends on a set of sensors and positive and negative regulators whose balance will determine cell fate and whether apoptosis is initiated or not. The mitochondria play major roles in these mechanisms. There may be no linear apoptosis pathways, but grouping apoptosis into intrinsic mechanisms, which are linked to the mitochondria, and extrinsic mechanisms, which are linked to death receptor complexes in the plasma membrane, provides some structure for discussion and analysis. There also appears to be an intrinsic mechanism that originates in the endoplasmic reticulum and may or may not be linked to the mitochondria. The intrinsic pathway is regulated through pro- and anti-apoptotic Bcl-2 family members in response to intracellular stresses with mitochondria-dependent release of cytochrome *c* and other factors causing activation of apical initiator caspase-9 through formation of the apoptosome with APAF-1. This then leads to activation of downstream execution caspases -3, -6, and/or -7. The regulation of mitochondria-dependent mechanisms is complex. Activators of this pathway include endoplasmic reticulum stress, as discussed earlier, DNA damage, hypoxia, and reactive oxygen species and growth factor deprivation, among others. Caspase activation is controlled by inhibitors of apoptosis (IAP), which can be inactivated by pro-apoptotic factors released from the mitochondria such as Smac/Diablo and Omi/OtrA. P53, the "guardian of the genome" senses potential apoptotic signals and leads to increases in factors such as Puma, Nova, and Bax, which lead to release of cytochrome *c*. However, these factors are opposed by anti-apoptotic factors such as Bcl-2 and Bcl-xl.

The extrinsic pathway is initiated by death receptor ligands that bind and trimerize death receptors such as Fas, TNF or TRAIL at the plasma membrane. This signals the recruitment of intracellular adaptor proteins and the apical initiator caspase-8 to the plasma membrane and the formation of a death-induced signaling complex (DISC). In type I cells, caspase-8 directly activates the executioner caspase-3. The formation of DISC is also regulated by positive (caspase-8) and negative (FLIP) regulators. In some cells (type II), formation of the DISC is insufficient to signal caspase-8 and caspase-3 directly. Instead caspase-8 cleaves a BH-3 only Bcl-2 pro-apoptotic protein Bid, forming a truncated Bid (t-Bid) that signals through the mitochondria, releasing cytochrome *c* causing activation of caspase-9, like that occurring in the intrinsic mechanism. In this way, the extrinsic pathway is connected to the intrinsic pathway through mitochondria-mediated mechanisms in type II cells.

Mechanisms for nsPEF-induced apoptosis induction appear to be dependent on the pulse conditions and/or on cell type. For example, pulse power-induced Jurkat cell apoptosis, in response to three 60ns 60kV/cm pulses, involved coincident release of cytochrome *c* and activation of caspases within the first 30-45 minutes after pulse delivery [Beebe et al., 2003a]. However, it is not yet clear if this mitochondria-dependent response occurs through the intrinsic pathway due to intracellular effects on the endoplasmic reticulum or mitochondria or occurs through the type II cell extrinsic pathway. In contrast, nsPEF-induced apoptosis in HCT116 colon carcinoma cells involves caspase activation in the first 45-60 minutes post-pulse with cytochrome *c* release as a later event [Hall et al., 2007a].

When B16f10 cells were suspended in Dulbecco's PBS (DPBS) solution and exposed to ten 300ns pulses with increasing electric fields, an increasing number of cells exhibit active caspases as determined 1 hour after treatment using the cell permeable pan caspase irreversible inhibitor z-VAD-fmk [Ford et al., 2010]. This is opposed to elevating caspase levels in a given population of cells. Thus this increase in the numbers of cells with active caspases occurred in an electric field-dependent increments. About 10% of cells were positive for active caspases in untreated cells and that number increased to greater than 75% when treated with ten 300ns pulses at 60 kV/cm. The analysis by flow cytometry indicated an increasing population of cells shifting to the right with increased fluorescence with the FITC- labeled pan caspase probe. This indicates that cells become positive for this probe in an all or none manner. This is consistent with the concept that once caspases are active they reach a point-of-no-return with a positively reinforced cascade of caspase activation leading to cell death. In addition, this behavior indicates that the B16f10 cell population responded in a heterogeneous manner with only a subpopulation of cells showing positive responses with each increasing electric field increment. Also when cells were treated with 20% ethanol they become positive for active caspases.

In another experimental approach, cells were treated as in Figure 5 with ten 300ns pulses at 60 kV/cm and analyzed by fluorescent microscopy. DAPI was used to identify the nuclei and a cell permeable, irreversible inhibitor or pseudosubstrate (Sulforhodamine-DEVD-fmk with red fluorescence) was used to identify caspase-3/7 (Figure 5). In controls that were sham treated without exposure to electric fields (0 kV/cm), cell nuclei were stained blue with DAPI, but caspase-3/7 cells were essentially absent {or in few cells (<10%)} and therefore exhibited little of no red fluorescence. Cells that were treated with nsPEFs ultra-high pulse power as indicated above exhibited a large population of red fluorescence with the presence of active caspase-3/7.

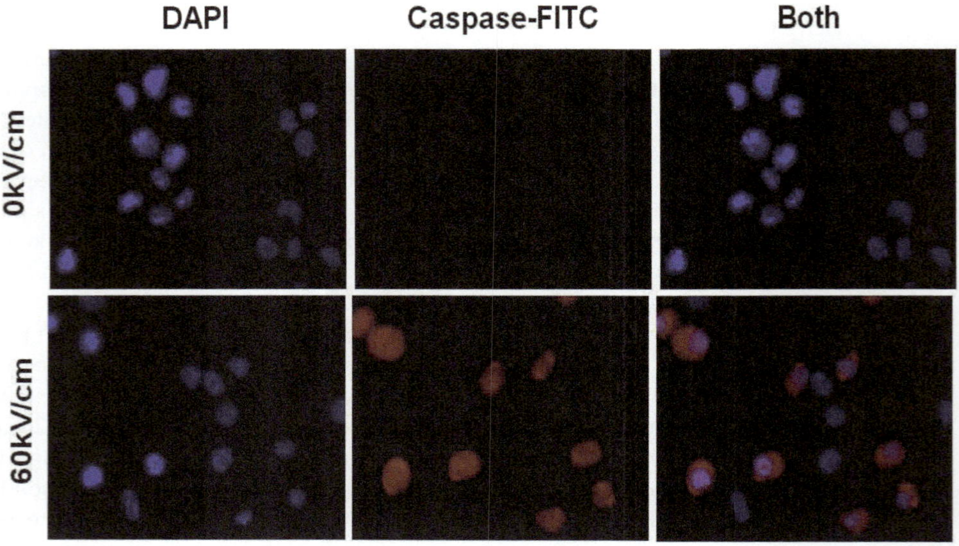

Fig. 5. nsPEF treated b16f10 cells exhibit increased binding of a cell permeable, irreversible caspase inhibitor.

Based on available evidence, it appears that nsPEF-induced apoptosis in B16f10 cells mimics the extrinsic pathway because active caspase-3-7 were present without concomitant cytochrome *c* release from B16f10 cells. Thus, pulse power induced apoptosis in these cells by mechanism(s) that were mitochondria-independent. Of interest here it the possibility for these pulses to activate mechanisms that bypass mutations that are common in cancer and resistances to treatment through mutations in mitochondria-mediated apoptosis mechanisms. For example [see Soengas and Lowe, 2003 for a review], Bcl-2 is often upregulated in melanoma to protect cells from apoptosis by inhibiting cytochrome *c* release from mitochondria. In addition, MitF is a factor that may also contribute to melanocyte survival by the transactivation of Bcl-2, which supports melanocyte survival. In addition, Apaf-1 protein and mRNA expression are frequently downregulated in metastatic cell lines and tumor specimens. Neither of these mutations would deter nsPEFs from preventing melanoma ablation. Thus, there may be advantages for applying pulse power ablation for eliminating melanoma at early stages (see below).

11. Multiple mechanisms for nsPEFs to eliminate cancer cells *in vitro*

Effects of nsPEF conditions have been observed that are coincident with a number of cellular responses from plasma membranes, intracellular cell membrane, proteases, and Bcl-2 family member proteins. Cell responses that seem to happen rapidly are likely direct actions of membrane charging and/or energy density "dose" effects are decreases in the plasma cell membrane potential as well as the mitochondria membrane potential. Phosphatidylserine externalization can also occur as a direct effect of pulse power. The best explanations for these phenomena are the formation of nanopores in those membranes. Likewise, increases in intracellular calcium occur by mobilization from extracellular and intracellular sources, which are relatively rapid and sensitive responses that could also be due to nanopores in the plasma membrane and endoplasmic reticulum. Other pulse-power-induced cellular responses include cytochrome *c* release, cytoskeletal changes, disruption of pre-messenger RNA splicing mechanisms, changes in nuclear shape and morphology, DNA double stranded breaks and general DNA damage, depending on pulse power conditions and the cell type. Other changes include increases in active caspases and calpains, cleavage of Bid to t-Bid and changes in other Bcl-2 proteins. There appears to be different thresholds and some of these changes appear to be dependent on the cell type. Under intense pulse power conditions, cells die by different mechanisms that may or may not be related to programmed cell death such as apoptosis and other death responses may be due to caspase-independent mechanisms including necrosis. Since many of these responses have been observed in different cell types, under different pulse power conditions and cell concentrations, in different buffers and by different assay procedures, it is difficult to determine specific cell death mechanisms. Just as difficult to determine is whether cell death is due to direct electric field effects or subsequent biological effects and whether cell death or sub-lethal effects are due to plasma membrane or intracellular membrane charging or energy density-related effects. Based on our present understanding of these numerous complex events, it is safe to conclude that given the plethora of cell responses that cell death is due to multiple mechanisms that depend on a variety of conditions. Given these complex scenarios, it could be simply proposed that when pulse durations are short and electric fields are low a minimal number of cellular "targets" respond. As the pulse durations become longer and electric fields higher, increasing numbers of "targets"respond. Where these targets are located and how sensitive they are or what their thresholds are appears to be dependent on the cell type.

12. Multiple mechanisms for nsPEFs to eliminate tumors *in vivo*

Treatment of melanoma requires new modalities to those presently available. Presently available melanoma therapy has significant limitations due to poor efficacy, quasi-tolerable toxicity and limited enhancement in survival and life quality. Here we discuss encouraging successes in applications of nsPEF for the treatment of cancer. *In vitro*, pulse power ablation induces cell death through multiple mechanisms that appear to be cell type-dependent. As discussed above, effects are evident on the plasma membrane, endoplasmic reticulum, cytoskeletal structure, mitochondria and nucleus. Coincident with cell death are events that are dependent and independent of calcium, caspases and cytochrome *c* release depending on the cell type. In murine B16f10 melanoma *in vitro*, nsPEFs induce caspase activation without cytochrome *c* release and with limited effects on phosphatidylserine externalization. The first studies demonstrating the possibility that nsPEFs could kill cancer cells used a B10.2 fibrosarcoma tumor in mice [Beebe et al., 2002, 2003b, 2004]. These studies used the first developed electrode design for *in vivo* applications of pulse power to tumors. Since then significant advances with a number of electrode designs have been used [Beebe et al., 2010; Kolb et al., 2009; Garon et al., 2007; Nuccitelli et al., 2006, 2010]. The fibrosarcoma studies followed studies showing that pulse power with nanosecond pulsed electric fields induced markers for apoptosis in Jurkat and HL-60 cells [Beebe et al., 2002]. In initial fibrosarcoma tumor studies, nsPEFs reduced tumor size *in vivo*, induced activation of caspase catalytic activity and demonstrated the presence of TUNEL positive cells when tumors were treated *ex vivo* [Beebe et al., 2003b, 2004]. Since then, nsPEFs were shown to eliminate B16f10 melanoma tumors *in vivo* without recurrence using two different electrode designs [Nuccitelli et al., 2006, 2009]. These studies demonstrated calcium mobilization and confirmed the possibility for DNA damage using the comet assay in B16f10 cells *in vitro* and decreased microvascular density using CD34 as a marker *in vivo*. Chen et al. [2010] revealed apoptosis initiation using active caspase-specific antibodies and the expression of TUNEL positive cells confirming DNA damage *in vivo*. In addition, this study also showed that nsPEFs could induce DNA double strand breaks using antibodies specific for phosphorylated Histone 2AX, an early and sensitive marker for this trait [Bonner et al., 2008]. These DNA damage and DNA double strand break markers peaked before caspases were fully active, suggesting that they might not be due to apoptosis. This study also indicated that nsPEFs may be responsible for anti-angiogenesis mechanisms showing decreases in vascular endothelial cell growth factor (VEGF), which is required for the angiogenic switch, a limiting factor for multistage carcinogenesis [Hanahan and Weinberg, 2000, 2011] and platelet derived endothelial growth factor (PD-ECGF). Decreases in several microvascular density factors, including CD-31, CD-34 and CD-105, were also demonstrated. CD-31 (PECAM-1), a platelet-endothelial cell adhesion molecule used as a pan-endothelial cell marker, and CD-34, an endothelial cell marker, were decreased by 65-70%. CD-105 (endoglin) was decreased >40%. CD-105, which is part of the TGFβ receptor complex, is an important angiogenic factor that is strongly expressed in tumors and is an independent prognostic indicator, wherein increased MVD correlates with shorter survival [Duff et al., 2003].

The results indicate that pulse power ablation target two of the seven common cancer hallmarks (Hanahan and Weinberg, 2000, 2011; Kroemer and Pouyssegur 2008) on solid B16f10 melanoma tumors, including apoptosis evasion and sustained angiogenesis. The latter is critical for a third hallmark, invasion and metastasis. The study concluded that apoptosis was initiated but most likely did not go to completion as suggested by the absence of DNA fragmentation ladders but the presence of large molecular weight DNA fragments on agarose gels [Chen et al., 2010]. It was suggested that the initiation of apoptosis without completion was likely due to loss of vascular viability contributing to infarctive tumor death. However, the presence of active caspases for several hours after nsPEF treatment could help disassemble tumors to initiate the removal of dead tumor cells. Consequently, nsPEF ablation induces B16f10 tumor elimination by multiple mechanisms that can bypass common cancer mutations that frequently result in chemotherapeutic resistances and metastasis. The application of nsPEF ablation is safe, has no systemic side effects, is non- or minimally invasive, leaves no scars, and provides an inexpensive and effective method to the arsenal for cancer treatment strategies [Chen et al., 2010; Nuccitelli et al., 2006, 2009, 2010]

13. Advantages for nsPEF ablation as a cancer therapy

There are a number of advantages for using nsPEF ablation as a means for cancer therapy as opposed to other physical methods that rely on overt necrosis for tumor cell death. These advantages include (1) targeting multiple programmed cell death mechanisms including apoptosis induction and anti-angiogenesis, two well known cancer hallmarks, the latter necessary for a third cancer hallmark, invasion and metastasis; (2) targeting rapid death induction with minimal treatment exposures, which reduces chances for resistances and recurrences; (3) targeting non-mitochondria-mediated programmed cell death in melanoma, which can bypass many melanoma and other cancer-causing mutations; (4) an apparent broad specificity for cell death induction, effective for all cells within electric fields, including rapidly growing tumor cells, slower growing host cells that have been hijacked by tumors and cancer stem cells, all constituting the tumor mass and the microenvironment; (5) small vessel, local infarction, which deprives tumors of feeder vessels that are important for immediate oxygenation and nutrition, which provides local stresses; (6) minimal local and systemic side effects and (7) the potential for enhancing immune surveillance from cells undergoing apoptotic.

NsPEF ablation provides a local targeted treatment at the level of the entire tumor without systemic effects, affecting multiple molecular structures and functions in plasma membranes and intracellular organelles. All tumor cells exposed to conditions of pulse duration, number and electric field that are above the threshold for cell death are subject to programmed and other forms of cell death. The foremost targets bypass two important hallmarks of cancer causing apoptosis-like appearances and anti-angiogenesis. In its full capacity, this should lead to inhibition of invasion and metastasis, another cancer hallmark. The multi-mechanisms for nsPEF interactions with tumors are similar to using a combination of at least two chemotherapeutic agents and/or molecular targeted drugs that induce apoptosis-like characteristics and limit angiogenesis; both well defined sites for cancer targeted drugs. The observed decreases in vessel numbers and angiogenic factors (VEGF and PD-ECGF) prevent the possibility for re-vascularization and reduce chances for tumor cells to continue to proliferate [Chen et al., 2010]. Sustained hypoxia has been implicated in metastasis and hypoxia induced factor (HIF) transcriptional activity that is beyond that of normal tissue [Cairns et al., 2001; Peng et al., 2006]. The combination of apoptosis-like qualities and anti-angiogenesis as sites of nsPEF action makes this an attractive cancer therapeutic modality [Chen et al., 2010].

Another advantage to nsPEF interactions with tumors is the rapid onset of apoptosis-like features and some level of tumor infarction. Caspase activation *in vitro* is seen within 30-45 minutes [Beebe et al., 2002, 2003a] and within the first hours after treatment *in vivo* [Chen et al., 2010]. This rapid caspase activation is likely to rapidly induce cell death mechanisms. In contrast, chemotherapeutic agents, ionizing radiation and molecular targeting drugs are administered over weeks or months and often do not eliminate cancer but reduce tumor size or stabilize it. This provides a potential for mechanisms to allow tumor cells to escape therapeutic action and increases the possibility for treatment resistances and recurrences. Examples include upregulation of drug efflux transporters and tumor immune evasion in chemoresistant melanomas [Schatton et al., 2009] and the chemotherapy-induced upregulation of factors like clusterin, an anti-apoptotic protein conferring resistances to several cell death agonists [Wei et al., 2009]. As indicated earlier, two mechanisms of resistance to PLX4220 treated melanoma tumors include creating alternative survival pathways by overexpressing a cell surface Beta-type protein platelet derived growth factor receptor or by reactivating the normal BRAF survival pathway [Nazarian et al., 2010]. Ultra-high pulse power-induced interruption of the tumor small vessel blood supply is also rapid, limiting blood flow to the tumor as it is being dismantled, at least in part by apoptosis-like mechanisms. NsPEF ablation has rapid therapeutic onset, which should reduce the potential for resistances and recurrences as all tumor cells are affected by conditions above the threshold for cell death.

Many mutations that lead to cancers often occur in mitochondria-mediated mechanisms and pathways, most likely because there are more regulatory sites through intrinsic and Bid-dependent extrinsic pathways than in mitochondria-independent apoptosis pathways [Hanahan and Weinberg, 2011]. Consequently, many chemotherapeutic agents and ionizing radiation have significant effects on mitochondria-dependent apoptotic mechanisms [Latai, 2008]. NsPEF ablation has both mitochondria-dependent and -independent sites of action that appear to be cell type-dependent. In melanoma, the apparent exclusive recruitment of cytochrome c-independent extrinsic mechanisms provides an alternative mechanism to many cancer therapeutic treatments that act on mitochondria-dependent pathways. A simple, bistable rate-equation-based model of apoptosis pathways predicted that the extrinsic caspase-8 mechanism was more sensitive than the mitochondrial intrinsic pathway for electric pulse induced cell apoptosis [Song et al., 2010], which is in keeping with results from B16F10 melanoma studies [Ford et al., 2010] as well as HCT116 colon carcinoma [Hall et al., 2007a] and E4 squamous cell carcinoma studies [Ren and Beebe, 2011]. Thus, by favoring the extrinsic apoptosis pathway, nsPEFs may bypass many cancer causing mutations in mitochondria-mediated apoptosis mechanisms, which are often involved in resistances and recurrences.

Another potential advantage of nsPEF ablation for cancer therapy is related to considerations for cell type specificity. Chemotherapeutic drugs and ionizing radiation primarily affect rapidly dividing cells. Effects of nsPEFs appear to be cell-type specific for a number of cell responses suggesting some cell type specificity; however, it remains to be determine if this has therapeutic relevance. Cultured cells that grow attached as opposed to cells in suspension require longer pulse durations, greater numbers and/or higher electric fields to elicit cell responses [Stacey et al., 2003], including cell death [Beebe et al., 2002; Hall et al., 2007a]. In contrast to conventional electroporation, which affects larger cells more readily than smaller ones, cell size did not matter for plasma membrane permeabilization with nsPEF ablation [Hair et al., 2003]. However, there is no evidence that nsPEF ablation preferentially affect only rapidly proliferating cells. S phase synchronized cells under limiting pulse power conditions exhibited greater membrane integrity and maintained cytoskeletal structure but did not differ in survival compared to unsynchronized cells [Hall et al., 2007b]. Thus, within a heterogeneous tumor mass, nsPEF therapy is expected to induce cell death in rapidly proliferating tumor cells as well as slower proliferating host cells that are collaborating with tumor cells regardless of their size. This suggests an alternative to almany therapeutic regiments that predominantly target rapid proliferating cells. Melanoma tumors also can contain cancer stem cells or other slower cycling cells, which possess characteristics common to normal stem cells, including self renewal capacity, high tumorigenicity and potential to differentiate into multiple cell types [Fang et al., 2005; Grichnik et al., 2006; Roesch et al., 2010; Zabierowski and Herlyn; 2008a, b]. Cancer stem cells or other slower cycling cells may be more prevalent in tumors than initially considered as demonstrated with melanomas from 12 different patients [Quintana et al., 2008]. Herlyn and colleagues have suggested an alternative to the unidirectional stem cell model in melanoma proposing a dynamic temporarily distinct subpopulation of slow cycling melanoma cells that are responsible for tumor maintenance [Roesch et al., 2010]. The existence of these slow cycling cells is clinically relevant because they would be less resistant to most therapeutic regimens; however, they would probably not be resistant to nsPEF ablation. Cancer stem cells or slow cycling cells have been reported to be responsible for recurrences after chemotherapy and ionizing radiation therapy through multiple mechanisms [Weissman and Clarke, 2009]. One of these mechanisms is to minimize therapy-induced DNA damage that is produced by free radical scavengers to minimize the effects of reactive oxygen species (ROS). Cancer stem cells had significantly lower levels of ROS and enhanced ROS defenses compared to non-tumorigenic cells [Diehn et al., 2009]. NsPEF ablation is non-ionizing and it does not appear to induce cell death by generating measurable ROS in B16F10 melanoma cells [Ford et al., 2010] or in E4 squamous cell carcinoma [Ren and Beebe, 2011]. Thus, this mechanism would not provide survival advantages to cancer stem cells exposed to nsPEF ablation. Another mechanism that may be responsible for resistance and recurrences with conventional treatments is to preferentially activate DNA damage checkpoint response and increases in DNA repair capacity [Bao et al., 2006]. NsPEF ablation does cause DNA damage in B16F10 melanoma cells [Nuccitelli et al., 2009] and tumors [Chen et al., 2010]. However, DNA damage may not be a major cause of cell death in these tumors. Furthermore, DNA damage induces apoptosis through release of pro-apoptotic factors from mitochondria [Gross et al., 1999; Hengartner et al., 2000; Korsmeyer et al., 2000] and nsPEF ablation induces melanoma cell death with minimal release of pro-apoptotic factors [Figure 3; Ford et al., 2010]. Thus, minimizing DNA damage and enhancing repair would not provide survival advantages to cancer stem cells or slow cycling cells exposed to nsPEF ablation.

An early study investigating local tissue affects at tumor treatment sites indicated that blood flow to the tumor was disrupted as blood cell leaked out of the tumor around small vessels [Nuccitelli et al., 2006]. This local tumor infarction with an absence of local blood flow for about two weeks appears to be sufficient to deprive tumors of needed oxygenation and nutrition to facilitate tumor demise. A subsequent analysis also demonstrated the presence of iron stain suggesting nsPEF caused slight hemorrhage in the treated tissue [Chen et al., 2010]. Other studies demonstrated that microvessel density markers were significantly reduced, indicating that angiogenesis and/or vasculogenesis were significantly thwarted [Chen et al., 2010; Nuccitelli et al., 2009].

An important benefit to local treatment with nsPEFs is an absence of chemical side effects and toxicities, which are common with nearly all systemic treatments, especially chemotherapy and ionizing radiation. In studies with mice, nsPEF ablation has minimal and resolvable effects on skin. With parallel plate electrodes that eliminated B16F10 melanoma, the stratum corneum showed signs of necrosis and hemorrhage with accompanying superficial erosion of the epidermis [Nuccitelli et al., 2006]. However, these characteristics appeared two days after treatment, differentiating the effect from burn or heat related injuries, which occur immediately. With a four plus one needle array electrode, nsPEF ablation caused some edema and bleeding, but the damage was resolved within a week [Chen et al., 2009]. Small scabs formed but were resolved within two weeks and did not leave a scar. However, mice do not readily scar. In an unpublished clinical study observing effects of nsPEFs on human skin, treatments with two parallel needle electrodes caused some irritation, redness and itching at insertion / treatment sites, which were readily relieved by anti-histamines, local anti-inflammatory ointment and protection from scratching. The treatments caused no permanent scars or discoloration of skin regardless of pigmentation. While there was some pain and discomfort with applications of nsPEF without anesthesia, they were eliminated when a local anesthetic was injected at treatment sites. In addition, application of nsPEFs resulted in few/no muscle contractions, when applied appropriately, which are common with conventional electroporation and irreversible electroporation. In addition, studies monitoring general reactions to nsPEF ablation with parallel plate electrodes, mice had slightly higher heart rates and respiratory rates, but body temperature and systolic blood pressure did not change significantly [Chen et al., 2009]. Thus, as tested so far, applications of nsPEF ablation are generally safe, non-toxic and without scarring or other permanent effects on skin in mice and humans. While pulse power treatments can now be used for surface tumors using needle or plate electrodes, applications to internal tumors will likely be possible as catheter electrodes are developed for laparoscopic surgeries. For all nsPEF treatments, multi-needle electrode systems with adjustable field orientations would likely enhance apoptosis in the context of pulsed voltage-induced inactivation of tumor cells [Song et al., 2010].

An ending argument for applications of nsPEF ablation involves a significant question for the treatment of melanoma and other cancers: Can pulse power ablation with nsPEF effectively treat metastatic melanoma as a systemic disease? This question has begun to be addressed in an experimental protocol, not with B16f10 melanoma cells, but with Hepa 1-6 hepatocellular carcinoma (HCC) cells [Chen and Beebe, unpublished]. When Hepa 1-6 tumors were treated with 900 pulses at 100ns and 55kV/cm, tumors were eliminated in 6 of the 8 mice, while all control mice were humanely euthanized due to tumor burden 14-18 days after tumor initiated. When the 6 successfully treated mice were tumor free for 60 days, tumors cells were injected in the opposite flank as before. None of these animals grew tumors for 49 days before the experiment was terminated. In naïve age-match control HCC tumors grew to treatable sizes in less than two weeks. These results suggest that nsPEF ablation allows a host cell immune response. While these studies must be repeated and the mechanisms of this resistance further investigated, these results suggest that nsPEF ablation addresses another cancer hallmark, evasion of immune surveillance.

It is generally accepted that an ultimate outcome of apoptosis is the removal of aberrant cells without inflammation. This is certainly true for during development and the clearance of immune cells, but it is likely not completely true for cancer therapeutic agents that induce apoptosis in tumors. The tumor masses are likely not cleared before some tumor cells are functionally dead. Many chemotherapeutic agents, as well as nsPEF ablation, induce cell death by apoptosis. However, it is generally considered, but not universally, that apoptosis is immunologically silent. Most chemotherapeutic agents, many of which induce apoptosis, are immunosuppressive. Conversely, considering the challenge experiments of HCC tumors presented above, nsPEF ablation may not be immunologically silent or immunosuppressive. Thus, it is possible for immune cells to present antigens from apoptotic cells. Alberts et al., [1998] demonstrated that human dendritic cells efficiently present antigen derived from apoptotic cells that stimulated class I-restricted CD8+ cytotoxic T-cells. When Chattergoon and co-workers [2000] engineered Fas-mediated apoptotic death of antigen-bearing cells *in vivo* by co-expressing the immunogen and Fas in the same cells, they observed that the death of antigen-bearing cells resulted in increased antigen acquisition by antigen presenting cells including dendritic cells (DCs). Casares et al., [2005] demonstrated that caspase inhibition did not inhibit doxorubicin (DX)-induced cell death, yet suppressed the immunogenicity of dying tumor cells in several rodent models of neoplasia. Further, depletion of DCs or CD8+T cells abolished the immune response against DX-treated apoptotic tumor cells *in vivo*. Russo et al., [2000] showed that irradiated vector-producing cells undergoing apoptosis were phagocytosed by dendritic cells (DCs). They then took lymphocytes obtained from a patient affected by a MAGE-3(+) melanoma, stimulated them *in vitro* with autologous DCs previously exposed to irradiated MAGE-3-expressing cells, which led to induction of MAGE-3-specific cytotoxic effectors, directed against a yet unknown MAGE-3 epitope. These results indicate not only that apoptotic cells and perhaps the presence of active caspases can be immunogenic, it is suggested that they may have immunogenicity. Finally, these results not only indicate that apoptotic cells can stimulate anti-neoplastic immune responses, but that they could generate cancer vaccines, having important implication for gene therapy for melanoma and other cancers.

14. Acknowledgements

The authors thank Mr. Frank Reidy whose financial generosity supported these studies and to Dr. Helen Fillmore for reviewing the manuscript.

15. References

Albert, M.L.; Sauter, B.; Bhardwaj, N. (1998). Dendritic cells acquire antigen from apoptotic cells and induce class I-restricted CTLs. *Nature*, Vol. 392, pp. (86-89), print ISSN 0028-0836, online ISSN 1476-4687

Al-Sakere, B.; André, F.; Bernat, C.; Connault, E.; Opolon, P.; Davalos, R.V.; Rubinsky, B.; Mir, L.M. (2007). Tumor ablation with irreversible electroporation. *PLoS One*, Vol. 2, No. 11, (Nov. 2007), pp. (e1135), ISSN 1932-6203

Amaravadi, R.K.; & Flaherty, K.T. (2007). Targeted therapy for metastatic melanoma. *Clinical Advances in Hematology and Oncology*, Vol.5, No.5, (May 2007) pp. (386-394), ISSN 1543-0790

Bao, S.; Wu, Q.; McLendon, R.E.; Hao, Y.; Shi. Q.; Hjelmeland, A.B.; Dewhirst, M.W.; Bigner, D.D.; Rich, J.N. (2006) Glioma stem cells promote radioresistance by preferential activation of the DNA damage response. *Nature*, Vol.444, (Dec. 2006), pp. (756–760), print ISSN 0028-0836, online ISSN 1476-4687

Beebe, S.J.; Fox, P.M.; Rec, L.J.; Buescher, E.S.; Somers, K; Schoenbach, K.H. (2002). Nanosecond Pulsed Electric Field (nsPEF) Effects on Cells and Tissues: Apoptosis Induction and Tumor Growth Inhibition. *IEEE Transactions in Plasma Science*, Vol.30, No.1, (Feb. 2002), pp. (286-292), ISSN 0093-3813

Beebe, S.J.; Fox, P.M.; Rec, L.J.; Willis, E.L.; Schoenbach, K.H. (2003a). Nanosecond, high-intensity pulsed electric fields induce apoptosis in human cells. *FASEB Journal*, Vol.17, No.11, (Aug. 2003), pp. (1493-1495), print ISSN 0892-6638, online ISSN: 1530-6860

Beebe, S.J.; White, J.; Blackmore, P.F.; Deng, Y.; Somers, K.; Schoenbach, K.H. (2003b). Diverse effects of nanosecond pulsed electric fields on cells and tissues. *DNA Cell Biology*, Vol.22, No.12, (Dec. 2003), pp. (785-796), print ISSN 1044-5498, online ISSN 1557-7430

Beebe, S.J.; Blackmore, P.F.; White, J.; Joshi, R.P.; Schoenbach, K.H. (2004). Nanosecond pulsed electric fields modulate cell function through intracellular signal transduction mechanisms. *Physiological Measurements*, Vol.25, No.4, (Aug. 2004), pp. (1077-1093), ISSN 1361-6579

Beebe, S.J.; Schoenbach K.H. (2005). Nanosecond pulsed electric fields: a new stimulus to activate intracellular signaling. *Journal of Biomedicine and Biotechnology*, Vol.2005, No.4, pp. (297-300), ISSN 1110-7251

Beebe, S.J.; Schoenbach, K.H.; Heller, R. (2010). Bioelectric applications for treatment of melanoma. *Cancers*, Vol.2, pp. (1731-1770), ISSN 2072-6694

Berridge, M.J.; Lipp, P.;& Bootman, M.D. (2000). The versatility and universality of calcium signalling. *Nature Reviews Molecular and Cell Biology*, Vol. 1, No. 1, (Oct. 2000), pp. (11-21), 1471-0072, print ISSN 1471-0072, online ISSN 1471-0080

Bonner, W.M.; Redon, C.E.; Dickey, J.S.; Nakamura, A.J.; Sedelnikova, O.A.; Solier, S.; and Pommier, Y. (2008). Gamma H2AX and cancer. *Nature Reviews Cancer*, Vol. 8, No.12, (Dec. 2000), pp. (957-967), print ISSN 1474-175X, online ISSN 1474-1768

Blume-Jensen, P.; Hunter,T. (2001). Oncogenic kinase signaling. *Nature*, Vol. 411 No. 6835, (May 2001), pp. (355–365), print ISSN 0028-0836, online ISSN 1476-4687

Bowman AM, Nesin OM, Pakhomova ON, Pakhomov AG. (2008). Analysis of plasma membrane integrity by fluorescent detection of Tl(+) uptake. *Journal of Membrane Biology*, Vol.236, No. 1, (Jul. 2010), pp. (15-26), ISSN 0022-2631

Brown, D.A.; London, E. (1998). Functions of lipid rafts in biological membranes. *Annual Reviews Cell and Developmental Biology*, Vol.4, pp. (111–136), print ISSN 1081-0706, online ISSN 1530-8995

Buescher, E.S.; Schoenbach, K.H. (2003). Effects of Submicrosecond, High Intensity Pulsed Electric Fields on Living Cells - Intracellular Electromanipulation. *IEEE Transactions on Dielectrics and Electrical Insulation*, Vol. 10, No. 5, (Oct. 2003), pp. (788–794), ISSN 1070-9878

Cairns, R.A.; Kalliomaki, T.; Hill, R.P. (2001) Acute (cyclic) hypoxia enhances spontaneous metastasis of KHT murine tumors. *Cancer Research*, Vol. 61, No. 24, (Dec. 2001), pp. (8903–8908), print ISSN 0008-5472, online ISSN: 1538-7445

Callahan, M.K.; Wolchok, J.D.; Allison, J.P. (2010). Anti-CTLA-4 antibody therapy: immune monitoring during clinical development of a novel immunotherapy. *Seminars in Oncology*, Vol.37, No.5, (Oct. 2010), pp. (473-484), ISSN 0093-7754

Casares N, Pequignot MO, Tesniere A, Ghiringhelli F, Roux S, Chaput N, Schmitt E, Hamai A, Hervas-Stubbs S, Obeid M, et al. (2005). Caspase-dependent immunogenicity of doxorubicin-induced tumor cell death. *Journal Experimental Medicine*, Vol. 202, No. 12, (Dec. 2005), pp. (1691-1701), print ISSN 0022-1007, online ISSN 1540-9538

Chattergoon, M.A.; Kim, J.J.; Yang. J.S.; Robinson, T.M.; Lee, D.J.; Dentchev, T.; Wilson, D.M.; Ayyavoo, V.; Weiner, D.B. (2000).Targeted antigen delivery to antigen-presenting cells including dendritic cells by engineered Fas-mediated apoptosis. *Nature Biotechnology*, Vol. 18, No. 9, (Sept. 2000), pp. (974-979), print ISSN 1087-0156, online EISSN 1546-1696

Chen, N.; Schoenbach K.H.; Kolb, J.F.; Swanson,R.J; Garner, A.L.; Yang, J.; Joshi, R.P.; Beebe, S.J. (2004). Leukemic cell intracellular responses to nanosecond electric fields. *Biochemical Biophysical Research Communications*, Vol.317, No.2, (April 30, 2004), pp. (421-427), print ISSN 0006-291X, online ISSN 1090-2104

Chen N, Garner AL, Chen G, Jing Y, Deng Y, Swanson RJ, Kolb JF, Beebe SJ, Joshi RP, Schoenbach KH. (2007). Nanosecond electric pulses penetrate the nucleus and enhance speckle formation. *Biochemical Biophysical Research Communications*, Vol. 364, No. 2, (Dec. 2007), pp. (220-225), print ISSN 0006-291X, online ISSN 1090-2104

Chen, X.; Swanson, J.R.; Kolb, J.F.; Nuccitelli, R.; Schoenbach, K.H. (2009). Histopathology of normal skin and melanomas after nanosecond pulsed electric field treatment. *Melanoma Research*, Vol. 19, No. 6, (Dec. 2009), pp. (361-371), print ISSN 0960-8931, online ISSN 1473-5636

Chen, X.; Kolb, J.F.; Swanson, R.J.; Schoenbach, K.H.; Beebe, S.J. (2010). Apoptosis initiation and angiogenesis inhibition: melanoma targets for nanosecond pulsed electric fields. *Pigment Cell & Melanoma Research*, Vol. 23, No. 4, (Aug. 2010), pp. (554-563), print ISSN: 1755-1471, online ISSN 1755-148X

Chenga, H.; Force, T. (2010). Why do Kinase Inhibitors Cause Cardiotoxicity and What can be Done About It? *Progress in Cardiovascular Diseases* Vol. 53, No. 2, (Sept.-Oct. 2010), pp. (114-120), print ISSN 0033-0620, online ISSN 1532-8643

Craviso, G.L.; Choe, S.; Chatterjee, P.; Chatterjee, I.; Vernier, P.T. (2010). Nanosecond electric pulses: a novel stimulus for triggering Ca2+ influx into chromaffin cells via voltage-gated Ca2+ channels. *Cellular & Molecular Neurobiology*, Vol. 30, No. 8, (Nov. 2010), pp. (1259-1265), print ISSN 0272-4340, online 1573-6830

Daud, A.I.; DeConti, R.C.; Andrews, S.; Urbas, P.; Riker, A.I.; Sondak, V.K.; Munster, P.N.; Sullivan, D.M.; Ugen, K.E.; Messina, L.; Heller, R. (2008). Phase I trial of interleukin-12 plasmid electroporation in patients with metastatic melanoma. *Journal of Clinical Oncology*, Vol. *26*, No. 36, (Dec. 2008), pp. (5896-5903), print ISSN 0732-183X, online ISSN 1527-7755

Deng, J.; Schoenbach, K.H.; Buescher, E.S.; Hair, P.S.; Fox, P.M.; Beebe, S. J. (2003). The Effects of Intense Submicrosecond Electrical Pulses on Cells. *Biophysical Journal*, Vol.84, No.4, (April 2003), pp. (2709-2714), print ISSN 0006-3495, online ISSN 1542-0086

Davalos, R.V.; Mir, I.L.; Rubinsky. B.; (2005). Tissue ablation with irreversible electroporation. *Annals of Biomedical Engineering*, Vol. 33, Vol. 33, No. 2, (Feb. 2005), pp. (223-231), print ISSN 0090-6964, online ISSN 1573-9686

Diehn, M.; Cho, R.W.; Lobo, N.A.; Kalisky, T.; Dorie, M.J.; Kulp, A.N.; Qian, D.; Lam, J.S.; Ailles, L.E.; Wong, M.; et. al. (2009). ssociation of reactive oxygen species levels and radioresistance in cancer stem cells. *Nature*, Vol. 458, No. 7239, (Apr. 9, 2009), pp. (780-783), print ISSN 0028-0836, online ISSN 1476-4687

Duff, S.E.; Li, C.; Garland, J.M.; Kumar, S. (2003). CD105 is important for angiogenesis: evidence and potential applications. *FASEB Journal*, Vol. 17, No 9, (Jun. 2003), pp. (984-992), print ISSN 0892-6638, online ISSN: 1530-6860

Esser, A.T.; Smith, K.C.; Gowrishankar, T.R.; Vasilkoski, Z.; Weaver J.C. (2010). Mechanisms for the intracellular manipulation of organelles by conventional electroporation. *Biophysical Journal*, Vol. 98, No. 11, (Jun. 2010), pp. 1–9, print ISSN 0006-3495, online ISSN 1542-0086

Fang, D.; Nguyen, T.K.; Leishear, K.; Finko. R.; Kulp, A.N.; Hotz, S.; Van Belle, P.A.; Xu, X.; Elder, D.E.; Herlyn, M.A. (2005). A tumorigenic subpopulation with stem cell properties in melanomas. *Cancer Research*, Vol. 65, No. 20, (Oct. 2005), pp. (9328-9337), print ISSN 0008-5472, online ISSN: 1538-7445

Flaherty, K.T.; Puzanov, I.; Kim, K.B.; Ribas, A.; McArthur, G.A.; Sosman, J.A.; O'Dwyer, P.J.; Lee, R.J.; Grippo, J.F.; Nolop, K.; et al. (2010). Inhibition of Mutated, Activated BRAF in Metastatic Melanoma. *New England Journal of Medicine*, Vol. 363, No. 9, (Aug. 2010) pp. (809-819), print ISSN 0028-4793, online ISSN 1533-4406

Ford, W.E.; Ren, W.; Blackmore, P.F.; Schoenbach, K.H.; Beebe. S.J. (2010). Nanosecond pulsed electric fields stimulate apoptosis without release of pro-apoptotic factors from mitochondria in B16f10 melanoma. *Archives of Biochemistry and Biophysics*, Vol. 497, No. 1-2, (May 2010), pp. (82-89), print ISSN 0003-9861, online ISSN 1096-0384

Fulda, S.; Debatin, K.M. (2006). Extrinsic versus intrinsic apoptosis pathways in anticancer chemotherapy. *Oncogene*, Vol. 25, No. 34, (Aug. 2006), pp. (4798-4811), print ISSN 0950-9232, online ISSN 1476-5594

Garon, E.B; Sawcer, D.; Vernier, P.T.; Tang, T.; Sun, Y.; Marcu, L.; Gundersen, M.A.; Koeffler. H.P. (2007). In vitro and in vivo evaluation and a case report of intense nanosecond pulsed electric field as a local therapy for human malignancies. *International Journal of Cancer*, Vol. 121, No. 3, (Aug. 2007), pp. (675-82), print ISSN 0020-7136, online ISSN 1097-0215

Gogas, H.J.; Kirkwood, J.M.; Sondak, V.K. (2007). Chemotherapy for metastatic melanoma: time for a change? *Cancer*, Vol. 109, No. 3, (Feb. 2007), pp. (455-464), online ISSN 1097-0142

Gowrishankar, T.R.; Esser, A.T.; Vasilkoski, Z.; Smith, K.C.; Weaver, J.C. (2006). Microdosimetry for conventional and supra-electroporation in cells with organelles. *Biochemical Biophysical Research Communications*, Vol. 341, No. 4, (Mar. 2006), pp., (1266-1276), print ISSN 0006-291X, online ISSN 1090-2104

Granot, Y.; Ivorra, A.; Maor, E.; Rubinsky, B. (2009). In vivo imaging of irreversible electroporation by means of electrical impedance tomography. *Physics in Medicine & Biology*, Vol. 54, No. 16, (Aug. 2009), pp. (4927-4943),

Grichnik, J.M.; Burch, J.A.; Schulteis, R.D.; Shan, S.; Liu, J.; Darrow, T.L.; Vervaert, C.E.; Seigler, H.F. (2006). Melanoma, a tumor based on a mutant stem cell? *Journal Investigative Dermatology*, Vol. 126, No. 1, (Jan. 2006), pp. (142-153), print ISSN 0022-202X, online ISSN 1523-1747

Gross, A.; Yin, X.M.; Wang, K.; Wei, M.C.; Jockel, J.; Milliman, C.; Erdjument-Bromage, H.; Tempst, P,; Korsmeyer, S.J. (1999). Caspase cleaved BID targets mitochondria and is required for cytochrome c release, while BCL-XL prevents this release but not tumor necrosis factor-R1/Fas death. *Journal Biological Chemistry*, Vol. 274, No. 2, (Jan. 1999), pp. (1156-11563), print ISSN 0021-9258, online ISSN 1083-351X

Guo, Y.; Zhang, Y.; Klein, R.; Nijm, G.M,; Sahakian, A.V,; Omary, R.A.; Yang, G,Y.; Larson, A.C. (2010). Irreversible electroporation therapy in the liver: longitudinal efficacy studies in a rat model of hepatocellular carcinoma. *Cancer Research*, Vol. 70, No. 4, (Feb. 2010), pp. (1555-1563), print ISSN 0008-5472, online ISSN: 1538-7445

Haest, C.W.; Kamp, D.; Deuticke, B. (1997). Transbilayer reorientation of phospholipid probes in the human erythrocyte membrane: Lessons from studies on electroporated and resealed cells. *Biochimica Biophysica Acta*, Vol. 1325, No. 1, (Apr. 1997), pp. (17-33), print ISSN 0005-2736

Hair, P.S.; Schoenbach, K.H.; Buescher, E.S. (2003). Sub-microsecond, intense pulsed electric field applications to cells show specificity of effects. *Bioelectrochemistry*, Vol. 61, No. 1-2, (Oct. 203), pp. (65-72), print ISSN 1567-5394, online ISSN 1878-562X

Hall, E.H.; Schoenbach, K.H.; Beebe, S.J. (2005). Nanosecond pulsed electric fields (nsPEF) induce direct electric field effects and biological effects on human colon carcinoma cells. *DNA and Cell Biology*, Vol. 24, No. 5, (May 2005), pp. (283-291), print ISSN 1044-5498, online ISSN 1557-7430

Hall, E.H.; Schoenbach, K.H.; Beebe, S.J. (2007a). Nanosecond pulsed electric fields induce apoptosis in p53-wildtype and p53-null HCT116 colon carcinoma cells. *Apoptosis*, Vol. 12, No. 9, (Sept. 2007), pp. (1721-1731), ISSN 1360-8185

Hall, E.H.; Schoenbach, K.H.; Beebe, S.J. (2007b). Nanosecond pulsed electric fields have differential effects on cells in the S-phase. *DNA Cell Biology*, Vol. 26, No. 3, (Mar. 2007), pp. (160-171), print ISSN 1360-8185, online ISSN 1573-675X

Hanahan, D.; Weinberg, R.A. (2000). The hallmarks of cancer. *Cell*, Vol. 100, No. 1, (Jan. 2000), pp. (57-70), print ISSN 1097-4172, online ISSN 0092-8674

Hanahan, D.; Weinberg, R.A. (2011). Hallmarks of cancer: the next generation. *Cell*, Vol. 144, No. 5, (Mar. 2011), pp. (646-674), print ISSN 1097-4172, online ISSN 0092-8674

Heller, R.; Jaroszeski, M. J.; Glass, L. F.; Messina, J. L. Rapaport, D. P.; DeConti, R. C.; Fenske, N. A.; Gilbert, R. A.; Mir, L. M. Reintgen, D. S. (1996). Phase I/II trial for the treatment of cutaneous and subcutaneous tumors using electrochemotherapy. *Cancer*, Vol. 77, No. 5, (Mar. 1996), pp. (964–971), print ISSN 0008-543X, online ISSN 1097-0142

Hengartner, M.O. The biochemistry of apoptosis. (2000) *Nature*, Vol. 407, No. 6805, (Oct. 2000), pp. (770-776), print ISSN 0028-0836, online ISSN 1476-4687

Hodi, F.S.; O'Day, S.J.; McDermott, D.F.; Weber, R.W.; Sosman, J.A.; Haanen, J.B.; Gonzalez, R.; Robert, C.; Schadendorf, D.; Hassel, J.C.; et al. (2010). Improved survival with ipilimumab in patients with metastatic melanoma.(2010). *New England Journal of*

Medicine, Vol. 363, No. 8, (Aug. 2010), pp. (711-723),. Erratum in *ibid* Vol. 363, No. 13, pp. (1290). Comment in: *ibid*. Vol. 363, No. 8, pp. (779-781), print ISSN 0028-4793, online ISSN 1533-4406

Holcik, M.; Sonenberg, N. (2005). Translational control in stress and apoptosis. *Natures Reviews Molecular Cell Biology*, Vol. 6, No. 4, (Apr. 2005), pp. (318-327), print ISSN 1471-0072, online ISSN 1471-0080

Hu, Q., Joshi, R.P., Schoenbach, K.H., 2005. Simulations of nanopore formation and phosphatidylserine externalization in lipid membranes subjected to a high-intensity, ultrashort electric pulse. *Physical Review E - Statistical, Nonlinear and Soft Matter Physics*, Vol. 72, No. 3 pt 1, (Sept. 2005) pp. 031902, print ISSN 1539-3755, online ISSN 1550-2376

Hu, Q.; Sridhara, V.; Joshi, R.P.; Kolb, J.F.; Schoenbach, K.H. (2006). Molecular Dynamics Analysis of High Electric Pulse Effects on Bilayer Membranes Containing DPPC and DPPS. *IEEE Transactions on Plasma Science*, Vol. 34, No. 4 Pt 2, (2006), pp. 1405-1411, ISSN 0093-3813

Ibey, BL.; Xiao, S.; Schoenbach, K.H.; Murphy, M.R.; Pakhomov, A.G. (2009). Plasma membrane permeabilization by 60- and 600-ns electric pulses is determined by the absorbed dose. *Bioelectromagnetics*, Vol.30, No.2, (February 2009), pp. 92-99, ISSN 0197-8462

Ibey, B.L.; Pakhomov, A.G.; Gregory, B.W.; Khorokhorina, V.A.; Roth, C.C.; Rassokhin, M.A.; Bernhard, J.A.; Wilmink, G.J.; Pakhomova, O.N. (2010). Selective cytotoxicity of intense nanosecond-duration electric pulses in mammalian cells. *Biochimica Biophysica Acta*, Vol.1800, No.11, (November 2010), pp. 1210-1219, print ISSN 0006-3002

Ivorra, A.; Al-Sakere, B.; Rubinsky, B.; Mir, L.M. (2009). In vivo electrical conductivity measurements during and after tumor electroporation: conductivity changes reflect the treatment outcome. *Physics in Medicine & Biology*, Vol. 54, No. 19, (Oct. 2009), pp. (5949-5963), print ISSN 0031-9155, online ISSN 1361-6560

Joshi, R.P.; Schoenbach, K. H. (2000). Electroporation dynamics in biological cells subjected to ultrafast electrical pulses: A numerical simulation study. *Physical Review E, - Statistical, Nonlinear and Soft Matter Physics*, Vol.62, No.1, (Jul. 2000), pp.1025–1033, print ISSN 1539-3755, online ISSN 1550-2376

Joshi, R.P.; Hu, Q.; Schoenbach, K.H.; Hjalmarson H.P. (2002). Improved energy model for membrane electroporation in biological cells subjected to electrical pulses. *Physical Review E - Statistical, Nonlinear and Soft Matter Physics*, Vol. 65, No. 4 pt 1, (Apr. 2002), pp. (041920), ISSN 1539-3755, online ISSN 1550-2376

Kolb, J.F.; Chen, X.; Zhuang, J.; Ren, W.; Scully, N; Swanson, R.J.; Beebe, S.J; Schoenbach KH. (2009). Tumor treatment with nanosecond pulsed electric fields. *IEEE Pulse Power Conference* Jun.-Jul. 2009; pg.880-885.

Korsmeyer, S.J.; Wei, M.C.; Saito, M.; Weiler, S.; Oh, K.J.; Schlesinger, P.H. (2000). Pro-apoptotic cascade activates BID, which oligomerizes BAK or BAX into pores that result in the release of cytochrome c. *Cell Death & Differentiation*, Vol. 7, No. 12, (Dec. 2002), pp. (1166-1173), ISSN print 1350-9047, online 1476-5403

Kotnik, T.; Miklavcic, D. (2006). Theoretical Evaluation of Voltage Inducement on Internal Membranes of Biological Cells Exposed to Electric Fields. *Biophysical Journal,* Vol. 90, No. 2, (Jan. 2006), pp. 480-491, print ISSN 0006-3495, online ISSN 1542-0086

Kroemer, G.; Pouyssegur, J. (2008). Tumor cell metabolism: cancer's Achilles' heel. *Cancer Cell,* Vol. 13, No. 6, (Jun. 2006), pp. (472-482), print ISSN 1535-6108

Lee, E.W.; Chen, C.; Prieto, V.E.; Dry, S.M.; Loh, C.T.; Kee, S.T. (2010). Advanced hepatic ablation technique for creating complete cell death: irreversible electroporation. *Radiology,* Vol. 255, No. 2, (May 2010), pp. (426-433), print ISSN 0033-8419, online ISSN 1527-1315

Letai, AG. (2008). Diagnosing and exploiting cancer's addiction to blocks in apoptosis. *Nature Reviews Cancer,* Vol. 8, No. 2, (Feb. 2008), pp. (121-132), print ISSN 1474-175X, online ISSN 1474-1768

Long, G.; Shires, P.; Plescia, D.; Beebe, S.J.; Kolb, J. F.; Schoenbach, K.H. (2011) Targeted Tissue Ablation with nanosecond pulsed electric fields. *IEEE Engineering in Medicine and Biology,* in press

Maor, E.; Ivorra, A.; Leor, J.; Rubinsky, B. (2007). The effect of irreversible electroporation on blood vessels. *Technology in Cancer Research and Treatment,* Vol. 6, No. 4, (Aug. 2007), pp. (307-312), print ISSN 1533-0346

Mir, L.M.; Orlowski, S.; Belehradek, J. Jr.; Paoletti, C. (1991). Electrochemotherapy potentiation of antitumour effect of bleomycin by local electric pulses. *European Journal of Cancer,* Vol. 27, No. 1, pp. (68-72), print ISSN 0961-5423, online ISSN 1365-2354

Momoi, T. (2004). Caspases involved in ER stress-mediated cell death. *Journal of Chemical Neuroanatomy,* Vol. 28, No. 1-2, (Sept. 2004), pp. (101-105), print ISSN 0028-3835, online ISSN: 0891-0618

Nazarian, R.; Shi, H.; Wang, Q.; Kong, X.; Koya, R.C.; Lee, H.; Chen, Z.; Lee, M.K.; Attar, N.; Sazegar, H.; et al. (2010). Melanomas acquire resistance to B-RAF(V600E) inhibition by RTK or N-RAS upregulation. *Nature,* Vol. 468, No. 7326, (Dec. 2010), pp. (973-977), print ISSN 0028-0836, online ISSN 1476-4687

Neumann, E.; Schaefer-Ridder,M.; Wang, Y.; Hofschneider, P.H. (1982). Gene transfer into mouse lyoma cells by electroporation in high electric fields. *EMBO Journal,* Vol. 1, No. 7, pp. (841-845), Online ISSN : 0261-4189

Nuccitelli, R.; Pliquett, U.; Chen, X.; Ford, W.; Swanson, J.R.; Beebe, S.J.; Kolb, J.F.; Schoenbach, K.H. (2006). Nanosecond pulsed electric fields cause melanomas to self-destruct. *Biochemical Biophysical Research Communications,* Vol. 343, No. 2, (May 2006), pp. (351-360), print ISSN 0006-291X, online ISSN 1090-2104

Nuccitelli, R.; Chen, X.; Pakhomov, A.G.; Baldwin, W.H.; Sheikh, S.; Pomicter, J.L.; Ren, W.; Osgood, C.; Swanson, R.J.; Kolb, J.F.; Beebe, S.J.; Schoenbach, K.H. (2009). A new pulsed electric field therapy for melanoma disrupts the tumor's blood supply and causes complete remission without recurrence. *International Journal Cancer,* Vol. 25, No. 2, pp. (Jul. 2009), (438-445), print ISSN 0020-7136, online ISSN 1097-0215

Nuccitelli, R.; Tran, K.; Sheikh, S.; Athos, B.; Kreis, M.; Nuccitelli, P. (2010). Optimized nanosecond pulsed electric field therapy can cause murine malignant melanomas to self-destruct with a single treatment. *International Journal of Cancer*, Vol. 127, No. 7, (Oct. 2010), pp. (1727-1736), print ISSN 0020-7136, online ISSN 1097-0215

Onik, G.; Mikus, P.; Rubinsky, B. (2007). Irreversible electroporation: implications for prostate ablation. *Technology in Cancer Research and Treatment*, Vol. 6, No. 4, (Aug. 2007), pp. (295-300), print ISSN 1533-0338

Pakhomov, A.G.; Phinney, A.; Ashmore, J.; Walker, K., III; Kolb, J.F.; Kono, S.; Schoenbach, K.H.; Murphy, M.R. (2004). Characterization of the cytotoxic effect of high-intensity, 10-ns duration electrical pulses. *IEEE Transactions on Plasma Science*, Vol.32, No. 4, (August 2004), pp. 1579-1586, ISSN: 0093-3813.

Pakhomov, A.G.; Shevin, R.; White, J.A.; Kolb, J.F.; Pakhomova, O.N.; Joshi, R.P.; Schoenbach, K.H. (2007a). Membrane permeabilization and cell damage by ultrashort electric field shocks. *Archives Biochemistry and Biophysics*, Vol. 465, No. 1, (Sept. 2007), pp (109-118), print ISSN 0003-9861, online ISSN 1096-0384,

Pakhomov, A.G.; Kolb, J.F.; White, J.A.; Joshi, R.P.; Xiao, S.; Schoenbach, K.H. (2007b). Long-lasting plasma membrane permeabilization in mammalian cells by nanosecond pulsed electric field (nsPEF). *Bioelectromagnetics*, Vol.28, No. 8, (Dec. 2001), pp. ISSN 0197-8462

Pakhomov, A.G.; Bowman, A.M.; Ibey, B.L.; Andre, F.M.; Pakhomova, O.N.; Schoenbach, K.H. (2009). Lipid nanopores can form a stable, ion channel-like conduction pathway in cell membrane. *Biochemical Biophysical Research Communications*, Vol. 385, No. 2, (Jul. 2009), pp. (181-186), print ISSN 0006-291X, online ISSN 1090-2104

Peggs, K.S.; Quezada, S.A. (2010). Ipilimumab: attenuation of an inhibitory immune checkpoint improves survival in metastatic melanoma. *Expert Reviews of Anticancer Therapy*, Vol. 10, No. 11, (Nov. 2010), pp. (1697-1701), ISSN: 1473-7140, 1744-8328

Peng, Y.J.; Yuan, G.; Ramakrishnan, D.; Sharma, S.D.; Bosch-Marce, M.; Kumar, G.K.; Semenza, G.L.; Prabhakar, N.R. (2006). Heterozygous HIF-1alpha deficiency impairs carotid body-mediated systemic responses and reactive oxygen species generation in mice exposed to intermittent hypoxia. *Journal of Physiology*, Vol. 577, No. Pt 2, (Dec. 2006), pp. (705–716), print ISSN 0022-3751, online ISSN 1469-7793

Phillips, M.; Maor, E.; Rubinsky, B.; (2010). Nonthermal irreversible electroporation for tissue decellularization. *Journal Biomechanical Engineering*, Vol. 132, No. 9, (Sept. 2010), pp. (091003),

Quintana, E.; Shackleton, M.; Sabel, M.S.; Fullen, D.R.; Johnson, T.M.; Morrison, S.M. (2008). Efficient tumor formation by single melanoma cells. *Nature*, Vol. 456, No. 7222, (Dec, 2008), pp. (593–599), print ISSN 0028-0836, online ISSN 1476-4687

Ren, W.; Beebe, S.J. (2011). An Apoptosis Targeted Stimulus with Nanosecond Pulsed Electric Fields (nsPEFs) in E4 Squamous Cell Carcinoma, *Apoptosis*, Vol. 16, No. 4 (Apr. 2011), pp. (382-393), print ISSN 1360-8185

Reuben, J.M.; Lee, B.N.; Li, C.; Gomez-Navarro, J.; Bozon, V.A.; Parker, C.A.; Hernandez, I.M.; Gutierrez, C.; Lopez-Berestein, G.; Camacho, L.H. (2006). Biologic and immunomodulatory events after CTLA-4 blockade with ticilimumab in patients with advanced malignant melanoma. *Cancer*, Vol. 106, No. 11, (Jun. 2006), pp. (2437-2244), print ISSN 0008-543X, online ISSN 1097-0142

Riker, A.I.; Radfar, S.; Liu, S.; Wang, Y.; Khong, H.T. (2007). Immunotherapy of melanoma: a critical review of current concepts and future strategies. *Expert Opinions Biological Therapy*, Vol. 7, No. 3, (Mar. 2007), pp. (345-358), print ISSN 1471-2598, online ISSN 1744-7682

Roesch, A.; Fukunaga-Kalabis, M.; Schmidt, E.C.; Zabierowski, S.E.; Brafford, P.A.; Vultur, A.; Basu, D.; Gimotty, P.; Vogt, T.; Herlyn, M.A (2010) Temporarily distinct subpopulation of slow-cycling melanoma cells is required for continuous tumor growth. *Cell*, Vol. 141, No. 4, (May 2010), pp. (583-594), print ISSN 0092-8674

Rogakou EP, Pilch DR, Orr AH, Ivanova VS, Bonner WM (1998). DNA double-stranded breaks induce histone H2AX phosphorylation on serine 139. *Journal of Biological Chemistry*, Vol. 273, No. 10, (Mar. 1998), pp. (5858–5868), print ISSN 0021-9258, 1083-351X

Rózanowska, M.; Sarna, T.; Land, E.J.; Truscott, T.G. (1999). Free radical scavenging properties of melanin interaction of eu- and pheo-melanin models with reducing and oxidising radicals. *Free Radicals in Biology and Medicine*, Vol. 26, No. 5-6, (Mar. 1999), pp. (518-525), ISSN: 0891-5849

Russo, V.; Tanzarella, S.; Dalerba, P.; Rigatti, D.; Rovere, P.; Villa, A.; Bordignon, C.; Traversari, C. (2000). Dendritic cells acquire the MAGE-3 human tumor antigen from apoptotic cells and induce a class I-restricted T cell response. *Proceeding National Academy of Science* USA, Vol. 97 No. 5, (Feb. 2000) pp. (2185-2190), print ISSN 0027-8424, online ISSN 1091-6490

Satzger, I.; Küttler, U.; Völker, B.; Schenck, F.; Kapp, A.; Gutzmer, R. (2010). Anal mucosal melanoma with KIT-activating mutation and response to imatinib therapy--case report and review of the literature. *Dermatology*, Vol. 220, No. 1, (Jan. 2010), pp. (77-81), online ISSN: 1087-2108

Savill, J.; Dransfield, I.; Gregory, C.; Haslett, C. (2002). A blast from the past: clearance of apoptotic cells regulates immune responses. *Nature Reviews in Immunology*. Vol. 2, No. 12, (Dec. 2002), pp. (965-675), print ISSN 1474-1733, online ISSN 1474-1741

Schatton, T.; Frank, M.H. (2009). Antitumor immunity and cancer stem cells. *Annals New York Academy of Science*, Vol. 1176, Hematopoietic Stem Cells VII, (Sept. 2009), pp. (154-169), print ISSN 0077-8923, online ISSN 1749-6632

Schoenbach, K.H.; Beebe, S.J.; Buescher, E.S. (2001). Intracellular effect of ultrashort electrical pulses. *Bioelectromagnetics*, Vol. 22, No. 6, (Sept. 2001), pp. (440-448), ISSN 0197-8462

Schoenbach, K.H.; Joshi, R.P.; Kolb, J.F.; Chen, N.; Stacey, M.; Blackmore, P.F.; Buescher, E.S.; Beebe, S.J. (2004). Ultrashort electrical pulses open a new gateway into biological cells. *Proceedings of IEEE*, Vol. 92, No. 7, (Jun. 2004), pp. (1122–1137), ISSN: 0018-9219

Schoenbach, K.H.; Xiao, S.; Joshi, R.P.; Camp, J.T.; Heeren, T.; Kolb, J.F.; Beebe, S.J. (2008). The Effect of Intense Subnanosecond Electrical Pulses on Biological Cells. *IEEE Transactions in Plasma Science*, Vol. 36, No. 6, (Apr. 2008), pp. (414-424), ISSN 0093-3813

Schoenbach, K.H.; Joshi, R.P.; Beebe, S.J.; Baum, C.E. (2009). A Scaling Law for Bioelectric Effects of Nanosecond Pulses. *IEEE Transactions in Dielectrics and Electrical Insulation* Vol. 16, No. 5, (Oct. 2009) pp. (1224-1235), ISSN: 1070-9878.

Schwarz, S, Deuticke B, Haest CW. (1999). Passive transmembrane redistributions of phospholipids as a determinant of erythrocyte shape change: Studies on electroporated cells. *Molecular Membrane Biology*, Vol. 16, No. 3, (Sept. 1999), pp. (247-255), print ISSN 0968-7688, online ISSN 1464-5203

Smith, R.C.; Gowrishankar, T.R.; Esser, A.T.; Stewart D.A.; Weaver J.C. (2006). The Spatially Distributed Dynamic Transmembrane Voltage of Cells and Organelles due to 10 ns Pulses: Meshed Transport Networks. *IEEE Transactions on Plasma Science*, Vol. 34, No. 4, (Aug. 2006), pp. (1394-1404), ISSN 0093-3813

Soengas, M.S.; Lowe, S.W. (2003). Apoptosis and melanoma chemoresistance. *Oncogene*, Vol. 22, No. 20, (May 2003), pp. (3138-3151), print ISSN 0950-9232, online 1476-5594

Song, J.; Joshi, R.P.; Beebe, S.J. (2010). Cellular apoptosis by nanosecond, high-intensity electric pulses: Model evaluation of the pulsing threshold and extrinsic pathway. *Bioelectrochemistry*, Vol. 79, No. 2, (Oct. 2010), pp. (179-186), print ISSN 1567-5394, online ISSN 1878-562X

Stacey, M.; Stickley, J.; Fox, P.; Statler, V.; Schoenbach, K.H.; Beebe, S.J.; Buescher, E.S. (2003). Differential effects in cells exposed to ultra-short, high intensity electric fields: cell survival, DNA damage, and cell cycle analysis. *Mutation Research*, Vol. 542, No. 1-2, (Dec. 2003), pp. (65-75), print ISSN 1383-5718

Stewart, D.A.; Gowrishankar, T.R.; Weaver, J.C. (2004). Transport lattice approach to describing electroporation: use of local asymptotic model. *IEEE Transactions on Plasma Science*, Vol. 32, No. 4, (Aug. 2004), pp. (1696-1708), ISSN 0093-3813

Szegezdi, E.; Fitzgerald, U.; Samali A. (2006). Caspase-12 and ER-stress-mediated apoptosis: the story so far. *Annals of the New York Academy of Science*, Vol.1010, (Dec. 2006), pp. (186-194), print ISSN 0077-8923, online ISSN 1749-6632

Tarhini, A.A.; Agarwala, S.S. (2006). Cutaneous melanoma: available therapy for metastatic disease. *Dermatological Therapy*, Vol. 19, No. 1, (Jan.-Feb., 2006), pp. (19-25), print ISSN: 1396-0296, online ISSN 1529-8019.

Tekle, E.; Wolfe, M.D.; Oubrahim, H.; Chock, P.B. (2008). Phagocytic clearance of electric field induced apoptosis-mimetic' cells. *Biochemical Biophysical Research Communications*, Vol. 376, No. 2, (Nov. 2008), pp. (256-260), print ISSN 0006-291X, online ISSN 1090-2104

Tekle, E.; Oubrahim, H.; Dzekunov, S.M.; Kolb, J.F.; Schoenbach, K.H.; Chock, P.B. (2005) Selective field effects on intracellular vacuoles and vesicle membranes with nanosecond electric pulses. *Biophysical Journal*, Vol. 89, No. 1, (Jul. 2005), pp. (274-284), print ISSN 0006-3495, online ISSN 1542-0086

Tieleman, D.; Leontiadou, H.; Mark, A.E.; Marrink S.J. (2003). Simulation of Pore Formation in Lipid Bilayers by Mechanical Stress and Electric. Fields. *Journal of the American Chemical Society*, Vol. 125, No. 21, (May, 2003), pp. (6382-6383), print ISSN 0002-7863

Tsatmalia, M.; Ancansa, J.; Thodya, A.J. (2002). Melanocyte Function and Its Control by Melanocortin Peptides. *Journal of Histochemistry and Cytochemistry*, Vol. 50, No. 2, (Feb. 2002), pp. (125-134), print ISSN 0022-1554, online ISSN 0022-1554

Vernier, P.T.; Sun, Y.; Marcu, L.; Salemi, S.; Craft, C.M.; Gundersen, M.A. (2003a). Calcium bursts induced by nanosecond electric pulses. *Biochemical Biophysical Research*

Communications, Vol. 310, No. 2, (Oct. 2003), pp. (286-295), print ISSN 0006-291X, online ISSN 1090-2104

Vernier, P.T.; Li, A.; Marcu, L.; Craft, C.M.; Gundersen, M.A. (2003b), Ultrashort Pulsed Electric Fields Induce Membrane Phospholipid Translocation and Caspase Activation: Differential Sensitivities of Jurkat T Lymphoblasts and Rat Glioma C6 Cells. *IEEE Transactions in Dielectrics and Electrical Insulation*, Vol. 10, No. 5, (Oct. 2003), pp. (795-809), print ISSN 1070-9878

Vernier, P.T.; Ziegler, M.J.; Sun, Y.; Gundersen, M.A.; Tieleman, D.T. (2006a). Nanopore-facilitated, voltage-driven phosphatidylserine translocation in lipid bilayers - in cells and in silico. *Physical Biology*, Vol. 3, No. 4, (Nov. 2006), pp. (233-247), print ISSN 1478-3967, online 1478-3975

Vernier, P.T., Ziegler, M.J., Sun, Y.; Chang, V.T., Gundersen, M.A., Tieleman, D.P., 2006b. Nanopore Formation and Phosphatidylserine Externalization in a Phospholipid Bilayer at High Transmembrane Potential. *Journal of the American Chemical Society*, Vol. 128, No. 4, (Nov. 2006), pp. (6288-6289), print ISSN 0002-7863, online ISSN 1520-5126

Vernier, P.T.; Sun, Y.; Chen, M.T.; Gundersen, M.; Craviso, G.L. (2008). Nanosecond electric pulse-induced calcium entry into chromaffin cells. *Bioelectrochemistry*, Vol. 73, No. 1, (Jul. 2008), pp. (1-4), print ISSN 1567-5394, online ISSN 1878-562X

Wang, S.; Chen, J.; Chen, M.T.; Vernier, P.T.; Gundersen, M.A.; Valderrábano, M. (2009). Cardiac myocyte excitation by ultrashort high-field pulses. *Biophysical Journal*, Vol. 96, No. 4, (Feb. 2009), pp. (1640-1648), print ISSN 0006-3495, online ISSN 1542-0086

Waterhouse, N.J.; Trapani, J.A. (2003). A new quantitative assay for cytochrome c release in apoptotic cells. *Cell Death and Differentiation*, Vol.10, No. 7, (Jul., 2003), pp. 853–855, ISSN print 1350-9047, online 1476-5403

Wei, L.; Xue, T.; Wang, J.; Chen, B.; Lei, Y.; Huang, Y.; Wang, H.; Xin, X. (2009). Roles of clusterin in progression, chemoresistance and metastasis of human ovarian cancer. *International Journal of Cancer*, Vol. 125, No. 4, (Aug. 2009), pp. (791-806), print ISSN 0020-7136, online ISSN 1097-0215

Weissman, I.L.; Clarke, M.F. (2009). Association of reactive oxygen species levels and radioresistance in cancer stem cells. *Nature*, Vol. 458, No. 7239, (Apr. 2009), pp. (780–783), print ISSN 0028-0836, online ISSN 1476-4687

White, J.A.; Blackmore, P.F.; Schoenbach, K.H.; Beebe, S.J. (2004). Stimulation of capacitative calcium entry in HL-60 cells by nanosecond pulsed electric fields. *Journal Biological Chemistry*, Vol. 279, No. 22, (May 2004), pp. (22964-22972), print ISSN 0021-9258, online ISSN 1083-351X

White, R.M.; Zon, L.I. (2008). Melanocytes in development, regeneration, and cancer. *Cell Stem Cell*, Vol. 3, No. 3, (Sept. 2008), pp. (242-252), print ISSN 1934-5909, online 1875-9777

Zabierowski, S.E.; Herlyn, M. (2008a). Melanoma stem cells: the dark seed of melanoma. *Journal of Clinical Oncology*, Vol. 26, No. 17, (Jun 2008), pp. (2890-2894), print ISSN 0732-183X, online ISSN 1527-7755

Zabierowski, S.E., Herlyn, M., (2008b). Learning the ABCs of melanoma-initiating cells. *Cancer Cell,* Vol. 13, No. 3, (Mar. 2008), pp. (185-187), print ISSN 1535-6108

Zhang, J.; Blackmore, P.F.; Hargrave, B.;, Xiao, S.; Beebe, S.J.; Schoenbach, K.H. (2008). Nanosecond pulse electric field (nanopulse): a novel non-ligand agonist for platelet activation. *Archive Biochemistry and Biophysics*, Vol. 471, No. 2, pp. (240-248), print ISSN 0003-9861, online ISSN 1096-0384

11

The Role of Electrochemotherapy in the Treatment of Malignant Melanoma

Mecker G. Möller[1], Slawomir Salwa[2],
Declan M. Soden[2] and Gerald C. O'Sullivan[2]
[1]*Division of Surgical Oncology, Department of Surgery, University of Miami, Miller School of Medicine, Miami, Florida*
[2]*Cork Cancer Research Centre, Leslie C. Quick Laboratory, BioSciences Institute, University College Cork and Department of Surgery, Mercy University Hospital, Cork,*
[1]*USA*
[2]*Ireland*

1. Introduction

About 68,130 new melanomas will be diagnosed in the United States during 2010 (38,870 men: 29,260 women) and of those 8,700 people will die of the disease (5,670 men; 3,030 women). The death rate has been dropping since the 1990s for those younger than 50, but has remained stable or is rising for older individuals. However, the incidence of melanoma has been increasing for at least 30 years, and this trend has become more pronounced in young white females and in older white men[1].

Malignant Melanoma is the seventh most common type of cancer, but it is the first cause of death from cutaneous skin cancers[2]. It has been estimated that the lifetime risk of developing malignant melanoma is 2% (1 in 50) for Caucasians, 0.1% (1 in 1,000) for those of black descent, and 0.5% (1 in 200) for Hispanics[3] .

When melanoma is detected in advanced stages, it carries a dismal prognosis, with a mean survival of about 8 months and a 5-year survival as low as 5% [4-6]. The disease spreads both by the lymphogenous and the haematogenous routes and can metastasize to virtually any organ in the body. When secondary tumours emerge, these usually follow a sequential pattern to regional lymph node basins, followed by distant sites including skin, subcutaneous tissue, lung, liver, brain, bone and other viscera[5-6]. Local recurrence, in-transit metastases and satellitosis (cutaneous metastases within 2 cm of original lesion) represent the same dissemination process[4] in the dermal lymphatics. When the patients present with cutaneous metastases, they are considered to have stage IIIB disease[7]. Cutaneous metastases occur in 2-20% of patients, depending on tumor thickness [6, 8-9] and can occur either during the early or late phase of the disease [10]. In many instances they can represent the first site of recurrence after surgical excision of the primary tumor [11] . The majority (70-80%) of recurrences are diagnosed within the first 3 years of initial diagnosis, and the median time to the presence of in-transit disease could range between 3 to 16 months[4]. The recurrences present as local or in-transit disease in 20-28%, regional disease in 26-60% and as distant metastases in 15-50% of patients. Even though local recurrence is not yet considered stage IV disease, the prognosis is poor with 5 year survival rates of less than 50% [9,12]. The risk of developing metastases may be predicted at excision of the primary lesion and determinants include, increasing thickness of the tumour, the anatomical location, histological subtype and gender [13]. In general tumours of the trunk, non cutaneous and subungual regions behave more aggressively than those of the extremity [14-16] .

2. Treatment limitations for recurrent or in-transit melanoma

Treating extensive cutaneous/subcutaneous nodules or in-transit disease is a clinical challenge because of common unresectability and relative insensitivity to conventional systemic therapies[6]. These recurrences provide a significant psychological burden for patients whose quality of life is negatively affected by the symptoms caused by the tumor, such as pain, bleeding, ulceration, and malodorous discharge [4, 17-18]. Many patients suffering from in-transit disease also manifest with systemic disease, within 6-13 months of the onset of the local lesions. Their life expectancy is foreshortened and is determined by factors such as the burden of the loco-regional disease, the interval from initial treatment and their immune status [4].

The aim of the treatment should be the elimination of both local and systemic disease with the benefit of improved life expectancy and quality of life, while minimizing toxicities or deformities. It is important to note that metastatic cells have disseminated prior to surgical intervention, outlining the critical need for the development of adjuvant therapeutic strategies[19]. Thus the treatment of unresectable and in-transit disease is both systemic and loco/regional. The options include surgery, which is the most effective method for limited recurrent or in-transit disease, systemic chemotherapy[12,21], radiation therapy[22], cryosurgery[23]; carbon dioxide laser ablation,[12,24-26], intralesional therapies[12,21] with the Bacille Calmette-Guerin vaccine[27], TNFerade a non replicant adenovirus complex, expressing the Tumor Necrosis Factor alpha (TNF-α) gene (hTNF-α cDNA)[12,28], and Interleukin-2[29], Cell Vaccine and Immunotherapy [30-33], Interferon alpha[34-36], Regional therapies such as hyperthermic isolated limb perfusion (HILP) and Isolated limb infusion (ILP)[37], Novel Molecular Therapies with c-Kit inhibitors (Imatinib), C-RAF-inhibitors (Sorafenib) [38], and blocking B-RAF regulation of mitogen-activated protein kinase pathway (MAPK) [38]. In more recent years electroporation with anticancer drugs which is termed electrochemotherapy (ECT) has been successfully applied for local tumour control [17, 19, 39]. In general malignant melanoma is refractory to systemic treatments and survival after treatment of regional cutaneous metastases has been reported to be between 20-28% at 10 years[6,9,40]. However all current treatment modalities have individual limitations and variable response rates [4, 12, 19, 41-42].

3. Electrochemotherapy (ECT)

Definition and physiological effect:

The cell membrane represents a physical barrier to the intracellular transfer of hydrophilic drugs, macromolecules, nucleotides and peptides. The movement of polar and hydrophilic molecules across the membrane is restricted by the phospholipid bilayer[18] Studies suggest that exposure to sufficiently strong and long electrical fields, could rearrange the lipid bilayer, by reorienting the hydrophillic heads in pore-like fashion, while the hydrophobic tails are embedded within the plasma membrane. This porosity is transient and reversible if short duration high amplitude square wave electrical pulses are optimized.[18]

Electroporation (EP) of tumour nodules allow the permeation, into the cancer cells, of poorly permeable antineoplastic drugs, such as bleomycin or cisplatin which are given either systemically or intratumorally (IT)[18, 39, 43-46]

The temporary permeability of the cell membrane caused by the electric pulses facilitates a potent localized effect and magnifies the drugs cytotoxicity by orders of magnitude [18, 39, 46-50].

Types of Drugs

After several studies of different cytotoxic drugs, two have been identified as the best candidates for ECT: Bleomycin and Cisplatin [17, 45]. Of importance in these studies EP or the drugs on their own do not influence the growth of tumours, yet their combination have potent tumoricidal effects[18, 51-53] (See Figure 1). An advantage of ECT is that it requires much lower doses of the cytotoxic drug for optimal effects than those usually used for systemic treatments. In addition there is little in the way of collateral damage or complications, since the the cell killing is confined to the tissues affected by the electric field. Bleomycin intercalates into the cellular chromatin causing single and double stranded breaks in DNA resulting in a mitotic cell death by pseudoapoptosis. (Figure 1 B,C & D). On the other hand, Cisplatin creates an apoptosis effect on the cell [18, 46]. This cytolytic activity is potentiated more than 1,000 fold for Bleomycin and 100 fold for Cisplatin by the addition of EP [12, 19, 48-49].

The Vascular Lock

The electric pulses produce a transient state of hypoperfusion by local reflex vasoconstriction at the arteriolar level (lasting 1-2 minutes) and a phase of interstitial edema (that resolves with membrane resealing). However the effect may last longer (12 hours to 5 days) in rapidly dividing tumor cells and is more prominent in tumours with a less mature endothelial lining and higher interstitial pressure. This phenomenon mediated by the sympathetic nervous system is termed the "vascular lock" and it has implications for timing of drug administration[18-19]. After application of the electric current, there is a retention of drugs already in the tumour but there is also an impairment of entry of drugs from the circulation. Thus when the cytotoxic drugs are administered systemically sufficient time should be allowed to achieve optimal intratumoral drug concentration prior to application of EP. ECT produces other vascular influences, which are believed to be secondary to a reduction in local angiogenic factor production, such as endothelial cell destruction and neovascular reorganization [46, 54-55]. The combined vascular influences have been successfully exploited in the treatment of bleeding melanomas [56-57]– which may be a difficult to manage problem, sometimes refractory and fatal, in patients with unresectable disease.

4. Technique of electrochemotherapy

1. The Equipment

The electric pulses may be applied to the tumors either by plate electrodes on the skin surface or by needle electrodes inserted into the lesion (figure2). The electric field distribution is determined by the geometry of the electrodes. Regardless of the type of electrode the electric field is highest around and between the electrodes [17-18]. The current pulse generators in use are the Cliniporator (IGEA, Carpi, Italy) (FIG 2) and the Medpulser™ (Inovio Biomedical Corporation, CA, USA). It appears that plate electrodes are

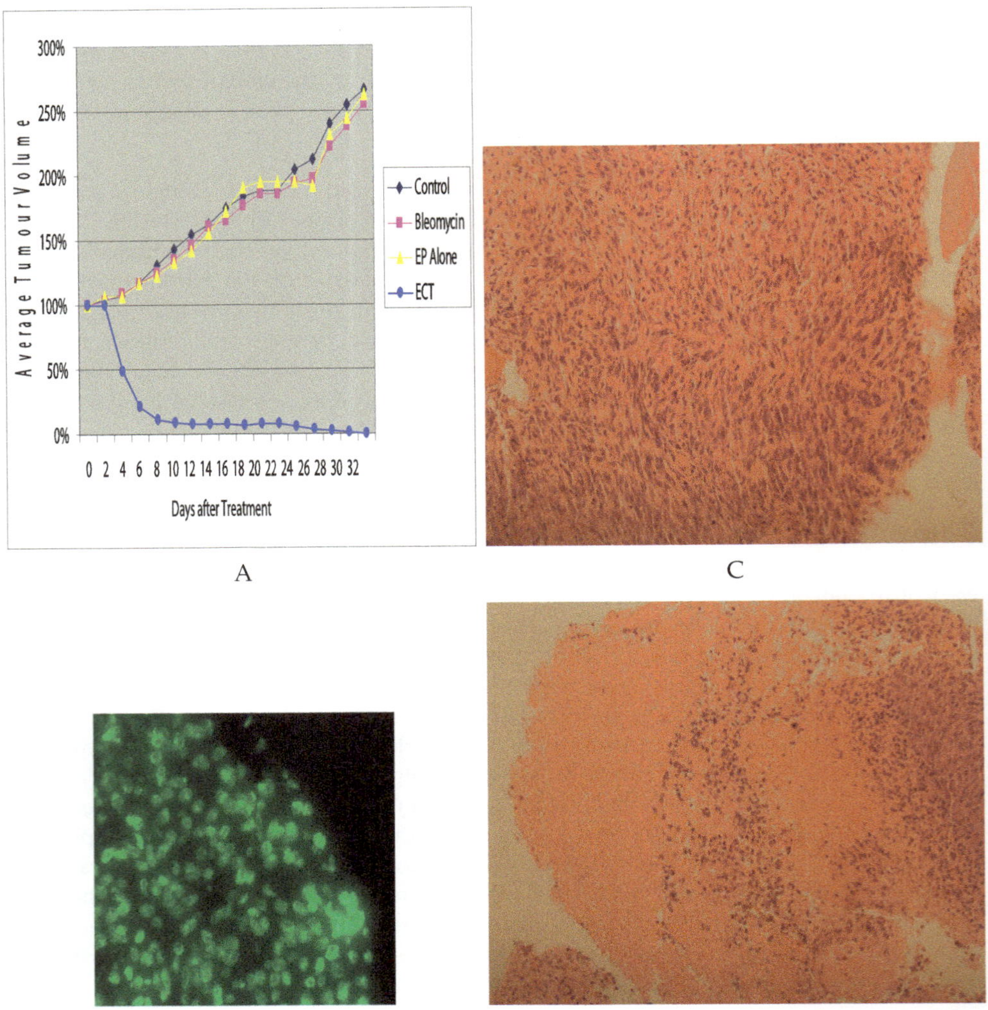

Fig. 1. A. Growth curves of experimental cancers in mice, which demonstrate that electropermeabilisation or intratumoural bleomycin alone, have no influence on tumour growth but when used together completely ablate the tumour. B) Positive Tunel stain 48 hrs post ECT indicating tumor cell death by apoptosis. C &D Tumour before showing normal cellularity and D 48 hrs post ECT showing regions of denucleation

more suitable for use in superficial skin lesions, while needle electrodes are used for deeper seated lesions, such as exophytic and thick lesions (maximum depth 3 cm)[52]. A disadvantage of plate electrodes over the needle type is the potential skin damage that may be generated by the higher impedance/resistance of the skin, especially when treating larger affected areas[19, 58]. Care must be taken to avoid inserting the needle electrodes into the healthy tissue surrounding the tumors, which may also result in local subcutaneous burns [39]. There are three types of electrodes in common usage *(FIG 2)*. Type I electrodes consist of two parallel stainless-steel plate electrodes, used for superficial lesions and do not penetrate the skin. Type II electrodes are used for smaller lesions and consist of two rows of eight needles with 4 mm distance between them, while Type III electrodes are recommended for larger lesions (>1cm), with the needles in a hexagonal configuration. The needles are inserted encircling the tumor and down to the subcutaneous tissue, slightly deeper than tumor depth [17, 19, 52, 59]. It is recommended to elevate or tent the skin at the time of delivering the electric current , if the electrodes are to be inserted in a superficial or shallow subcutaneous areas such as near the knees, tibial tuborosities, the scalp, or close to any other osseous structures[52]

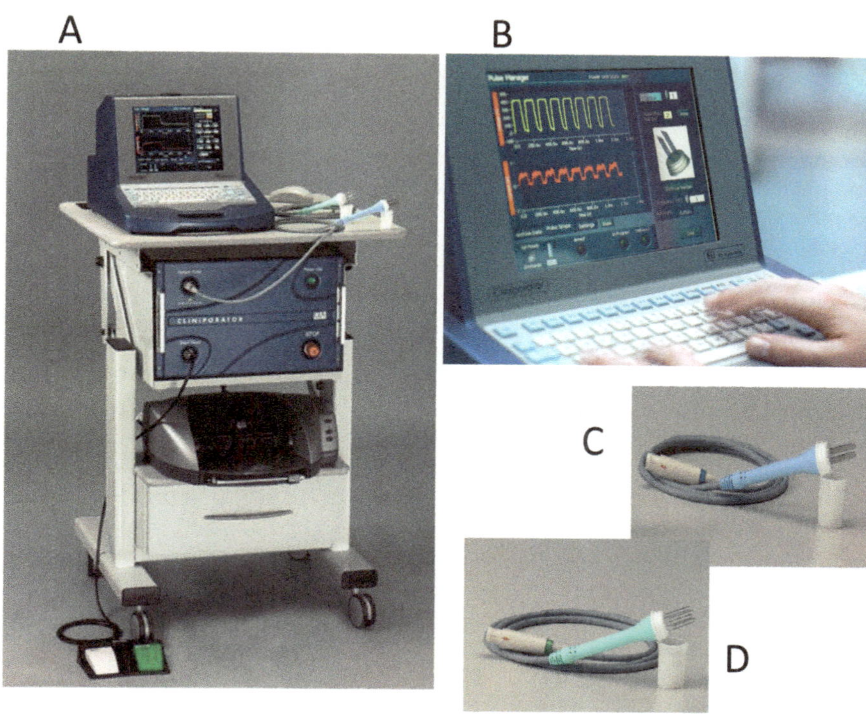

Fig. 2. (A) The ECT pulse generator. B) Note an entrainment of 8 square wave pulses. C) Electrodes type1 (plates) and (D) type 3 (Needle array).

2. Anesthesia

The procedure can be performed in the outpatient or ambulatory setting, under local anesthesia in association with conscious sedation. General anesthesia may be preferred for larger tumors, or tumors located in prior irradiated or fibrotic tissues where infiltration of local anesthetic may be painful and less likely to diffuse and thus achieve adequate pain control and for those located too close to vascular or bony structures. The dose of local anesthetic should be recorded and should not exceed the maximum allowed per body weight for Lidocaine without epinephrin (3 mg/kg) [52, 59-60]. In addition, a mixture of 0_2/air with $Fi0_2$ of 40 % is administered to the patients during conscious sedation.

3. The Electric Current

Permeabilization occurs in the cell when the internal transmembrane potential has surpassed the critical value between 200-300mV. The extent of the electroporative effect depends on the number and duration of the electric pulses[18,55]. Two pulse parameters have been evaluated - exponentially decaying pulses and square wave pulses. Of the two, square wave pulses are preferred as they permit independent control of the length and amplitude. The pulse parameters selected for treatment depend on the type of electrode [18, 52].

Pulse parameters

Ideally for Type I (plate) electrodes, pulse parameters of 8 square waves with amplitude of 1300 V/cm, duration of 100 μs, and frequency of 1Hz are used. The current should be delivered in two perpendicular directions.

For type II (needle) electrodes the voltage amplitude may be reduced to 1000V/cm. The pulses are administered simultaneously between the needle pairs.

For Type III, the needles are positioned hexagonally and 96 pulses are given together (12 pairs x 8 pulses) at a frequency of 5 kHz [61].

Due to the already described vascular lock phenomenon, it is recommended that the electric current is applied between 8 to 28 minutes after IV administration of the drug[62], or immediately (within 2-10 minutes) after intratumoral administration [19, 59, 63-64].

4. Drug Dosage Recommendations

Initial studies compared the routes of administration of Bleomycin suggested advantages for the intralesional over intravenous administration (77% vs. 45 % complete responses) [45] but later the prospective multi-institutional ESOPE (European Standard Operating Procedures of Electrochemotherapy) study in 2006, concluded that IV or IT Bleomycin were comparable when given to tumors of volumes less than 0.5 cm^3 [52]. For Cisplatin, the studies have shown that IT is more effective than the IV route, with CR rates of 82% vs. 48% respectively[19, 45]. In the ESOPE study local tumor control was achieved in up to 88% of tumors treated with IV Bleomycin, 73% with IT Bleomycin and 75% with IT Cisplatin[52].

If a lack of uniformity of drug distribution within the tumor is anticipated either by the presence of large and extensive disease, harder fibrotic tumor nodules, lymphedema or limb fibrosis, the IV route would be more suitable [52]. The Intratumoral route is more feasible for those less perfused nodules located in previously pretreated areas[19].

When Bleomycin is given IV the dose is 15,000 IU/m2 of body surface area in a bolus lasting 30-45 seconds. But when the IT route is chosen, both drugs are given in a dose calculation based on tumor burden. The IT dose of Bleomycin based on tumor size is calculated as follows: for tumor nodules less than 0.5 cm^3 a dose of 1000 IU/cm^3, tumor nodules between 0.5 and 1 cm^3 a dose of 500 IU/cm^3 and for tumors larger than 1 cm^3 a dose of 250IU/cm3 is administered. The cumulative dose should not exceed 400,000 IU/m^2 due to the cumulative risk of lung fibrosis[46,52]. If the cumulative dose surpasses 60,000 IU /m2, objective respiratory function tests should be made at intervals and the drug discontinued if the respiratory diffusion capacity is abnormal[60]. The IT dose of Cisplatin is given as follow: for nodules less than 0.5 cm^3 a dose of 2mg/cm^3, for nodules between 0.5-1 cm^3, a dose of 1mg/cm^3 and for nodules larger than 1 cm^3 a dose of 0.5mg/cm^3 is given. (Table 1)

Tumor Volume ($V=ab^2\pi/6$)	**Bleomycin dose (1000 IU/mL concentration)**	**Cisplastin dose (2mg/mL concentration)**
<0.5 cm^3	1 mL/cm^3 tumor	
>0.5 < 1 cm^3	0.5 mL/ cm^3 tumor	
>1 cm^3	0.25 mL/ cm^3 tumor	

Table 1. Tumor volume and IT drug dose concentration

The rationale for reducing the intralesional dose per cm^3 when treating areas with larger tumor burdens is to reduce the risk of systemic toxicities of the absorbed drug without compromising local efficacy[19].

Prophylactic antibiotics against skin flora should be given intravenously prior to the start of the procedure, especially when lesions are ulcerated or necrotic.

The required time for the procedure is short, with a median treatment duration of 25 minutes[32]. Repeated treatments are usually well tolerated by the patients [11, 65-66] and these can usually be performed at 1-6 weekly intervals, without evident resistance [45].

5. Patient monitoring

Prior to each treatment session patients should have an electrocardiogram (ECG), blood work for evaluation of renal function, coagulation and electrolyte values. All lesions should be photographed and the tumor burden documented. Cellular debris may be released from the tumour during electroporation and these may interfere with the clearance of cytotoxic drugs by the kidney. Thus, when using IV Bleomycin, the serum creatinine should be maintained at less than 150mol/L to ensure proper renal clearance. Physiological monitoring includes visual display of O2 saturation, pulse rate, blood pressure, continuous ECG tracing and respiratory parameters. Acetominophen or an anti-histaminic medication may be given to prevent the mild febrile reaction that may occur in the early post procedural period when Bleomycin is administered [46, 59].

Technical pearls

1. Test the device and the electrodes prior to beginning the procedure
2. Prep and drape following sterile technique principles
3. Keep in mind correct timing of drug administration and application of the electric current
4. Protect osseous surfaces by tenting the skin
5. Communicate with awake patients and assisting staff, prior to delivery of electric current
6. Check electroporator traces and waves to confirm proper current delivery
7. Do not overlap treating fields with normal tissue
8. Dress wounds according to presenting symptoms

5. ECT development and clinical applications in melanoma

Neumann in 1982[67] published the first paper regarding EP as a method to transfer genes into mammalian and bacterial cells. There were other *in vitro* [65, 68] and *in vivo* studies in early and late 1980's using EP in combination with drugs[69], but the first clinical trials demonstrating its effectiveness over Bleomycin alone for the treatment of a diversity of cutaneous tumors of the head and neck region, were published in early 90's by Mir et al[47] and Belehradek et al.[70] from the Institute Gustave Roussy, in Villejuif France. These first 8 patients were treated for squamous cell carcinoma tumors and a complete response (CR) was observed in 57% of the lesions. These early publications encouraged other investigators to expand the principles of this technique to other tumor types including basal cell carcinomas, Kaposi sarcoma, and melanoma metastases [6, 62, 71-74]. By the mid 90's, Rudolf et al.[71] and Heller et al. [73] published the results of an initial small group (5) of melanoma patients that underwent treatment with ECT and IV Bleomycin. They reported overall response rates (OR) in 92% and 50% of 24 and 10 metastatic nodules respectively[19]. That same year, Glass et al. [75] from the University of South Florida in Tampa, USA, reported on the first study using ECT with IT Bleomycin in melanoma metastases obtaining OR rates of 92% (78% CR and 14 % PR) in 20 metastatic lesion - results similar to those obtained by the IV route in the previous studies. Later in 1998, the same group of investigators published the results of a bigger cohort of patients with a variety of cutaneous and subcutaneous malignant nodules. Twelve of 34 patients had 84 metastatic melanoma nodules with documented OR rates up to 99% (89% complete response (CR) and 10 % partial response (PR))[76]. That same year, the combined data produced by five institutions in USA, France and Slovenia was published by Mir et al.[39] In this study, twenty patients with metastatic melanoma lesions showed responses in 131 (92%) of 142 lesions, with CR of 53% and PR of 39%. A major finding of this study was that the results were comparable among the institutions even though their treatment protocols and the route used for administering the Bleomycin were not standardized. Additional small studies [56, 77-79] using ECT with IT Bleomycin for melanoma lesions continued to show good responses, with OR rates of 71 to 100% (CR 23%-100% and PR 0%-62%). Rols et al.[80] in 2000 continued to demonstrate OR's of 93% using ECT and IV Bleomycin in the treatment of 54 metastatic melanoma nodules.

Sersa et al.[81-82] introduced Cisplatin as a therapeutic option in 1998. In their studies they reported CR rates of 100% for 2 patients with 13 lesions treated with IT Cisplatin, but low CR rates of 11 % in 9 patients with 27 lesions treated using the IV route. Additional studies were published using this drug by the IT route only [61, 82-83] with OR rates ranging from 81% to 100% (CR 0%-70 % and PR 6%-100%).

The main issue with most of the studies of the 1990's and early 2000's was the utilization of a variety of treatment protocols with different pulse parameters and pulse generators in combination with different electrode types and drug administration routes [6, 39, 44, 47, 52, 56, 58, 63, 70, 72-73, 75-78, 81-88]. But in 2006 the results of a pivotal prospective non-randomized multicenter ESOPE study [52] were published, thus providing recommendations for a standardized protocol for the procedure. The study included 102 patients, 61 evaluated for response and 41 for toxicity respectively. The protocol allowed for administration of Bleomycin either IV or IT, or with Cisplatin IT, and included several histological types of lesions. Ninety-eight lesions from 20 melanoma patients were evaluated - The OR rates were 81% with a CR of 66%. The results confirmed the effectiveness of ECT in the treatment of lesions of different histology, demonstrating an 85% objective response rate and a CR rate of 74% for all lesions.

These results were independent of the drug used or the route of administration chosen. Additionally subsequent studies [11, 49, 66, 89-92] of ECT evaluating its effect in the treatment of melanoma and other skin cancers continue to demonstrate the efficacy of the treatment, with response rates comparable to the earlier studies, ranging from 46-100%.

Repeated treatments are feasible as demonstrated by Campana et al.[90] and Quaglino et al.[11] producing additional clinical responses in patients who had initial non or partial responses or who presented with new recurrent lesions. In the Campana[90] study 34 patients out of 52 were diagnosed with unresectable melanoma, but the response rate for the entire cohort of patients treated with either IT or IV Bleomycin improved significantly from a CR of 50%, up to 83 % after the third ECT treatments.

There are approximately 60 institutions in Europe and in the United States that continue to investigate and offer ECT as a palliative treatment for a variety of unresectable tumors, including melanoma; and in an occasional report it has been used as an alternative curative therapy [93].

6. ECT in the treatment of advanced melanoma

In patients with unresectable recurrent or in-transit melanoma disease who are not candidates for standard surgical or medical treatment, ECT is now an important therapeutic option[18,43,49,75,84,94]. These cases include those with unresectable disease due to the extensive number of nodules or lesions located in compromising anatomic areas, such as those around joints, nerves, distal leg and in previously operated fields. Encouraging results with long term remissions have been documented [17, 45, 78, 93, 95-96]. (Figure 3)

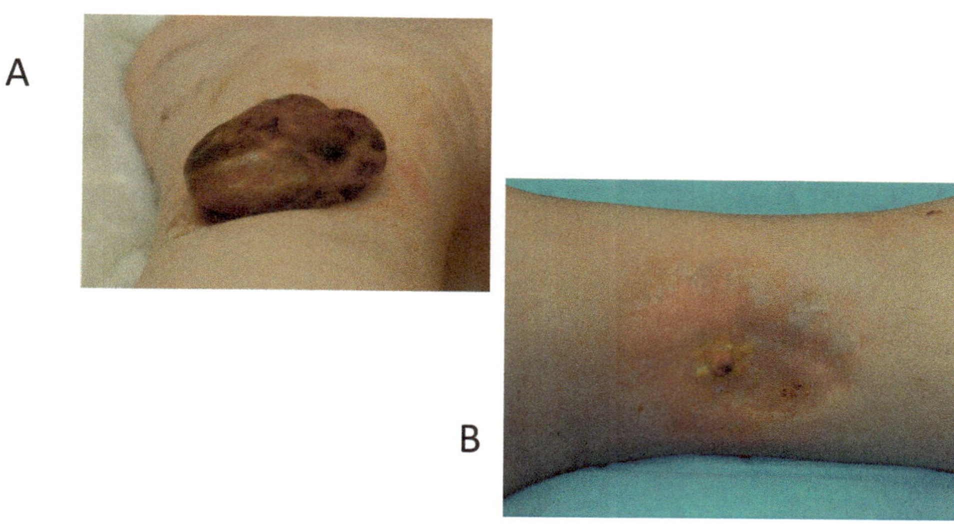

Fig. 3. A) An Exophytic type recurrent malignant melanoma after isolated limb perfusion. B) Six months following treatment by ECT .

Author	No. Patients	Nodules	Drug/route	CRR %	ORR (PR+CR)%
Rudolf 1995[135]	2	24	Bleomycin IV	92	92
Heller 1996[137]	3	10	Bleomycin IV	30	50
Glass 1996[140]	5	23	Bleomycin IT	78	96
Heller 1998[141]	12	84	Bleomycin IT	75	99
Kubota 1998[144]	1	8	Bleomycin IT	100	100
Mir 1998[27]	20	142	Bleomycin IV	53	92
Sersa 1998[146]	2	13	Cisplastin IT	100	100
Sersa 2000[147]	9	27	Cisplastin IV	11	48
Sersa 2000[153]	10	82	Cisplastin IT	80	87
Rols 2000[145]	4	55	Bleomycin IV	9	93
Gehl 2000[128]	1	9	Bleomycin IT	100	100
Rodriguez 2001[143]	2	13	Bleomycin IT	23	85
Sersa 2003[149]	14	211	Cisplastin IT	70	81
Byrne 2005[144]	21	52	Bleomycin IT	63	71
Snoj 2005[148]	1	1	Cisplastin IT	0	100
Marty 2006[124]	20	98	Bleomycin IT/IV* larger 3 cm	66	81
Gaudy 2006[159]	12 *(7 per protocol)*	30 23	Bleomycin IT	36 74	46 82
Snoj 2006[165]	1	16	Cisplastin IT	100	100
Larkin 2007[121]	4 *(2 pts LTF)*	56	Bleomycin IT or IV for nodules > 3 cm	0	50
Snoj 2007[164]	1 *(RETC x4)*	224	Bleomycin IV	100	100
Tauceri 2007[157]	3	ns	Bleomycin IT	ns	ns
Qualigno 2008[12]	14 *(7 pts RETC)*	160 73	Bleomycin IV	50 58	93 93
Campana 2009[158]	34 MM **(52 cohort 27 RETC)*	373 608 257	Bleomycin IT/IV	ns 50 66	ns 74 90

IV: Intravenous, IT: Intratumoral, CRR: Complete Response Rate, ORR: Overall Response Rate, PR: Partial Response, CR: Complete Response

RETC: Repeated Electrochemotherapy, LTF: Lost to follow up, ns: No specified, MM: Malignant melanoma

*: Patients with different histological types

Table 2. Summary of most relevant studies using ECT for unresectable or In-Transit Melanoma

Its effectiveness has been proven when providing palliative treatment for hemorrhagic and painful tumor nodules [56-57, 79, 97-98]. This is a benefit believed to be secondary to the "vascular lock" phenomenon The vasoconstriction at the arteriolar level produces an imediate and dramatic reduction of perfusion of the malignant lesions, thus controlling the bleeding [18, 45, 98]. ECT can also be useful as a neoadjuvant treatment for cytoreduction and organ sparing treatment. Its benefits has been reported in patients with perineal melanoma treated with Cisplatin [85] and for a sphincter saving procedure in anal melanoma [83].

ECT can also be suitable for and more tolerable by those patients with a prohibitive surgical risk due to significant comorbidities[52] because the length of the procedure is relatively short [52] and patients are able to tolerate multiple sessions. In some anatomical locations ECT could provide good and sometimes better cosmetic results than surgery [93].

ECT in combination with cytokine therapy or gene coding immunotherapies has advanced to clinical trials in advanced melanoma. In a phase II study, patients treated with injections of low dose perilesional IL-2 and ECT with Bleomycin, the cytotoxic T lymphocytes response against the known melanoma antigens initially decreased after treatment to reappear when IL-2 was stopped. The tumor-specific peripheral T cells could be detected later in the lesions. The authors theorized that cell death produced by ECT may have attracted and primed denditric cells with the tumor antigens, which later migrated to the draining lymph node basin, and elicited a T cell response against those antigens expressed by the melanoma[100].

The first Human phase I trial of in vivo DNA electroporation of recurrent malignant melanoma was published in the USA in 2009[101]. EP with dose escalation of the interleukin-12 plasmid (in vivo DNA EP) was used in the treatment of 24 patients with stage III B/C or IV disease. It resulted in significant necrosis of melanoma cells and regression of the majority of treated lesions. In addition, clinical regression of untreated lesions suggested the induction of systemic anti tumor immune responses. The treatment was found to be safe with no significant reported toxicities . While additional studies in larger cohorts of patients are still necessary, to obtain reproducibility of these results, these data show a new method of inducing potent tumour specific immune responses individual to the patient.

There are no studies comparing ECT with other surgical modalities, however when taking into consideration the learning curve of other complex regional treatment modalities, the techniques of ECT are considered to be "user friendly" and easy to teach and learn. This technique can also be highly advantageous and useful in countries or hospitals where other modalities or resources are limited.[45]

7. Advantages of ECT

1. Excellent local tumor control rates (80-90%)
2. Minimal risk of damage to healthy surrounding tissue
3. Lower chemotherapy doses needed, minimizing the toxicity profile of the drug
4. There is no protein denaturation, which may elicit an undesireable immune response against self antigens
5. High safety profile without severe side effects
6. Good cost/benefit ratio profile: ambulatory setting, lower cost for drugs, and minimal equipment needed.
7. Treatments are well tolerated by patients
8. Improvement in the perceived quality of life

8. Patient selection and limitations of the procedure

The contraindications of the ECT could be divided into drug and procedure related.

A. Drug related contraindications[60]:

1. Known allergy to the drug to be administered
2. Interstitial lung fibrosis, if Bleomycin is going to be used
3. Kidney failure or limited renal function
4. When the cumulative dose of Bleomycin has reached >400,000 UI/m^2

B. Procedure related contraindications[43]:

1. For safety reasons ECT should not be used in patients with implanted electric devices such as pacemakers
2. In patients who may carry a higher risk of bleeding such as those on anticoagulants or with increased INR and platelets count < 70,000.

9. Limitations

With the current available electrodes, ECT has limitations when treating deep seated tumors[43]. Tumors larger than 3 cm^2 appear to have lower response rates (CR 73 %) to ECT [11,49,90] as compared to nodules smaller than 1cm^2 (CR 98%). These findings were not affected by either the cutaneous or subcutaneous location of the nodules [11].

When tumor nodules are located in irradiated or fibrotic tissues the needle electrode penetration may be problematic with a suboptimal delivery of the electrical current or drugs [90]. Nonetheless, if optimal needle penetration is achieved, ECT is equally effective in irradiated as in non-irradiated tissue[52]. If extensive disease (more than 15 lesions) is present repeated sessions may be necessary. In aggressive disease - while undergoing ECT new cutaneous nodules may emerge but palliative retreatment is worthwhile eventhough the systemic disease progresses rapidly[60].

This treatment modality has not been studied in randomized trials with other treatment techniques, such as ablative and perfusion or infusion procedures, or radiation therapy. More studies with longer follow up are still needed to evaluate disease free survival and to compare ECT to surgical excision, not only in the palliative setting but as a curative alternative in those patients unsuitable or unfit for a surgical procedure[19].

10. Toxicity and side effects

ECT has a low toxicity profile with limited side effects as compared to other regional therapies such as HILP or ILP [41]. However one of the limitations of fully assessing the toxicities of the treatment is the inconsistency of the large majority of the published studies documenting complications.

The systemic dose of Bleomycin is one twentieth of that used in the majority of chemotherapeutic regimens and thus the systemic side effects appear to be limited to nausea [18, 90]. There has been two reported cases of post procedure lypothymia[90].

The most common local side effects reported by the majority of patients are pain (75%) and erythema limited to the tumor and surrounding treated tissue [11, 45, 52, 66]. Most of the patients considered those symptoms tolerable as documented by the ESOPE study [52]. The erythematous reaction usually recedes within a few days[11]. Local tumor necrosis has been reported in 42% of cases[66]. Delayed wound healing that may take several weeks or months to resolve, and epidermal erosions, and hematomas have been reported as rare events[66,73,75]. The injection site reactions appear to be low (Type I and II) in the Wiebendirk toxicity scale[90].

Transient muscle spasms myoclonus, secondary to muscle stimulation by the electrical pulses, have been reported in 25% with lower intensity contractions in up to 78% of patients[52,66]. Some authors advocate the administration of diazepam to alleviate these particular symptoms[73,75]. Interestingly the majority of patients are willing to continue treatment if indicated, since the side effects are tolerable[19].

11. What the future holds

Equipment evolution

Bioengineering developments and evolution of the technique continue to expand the applications of ECT as an alternative treatment for tumors that are inaccessible to current electrical probes. A redeveloped electroporator generator provides more flexibility to deliver the electric current at different phases of the cardiac cycle and the facility to connect several electrode probes around the tumor to deliver the electric pulses in synchrony. The other development is related to the type of electrodes. Longer array electrodes are now available to treat larger and deeper seated tumors, which in the past was a limitation of the procedure. These longer electrodes are insulated proximally to prevent short circuiting of current and to protect the normal tissues that are transgressed en-route to the tumor. These new devices have recently been applied clinically[19, 102-103]. Kos et al. [103] have proposed an algorithmic computer optimized analysis to treat deeper tumors, to minimize errors and to maximize treatment benefits.

Another novelty is the creation of finger applicators which allows the application of electrodes into lesions located in difficult to reach anatomic locations, such as the inside of the oral cavity. These finger electrodes have been already tested in the treatment of melanoma of the oral mucosa, and head and neck regions, with complete tumor regression [90].

New endoluminal electrodes to reach internal lesions within the gastrointestinal tract have been used in animal models, as well as tumors transplanted into rabbit liver and murine models [87, 104-106]. These studies are encouraging and have demonstrated both *in vitro* and *in vivo* (human solid tumor masses in nude mouse models), that the use of flexible electrodes is safe, feasible and reproducible.

There is still the need to create harder needle probes for use in those difficult to treat subcutaneous and cutaneous tumors. These needles must be capable of penetrating into hard fibrotic tissue, while minimizing the bleeding risks and maintaining an adequate electrical distance between the probes.

Nanopulses

Higher amplitude electric pulses or "nanopulses" are currently being evaluated. The use of shorter pulse durations in the nanosecond range are believed to create smaller pores that allow ions but not large molecules to penetrate the membrane. These higher electric fields increase the possibility of producing non resealable pores, thus producing the effect of irreversible electroporation, and consequently allowing the cells to lose their cytoplasm with concomitant cell death. This principle is being used for tumor ablation, palliation or both [43,

[107-109]. However in the treatment of melanoma, the advantages of these higher electric fields are not immediately evident.

ECT combination with Gene transfer, immunology and nanomolecules

Several studies suggest that the immune system is also involved in the mechanisms of response to ECT treatment and that this could be exploited for systemic disease control.
In a murine model [114], ECT followed by CpG oligonucleotide injection locally, produced an enhancement of the complete regression responses of tumors from 43 to 100 % , while also triggering systemic antitumor phenomenon with specific immune memory. Activation of dendritic cells released from the tumors are believed to be involved in this response with a recruitment of CD11c and CD11b receptors and an increase of TLR9 expression .
EP in combination with gene transfer is termed "Gene Electrotransfer ". It uses gene coding plasmids in order to transfer intracellularly a combination of genes, to either knock down the expression of a particular gene, or to stimulate temporary patterns of gene expression). The technique allows for avoidance of the biohazard issues intrinsic to viral vectors [101, 115-116]. Scientists at the Cork Cancer Research Centar in Ireland have investigated in an *in vivo* murine model, the application of EP and local gene therapy for malignant tumors. A plasmid coding for two immunogenes, granulocyte-macrophage colony-stimulating factor (GM-CSF) and the B7-1 co-stimulatory immune molecule were delivered by EP. This resulted in the complete regression of the majority (60%) of non immunogenic tumors, while eliciting a tumour specific systemic response that hindered the metastatic growth in the liver in a 100 % of the mice. This was a durable potent response with tumor specificity. When the remaining non responders non responders tumors were excised, an improved survival was observed when compared to the control groups, thus suggesting that the use of neoadjuvant electroporation and gene therapy given at an appropriate time interval prior to tumour excision or ablation could prevent the surfacing of metastatic disease [117-119]. Regulatory T cell depletion at the time of electrogenetherapy stimulated improved complete response rates from 60 to near 100% suggesting a potential for improving efficacy of electroporation based immunogene therapy.
ECT with injection of TNF-α intra or peritumorally and suboptimal doses of Bleomycin in mice might have a positive immunomodulatory effect, and possibly adds a systemic component to the localized ECT treatment[120] . It has been noted that EP with INF-α used to treat Mycosis Fungoides (subcutaneous lymphoma) lesions produced a 100 % CR [121] The cytotoxic action of INF-α was attributed to its increased tumoral concentration and the prolonged time of action produced by the EP. ECT either with INF-α or TNF-α might permit the usage of less toxic doses, while enhancing clinical local and systemic immunological response rates and minimizing systemic side effects[19].

ECT, radiotherapy and activation of bioreductive drugs

The "vascular lock" principle of EP has the potential to be used to "activate" bioreductive drugs such as Tirapazamine against neoplastic cells [43], due to its vascular disrupting effect of tumor blood supply. In addition ECT has been shown to have a synergistic effect with radiotherapy in preclinical investigations, opening the possibility to use it as a radiosensitising tool for the palliation of subcutaneous lesion[43, 122].
The continued development of improved diagnostic methods will allow for earlier diagnosis of metastases, and possibly open the opportunities for *in situ* neoadjuvant treatment of

higher risk malignant melanomas by means of immunogene or cytokine therapies, hence establishing tumour specific responses which could prevent recurrence and eradicate disseminated micometastases.

12. Summary

ECT with Bleomycin or Cisplatin is an effective treatment in the palliative management of unresectable recurrent cutaneous or subcutaneous melanoma metastases or in-transit disease, with OR rates of approximately 80-90%. ECT should now be considered as part of the armamentarium for treatment of loco regional advanced melanoma. The technology of ECT continues to evolve allowing for the treatment of metastatic lesions in other organs or anatomic regions. The principles of EP are already being applied in the clinical setting for the delivery of targeted therapies such as gene transfer and immunotherapy. These therapies along with ECT have the potential not only for local, but for distant treatment of tumors such as those of malignant melanoma, by stimulating a self-driven immune response to achieve systemic control of the disease

However studies evaluating long term follow up results of ECT in melanoma are still needed prior to considering it as an option for curative intent. ECT has been proven to be an excellent palliative option in treatment of recurrent unresectable or in-transit disease.

13. References

[1] Institute NC. (http://www.cancer.gov/cancertopics/pdq/treatment/melanoma/HealthProfessional/. Accessed 18 March 2011.

[2] American Cancer Society: Cancer facts and figures 2010. 2010; http://www.cancer.org/Research/CancerFactsFigures/CancerFactsFigures/cancer-facts-and-figures-2010. Accessed 21 March, 2011.

[3] American Cancer Society: Detailed Guide: Skin Cancer - Melanoma. What Are the Key Statistics About Melanoma? . 2009; http://www.cancer.org/docroot/CRI/content/CRI_2_4_1X_What_are_the_key_statistics_for_melanoma_50.asp?sitearea=.

[4] Hoekstra HJ. The European approach to in-transit melanoma lesions. *Int J Hyperthermia.* May 2008;24(3):227-237.

[5] Yeatman TJ, Nicolson GL. Molecular basis of tumor progression: mechanisms of organ-specific tumor metastasis. *Semin Surg Oncol.* May-Jun 1993;9(3):256-263.

[6] Glass LF, Fenske NA, Jaroszeski M, et al. Bleomycin-mediated electrochemotherapy of basal cell carcinoma. *J Am Acad Dermatol.* Jan 1996;34(1):82-86.

[7] Balch CM, Buzaid AC, Soong SJ, et al. Final version of the American Joint Committee on Cancer staging system for cutaneous melanoma. *J Clin Oncol.* Aug 15 2001;19(16):3635-3648.

[8] Karakousis CP, Choe KJ, Holyoke ED. Biologic behavior and treatment of intransit metastasis of melanoma. *Surg Gynecol Obstet.* Jan 1980;150(1):29-32.

[9] Ross MI, Balch CM. The current management of cutaneous melanoma. *Adv Surg.* 1991;24:139-200.

[10] Meier F, Will S, Ellwanger U, et al. Metastatic pathways and time courses in the orderly progression of cutaneous melanoma. *Br J Dermatol.* Jul 2002;147(1):62-70.

[11] Quaglino P, Mortera C, Osella-Abate S, et al. Electrochemotherapy with intravenous bleomycin in the local treatment of skin melanoma metastases. *Ann Surg Oncol.* Aug 2008;15(8):2215-2222.

[12] Gimbel MI, Delman KA, Zager JS. Therapy for unresectable recurrent and in-transit extremity melanoma. *Cancer Control.* Jul 2008;15(3):225-232.

[13] Balch CM, Soong SJ, Gershenwald JE, et al. Prognostic factors analysis of 17,600 melanoma patients: validation of the American Joint Committee on Cancer melanoma staging system. *J Clin Oncol.* Aug 15 2001;19(16):3622-3634.

[14] Weinstock MA. Epidemiology and prognosis of anorectal melanoma. *Gastroenterology.* Jan 1993;104(1):174-178.

[15] Garbe C, Buttner P, Bertz J, et al. Primary cutaneous melanoma. Prognostic classification of anatomic location. *Cancer.* May 15 1995;75(10):2492-2498.

[16] Garbe C, Buttner P, Bertz J, et al. Primary cutaneous melanoma. Identification of prognostic groups and estimation of individual prognosis for 5093 patients. *Cancer.* May 15 1995;75(10):2484-2491.

[17] Byrne CM, Thompson JF. Role of electrochemotherapy in the treatment of metastatic melanoma and other metastatic and primary skin tumors. *Expert Rev Anticancer Ther.* May 2006;6(5):671-678.

[18] Sadadcharam M, Soden DM, O'Sullivan G C. Electrochemotherapy: an emerging cancer treatment. *Int J Hyperthermia.* May 2008;24(3):263-273.

[19] Moller MG, Salwa S, Soden DM, O'Sullivan GC. Electrochemotherapy as an adjunct or alternative to other treatments for unresectable or in-transit melanoma. *Expert Rev Anticancer Ther.* Nov 2009;9(11):1611-1630.

[20] Testori A, Rutkowski P, Marsden J, et al. Surgery and radiotherapy in the treatment of cutaneous melanoma. *Ann Oncol.* Aug 2009;20 Suppl 6:vi22-29.

[21] Atkins MB, Hsu J, Lee S, et al. Phase III trial comparing concurrent biochemotherapy with cisplatin, vinblastine, dacarbazine, interleukin-2, and interferon alfa-2b with cisplatin, vinblastine, and dacarbazine alone in patients with metastatic malignant melanoma (E3695): a trial coordinated by the Eastern Cooperative Oncology Group. *J Clin Oncol.* Dec 10 2008;26(35):5748-5754.

[22] Barranco SC, Romsdahl MM, Humphrey RM. The radiation response of human malignant melanoma cells grown in vitro. *Cancer Res.* Jun 1971;31(6):830-833.

[23] Scala M, Gipponi M, Queirolo P, et al. Cryosurgery for advanced malignant melanoma of the facial skin. A case report. *In Vivo.* Jan-Feb 2006;20(1):153-156.

[24] Hill S, Thomas JM. Use of the carbon dioxide laser to manage cutaneous metastases from malignant melanoma. *Br J Surg.* Apr 1996;83(4):509-512.

[25] Kandamany N, Mahaffey P. Carbon dioxide laser ablation as first-line management of in-transit cutaneous malignant melanoma metastases. *Lasers Med Sci.* May 2009;24(3):411-414.

[26] Hayes AJ, Clark MA, Harries M, Thomas JM. Management of in-transit metastases from cutaneous malignant melanoma. *Br J Surg.* Jun 2004;91(6):673-682.

[27] Morton DL, Eilber FR, Holmes EC, et al. BCG immunotherapy of malignant melanoma: summary of a seven-year experience. *Ann Surg.* Oct 1974;180(4):635-643.

[28] Rasmussen H, Rasmussen C, Lempicki M, et al. TNFerade Biologic: preclinical toxicology of a novel adenovector with a radiation-inducible promoter, carrying the human tumor necrosis factor alpha gene. *Cancer Gene Ther.* Nov 2002;9(11):951-957.

[29] Atkins MB, Lotze MT, Dutcher JP, et al. High-dose recombinant interleukin 2 therapy for patients with metastatic melanoma: analysis of 270 patients treated between 1985 and 1993. *J Clin Oncol.* Jul 1999;17(7):2105-2116.
[30] Terando AM, Faries MB, Morton DL. Vaccine therapy for melanoma: current status and future directions. *Vaccine.* Sep 27 2007;25 Suppl 2:B4-16.
[31] Yun CO, Nolan KF, Beecham EJ, Reisfeld RA, Junghans RP. Targeting of T lymphocytes to melanoma cells through chimeric anti-GD3 immunoglobulin T-cell receptors. *Neoplasia.* Sep-Oct 2000;2(5):449-459.
[32] Lotem M, Machlenkin A, Hamburger T, et al. Autologous melanoma vaccine induces antitumor and self-reactive immune responses that affect patient survival and depend on MHC class II expression on vaccine cells. *Clin Cancer Res.* Aug 1 2009;15(15):4968-4977.
[33] Gilboa E. DC-based cancer vaccines. *J Clin Invest.* May 2007;117(5):1195-1203.
[34] Eggermont AM, Testori A, Marsden J, et al. Utility of adjuvant systemic therapy in melanoma. *Ann Oncol.* Aug 2009;20 Suppl 6:vi30-34.
[35] Sondak VK, Flaherty LE. Adjuvant therapy of melanoma: is pegylated interferon alfa-2b what we've been waiting for? *Lancet.* Jul 12 2008;372(9633):89-90.
[36] Schadendorf D, Algarra SM, Bastholt L, et al. Immunotherapy of distant metastatic disease. *Ann Oncol.* Aug 2009;20 Suppl 6:vi41-50.
[37] Creech O, Jr., Krementz ET, Ryan RF, Winblad JN. Chemotherapy of cancer: regional perfusion utilizing an extracorporeal circuit. *Ann Surg.* Oct 1958;148(4):616-632.
[38] Smalley KS, Nathanson KL, Flaherty KT. Genetic subgrouping of melanoma reveals new opportunities for targeted therapy. *Cancer Res.* Apr 15 2009;69(8):3241-3244.
[39] Mir LM, Glass LF, Sersa G, et al. Effective treatment of cutaneous and subcutaneous malignant tumours by electrochemotherapy. *Br J Cancer.* Jun 1998;77(12):2336-2342.
[40] Ross MI. Surgery and other local-regional modalities for all stages of melanoma. *Curr Opin Oncol.* Mar 1994;6(2):197-203.
[41] Moller MG, Lewis JM, Dessureault S, Zager JS. Toxicities associated with hyperthermic isolated limb perfusion and isolated limb infusion in the treatment of melanoma and sarcoma. *Int J Hyperthermia.* May 2008;24(3):275-289.
[42] Eggermont AM, Gore M. Randomized adjuvant therapy trials in melanoma: surgical and systemic. *Semin Oncol.* Dec 2007;34(6):509-515.
[43] Sersa G, Miklavcic D, Cemazar M, Rudolf Z, Pucihar G, Snoj M. Electrochemotherapy in treatment of tumours. *Eur J Surg Oncol.* Feb 2008;34(2):232-240.
[44] Glass LF, Jaroszeski M, Gilbert R, Reintgen DS, Heller R. Intralesional bleomycin-mediated electrochemotherapy in 20 patients with basal cell carcinoma. *J Am Acad Dermatol.* Oct 1997;37(4):596-599.
[45] Sersa G. The state-of-the-art of electrochemotherapy before the ESOPE study; advantages and clinical uses. *Eur J Cancer. Supplement.* 2006(4):8.
[46] Mir LM. Bases and rationale of electrochemotherapy. *European Journal of Cancer. Supplement.* 2006;4:38-44.
[47] Mir LM, Belehradek M, Domenge C, et al. [Electrochemotherapy, a new antitumor treatment: first clinical trial]. *C R Acad Sci III.* 1991;313(13):613-618.
[48] Orlowski S, Belehradek J, Jr., Paoletti C, Mir LM. Transient electropermeabilization of cells in culture. Increase of the cytotoxicity of anticancer drugs. *Biochem Pharmacol.* Dec 15 1988;37(24):4727-4733.

[49] Larkin JO, Collins CG, Aarons S, et al. Electrochemotherapy: aspects of preclinical development and early clinical experience. *Ann Surg.* Mar 2007;245(3):469-479.

[50] Weaver JC. Electroporation theory. Concepts and mechanisms. *Methods Mol Biol.* 1995;55:3-28.

[51] Belehradek J, Jr., Orlowski S, Poddevin B, Paoletti C, Mir LM. Electrochemotherapy of spontaneous mammary tumours in mice. *Eur J Cancer.* 1991;27(1):73-76.

[52] Marty M SG, Garbay JM, Gehl J, .Collins CG, Snoj M, Billard V, Geertsen PF, Larkin JO, Miklavcic D, Paulovic I, Pavlin-Kosir SM, Cemazar M, Morsli N, Soden DM, Rudolf Z, Robert C , O'Sullivan GC, Mir LM. Electrochemotherapy -An easy, highly effective and safe treatment of cutaneous and subcutaneous metastases : Results of ESOPE (european standard operating procedures of electrochemotherapy) study. *European Journal of Cancer. Supplement.* 2006;4(11):3-13.

[53] Sersa G, Cemazar M, Miklavcic D. Antitumor effectiveness of electrochemotherapy with cis-diamminedichloroplatinum(II) in mice. *Cancer Res.* Aug 1 1995;55(15):3450-3455.

[54] Gehl J. Electroporation for drug and gene delivery in the clinic: doctors go electric. *Methods Mol Biol.* 2008;423:351-359.

[55] Gehl J. Electroporation: theory and methods, perspectives for drug delivery, gene therapy and research. *Acta Physiol Scand.* Apr 2003;177(4):437-447.

[56] Gehl J, Geertsen PF. Efficient palliation of haemorrhaging malignant melanoma skin metastases by electrochemotherapy. *Melanoma Res.* Dec 2000;10(6):585-589.

[57] Snoj M, Cemazar M, Srnovrsnik T, Kosir SP, Sersa G. Limb sparing treatment of bleeding melanoma recurrence by electrochemotherapy. *Tumori.* May-Jun 2009;95(3):398-402.

[58] Hofmann GA, Dev SB, Nanda GS, Rabussay D. Electroporation therapy of solid tumors. *Crit Rev Ther Drug Carrier Syst.* 1999;16(6):523-569.

[59] Mir L, Gehl J, Sersa G, Collins CG, Garbay J, Billard V, Geertsen PF, Rudolf Z, OSullivan GC, Marty M. Standard operating procedures of hte electrochemotherapy: Instructions for the use of bleomycin and cisplastin administered either systemically or locally and electric pulses delivered by Cliniporator™ by means of ivansive or non-invasive electrodes. *European Journal of Cancer. Supplement.* 2006;4:14-25.

[60] Testori A, Tosti G, Martinoli C, et al. Electrochemotherapy for cutaneous and subcutaneous tumor lesions: a novel therapeutic approach. *Dermatol Ther.* Nov 2010;23(6):651-661.

[61] Sersa G CM, Rudolf Z. . Electrochemotherapy: advantages and drawbacks in treatment of cancer patients. *Cancer Therapy.* 2003;1:133-142.

[62] Domenge C, Orlowski S, Luboinski B, et al. Antitumor electrochemotherapy: new advances in the clinical protocol. *Cancer.* Mar 1 1996;77(5):956-963.

[63] Heller R, Jaroszeski M, Perrott R, Messina J, Gilbert R. Effective treatment of B16 melanoma by direct delivery of bleomycin using electrochemotherapy. *Melanoma Res.* Feb 1997;7(1):10-18.

[64] Cemazar M, Milacic R, Miklavcic D, Dolzan V, Sersa G. Intratumoral cisplatin administration in electrochemotherapy: antitumor effectiveness, sequence dependence and platinum content. *Anticancer Drugs.* Jul 1998;9(6):525-530.

[65] Mir LM, Banoun H, Paoletti C. Introduction of definite amounts of nonpermeant molecules into living cells after electropermeabilization: direct access to the cytosol. *Exp Cell Res.* Mar 1988;175(1):15-25.

[66] Gaudy C, Richard MA, Folchetti G, Bonerandi JJ, Grob JJ. Randomized controlled study of electrochemotherapy in the local treatment of skin metastases of melanoma. *J Cutan Med Surg.* May-Jun 2006;10(3):115-121.

[67] Neumann E, Schaefer-Ridder M, Wang Y, Hofschneider PH. Gene transfer into mouse lyoma cells by electroporation in high electric fields. *EMBO J.* 1982;1(7):841-845.

[68] Melvik JE, Pettersen EO, Gordon PB, Seglen PO. Increase in cis-dichlorodiammineplatinum (II) cytotoxicity upon reversible electropermeabilization of the plasma membrane in cultured human NHIK 3025 cells. *Eur J Cancer Clin Oncol.* Dec 1986;22(12):1523-1530.

[69] Okino M, Mohri H. Effects of a high-voltage electrical impulse and an anticancer drug on in vivo growing tumors. *Jpn J Cancer Res.* Dec 1987;78(12):1319-1321.

[70] Belehradek M, Domenge C, Luboinski B, Orlowski S, Belehradek J, Jr., Mir LM. Electrochemotherapy, a new antitumor treatment. First clinical phase I-II trial. *Cancer.* Dec 15 1993;72(12):3694-3700.

[71] Rudolf Z, Stabuc B, Cemazar M, Miklavcic F, Vodovnik L, Sersa G. Electrochemotherapy with bleomycin: the first clinical experiencie in malignant melanoma patients. *Radiol Oncol.* 1995(29):6.

[72] Rols MP, Bachaud JM, Giraud P, Chevreau C, Roche H, Teissie J. Electrochemotherapy of cutaneous metastases in malignant melanoma. *Melanoma Res.* Oct 2000;10(5):468-474.

[73] Heller R, Jaroszeski MJ, Glass LF, et al. Phase I/II trial for the treatment of cutaneous and subcutaneous tumors using electrochemotherapy. *Cancer.* Mar 1 1996;77(5):964-971.

[74] Sersa G, Cufer T, Cemazar M, Rebersek M, Zvonimir R. Electrochemotherapy with bleomycin in the treatment of hypernephroma metastasis: case report and literature review. *Tumori.* Mar-Apr 2000;86(2):163-165.

[75] Glass LF, Pepine ML, Fenske NA, Jaroszeski M, Reintgen DS, Heller R. Bleomycin-mediated electrochemotherapy of metastatic melanoma. *Arch Dermatol.* Nov 1996;132(11):1353-1357.

[76] Heller R, Jaroszeski MJ, Reintgen DS, et al. Treatment of cutaneous and subcutaneous tumors with electrochemotherapy using intralesional bleomycin. *Cancer.* Jul 1 1998;83(1):148-157.

[77] Rodriguez-Cuevas S, Barroso-Bravo S, Almanza-Estrada J, Cristobal-Martinez L, Gonzalez-Rodriguez E. Electrochemotherapy in primary and metastatic skin tumors: phase II trial using intralesional bleomycin. *Arch Med Res.* Jul-Aug 2001;32(4):273-276.

[78] Byrne CM, Thompson JF, Johnston H, et al. Treatment of metastatic melanoma using electroporation therapy with bleomycin (electrochemotherapy). *Melanoma Res.* Feb 2005;15(1):45-51.

[79] Kubota Y, Mir LM, Nakada T, Sasagawa I, Suzuki H, Aoyama N. Successful treatment of metastatic skin lesions with electrochemotherapy. *J Urol.* Oct 1998;160(4):1426.

[80] Giraud P, Bachaud JM, Teissie J, Rols MP. Effects of electrochemotherapy on cutaneous metastases of human malignant melanoma. *Int J Radiat Oncol Biol Phys.* Dec 1 1996;36(5):1285.

[81] Sersa G, Stabuc B, Cemazar M, Jancar B, Miklavcic D, Rudolf Z. Electrochemotherapy with cisplatin: potentiation of local cisplatin antitumour effectiveness by

application of electric pulses in cancer patients. *Eur J Cancer.* Jul 1998;34(8):1213-1218.
[82] Sersa G, Stabuc B, Cemazar M, Miklavcic D, Rudolf Z. Electrochemotherapy with cisplatin: clinical experience in malignant melanoma patients. *Clin Cancer Res.* Mar 2000;6(3):863-867.
[83] Snoj M, Rudolf Z, Cemazar M, Jancar B, Sersa G. Successful sphincter-saving treatment of anorectal malignant melanoma with electrochemotherapy, local excision and adjuvant brachytherapy. *Anticancer Drugs.* Mar 2005;16(3):345-348.
[84] Heller R. Treatment of cutaneous nodules using electrochemotherapy. *J Fla Med Assoc.* Feb 1995;82(2):147-150.
[85] Kubota Y, Tomita Y, Tsukigi M, Kurachi H, Motoyama T, Mir LM. A case of perineal malignant melanoma successfully treated with electrochemotherapy. *Melanoma Res.* Apr 2005;15(2):133-134.
[86] Sersa G, Stabuc B, Cemazar M, Miklavcic D, Rudolf Z. Electrochemotherapy with cisplatin: the systemic antitumour effectiveness of cisplatin can be potentiated locally by the application of electric pulses in the treatment of malignant melanoma skin metastases. *Melanoma Res.* Aug 2000;10(4):381-385.
[87] Soden DM, Larkin JO, Collins CG, et al. Successful application of targeted electrochemotherapy using novel flexible electrodes and low dose bleomycin to solid tumours. *Cancer Lett.* Feb 8 2006;232(2):300-310.
[88] Rabussay DP, Nanda GS, Goldfarb PM. Enhancing the effectiveness of drug-based cancer therapy by electroporation (electropermeabilization). *Technol Cancer Res Treat.* Feb 2002;1(1):71-82.
[89] Tauceri F, Mura G, Roseano M, Framarini M, Ridolfi L, Verdecchia GM. Surgery and adjuvant therapies in the treatment of stage IV melanoma: our experience in 84 patients. *Langenbecks Arch Surg.* Mar 4 2008.
[90] Campana LG, Mocellin S, Basso M, et al. Bleomycin-based electrochemotherapy: clinical outcome from a single institution's experience with 52 patients. *Ann Surg Oncol.* Jan 2009;16(1):191-199.
[91] Landstrom FJ, Nilsson CO, Crafoord S, Reizenstein JA, Adamsson GB, Lofgren LA. Electroporation therapy of skin cancer in the head and neck area. *Dermatol Surg.* Aug 2010;36(8):1245-1250.
[92] Landstrom FJ, Nilsson CO, Reizenstein JA, Nordqvist K, Adamsson GB, Lofgren AL. Electroporation therapy for T1 and T2 oral tongue cancer. *Acta Otolaryngol.* Dec 29 2010.
[93] Sersa G, Cemazar M, Snoj M. Electrochemotherapy of tumours. *Curr Oncol.* Mar 2009;16(2):34-35.
[94] Heller R, Gilbert R, Jaroszeski MJ. Clinical applications of electrochemotherapy. *Adv Drug Deliv Rev.* Jan 4 1999;35(1):119-129.
[95] Snoj M, Cemazar M, Slekovec Kolar B, Sersa G. Effective treatment of multiple unresectable skin melanoma metastases by electrochemotherapy. *Croat Med J.* Jun 2007;48(3):391-395.
[96] Snoj MR, Z. Paulin-Kosir, S. Cemanzar, M, Snoj, R. Sersa, G. . Long lasting complete response in melanoma treated by electrochemotherapy. *Eur J Cancer Suppl.* 2006;4(11):2.

[97] Giardino R, Fini M, Bonazzi V, Cadossi R, Nicolini A, Carpi A. Electrochemotherapy a novel approach to the treatment of metastatic nodules on the skin and subcutaneous tissues. *Biomed Pharmacother.* Sep 2006;60(8):458-462.
[98] Kaehler KC, Egberts F, Hauschild A. Electrochemotherapy in symptomatic melanoma skin metastases: intraindividual comparison with conventional surgery. *Dermatol Surg.* Jul 2010;36(7):1200-1202.
[99] Heller LC, Heller R. Electroporation gene therapy preclinical and clinical trials for melanoma. *Curr Gene Ther.* Aug 2010;10(4):312-317.
[100] Andersen MH, Gehl J, Reker S, et al. Dynamic changes of specific T cell responses to melanoma correlate with IL-2 administration. *Semin Cancer Biol.* Dec 2003;13(6):449-459.
[101] Daud AI, DeConti RC, Andrews S, et al. Phase I trial of interleukin-12 plasmid electroporation in patients with metastatic melanoma. *J Clin Oncol.* Dec 20 2008;26(36):5896-5903.
[102] Miklavcic D, Snoj M, Zupanic A, et al. Towards treatment planning and treatment of deep-seated solid tumors by electrochemotherapy. *Biomed Eng Online.* 2010;9:10.
[103] Kos B, Zupanic A, Kotnik T, Snoj M, Sersa G, Miklavcic D. Robustness of treatment planning for electrochemotherapy of deep-seated tumors. *J Membr Biol.* Jul 2010;236(1):147-153.
[104] Orlowski S, An D, Belehradek J, Jr., Mir LM. Antimetastatic effects of electrochemotherapy and of histoincompatible interleukin-2-secreting cells in the murine Lewis lung tumor. *Anticancer Drugs.* Jul 1998;9(6):551-556.
[105] Ramirez LH, Orlowski S, An D, et al. Electrochemotherapy on liver tumours in rabbits. *Br J Cancer.* Jun 1998;77(12):2104-2111.
[106] Soden D, Larkin J, Collins C, et al. The development of novel flexible electrode arrays for the electrochemotherapy of solid tumour tissue. (Potential for endoscopic treatment of inaccessible cancers). *Conf Proc IEEE Eng Med Biol Soc.* 2004;5:3547-3550.
[107] Edd JF, Horowitz L, Davalos RV, Mir LM, Rubinsky B. In vivo results of a new focal tissue ablation technique: irreversible electroporation. *IEEE Trans Biomed Eng.* Jul 2006;53(7):1409-1415.
[108] Nuccitelli R, Pliquett U, Chen X, et al. Nanosecond pulsed electric fields cause melanomas to self-destruct. *Biochem Biophys Res Commun.* May 5 2006;343(2):351-360.
[109] Frey W, White JA, Price RO, et al. Plasma membrane voltage changes during nanosecond pulsed electric field exposure. *Biophys J.* May 15 2006;90(10):3608-3615.
[110] Mir LM, Orlowski S, Belehradek J, Jr., Paoletti C. Electrochemotherapy potentiation of antitumour effect of bleomycin by local electric pulses. *Eur J Cancer.* 1991;27(1):68-72.
[111] Mir LM, Orlowski S, Poddevin B, Belehradek J, Jr. Electrochemotherapy tumor treatment is improved by interleukin-2 stimulation of the host's defenses. *Eur Cytokine Netw.* May-Jun 1992;3(3):331-334.
[112] Mir LM, Roth C, Orlowski S, et al. [Potentiation of the antitumoral effect of electrochemotherapy by immunotherapy with allogeneic cells producing interleukin 2]. *C R Acad Sci III.* 1992;314(12):539-544.
[113] Heller L, Pottinger C, Jaroszeski MJ, Gilbert R, Heller R. In vivo electroporation of plasmids encoding GM-CSF or interleukin-2 into existing B16 melanomas

combined with electrochemotherapy induces long-term antitumour immunity. *Melanoma Res.* Dec 2000;10(6):577-583.

[114] Roux S, Bernat C, Al-Sakere B, et al. Tumor destruction using electrochemotherapy followed by CpG oligodeoxynucleotide injection induces distant tumor responses. *Cancer Immunol Immunother.* Sep 2008;57(9):1291-1300.

[115] Heller LC, Heller R. In vivo electroporation for gene therapy. *Hum Gene Ther.* Sep 2006;17(9):890-897.

[116] Cemazar M, Golzio M, Sersa G, Rols MP, Teissie J. Electrically-assisted nucleic acids delivery to tissues in vivo: where do we stand? *Curr Pharm DRes*2006;12(29):3817-3825.

[117] Cashman JP,. Larkin JO,. Casey G,. et als. Immune gene therapy as a neoadjuvant to surgical excision to control metastatic cancers. *Cancer Lett.* Jan 5 2008.

[118] Collins CG, Tangney M, Larkin JO, et al. Local gene therapy of solid tumors with GM-CSF and B7-1 eradicates both treated and distal tumors. *Cancer Gene Ther.* Dec 2006;13(12):1061-1071.

[119] Tangney M, Casey G,. Larkin JO,. et al. Non-viral in vivo immune gene therapy of cancer: combined strategies for treatment of systemic disease. *Cancer Immunol Immunother.* Nov 2006;55(11):1443-1450.

[120] Sersa G, Cemazar M, Menart V, Gaberc-Porekar V, Miklavcic D. Anti-tumor effectiveness of electrochemotherapy with bleomycin is increased by TNF-alpha on SA-1 tumors in mice. *Cancer Lett.* Jun 3 1997;116(1):85-92.

[121] Peycheva E, Daskalov I, Tsoneva I. Electrochemotherapy of Mycosis fungoides by interferon-alpha. *Bioelectrochemistry.* May 2007;70(2):283-286.

[122] Kranjc S, Cemazar M, Grosel A, Sentjurc M, Sersa G. Radiosensitising effect of electrochemotherapy with bleomycin in LPB sarcoma cells and tumors in mice. *BMC Cancer.* 2005;5:115.

Websites:

[201] American Cancer Society: Cancer Facts and Figures 2009. Atlanta, Ga: American Cancer Society,. 2009. See a dermatologist. Skin cancer is very treatable when caught early. Also available online. 2009 [cited 2009 May 25, 2009]; Available from: http://www.cancer.org/docroot/PRO/content/PRO_1_1_Cancer_Statistics_2009_Presentation.asp

[202] American Cancer Society: Detailed Guide: Skin Cancer - Melanoma. What Are the Key Statistics About Melanoma? 2009 May 14, 2009 [cited 2009 May 25]; Available from: http://www.cancer.org/docroot/CRI/content/CRI_2_4_1X_What_are_the_key_statistics_for_melanoma_50.asp?sitearea=

[203] National Cancer Institute. Melanoma Treatment (PDQ)R. Staging Information. 2009 [cited August 4,. 2009.]; Available from: http://www.cancer.gov/cancertopics/pdq/treatment/melanoma/HealthProfessional/page4

[204] National Comprehensive Cancer Network. Melanoma 2009 [cited 2009 August 4,. 2009.]; Available from: http://www.nccn.org/professionals/physician_gls/PDF/melanoma.pdf

Part 5

Photodynamic Therapy

12

Can Photodynamic Therapy Be an Alternative Method in Melanoma Treatment?

Anna Choromańska, Julita Kulbacka, Agnieszka Chwiłkowska, Nina Skołucka, Andrzej Gamian and Jolanta Saczko
Wroclaw Medical University, Department of Medical Biochemistry, Wroclaw, Poland

1. Introduction

Photodynamic therapy (PDT) is an effective cancer treatment that is an alternative to local therapy including surgical treatment and radiotherapy or systemic treatment such as chemotherapy or some kinds of immunotherapy. In many patients with cancer these therapeutic methods are not efficient or put their life at serious risk.
The principle of PDT is based on a photochemical process involving the absorption of light by a photosensitizer and the subsequent generation of reactive oxygen species (ROS) that induces cytotoxicity.
In the body, photosensitizers accumulate particularly in cancer cells. The precise reason for this preferential uptake or retention by malignant tissue is still unclear, but properties that appear to be involved include activated cellular uptake by neoplastic cells, differences in proliferation rates between neoplastic and normal cells, leaky vasculature within neoplastic tissue, and variations in mitochondrial potential. Moreover, PDT is a selective treatment because light delivery can be restricted to specific regions, thereby limiting activation of the drug to cured areas. These conditions mean that PDT is a safe treatment in comparison with other local treatments such as ionizing radiation and thermal destruction of tissue.
Oxygen-dependent photodynamic reactions were first described by Oscar Raab (Allison, 2010). He noted that an acridine solution killed paramecia upon irradiation with light. There was no such effect observed in the absence of light. On the basis of this knowledge about photodynamic effects, H. Tappeiner and H. Jesionek performed the first PDT sessions on a patient with skin carcinoma, with eosin as a photosensitizer (Allison, 2010). Since that time PDT has made considerable progress; new photosensitizers have been discovered and the procedure of therapy has been established.

1.1 Mechanism of action

The procedure of PDT requires two steps: administration of a photosensitizer, and its activation by light in the presence of oxygen in the tissue. Photosensitizers used in PDT should be nontoxic in their native state, but after excitation they become cytotoxic and produce local tissue destruction through intercellular generation of ROS. The light induces excitation of the photosensitizer molecules to the singlet excited state, which can be converted into the triplet excited state. The triplet state may react with surrounding molecules in two types of photo-oxidative reaction. Type I involves electron or hydrogen atom transfer, producing radical forms of the substrate which may react with oxygen to form peroxides, superoxide ions, and hydroxyl radicals. Type II leads to the generation of singlet molecular oxygen ($^1O_2$). Both mechanisms may occur simultaneously (Lukšienė, 2003). It is known that $^1O_2$ can diffuse only 20 nm during its lifetime (Peng, 1996); hence the primary damage is closely related to the site of its formation. Therefore, cellular structures having both a high sensitizer and a high oxygen concentration will be preferentially damaged upon illumination.

In PDT also occurs a third type of reaction. In contrast to the other two it is independent on the dissolved oxygen in the tissue. In contrast to the other two it is independent of the dissolved oxygen in the tissue. The photosensitizer in the singlet excited state can react directly with biomolecules, inducing a process of photoadduct formation (Capella et al., 2003). However, this mechanism is often ignored because the electron transfer between a biomolecule and photosensitizer, and formation of free radicals, is not effective (Ochneser 1997).

1.2 Photosensitizers in PDT

The main features of an efficient photosensitizer are: low toxicity at therapeutic doses in darkness, highly tumor-targeting accumulation, homogeneous composition and stability, and absorption peaks in the low-loss transmission window of biological tissues (the far-red and near-infrared regions). An effective photosensitizer is characterized by a high quantum yield of singlet oxygen generation and/or electron transfer to substrate molecules (Granville, 2001, Lukšienė, 2003). Good photosensitizer qualities are high solubility in water, availability, uncomplicated manufacture and synthesis.

Most photosensitizers applied in PDT are based on porphyrins. The most common photosensitizers are haematoporphyrin derivatives (HPD). Its theirs purified version named Photofrin, has an absorption peak in the red wavelength region at about 630 nm. The first compound in the porphyrin synthesis pathway (5-aminolevulinic acid, 5-ALA) is also used in PDT. 5-ALA is converted in vivo into the photosensitizing compound protoporphyrin IX. The second generation of photosensitizers includes compounds from other chemical groups. Most of them are cyclic tetrapyrroles consisting of substituted derivatives of porphyrin, chlorin and bacteriochlorin. Many research centers are developing new and quite different molecular structures that can act as the ideal photosensitizer (Granville, 2001).

1.2.1 Light

The photodynamic reaction is dependent on the delivery of light of an appropriate wavelength to activate a photosensitizer. The light used for photosensitization is typically in the visible or near-infrared light range. In general, with increasing wavelength in the visible and near-infrared range the depth of penetration of light increases and the absorption by hemoglobin and other endogenous chromophores decreases (Smith, 2002).

Application in PDT of higher wavelengths of light enables treatment of heavily pigmented tissues (Woodburn, 1998). Good light sources in PDT are metal halogen lamps, which emit from 600 to 800 nm radiation at high power density, and short-arc xenon lamps, tunable over a bandwidth between 400 and 1200 nm (Lukšienė, 2003).

The popularization of laser technology with optical fibers facilitates photosensitization in clinical treatment. Lasers enable the precise endoscopic application of light to almost every site of the human body and allow the exact selection of wavelengths. Pulsed lasers, such as the gold vapor laser (GVL) and the copper vapor laser-pumped dye laser, produce brief light pulses of millisecond to nanosecond duration (Fisher 1995). Tunable solid-state lasers, such as the neodymium: YAG laser, are particularly useful for PDT. Portable semiconductor diode lasers, such as the gallium-aluminum-arsenide laser, produce light in the range from 770 to 850 nm, which corresponds to the absorption peaks of many new photosensitizers (Lukšienė, 2003).

2. Cell damage after PDT

The antitumor activity of PDT is based on four mechanisms: direct cytotoxicity, which is an intermediate reaction of singlet oxygen production with subsequent oxidation of the substrate, occlusion of blood vessels and lymphatics, and the impact on the immune response and inflammation of the body (Krawczyk-Krupka et al., 2001, Sieron &Adamek, 1999, Mazur et al., 2010). Generated reactive oxygen species (ROS) cause oxidative stress in the cells (Dellinger, 1996). The oxidative stress damage is targeted mainly at cellular macromolecules, such as lipids, nucleic acids and proteins. Hydrophobic photosensitizers accumulate mainly in cell membranes and they are primarily attacked by free radicals.

2.1 Oxidative stress

Oxidative stress is an imbalance between the formation of reactive oxygen species (ROS) and antioxidant mechanisms. Free radicals in living organisms may result from the action of endogenous factors (e.g. respiratory chain, activated leukocytes, inflammation, enzymes) or exogenous (e.g. cigarette smoke, alcohol, intense physical activity, UV radiation, ionizing radiation, car exhaust, contaminated air, physical and psychological stress). In physiological conditions the release of free radicals is controlled by the body's defense mechanisms (Sheu et al., 2006). Free radicals play a crucial role in cell functions including proliferation, apoptosis, inactivation of the growth of bacteria and viruses, intracellular signaling and intercellular communication. ROS have effects that augment or shrink the blood vessel walls, and stimulate glucose transport into cells. Disorder of the defense mechanisms under the influence of external factors or disease causes an increase in free radicals in the body, and consequently the occurrence of pathological reactions leading to damage to cells and tissues (Gałecka et al., 2008, Łagowska-Lenart et al., 2008). In vitro studies show that the destructive action of free radicals may include all biomolecules in the body, causing chemical modifications and damage to proteins (denaturation), lipids (peroxidation), carbohydrates and nucleotides, resulting in changes in the structure of DNA leading to mutations (Sheu et al., 2006, Bailey et al., 2005). The concentration of oxidation products (e.g. carbonyl groups) reflects the intensity of the reaction involving reactive oxygen species. An antioxidant barrier protects the organism from the damaging effects of reactive oxygen species.

2.2 Lipid peroxidation

Lipid peroxidation (LPO) is a free radical process of oxidation of polyunsaturated fatty acids or other lipids. Lipid peroxidation proceeds in three major steps: initiation, propagation, and termination. During the first stage a fatty acid radical is produced. The hydroxyl radical is identified as initiating lipid peroxidation by abstracting hydrogen atoms from fatty-acid side chains. Cell membranes contain unsaturated fatty acids that are readily attacked by

reactive oxygen species. LPO can be initiated by hydroxyl radical (•OH), superoxide radical (LOO•), alkoxy radical (LO•), alkyl radical (L•), as well as ozone (O_3), nitrogen monoxide and dioxide, sulfur dioxides, and hypochlorite (Shevchuk et al., 2002, Bartosz, 2003).
During the propagation phase, free alkyl radicals (L•) react with molecular oxygen to form peroxyl free radicals (LOO•). They may also detach hydrogen atoms from subsequent molecules of polyunsaturated fatty acids (LH). This cycle continues, as the new fatty acid radical reacts exactly in the same way until the termination reaction. The stage of termination occurs when a radical reacts with a non-radical. It is a "chain reaction mechanism" because a new radical is always produced. The radical reaction stops when there is such a high concentration of radical species that it can cause the impact of two radicals, forming a non-radical.
The final products of lipid peroxidation are hydroxy aldehydes (e.g. 4-hydroxynonenal), hydrocarbons (e.g. ethane and pentane) and aldehydes (e.g. malonic dialdehyde - MDA) - an endogenous genotoxic compound (Bartosz, 2003, Kessel et al., 1997, Hsieh et al., 2003). Increased production of reactive oxygen species induces an increase of lipid peroxidation products. These LPO products are able to modify the physical properties of cell membranes, leading to a loss of integrity of intracellular membranes by depolarization, increased permeability to H- ions, disruption and inhibition of the activity of the asymmetry of membrane enzymes and transport proteins (Hsieh et al., 2003).

2.3 Protein degradation under the influence of oxidative stress

Oxidative changes are an inherent effect of cellular metabolism and can not be eliminated. Accumulation of oxidized protein products impairs cell functions and can even induce cell death (Plaetzer 2003). ROS can induce oxidation of protein thiol groups (-SH) and form thiol radicals ($S^{\cdot}$). The most degenerating for the cell during oxidative stress is oxidation of thiols in the membrane. It can lead to membrane disintegration and increased permeability. Oxidative damage of –SH groups causes rapid loss of biological activity of protein. These radicals in turn oxidize to disulfides, forming intermolecular disulfide bridges. These reactions cause irreversible changes in membrane structures, which are dangerous to the life of the cell (Wang 2001).

2.4 Changes in DNA

DNA encodes genetic information, so any changes that occur in the genome are extremely dangerous for the cell. The number of daily incidents of DNA damage exceeds 10 000; therefore there are corrective mechanisms for sensing and correcting the damage. The mechanisms of DNA damage induced by photodynamic therapy are not well known. PDT can cause cross-linking of DNA strands (McNair et al., 1997, Haylett et al., 2003, Woods et al., 2004). DNA damage caused by photodynamic therapy may occur in cancer cells and normal cells surrounding the tumor. PDT generates through the photosensitizer reactive oxygen species. Singlet oxygen has a very limited range (< 0.1 µm) and life-span (less than 1 s). The probability of DNA damage is low, unless it is generated in the close proximity of a DNA strand. Current studies suggest that cell death after PDT is caused by damage to cytoplasmic proteins and mitochondria, and not damage to DNA (Miller et al., 2007). Normal cells are able to cope with the damage after PDT but this is dependent on the type of photosensitizer (Woods et al., 2004).

2.5 Antioxidative system

To protect against free radical damage the body uses a number of mechanisms to provide antioxidant protection of the body. Structural cell organization is one of these mechanisms. This specific formation enables isolation of those places where free radical reactions take place (Halliwell, 2000, Huang, 2000). In addition various metabolic mechanisms play an important role in protection against free radicals. The knowledge of oxidative damage caused by PDT is important in developing strategies for treating tumours and the potential reduction of side effects. They have been divided into the following categories (Santiard, 1995):

- Reactions with suppressive compounds (carotenoids, vitamin E);
- Non-enzymatic mechanisms: antioxidants, free radical scavengers, ions of transition metals, sequestration of metals, metallothioneins;
- Enzymatic mechanisms: superoxide dismutase, catalases, heme oxygenase, glutathione peroxidase, glutathione reductase, glutathione S-transferase and groups of secretory phospholipases A_2;
- Reactions with heat shock proteins - proteases and chaperone proteins.

2.5.1 MnSOD

MnSOD is a mitochondrial form with Mn in the active center. Human MnSOD is a tetrameric enzyme with four identical subunits each harboring a Mn^{+3} atom (McCord, 2002). It was demonstrated that transient transfection with the MnSOD gene resulted in decreased effectiveness of PDT. These results suggest that MnSOD plays a leading role in the response to PDT and that abnormal mitochondria may be a decisive factor in phototoxicity (Saczko et al., 2007). MnSOD is a critical antioxidant enzyme residing in mitochondria. Golab et al. observed that following PDT there was induction of MnSOD expression in tumor cells (Golab et al., 2003). The group of SODs is emerging as significant antioxidative enzymes that can regulate the sensitivity of cancer cells to different treatment modalities. Some authors have also observed that overexpression of MnSOD suppresses apoptosis (Kuroda et al., 2000).

2.5.2 Heme oxygenase-1 (HO-1)

Heme oxygenase exists in two isoforms: inducible (HO-1) and constitutively expressed (HO-2). Heme oxygenase-1 (HO-1) is an enzyme that catalyzes the degradation of heme to Fe^{2+} ion, carbon monoxide and biliverdin, and then biliverdin is converted to bilirubin by biliverdin reductase (Dulak & Jozkowicz, 2003). Biliverdin and bilirubin are antioxidants, and may therefore play a very important role in cytoprotection of cells exposed to the oxidative stress induced by PDT. Induction of HO-1 by PDT was described in the CHO (Chinese hamster ovary) cell line using Photofrin (Gomer, 1991). The photodynamic reaction induces HO-1 expression. HO-1 also plays a protective role in cells where PDT was applied. The removal of iron ions with desferrioxamine from cells after PDT resulted in increased cell death, which confirms the key role of ferrous ion generation in HO-1 mediated cytoprotection (Nowis et al., 2006).

2.5.3 Heat shock proteins

The heat shock proteins (HSPs) are a class of proteins whose expression is increased when cells are exposed to different kinds of stress such as heat shock, pH shift, hypoxia, osmotic and oxidative stress. Production of HSPs may also grow in response to infection, inflammation, effects of toxins, UV radiation, starvation, etc. HSPs work as chaperone proteins responsible for the proper folding of other proteins, translocation and degradation. They also participate in protein assembly, export, turnover and regulation. HSPs are found in virtually all living organisms. In normal conditions cellular levels of HSPs are stable and low, but if cells are exposed to any kind of stress, the levels of HSP quickly increase (Pockley, 2003). HSPs are generally classified according to their molecular weight, which can vary from 10 to 170 kDa, e.g. HSP70 (Hightower & Hendershot, 1997). PDT induces different HSPs including HSP27, HSP60, HSP70, HSP90, GRP78 and GRP94. A protective role in PDT-treated cells has been shown, for example survival of tumor cells exposed to PDT induced overexpression of HSP27 (Wang et al., 2002). When there are damaged proteins, HSP binds damaged molecules. This results in dissociation of HSF (heat shock factor), then migrates to the nucleus, where it binds with HSE (heat shock elements) leading to HSP overexpression (Morimoto, 1993). HSP90 inhibits formation of an active apoptosome whereas HSP70 prevents the recruitment of procaspase-9 to the apoptosome complex (Almeida et al., 2004).

2.5.4 GSTπ

Glutathione S-transferases (GSTs) are crucial in protection of cells against oxidation products. There are enzymes of the second phase of metabolism that counteract the process of carcinogenesis (L'Ecuyer 2004). This group of enzymes plays a key role in detoxification and reduction of reactive oxygen forms, especially the isoform GST-pi. This enzyme protects cells against DNA disintegration and drug toxicity. Genetic polymorphisms in glutathione S-transferase and its altered expression and activity are associated with oxidative DNA damage which in turn leads to increased susceptibility to cancer (L'Ecuyer al., 2004). A high level of GST-pi expression is related to the development of drug resistance in cancer cells not only by increased detoxification of anticancer agents, but also by suppression of cellular ROS which induce cell death. This means that a high level of GST-pi may be a prognostic factor in malignant diseases (Aliya et al., 2003).

2.5.5 Small molecule antioxidants

Molecular reactions of antioxidants with ROS are less specific than the effect of antioxidant enzymes, which means that these compounds are more versatile defenders. The body's antioxidant status is also dependent on the level of exogenous antioxidants, mainly supplied with food. An important role is played by vitamin E. Because of its lipophilic properties it may have a protective effect in relation to membrane phospholipids, protecting them from peroxidation. One free radical could trigger the whole cascade of reactions leading to oxidation of unsaturated fatty acids. This cascade proceeds until another formed fatty acid radical meets on their way vitamin E, which breaks the chain reaction. Reduced vitamin E can be regenerated by vitamin C that has the ability to stabilize the hydroxyl radical (Chow et al., 1999, Rahman, 2007, Sies et al., 1992). Vitamin C reacts with the hydroxyl radical and singlet oxygen. Vitamin C with glutathione coenzyme Q, cysteine, uric acid and bilirubin are among the active antioxidants in the aqueous phase. Vitamin C inhibits the peroxidation of hemoglobin and with coenzyme Q and reduced glutathione protects mitochondria from oxidative damage (Kurl et al., 2002). The effect of vitamin E supplements β-carotene and its metabolite, vitamin A. The precursors of vitamin A include carotenoids, the main dietary source of vitamin A in humans. In the gastrointestinal tract arises retinal, which is then converted to retinol (Rahman, 2007, Sies et al., 1992).

3. Mechanism of cell death

Oxidative stress is a factor which initiates cell death after photodynamic reaction (Almmeida et al., 2004, Castano et al., 2005, Kulbacka et al., 2010, Saczko et al., 2009). In this part of our review we will examine the mechanisms of cell death caused by ROS and related metabolites, which are stimulated during the photodynamic process. The type of cell death by PDT may be mainly apoptosis or necrosis depending on the properties and concentration of the photosensitizer connected with the irradiation dose. However, another mode of cell death was also observed after photodynamic treatment, i.e. autophagic. This type II cell death is characterized by an enormous increase of two-membrane autophagic vacuoles in the cytoplasm which are finally catalyzed by lysosomal hydrolases (Edinger et al., 2004, Kroemer et al., 2005, Golstein et al., 2006). Autophagy is a convertible process, which can provoke both survival and death pathways, in contrast to the apoptotic irreversible process leading only to cell death (Kessel et al., 2007). Apoptosis (type I cell death) is genetically and morphologically different from necrosis. Apoptosis represents a regulated, universal and perfectly efficient, strongly controlled energetic suicide pathway. This process requires the activation of some hydrolytic enzymes - proteases and nucleases - leading to DNA fragmentation and destruction of cell structures. The morphological changes connected with apoptosis include nuclear pyknosis, DNA fragmentation, membrane blebbing, cell shrinkage and production of apoptotic bodies which are removed by adjacent cells and resident phagocytes (Kroemer et al., 1998 and 2005, Ryter et al., 2007, Kroemer et al., 2007). Apoptotic cell death is the most preferable effect of various anticancer therapies which leads to destruction and elimination of pathological cells. Inflammation does not occur through apoptosis in cancer cells and surroundings tissue (Fiers et al., 1999). On the other hand, necrosis (type III cell death) appears in a negative way as death associated with gross membrane damage and cell outflow into the extracellular space. This characteristic modification may lead to local inflammation and injury of nearby tissue. The endpoint of necrosis is manifested in cell swelling or oncosis (Majno et al., 1995). However, a recent study showed that necrosis can also occur similarly to programmed cell death, which consists of induction, commitment and execution processes of necrosis triggering the cysteine cathepsin-mediated lysosomal death pathway (Leist et al., 2001, Bizik et al., 2004, Golstein et al., 2005, Golstein et al., 2006). In general, it can be observed that lower doses of PDT lead to apoptosis, while higher doses lead to necrosis in cells (Ketabchi et al., 1998, Kessel et al., 2000). A previous study showed that the three well-known types of cell death are dependent on the developmental stage, physiological conditions of cells and the nature of the death signal (Majno 1995). Mixed-type cell death forms, containing characteristic properties for both types, apoptosis and necrosis, have been noted (Wang et al., 2003).

3.1 Apoptosis following PDT

The photodynamic reaction activates different signal transduction pathways connected with transcription factors and cell cycle regulation, which often lead to cell death or survival (Pazos et al., 2007, Robertson et al., 2009). The different types of cell death-induced photodynamic processes are permanently under investigation. However, the majority of studies have shown that apoptosis is a rapid and dominant type of cell death following the photodynamic reaction, in different experimental conditions and a variety of sensitizers (Oleinick et al., 2001). On the other hand, cancer cells can die in other ways: necrosis or autophagy (Buytaret et al., 2006). Autophagic and programmed necrosis are rarely related to

PDT. There are a few commonly known significant factors which can induce necrosis: extra-mitochondrial location of photosensitizers, a high dose of PDT, and glucose starvation (Almeida et al., 2004, Kieslich et al., 2005, Nowis et al., 2005). Also the cells' sensitivity to PDT conditions and their genotype may control the type of cell death following PDT (Wyld et al., 2001, Bar et al., 2007, Saczko et al., 2005). The most significant factors determining the effect of PDT are the physicochemical properties, intracellular distribution of photosensitizers, and the interactions between different cellular organelles such as mitochondria, lysosomes, endoplasmic reticulum (ER), Golgi apparatus and plasma membranes. The uptake of photosensitizers into cancer cells plays a decisive function in increasing the efficiency of PDT (Pazos et al., 2007, Robertson et al., 2009). Numerous studies with various first and second generation photosensitizers have concluded that the induction of apoptotic cell death by PDT was connected with mitochondrial damage (Kessel et al., 1998, Saczko et al., 2005 and 2007, Chwiłkowska et al., 2006). Kessel and other researchers have demonstrated that sensitizers which localize in mitochondria are much more rapid inducers of apoptosis than photosensitizers localized in endoplasmic reticulum, Golgi apparatus, lysosomes and plasma membranes (Kessel et al., 1997, Dahle et al., 1990, Marchal et al., 2004). On the other hand, cationic photosensitizers or others accumulating in plasma membrane were associated with membrane photodamage and necrotic results (Kessel 1998, Luo 1996). Moreover, the availability of oxygen, the suitable wavelength and intensity of light, as well as the biological conditions and type of cancer cells can influence the mode of cell death (Rosa et al., 2000, Castano et al., 2004, Juzeniene et al., 2007, Plaetzer et al.,2003). Photodynamic therapy can induce apoptosis in two dissimilar pathways: intrinsic, mitochondria-dependent, and extrinsic, death receptor-dependent (Almeida et al., 2004).

3.2 Intrinsic pathway

Mitochondria play a crucial role in intrinsic pathways of apoptotic cell death, due to mitochondrial damage being the major object of photocytotoxicity. The mitochondrial pathway of apoptosis is often mediated when sensitizers are accumulated in these organelles, but it is not obligatory. The loss of mitochondrial transmembrane potential and the release of cytochrome c from the mitochondrial inner membrane space to the cytosol is a well-examined apoptotic occurrence, which has also been documented for numerous photosensitizers localized in mitochondria such as Photofrin, benzoporphin derivative, cyanine and phthalocyanine (Fabris et al., 2001, Pervaiz et al., 1999, Saczko et al., 2007). The present observation of apoptosis by the mitochondrial pathway shows that cytochrome c released to the cytoplasm forms a triple complex with the apoptosis-inducing factor (Apaf1) and procaspase 9, which leads to activation of procaspase 9 and following activation of executioner caspases. Uncontrolled generation of reactive oxygen species during PDT can lead to endoplasmic reticulum stress. It results in perturbation of the Ca^{2+} gradient, which can lead to the creation of a permeability transition complex and the involvement of Bcl-2 proteins (Grebenova et al., 2003, Buytaret et al., 2006, Nowis et al., 2005). Some data show that the endoplasmic reticulum as well as mitochondria may induce apoptosis and autophagy in cancer cells following the photodynamic reaction. Manipulation of the PDT conditions results in suppression of apoptosis with increasing autophagy in mouse L1210 leukemia cells (Kessel et al., 2007). The hydrophilic chlorine photosensitizers localize mainly in lysosomes and activate the mitochondrial apoptotic pathway following photodamage of lysosomes. The lysosomal proteases are released by lysosomal injury during the photodynamic reaction and activate caspases directly or indirectly through mitochondrial damage. However, the mechanisms by which lysosome-localizing sensitizers induce mitochondrial apoptotic cell death are not fully elucidated (Nakajima et al., 1992, Mori et al., 2000, Nagata et al., 2003, Reiners et al., 2002).

3.3 Activation of caspases

The apoptosis effectors contain intracellular proteases termed caspases. Caspases are a family of intracellular endopeptidases that are synthesized as zymogens and are converted into active enzymes. Caspases can be divided into two groups: initiators (numbers 1, 2, 4, 5, 8, 9, 10 and 12) and effectors (numbers 3, 6 and 7) (Castano et al., 2005). The properties of apoptotic cell death are dependent on proteolytic cleavage of cellular substrates by effector caspases and can be activated by three dissimilar pathways involving intrinsic apoptosis activated by caspase 9, an extrinsic way connected with caspase 8, and an endoplasmic reticulum stress one induced by caspase 12.

The mitochondrial pathway is associated with release of cytochrome c proteins by mitochondria into the cytoplasm involving establishment of caspase 9 and cleavage of executioner caspases 3, 6 or 7 (Ketabchi et al., 1998, Robertson et al., 2007). This leads to degradation of various proteins and DNA and finally cell death by apoptosis. Some investigations suggest that high doses of photodynamic therapy can photochemically inactivate crucial enzymes and other components of the apoptotic cascade such as caspases (Lavie et al., 1999). A previous study examined the level of expression of caspase 3, 8 and 9 after photodynamic reaction with Photofrin® (Ph) using immunocytochemical assay (ABC method) in MCF-7 (human breast adenocarcinoma cell line) and A549 (human lung carcinoma cells). Differentiated expression of caspases 3, 8 and 9 in A549 cells was observed. The intensity of immunocytochemical staining of caspases depends on the concentration of Photofrin®, the time of irradiation and the incubation time after irradiation. Detection of two initiators, caspases 8 and 9, after photodynamic reaction in human lung adenocarcinoma A549 cells may suggest that apoptosis activation occurs by two independent signal transduction pathways, which are relative (Fabris et al., 2001, Grebenova et al., 2003, Saczko et al., 2007). Also a mechanism has been documented in which caspase 8 cleaves Bid protein and there follows mitochondrial release of cytochrome c dependent activation of caspase 9 (Buggiani et al., 2008). Moreover, a variety of apoptosis activation pathways induced during the photodynamic reaction can result in a lot of alternatives and cross-link the apoptotic signal transduction pathway (Almeida et al., 2004, Mitsunga et al., 2007).

3.4 Bcl-2 family proteins and p53 status

The Bcl-2 family proteins are divided into two groups: antiapoptotic Bcl-2, Bcl-X_l, and Bcl-w, and proapoptotic Bax, Bak, Bad, and Bim, which respectively inhibit or support the execution of apoptotic cell death. Thus families of proteins control mitochondrial stability by maintaining the balance between proapoptotic proteins that translocate to the mitochondria and antiapoptotic ones that exist in the mitochondrial membrane (Ryter et al., 2007, Kelekar et al., 1998). The *Bcl-2* gene product is located in the membranes of the endoplasmic reticulum, nuclear envelope and the external membranes of the mitochondria (Ryter et al., 2007). The most significant objective of PDT in the cell signaling pathway is activation of the proapoptotic proteins belonging to the Bcl-2 family. Photodamage after photodynamic reaction provokes activation of these proteins and induces apoptosis in malignant cells. Bax protein expression has been linked to a beneficial reaction to PDT. It can be used to assess the cancer response to photodynamic reaction (Zhen-hui Peng et al., 2008, Roland et al., 2007, Robertson et al., 2007). Generally the role of Bax protein in the release of cytochrome c from mitochondria into the cytoplasm and activation of the apoptotic process has been established in many systems. Chiu and co-workers observed that phthalocyanine Pc-4-PDT induced Bax dislocation from the cytoplasm to mitochondria as early signaling for the mitochondrial pathway of apoptosis in human breast cancer MCF-7c3 cells (Chiu et al., 2003). Phthalocyanine Pc4 is a new generation sensitizer that localizes in intracellular membranes, particularly in mitochondria. Pc4-PDT photodamages antiapoptotic Bcl-2 and Bcl-xL proteins and activates apoptosis in cancer cells (Castano et al., 2005, Kessel et al., 2000, Xue et al., 2001). Usada et al. examined the cells with transfection and wild-type Bcl-2. Overexpression of Bcl-2 decreased apoptosis, which is connected with inhibition of the proapoptotic Bax protein. On the other hand, high doses of Pc4-PDT are necessary to activate Bax in cells with increasing expression of antiapoptotic Bcl-2 protein (Usada et al., 2003). The p53 tumor suppressor gene takes part in the response to DNA damage, connected with cell cycle regulation, DNA repair, and induction of apoptosis (el-Deiry et al., 1998, Bunz et al., 1999). Expression of wild-type p53 activated by chemotherapy, radiation or photodynamic reaction increases the sensitivity to apoptosis, whereas mutated p53 decreases the sensitivity. In many cases of cancer, mutated p53 was found (Lowe et al., 1994). P53 plays a crucial role in regulation of proapoptotic Bcl-2 proteins. Bax induced the mitochondrial pathway by outflow of apoptogenic proteins, such as cytochrome c. However, in different studies the involvement of Bax and p53 in PDT-mediated apoptosis was observed (Fisher et al., 1997, Fisher et al., 1998, Zhang et al., 1999). Some data indicate that p53 is required for caspase 3 activation, suggesting that p53 may play a role in PDT-activated early apoptosis in cancer cells (Mitsunga et al., 2007). Bar and co-workers examined the effect of Photofrin-PDT (Ph-PDT) on clear human ovarian carcinoma with a "silent" mutation in the p53 gene. The cells were dying in a necrotic way. They postulated that this mutation can inhibit apoptosis in these cells (Bar et al., 2007). The modification of Ph-PDT by 2-methoxyestradiol leads to activation of apoptotic cell death in these cells (unpublished data). Another study showed that PDT induced apoptosis in cancer cells independent on p53 (Almeida et al., 2004).

3.5 Extrinsic apoptosis pathway

This pathway is connected with initiation of the apoptotic process in response to induction of a cell surface receptor, such as the tumor-necrosis factor receptor (TNF-R) family of death receptor, or the apoptotic program can be initiated when a death ligand (Fas ligand - FasL) interacts with a cell surface receptor (Fas/APO-1/CD95) (Mupidi 2004). Death receptor mediated apoptosis occurs during photodynamic therapy when photosensitizers preferentially localize in the cell membrane. In human epidermoid carcinoma A431 treated photodynamic reaction with phthalocyanine 4 increasing levels of the surface death receptor Fas and of its ligand FasL were observed. Additionally, in the same conditions caspase-8 cleavage was increased in Pc4-sensitized A431 cells. The function of the Fas/FasL system in PDT was also observed in canine kidney cells and hamster lung fibroblast after photosensitization with Photofrin (Almeida 2004). PDT-induced apoptosis is dependent on many metabolic signals which have an influence on the apoptotic pathway. Many examinations suggest that both the intrinsic and extrinsic pathway were crosslinked during photosensitization.

4. PDT in melanoma treatment

Results from preclinical and clinical studies conducted worldwide over a 25-year period have established PDT as a useful treatment approach for some cancers (Mitton D, 2005). For more than 20 years scientists have maintained that PDT is not effective for pigmented melanomas (Ambrosone et al., 2005). Scientists focused on the improvement of inefficient PDT due to the competition between the absorbance of melanin from melanoma and the absorbance of photosensitizers at the photosensitizer excitation light wavelength. Melanin absorbs light over the entire wavelength region used for PDT (400-750 nm) (Ma et al., 2007). This was one reason why pigmented melanoma has been excluded in some PDT studies (Lim et al., 2004). It is well known that the longer wavelength of light absorption is, the deeper photosensitizer penetrates the skin (Woodburn et al., 1998). Since establishing the substantial heterogeneity of melanomas and their varying resistance to radio- and phototherapy, there have been intensive studies on the molecular processes occurring in these neoplasms during therapy (Kusmierz et al., 2009).

The limitations of the porphyrin-derived photosensitizers with regard to light penetration into tissues promoted the synthesis of longer wavelength absorbing photosensitizers (Kreimer- Birnbaum, 1989). PDT treatment with lutetium texaphyrin (PCI-0123) (excitation at 732 nm) promoted survival of mice bearing the highly pigmented B16F10 melanoma (Woodburn et al., 1998). Also in these studies tumor apoptosis was evident in the PDT-treated neoplasms after irradiation. PDT is a process with membranes being a principal target (Henderson et al., 1992). Woodburn et al. performed a confocal laser scanning microscopy studies with PDT and PCI-0123. Thre was proved that PDT destroys the melanosomal membrane, which leads to death due to oxidative stress of cells (Woodburn et al., 1997 and 1998).

An important aspect of the antitumour effectiveness of PDT is related to the distribution of the photosensitizer. The localization of the drug in cytoplasmic organelles during PDT plays a major role in cell death (Saczko et al., 2007). It was suggested that localization of photosensitizing drugs in the plasma membrane, or in lysosomes, leads to necrosis after PDT treatment. Localization in the mitochondrial membrane causes apoptosis (Chen et al., 2000). Intracellular accumulation of the photosensitizing drug is one of the most important factors to determine the efficacy of PDT (Saczko et al., 2007; Lam et al., 2001; Ogura et al., 2003). Photofrin (Ph) was the first photosensitizer used in PDT of cancer. This drug has proved to be effective in the treatment of many cancers (Almeida et al., 2004). Ph has been involved in several mechanisms in PDT, such as cytotoxicity and apoptosis (Konan et al., 2002). Saczko et al. showed that the intracellular localization of Ph in a cultured malignant melanoma (Me45) cell line is mainly intracellular compartments and mitochondrial membranes (Saczko et al., 2007). Ricchelli et al. also reported that Ph was localized in the mitochondria *in vitro* (Ricchelli et al., 1990). Mitochondria play an important role in the early events of apoptosis (Lam et al., 2001; Patito et al., 2001). Marchetti et al. demonstrated that Ph is a ligand for the mitochondrial peripheral benzodiazepine receptor, which is responsible for triggering pore transition (Saczko et al., 2007, Marchetti et al., 1996).

The mitochondrial apoptotic pathway was also shown by Chen et al. in therapy with methylene blue (MB) (Chen et al., 2008). It is a photosensitizer which has excellent photochemical properties. MB is well known to have a high quantum yield of intersystem crossing and singlet oxygen generation and can produce radical species in the presence of reducing agents (Gabrielli et al., 2004; Tardivo et al., 2005). This photosensitizing drug has affinity for melanocyte-produced melanin, which contributes to selective absorption of this compound by cutaneous melanomas (Link et al., 1989). MB showed enhanced penetration efficiency into melanoma cells and also in mitochondrial membranes, which induced apoptotic cell death by causing mitochondrial dysfunction (Ball et al., 1998). Chen et al. showed that MB-PDT could induce apoptotic cell death through the photochemical generation of reactive oxygen species that activate the caspase-9 and caspase-3 apoptosis pathway (Chen et al., 2008). A transplantable mouse melanoma model showed that the tumor size in treated mice decreased, which was associated with enhanced apoptotic cell death.

Nowak-Sliwinska et al. have tested several photosensitizers to evaluate their photoefficiency in the Cloudman S91/I3 mouse melanoma cell line (Nowak-Sliwinska et al., 2006). They compared the efficiency of the photodynamic effect using cyanine (MC540) and porphyrin derivative photosensitizers (Photofrin and verteporfin). Their study showed that verteporfin and Photofrin are effective compounds with the classical type II mechanism of photodynamic reaction, but verteporfin is the most potent photosensitizer against melanoma cells. Generation of singlet molecular oxygen by photo-activated verteporfin was more than twice as high as in the case of Photofrin. The LD50 light dose for verteporfin was four times lower than for Photofrin, in spite of the much lower concentration used (2 vs. 10 lg/ml) and 10 times higher for MC540 than for Photofrin. Busetti et al. described the pharmacokinetics of verteporfin in mice and showed that a single treatment inhibited growth of B16 tumor (Busetti et al., 1999).

Induction of apoptosis by PDT seemed to play an important role in the photodynamic treatment efficacy (Barge et al., 2004). Ph-PDT induces cell death in the human Beidegröm Melanoma (BM) cell line mainly through apoptosis (Saczko et al., 2005). The application of comet assay to study the influence of Ph-PDT on BM cells showed that some types of DNA damage depend on photosensitizer concentration, as well as on time and dose of irradiation. Similar results were obtained by Barge et al. (Barge et al., 2004) in human melanoma cells using a new silicon phthalocyanine photosensitizer and by Haddad et al. in murine malignant melanoma *in vitro* and *in vivo* using aluminum phthalocyanine (AlpcS4) (Haddad et al., 1998)

Higher doses of light and sensitizer lead to a dose-dependent augmentation of reaction oxygen species in melanoma cells (Kästle et al., 2011; Kolarova et al., 2007). A widely used photosensitizer is the protoporphyrin IX (PpIX) precursor 5-aminolevulinic acid (ALA). ALA is the first molecule in heme biosynthesis which is converted to the active photosensitizer PpIX in the mitochondria. Kästle et al. showed that WM451LU cells are more affected by ALA-PDT than non-tumorigenic keratinocytes (Kästle et al., 2011). The reason for this is elevated porphobilinogen deaminase activity and a significant decrease in ferrochelatase activity in cancer cells (Dailey et al., 1984; Kästle et al., 2011; Leibovici et al., 1988). What is more, PDT of melanoma with porphyrin and porphyrin derivatives is effective and well tolerated by patients (Szurko et al., 2003).

Kolarova et al. studied the effects of zinc-5,10,15,20-tetrakis(4-sulfonatophenyl) porphyrin ($ZnTPPS_4$) on human G361 melanoma cell line (Kolarova et al., 2005). Analysis of DNA damage in the cell line after PDT was proved by comet assay. This treatment method gave rise to DNA damage. Further studies demonstrated that $ZnTPPS_4$ induces the highest ROS production in the G361 cell line compared to other porphyrins - $TPPS_4$ and $PdTPPS_4$. A correlation was observed between ROS production and cell survival. The results

demonstrate that the photodynamic effect depends on sensitizer type, its concentration and light dose (Kolarova et al., 2007). Later research showed the most significant phototoxic effect of chloraluminium phthalocyanine disulfonate ($ClAlPcS_2$)-PDT in spite of significantly higher ROS production induced by $ZnTPPS_4$–PDT on G361 cells (Krestyn et al., 2010).
HO-1 has a number of potential protective effects against oxidative stress. Additionally, the last catalytic product of HO-1 is CO. CO acts as a second messenger. It has anti-inflammatory and anti-apoptotic effects (Bilban et al., 2008). Its expression is closely related to the oxidative stress levels in the cells (Saczko et al., 2007). An increase in expression of HO-1 following photodynamic therapy was observed by Gomer et al. (1991) and Nowis et al. (2006). They demonstrated that overexpression of HO-1 protects cancer cells against PDT with Photofrin. Other authors have also reported that PDT with 5-ALA resulted in increased formation of ROS and further enhancement of HO-1 induction (Frank et al., 2007). Kästle et al. applied inhibitors of HO-1 and PARP what improved the efficiency of photodynamic treatment (Kästle et al., 2011). Drastic reduction in viability by the addition of ZnPpIX is among other things the result of higher ROS levels (75% more than without ZnPpIX) after irradiation and inhibition of HO-I (Kästle et al., 2011). Also inhibition of the protein PARP-1 seems to be a plausible addition to anticancer treatment. PARP is a protein involved in a number of cellular processes. One of its important functions is to assist in the repair of single-strand DNA breaks. If one single-strand broken DNA is reduplicated, a double-strand broken DNA results. If PARP is inhibited, cell death occurs (D'Amours et al., 1999). In the co-culture 65% of WM451LU melanoma cells and 35% of HaCaT keratinocytes were present before PDT. After PDT the proportion was 41% of melanoma cells and 59% of HaCaT cells. Combination of both inhibitors with PDT improves these results to 16% of melanoma cells and 84% of HaCaT cells. Addition of HO-1 and PARP inhibitors significantly improves the efficiency of photodynamic treatment (Kästle et al., 2011).
A very interesting study was presented by Ma et al. (2007). In that work reflectance spectroscopy was applied to study depigmentation of human and murine skin with different melanin contents, and effects induced by PDT with topical application of methyl 5-aminolevulinate (MAL) on B16F10 melanotic melanomas transplanted to mice. Skin depigmentation leads to increase in reflectance. PDT with violet light (420 nm) bleached some of the melanin in the skin above the B16F10 melanomas. It was concluded that violet light in PDT can bleach melanin in melanotic tumors and therefore increase their sensitivity to red light (634 nm). This finding indicates a new PDT modality (Ma et al., 2007).
The direct effects of PDT are cytotoxic for cancer cells, but it also could induce an immune system response, what has been proved in vitro (Blom et al., 1997). Treatment of ocular melanoma cells with hematoporphyrin ester (HPE)-PDT temporally alters the expression of HLA class I and β2-microglobulin. This may affect anti-tumor-immune responses.

5. Conclusions

Photodynamic therapy, a minimally invasive therapeutic modality, has been shown to be effective in a number of oncological and non-oncological conditions. The advantages of PDT application are better cosmetic outcomes without surgical scars or the discoloration that is evident in surgery or cryotherapy. Moreover, PDT may be used to decrease the size of a large tumor, which can be subsequently removed with a smaller excision. The experience in the use of PDT in the treatment of other skin diseases, including psoriasis, sarcoidosis, acne and human papillomavirus infections, is preliminary and undergoing clinical testing.

Although the idea of PDT usage is rather simple, the procedure is complicated by several parameters such as the formulation of the photosensitizing agents, the mode of delivery and duration of application, as well as the multiple light-specific parameters, such as exact wavelength, duration and intensity of various light sources. With the application of second-generation, stable, lipophilic photosensitizers with optimized wavelengths, PDT may be a promising tool for therapy in skin cancer. Melanoma is the most severe of all skin neoplasms as it may grow rapidly and metastasize. For many years melanoma, mainly due to the presence of melanotic biopolymers and the presence of gene mutations which code pro-apoptotic proteins, has been included in the group of resistant irradiation cancers. However, the research in recent years has indicated high variation in sensitivity in melanoma cells. This information has led many researchers to focus on examining the potential use of photodynamic therapy (PDT) in the fight against this cancer. The application of photodynamic therapy opens new perspectives in treatment of this tumor. Photodynamic therapy is an effective local cancer treatment that induces cytotoxicity through intercellular generation of reactive oxygen species. There are three indispensable components in this therapy: a photosensitizer, light, and oxygen inside the diseased tissue. The photosensitizer is accumulated in the target cells and absorbs light of certain wavelength. The energy is transferred to oxygen and highly reactive oxygen species are generated. This is usually singlet oxygen. Potential cellular targets for photodynamic therapy are the cell membrane and membranous organelles such as mitochondria, lysosome and nuclei. The disintegration of cellular structures and modulation of genetic information induced by PDT leads cancer cells to a death pathway. Numerous studies suggest that the exposure of tumor cells to PDT can lead to cell death via two separate processes: apoptosis and necrosis. In contrast to necrosis, apoptosis is an energy-dependent, distinct form of cell death that follows a sequence of genetically programmed events and proceeds without inflammation. Morover there was also noticed that photodynamic therapy can increase the radical and the oxidant processes in oncological patients whose antioxidative mechanisms are overworked.

Potential targets for PDT in melanoma eradication include cell proliferation inhibition, activation of cell death, reduction in pro-survival autophagy and a decrease in the cellular melanocytic antioxidant system. As we have indicated, more research on PDT with melanoma is needed to determine the exact parameters optimal for the treatment of this disease. In our opinion PDT should be considered as a good candidate for treatment in malignant melanoma. This technique may be also a promising device for melanoma in combation with standard therapies.

6. Acknowledgment

This work was supported by a grant of the Ministry of Science and Higher Education, Poland, grant No. 5409/B/P01/2011/40 (A. Gamian).

7. References

Aliya, S.; Reddanna, P.; & Thyagaraju, K. (2003). Does glutathione S-transferase Pi (GST-Pi) a marker protein for cancer? *Molecular and Cellular Biochemistry*, Vol.253, No.1-2, pp. 319–27, ISSN 0300-8177

Allison, R.R.; Sibata, C.H. (2010) Oncologic photodynamic therapy photosensitizers: A clinical review. *Photodiagnosis and Photodynamic Therapy*, Vol.7, No.2 (April 2010), pp. 61-75, ISSN 1873-159

Almeida, R.D.; Manadas, B.J.; Carvalho, A.P.; Duarte, C.B. (2004). Intracellular signalling mechanism in photodynamic therapy. *Biochimica et Biophysica Acta*, Vol.1704, No.2 (June 2004), pp. 59-86, ISSN 0006-3002

Ambrosone, C.B.; Ahn, J.; Singh, K.K.; Rezaishiraz, H.; Furberg, H.; Sweeney, C.; Coles, B.; Trovato, A. (2005). Polymorphisms in Genes Related to Oxidative Stress (MPO, MnSOD, CAT) and Survival After Treatment for Breast Cancer. *Cancer Research*, Vol.65, No.3 (February 2005), pp. 1105-1111, ISSN 0008-5472

Bailey, M.S.; Landar, A.; & Darley-Usmar, V. (2005). Mitochondrial proteomics in free radical research. *Free Radical in Biology and Medicine*, Vol.38, No.2, pp. 175-188, ISSN 0891-5849

Ball, D.J.; Luo, Y.; Kessel, D.; Griffiths, J.; Brown, S.B. & Vernon, D.I. (1998). The induction of apoptosis by a positively charged methylene blue derivative. *Journal of Photochemistry and Photobiology*. B, Biology, Vol.42, No.2 (April 1998), pp. 159–63, ISSN 1011-1344

Bar, K.B.; Saczko, J.; Ziółkowski, P.; Chwiłkowska, A.; Słomska, I.; Drąg-Zalesińska, M.; Wysocka, T.; Duś, D. (2007). Photofrin II based photosensitization of human ovarian clear-cell carcinoma cell Line (OvBH-1). *Pharmacological Reports*, Vol.59, suppl.1, ISSN 1734-1140

Barge, J.; Decreau, R.; Julliard, M.; Hubaud, J.C.; Sabatier, A.S.; Grob, J.J.; Verrando, P. (2004). Killing efficacy of a new silicon phtalocyanine in human melanoma cells treated with photodynamic therapy by early activation of mitochondrion-mediated apoptosis. *Experimental Dermatology*, Vol.13, No.1 (January 2004), pp. 33-44, ISSN 0906-6705

Bartosz, G. (2003). Druga twarz tlenu, Wolne rodniki w przyrodzie, PWN, Warszawa

Bilban, M.; Haschemi, A.; Weigel, B.; Chin, B.Y.; Wagner, O.; Otterbein, L.E. (2008). Heme oxygenase and carbon monoxide initiate homeostatic signalling. *Journal of Molecular Medicine*, Vol.86, No.3 (October 2007), pp. 267–279, ISSN 0946-2716

Bizik, J.; Kankuri, E.; Ristimaki, A.; Taieb, A.; Vapaatalo, H.; Lubitz, W.; Waheri, A. (2004). Cell—cell contracts trigger programmed necrosis and induce cyclooxygenase-2 expression. *Cell Death and Differentiation*, Vol.11, No.4 (October 2003), pp. 183-95

Blom, D.J.; Schuitmaker, H.J.; de Waard-Siebinga, I.; Dubbelman, T.M.; Jager, M.J. (1997). Decreased expression of HLA class I on ocular melanoma cells following in vitro photodynamic therapy. *Cancer Letters*, Vol.112, No. 2 (January 1997), pp. 239-43, ISSN 0304-3835

Buggiani, G.; Trojano, R.; Rossi, R.; Lotti, T. (2008). Photodynamic therapy: off-label and alternative use in dermatological practice. *Photodiagnostic & Photodynamic Therapy*, Vol.1, pp. 1-5

Bunz, F.; Hwang, P.M.; Torrance, C..; Waldman, T.; Zhang, Y.; Dillehay, L.; Wiliams, J.; Lengauer, C.; Kinzler, W.; Vogelstein, B. (1999). Disruption of p53 in human cancer cells alters the responses to therapeutic agents. *Journal of Clinical Investigation*, Vol.104, No.3 (August 1999), pp. 263-269, ISSN 0021-9738

Busetti, A.; Soncin, M.; Jori, G.; Rodgers, M.A.J. (1999). High efficiency of benzoporphyrin derivative in the photodynamic therapy of pigmented malignant melanoma, *British Journal of Cancer*, Vol.79, No.5/6, pp. 821–824, ISSN 0007-0920

Buytaret, E.; Callewaert, G.; Hendrickx, N.; Scorrano, L.; Hartman, D.; Mssiaen, L.; Vandenheede, J.R.; Heirman, I.; Grotten, J.; & Agostinis, P. (2006) Role of endoplasmic reticulum depletion and multidomain proapoptotic BAX and BAK proteins in shaping cell death after hypericin-mediated photodynamic therapy. *The FASEB Journal*; 20: 756-758, ISSN: 0892-6638

Capella M. A. M., Capella, L. S. (2003) A light in multidrug resistance: photodynamic treatment of multidrug-resistant tumors, *Journal of Biomedical Science*; Vol. 10, No.4, pp: 361–366, ISSN 1021-7770

Castano, A.P.; Demidova, T.N.; Hamblin, M.R. (2004). Mechanisms in photodynamic therapy: Part two - photosensitizers, photochemistry and cellular localization. *Photodiagnosis and Photodynamic Therapy*, Vol.1, pp. 279-293, ISSN 1572-1000

Chen, J.Y.; Heung N.K.; Fung, M.C.; Wen, J.M.; Leung, W.N.; Mak, N.K. (2000). Subcellular localization of Merocyanine 540 (MC540) and induction of apoptosis in murine myeloid leukemia cells, *Photochemistry and Photobiology*, Vol.72, No.1 (May 2007), pp. 114–120, ISSN 0031-8655

Chen, Y.; Zheng, W.; Li, Y.; Zhong, J.; Ji, J.; Shen, P. (2008). Apoptosis induced by methylene-blue-mediated photodynamic therapy in melanomas and the involvement of mitochondrial dysfunction revealed by proteomics. *Cancer Science*, Vol.99, No.10 (October 2008), pp. 2019-2027,

Chiu, S.M.; Xue, L.Y.; Usada, J.; Azizuddin, K. & Oleinick, N.L. (2003). Bax is essential for mitochondrion-mediated apoptosis but not for cell death caused by photodynamic therapy. *British Journal of Cancer*, Vol.89, No.8 (October 2003), pp. 1590-1597, ISSN 0007-0920

Chow, C.K.; Ibrahim, W.; Wei, Z.; & Chan, A.C. (1999) Vitamin E regulates mitochondrial hydrogen peroxide generation. *Free Radical in Biology and Medicine*, Vol.27, No.5-6, pp. 580-587, ISSN 0891-5849

Chwiłkowska, A.; Saczko, J.; Kulbacka, J.; Ługowski, M.; Drąg-Zalesińska, M.; Wysocka, T.; Banaś, T. (2006). Influence of photofrin on survival and apoptosis of the Jurkat leukemic T-cell line undergoing photodynamic therapy. *Advances in Clinical and Experimental Medicine*, Vol.15, No.6, pp. 999-1002, ISSN 1230–025X

Dahle, J.; Steen, H.B.; Moan, J. (1999). The mode of cell death induced by photodynamic treatment depends on cell density. *Photochemistry and Photobiology*, Vol.70, No.3 (January 2008), pp. 363-367, ISSN 0031-8655

Dailey, H.A.; Smith, A. (1984). Differential interaction of porphyrins used in photoradiation therapy with ferrochelatase. *Biochemical Journal*, Vol.223, No.2, pp. 441–445, ISSN 0264-6021

D'Amours, D.; Desnoyers, S.; D'Silva, I.; Poirier, G.G. (1999). Poly(ADP-ribosylation) reaction in the regulation of nuclear functions. *Biochemical Journal*, Vol.342, No.2 (September 1999), pp. 249–268, ISSN 0264-6021

De Rosa, F.S.; Bently, M.V.L.B. (2000). Photodynamic therapy of skin cancers: sensitizers, clinical studies, and future directives. *Pharmaceutical Research*, Vol.17, No.12, pp. 1447-1455, ISSN 0724-8741

Dellinger, M. (1996). Apoptosis or necrosis following Photofrin photosensitization: Influence of the incubation protocol. *Photochemistry and Photobiology*, Vol.64, No.l, pp. 182-187, ISSN 0031-8655

Dulak, J.; & Jozkowicz, A. (2003). Carbon monoxide — a "new" gaseous modulator of gene expression. *Acta Biochimica Polonica*, Vol.50, No.1, pp. 31–47, ISSN 0001-527X

Edinger, A.L.; & Thompson, C.B. (2004). Death by design: apoptosis, necrosis and autophagy. *Current Opinion in Cell Biology*, Vol.16, No.6, pp. 663-669, ISSN 0955-0674

El-Deiry, W.S. (1998). Regulation of p53 downstream genes. *Seminars in Cancer Biology*. Vol.8, No.5, pp. 345-357, ISSN 1044-579X

Fabris, C.; Valduga, G.; Miotto, G.; Borsetto, L.; Jori, G.; Garbisa, S. & Reddi, E. (2001). Photosensitization with Zinc (II) Phthalocyanine as a switch in the decision between apoptosis and necrosis. *Cancer Research*, Vol.61 (October 2001), pp. 7495-7500, ISSN 0008-5472

Fiers, W.; Beyaert, R.; Declercq, W.; Vandenabeele, P. (1999). More than one way to die: apoptosis, necrosis and reactive oxygen damage. *Oncogene*, Vol.18, No.54 (December 1999), pp. 7719-7730, ISSN 0950-9232

Fisher, A.M.; Rucker, N.; Wong, S.; Gomer, C.J. (1998). Differential photosensitivity in wild type and mutant p53 human colon carcinoma cell lines. *Journal of Photochemistry and Photobiology. B, Biology*, Vol.42, No.2 (June 2005), pp. 104-107

Fisher, A.M.; Danenberg, K.; Benerjee, D.; Bertino, J.; Danenberg, P.; Gomer, CJ. (1997). Increased photosensitivity in HL60 cells expressing wild type p53. *Photochemistry and Photobiology*, Vol.66, No.2 (January 2008), pp. 265-270, ISSN 0031-8655

Fisher, A.M.R.; Murphree, A.L.; Gomer, C.J. (1995) Clinical and preclinical photodynamic therapy. *Lasers in Surgery and Medicine*, Vol.17, No.1, pp. 2-31, ISSN 0196-8092

Frank, J.; Lornejad-Schäfer, M. R.; Schöffel, H. (2007). Inhibition of heme oxygenase-1 increases responsiveness of melanoma cells to ALA-based photodynamic therapy. *International Journal of Oncology*, Vol.31. No.6 (January 2008), pp. 1539–1545, ISSN 1019-6439

Gabrielli, D.; Belisle, E.; Severino, D.; Kowaltowski, A.J.; Baptista, M.S. (2004). Binding, aggregation and photochemical properties of methylene blue in mitochondrial suspensions. *Photochemistry and Photobiology*, Vol.79, No.3 (May 2007), pp. 227–32, ISSN 0031-8655

Gałecka, E.; Mrowicka, M.; Malinowksa, K. et al.: (2008). Wybrane substancje nieenzymatyczne uczestniczące w procesie obrony przed nadmiernym wytwarzaniem wolnych rodników. *Polski Merkuriusz Lekarski*, Vol.147, No.25, pp. 269-272, ISSN 1426-9686

Golstein, P.; & Kroamer, G. (2005). Redundant cell death mechanisms as relics and backups. *Cell Death and Differentiation*, Vol.2, pp. 1490-1496, ISSN 1350-9047

Golstein, P. & Kroemer, G. (2006). Cell death by necrosis: towards a molecular definition. *Trends in Biochemical Sciences*, Vol.32, No.1, pp. 37-43, ISSN 0167-7640

Gomer, C.J.; Luna M.; Ferrario, A.; & Rucker, N. (1991). Increased transcription and translation of heme oxygenase in Chinese hamster fibroblasts following photodynamic stress or Photofrin II incubation. *Photochemistry and Photobiology*, Vol.53, No.2, pp. 275–279, ISSN 0031-8655

Granville, D.J.; McManus, B.M.; Hunt, D.W. (2001) Photodynamic therapy: shedding light on the biochemical pathways regulating porphyrin-mediated cell death. *Histology and Histopathology*, Vol.16, No. 1 (January 2001), pp. 309-17, ISSN 0213-3911

Grebenova, D.; Kuzelova, K.; Smetana, K. (2003). Mitochondrial and endoplasmic reticulum stress-induced apoptotic pathways are activated by 5-aminolevulinic acid-based photodynamic therapy in HL60 leukemia cells. *Journal of Photochemistry and Photobiology B: Biology*, Vol.69, No.2, pp. 71-85

Haddad, R.; Blumenfeld, A.; Siegal, A.; Kaplan, O.; Cohen, M.; Skornick, Y.; Kashtan, H. (1998). In vitro and in vivo effects of photodynamic therapy on murine malignant melanoma. *Annals of Surgical Oncology*, Vol.5, No.3, pp. 241-247, ISSN 1068-9265

Halliwell, B. (2000) A super way to kill cancer cells. *Nature Medicine*, 6(10): 1105-1106, ISSN: 1078-8956

Haylett, A.K.; Ward, T.H.; & Moore, J.V. (2003). DNA damage and repair in Gorlin syndrome and normal fibroblasts after aminolevulinic acid photodynamic therapy: a comet assay study. *Photochemistry and Photobiology*, Vol.78, No.4, pp. 337–341, ISSN 0031-8655

Henderson, B.W.; Doughtery, T.J. (1992) How does photodynamic therapy work? *Photochemistry and Photobiology*, Vol.55, No.1 (January 1992), pp. 145-157, ISSN 0031-8655

Hightower, L.E.; & Hendershot, L.M. (1997). Molecular chaperones and the heat shock response at Cold Spring Harbor. *Cell Stress and Chaperones*, Vol.2, No.1, pp. 1–11, ISSN 1355-8145

Hsieh, Y.J.; Wu, C.C.; Chang, H.C.; & Yu J.S. (2003). Subcellular localization of photofrin determines the death phenotype of human epidermoid carcinoma A431 cells triggered by photodynamic therapy: when plasma membranes are the main targets. *Journal of Cellular Physiology*, Vol.194, No.3, pp. 363-375, ISSN 0021-9541

Huang, P., Feng, L.I., Oldham, A., Keating, M.J., Plunkett, W. (2000) Superoxide dismutase as a target for the selective killing of cancer cells. *Nature*, 407: 390-395, ISSN: 0028-0836

Juzeniene, A.; Moan, J. (2007). The history of PDT in Norway. Part one - identification of basic mechanisms of general PDT. *Photodiagnosis and Photodynamic Therapy*, Vol.4, No.1, pp. 3-11, ISSN 1572-1000

Kästle, M.; Grimm, S.; Nagel, R.; Breusing, N.; Grune, T. (2010). Combination of PDT and inhibitor treatment affects melanoma cells and spares keratinocytes. *Free Radicals in Biology and Medicine*, Vol.50, No.2 (January 2011), pp. 305–312, ISSN 0891-5849

Kawczyk-Krupka, A. et al. (2001). Terapia fotodynamiczna i jej znaczenie immunomodulujące w leczeniu chorób skóry i leukoplakii jamy ustnej. *Acta Bio-Optica et Informatica Medica. Inżynieria Biomedyczna*, Vol. 7, pp. 67-72, ISSN 1234-5563

Kelekar, A.& Thompson, C.B. (1998). Bcl-2 family proteins: the role of the BH3 domain in apoptosis. *Trends in Cell Biology*, Vol.8, No.8 (October 2998), pp. 324-330

Kessel, D. & Arroyo, A.S. (2007). Apoptotic and autophagic responses to Bcl-2 inhibition and photodamage. *Photochemical & Photobiological Sciences*, Vol.6, No.12 (July 2007), pp. 1290-1295

Kessel, D. & Luo, Y. (1998). Mitochondrial photodamage and PDT-induced apoptosis. *Journal of Photochemistry and Photobiology B: Biology*, Vol.42, No.2 (April 1998), pp. 89-95

Kessel, D.; Luo, Y.; Deng, Y.; & Chang, C.K. (1997). The role of subcellular localization in initiation of apoptosis by photodynamic therapy. *Photochemistry and Photobiology*, Vol.65, No.3, pp.422-426, ISSN 0031-8655

Kessel, D.; Luo, Y.; Deng, Y.; Cheng, C.K. (1997). The role of subcellular localization in initiation of apoptosis by photodynamic therapy. *Photochemistry and Photobiology*, Vol.65, No.3 (March 1997), pp. 422-426, ISSN 0031-8655

Kessel, D.; Poretz, R.D. (2000). Sites of photodamage induced by photodynamic therapy with a chlorine e6 triacetoxymethyl ester (CAME). *Photochemistry and Photobiology*, Vol.71, No.1 (May 2007), pp. 94-6, ISSN 0031-8655

Ketabachi, A..; Macrobert, A.; Speight, P.M.; Benn, J.H. (1998). Induction of apoptotic cell death by photodynamic therapy in human keratinocytes. *Archives of Oral Biology*, Vol.43, No.2 (February 2008), pp. 143-149, ISSN 0003-9969

Khan, M.A.; Tania, M.; Zhang, D.; & Chen, H. (2010). Antioxidant enzymes and cancer. *Chinese Journal of Cancer Research*, Vol.22, No.2, pp. 87-92, ISSN 1000-9604

Kiesslich, T.; Plaetzer, K.; Oberdanner, C.B.; Berlanda, J.; Obermair, F.J.; & Krammer, B. (2005) Differential effects of glucose deprivation on the cellular sensitivity towards photodynamic treatment-based production of reactive oxygen species and apoptosis induction. *The FEBS Letters*, Vol. 579, No. 1 (3 January 2005), pp 185-190, ISSN 0014-5793

Kolarova, H.; Bajgar, R.; Tomankova, K.; Nevrelova, P.; Mosinger, J. (2007). Comparison of sensitizers by detecting reactive oxygen species after photodynamic reaction in vitro. *Toxicology in Vitro*, Vol.21, No.7,(May 2007), pp. 1287–1291

Kolarova, H.; Macecek, J.; Nevrelova, P.; Huf, M.; Tomecka, M.; Bajgar, R.; Mosinger, J.; Strnad, M. (2005). Photodynamic therapy with zinc-tetra(p-sulfophenyl)porphyrin bound to cyclodextrin induces single strand breaks of cellular DNA in G361 melanoma cells. *Toxicology in Vitro*, Vol.19, No.7 (August 2005), pp. 971-974

Konan, Y.N.; Gurny, R.; Allemann, E. (2002) State of the art in the delivery of photosensitizers for photodynamic therapy. *Journal of Photochemistry and Photobiology*, Vol.66, No.2 (December 2001), pp. 89-106, ISSN 1011-1344

Krestyn, E.; Kolarova, H.; Bajgar, R.; Tomankova, K. (2010). Photodynamic properties of ZnTPPS4, ClAlPcS2 and ALA in human melanoma G361 cells. *Toxicology in Vitro*, Vol.24, No.1 (August 2009), pp. 286-91

Kroemer, G. (2005). Classification of cell death: recommendations of the nomenclature committee on cell death. Cell Death and Differentiation, Vol.12, No.2, pp. 1463-1467, ISSN 1350-9047

Kroemer, G.; & Martin, S.J. (2005). Caspase independent cell death. *Nature Medicine*, Vol.11, No.7, pp. 725-730, ISSN 1078-8956

Kroemer, G.; Dallaporta, B.; & Resche-Rigon, M. (1998). The mitochondrial death/life regulator in apoptosis and necrosis. *Annual Review of Physiology*, Vol.60, pp. 619-642, ISSN 0066-4278

Kroemer, G.; Galluzzi, L.; & Brenner, C. (2007). Mitochondrial membrane permeabilization in cell death. *Physiological Reviews*, Vol.87, No.1, pp. 99-163, ISSN 0031-9333

Kulbacka, J.; Chwiłkowska, A.; Bar, J.; Poła, A.; Banaś, T.; Gamian, A.; & Saczko, J. (2010). Oxidative alterations induced in vitro by the photodynamic reaction in doxorubicin-sensitive (LoVo) and -resistant (LoVoDX) colon adenocarcinoma cells. *Experimental Biology and Medicine*, Vol.235, No.1, pp. 98-110, ISSN 1535-3699

Kurl, S.; Tuomainen, T.P.; Laukkanen, J.A.; Nyyssönen, K.; Lakka, T.; Sivenius, J.; & Salonen, J.T. (2002). Plasma vitamin C modifies the association between hypertension and risk of stroke. *Stroke*, Vol.33, No.6, pp. 1568-1573, ISSN 0039-2499

Kuroda, M., Himei, K., St. Clair, D. K., Urano, M., Yoshino, T., Akagi, T., Asaumi, J., Akaki, S., Takeda, Y., Kanazawa, S., and Hiraki, Y. (2000) Overexpression of manganese superoxide dismutase gene suppresses spontaneous apoptosis without a resultant alteration in in vivo growth of the mouse fibrosarcoma, FSa-II. *Anticancer Research*, 20, 7-10, ISSN : 0250-7005

Kusmierz, D.; Latocha, M.; Zielińska, A.; Nawrocka–Musial, D.; Sliupkas–Dyrda E. (2009). The expression of the melanogenesis pathway genes TYR, TYRP–1, and TYRP–2 and the synthesis of melanin in SH–4 melanoma cells after photodynamic therapy with photolon. (2009). *Advances in Clinical and Experimental Medicine*. Vol.18, No.5 (September 2009), pp. 449–459, ISSN 1230–025X

Łagowska-Lenard, M.; Bielewicz, J.; Raszewski, G. et al. (2008). Stres oksydacyjny w udarze mózgu. *Polski Merkuriusz Lekarski*, Vol.147, No.25, pp. 205-208, ISSN 1426-9686

Lam, M.; Oleinick, N.L.; Nieminien, A.L. (2001). Photodynamic therapy-induced apoptosis in epidermoid carcinoma cells: reactive oxygen species and mitochondrial inner membrane permeabilization. *Journal of Biological Chemistry*, Vol.276, No.50 (September 2001), pp. 47379-47386, ISSN 0021-9258

Lavie, G.; Kaplinsky, C.; Toren, A.; Aizman, I.; Meruelo, D.; Mazur, Y.; Mandel, M. (1999). A photodynamic pathway to apoptosis and necrosis induced by dimethyl tetrahydroxyhelianthrone and hypericin in leukaemic cells: possible relevance to photodynamic therapy. *British Journal of Cancer*, Vol. 79, No.3-4, 1pp. 423-32, ISSN 0007-0920

L'Ecuyer, T; Allebban, Z; Thomas, R; Vander Heide, R. Glutathione S-transferase overexpression protects against anthracycline-induced H9C2 cell death, *American Journal of Physiology, Heart Circulatory Physiology*, 2004; 286(6): 2057-2064, ISSN: 0363-6135

Leibovici, L.; Schoenfeld, N.; Yehoshua, H. A.; Mamet, R.; Rakowsky. E.; Shindel, A.; Atsmon, A. (1988). Activity of porphobilinogen deaminase in peripheral blood mononuclear cells of patients with metastatic cancer. *Cancer*, Vol.62, No.11 (June 2006), pp. 2297–2300, ISSN 0008-543X

Leist, M.; Jaattela, M. (2001). Triggering of apoptosis by cathepsins. *Cell Death and Differentiation*, Vol.8, No.4 (April 2001), pp. 324-326

Lim, D.S.; Ko, S.H.; Lee, W.Y. (2004). Silkworm-pheophorbide a mediated photodynamic therapy against B16F10 pigmented melanoma. *Journal of Photochemistry and Photobiology B: Biology*, Vol.74 (November 2003) pp. 1–6

Link, E.M.; Brown, I.; Carpenter, R.N.; Mitchell, J.S. (1989). Uptake and therapeutic effectiveness of 125I- and 211At-methylene blue for pigmented melanoma in an animal model system. *Cancer Research*, Vol.49, No.15, pp. 4332–4337, ISSN 1000-9604

Lowe, S.W.; Bodis, S.; McClatchey, A.; Remington, L.; Ruley, H.E.; Fisher, D.E.; Housman, D.E.; Jacks, T. (1994). P53 status and efficiency of cancer therapy in vivo. *Science*, Vol.266, No.5186 (November 1994), pp. 807-810, ISSN 0036-8075

Lukšienė, Ž. (2003) Photodynamic therapy: mechanism of action and ways to improve the efficiency of treatment. *Medicina (Kaunas)*, Vol.39, No.12 (August 2003), pp. 1137-1150, ISSN 1010-660X

Luo, Y.; Chang, C.K. & Kessel, D. (1996). Rapid initiation of apoptosis by photodynamic therapy. *Photochemistry and Photobiology*, Vol.63, No.4 (January 2008), pp. 528-534, ISSN 0031-8655

Ma, L.W.; Nielsen, K.P.; Iani, V.; Moan, J. (2007). A new method for photodynamic therapy of melanotic melanoma – effects of depigmentation with violet light photodynamic therapy. *Journal of Environmental Pathology, Toxicology and Oncology,* Vol.26, No.3, pp. 165-72, ISSN 0731-8898

Majno, G.; & Joris, I. (1995). Apoptosis, oncosis and necrosis. An overview of cell death. *American Journal of Pathology,* Vol.146, No.1, pp. 3-15, ISSN 0002-9440

Marchal, S.; Bezdetnaya, L.& Guillemin, F. (2004). Modality of cell death induced by Foscan®-based photodynamic treatment in human colon adenocarcinoma cell line HT29. *Biochemistry (Moscow),* Vol.69, No.1, pp. 45-49, ISSN 0006-2979

Marchetti, P.; Hirsch, T.; Zamzami, N.; Castedo, M.; Decaudin, D.; Susin, S.A.; Masse, B.; Kroemer, G. (1996). Mitochondrial permeability transition triggers lymphocyte apoptosis. *Journal of Immunology,* Vol.157, No.11 (December 1996), pp. 4830-4836, ISSN 0022-1767

Mazur, E.; Stołtny, D.; Kwiatek, S.; Kawczyk-Krupka, A.; Latos, W.; & Sieroń, A. (2010). Diagnostyka (PDD) i terapia fotodynamiczna (PDT) – wskazania i wykorzystanie PDD i PDT w leczeniu uzdrowiskowym. *Acta Balneologica,* LII, Vol.2, pp.107-111

McCord, J.M. (2002). Superoxide dismutase in aging and disease: an overview. *Methods in Enzymology,* Vol.349, pp. 331–341, ISSN 0076-6879

McNair, F.I.; Marples, B.; West, C.M.; & Moore, J.V. (1997). A comet assay of DNA damage and repair in K562 cells after photodynamic therapy using haematoporphyrin derivative, methylene blue and meso-tetrahydroxyphenylchlorin. *British Journal of Cancer,* Vol.75; No.12, pp. 1721–1729, ISSN 0007-0920

Miller, J.D.; Baron, E.D.; Scull, H.; Hsia, A.; Berlin, J.C.; McCormick, T.; Colussi, V.; Kenny, M.E.; Cooper, K.D.; & Oleinick, N.L. (2007). Photodynamic therapy with the phthalocyanine photosensitizer Pc4: the case experience with preclinical mechanistic and early clinical-translational studies. *Toxicology and Applied Pharmacology,* Vol.244, No.3, pp. 290-299, ISSN 0041-008X

Mitsunga, M.; Tsubota, A.; Nariai, K.; Sumi, M.; Yoshikawa, T. (2007). Early apoptosis and cell death induced by ATX-S10Na(II)-mediated photodynamic therapy are Bax- and p53 dependent in human colon cancer cells. World *Journal of Gastroenterology,* Vol.13, No.5 (February 2007), pp. 692-698

Mitton, D.; Ackroyd, R. (2005). History of photodynamic therapy in Great Britain. *Photodiagnosis and Photodynamic Therapy,* Vol.2, No.4 (December 2005), pp. 239-246

Mori, M.; Kuroda, T.; Obana, A.; Sakata, I.; Hirano, T.; Nakajima, S.; Hikida, M.; Kumagai, T. (2000). In vitro plasma protein binding and cellular uptake of ATX-S10(Na), a hydrophilic chlorin photosensitizer. *Japanese Journal of Cancer Research,* Vol.91, No.8, pp. 845-852, ISSN 0910-5050

Morimoto, R.I. (1993). Cells in stress: transcriptional activation of heat shock genes. *Science,* Vol.259, No.5100, pp. 1409–1410, ISSN 0036-8075

Mupidi, J.R.; Tschopp, J. & Siegel, RM. (2004). Life and death decisions: secondary complexes and lipid rafts in TNF-receptor family signal transduction. *Immunity,* Vol.21, No.4 (October 2004), pp. 461-465, ISSN 1074-7613

Nagata, S.; Obana, A.; Gohto, Y.; Nakajima, S. (2003). Necrotic and apoptotic cell death of human malignant melanoma cells following photodynamic therapy using an amphiphilic photosensitizer, ATX-S10(Na). *Lasers in Surgery and Medicine,* Vol.33, No.1, pp. 64-70, ISSN 0196-8092

Nakajima, S.; Sakata, I.; Takemura, T.; Maeda, T.; Hayashi, H.; Kubo, Y. (1992). Tumor localizing and photosensitization of photochlorin ATX-S10. In : *Photodynamic*

Therapy and Biomedical Lasers, S. Spinelli, D. Fante, R. Marchesanin (Ed.), 531-534, Elsevier Science, Amsterdam

Nowak-Sliwinska, P.; Karocki, A.; Elas, M.; Pawlak, A.; Stochel, G.; Urbanska, K. (2006). Verteporfin, Photofrin II and merocyanine 540 as PDT photosensitizers against melanoma cells. *Biochemical and Biophysical Research Communications*, Vol.349, No.2 (August 2006), pp. 549-555, ISSN 0006-291X

Nowis, D.; Legat, M.; Grzela, T.; Niderla, J.; Wilczek, E.; Wilczynski, G.M.; Glodkowska, E.; Mrowka, P.; Issat, T.; Dulak, J.; Jozkowicz, A.; Was, H.; Adamek, M.; Wrzosek, A.; Nazarewski, S.; Makowski, M.; Stoklosa, T.; Jakobisiak, M.; Golab, J. (2006). Heme oxygenase-1 protects tumor cells against photodynamic therapy-mediated cytotoxicity. *Oncogene,* Vol. 25, No.24 (February 2006), pp. 3365-3374, ISSN 0950-9232

Nowis, D.; Makowski, M.; Stokłosa, T.; Legat, M.; Issat, T.; & Gołąb, J. (2005). Direct tumor damage of photodynamic therapy. *Acta Biochimica Polonica*, Vol.52, No.2, pp. 339-352, ISSN 0001-527X

Ochsner, M. (1997) Photophysical and photobiological processes in the photodynamic therapy of tumours. *Journal of Photochemistry & Photobiology, B: Biology*, 1997, 39: 1–18, ISSN1011-1344

Ogura, M.; Sato, S.; Terakawa, M.; Wakisaka, H.; Uenoyama, M.; Ikeda, T.; Ashida, H.; Obara, M. (2003) Delivery of photosensitizer to cells by the stress wave induced by a single nanosecond laser pulse. *Japanese Journal of Applied Physics*, Vol.42, No.8A (August 2003), pp. 977- 979

Patito, I.A.; Rothman, C.H.; Malik, Z. (2001). Nuclear transport of photosensitizers during photosensitization and oxidative stress. *Biology of the Cell*, Vol.93, No.5 (November 2001), pp. 285-291, ISSN 0248-4900

Pazos, M.D.C.; & Nader, H.B. (2007). Effect of photodynamic therapy on the extracellular matrix and associated components. *Brazilian Journal of Medical and Biological Research*, Vol.40, No.8, pp. 1025-1035, ISSN 0100-879X

Peng, Q.; Moan, J.; Nesland, J.M. (1996). Correlation of subcellular and intratumoral photosensitizer localization with ultrastructural features after photodynamic therapy. *Ultrastructural Pathology*, Vol.20, No. 2 (March-April 1996), pp. 109-129, ISSN 0191-3123

Pervaiz, S.; Seyed, M.A.; Hirpara, J.L.; Clement, M.V.; Loh, K.W. (1999). Purified photoproducts of merocyanine 540 trigger cytochrome c release and caspase 8 dependent apoptosis in human leukemia and melanoma cells. *Blood*, Vol. 93, No.12 (June 1999), pp. 4096-4108, ISSN 0006-4971

Plaetzer, K.; Kiesslich, T.; Verwanger, T.; Krammer, B. (2003). The modes of cell death induced by PDT: an overview, *Medical Laser Application*, 2003, 18: 7-19, ISSN: 1615-1615

Plaetzer, K.; Krammer, B.; Berlanda, J.; Berr, F.; Kiesslich, T. (2008). Photophysics and photochemistry of photodynamic therapy: fundamental aspects. *Lasers in Medical Science*, Vol.24, No.2, pp. 259-268, ISSN 0268-8921

Pockley, A.G. (2003). Heat shock proteins as regulators of the immune response. *Lancet*, Vol.362, No.9382, pp. 469–476, ISSN 0140-6736

Rahman, K. (2007). Studies on free radicals, antioxidants, and co-factors. *Clinical Interventions in Aging*, Vol.2, No.2, pp. 219-236, ISSN 1176-9092

Rastogi, R.P.; Richa, & Sinha, R.P. (2009). Apoptosis: molecular mechanisms and pathogenicity. *EXLI Journal*, Vol.8, pp. 155-181, ISSN 1611-2156

Reiners, J.J.Jr.; Caruso, J.A.; Mathieu, P.; Chelladurai, B.; Yin, X.M.; Kessel, D. (2002). Release of cytochrome c and activation of procaspase-9 following lysosomal damage involves Bid cleavage. *Cell Death and Differentiation*, Vol.9, No.9 (September 2002), pp. 934-944

Ricchelli, F.; Jori, G.; Moreno, G.; Vinzens, F.; Salet, C. (1990). Factors influencing the distribution pattern of porphyrins in cell membranes. *Journal of Photochemistry and Photobiology. B, Biology*, Vol.6, No.1-2 (June 1990), pp. 69-77, ISSN 1011-1344

Robertson, C.A.; Hawkins, D.; & Abrahamse, E.H. (2009). Photodynamic therapy (PDT): A short review on cellular mechanisms and cancer research applications for PDT. *Journal of Photochemistry and Photobiology. B, Biology*, Vol.96, No.1, pp. 1-8, ISSN 1011-1344

Roland, C.L.; Harken, A.H.; Sarr, M.G.; Barnett, C.C. (2007). Evidence-based surgical hypothesis: ICAM-1 expression determines malignant potential of cancer. *Surgery*, Vol.141, No.6 (June 2007), pp. 705-707, ISSN 0039-6060

Ryter, S.W.; Kim, H.P.; Hoetzel, A.; Park, J.W.; Nakahira, K.; Wang, X.; & Choi, A.M.K. (2007). Mechanisms of cell death in oxidative stress. *Antioxidant & Redox signaling*, Vol.9, No.1, pp. 49-89, ISSN 1523-0864

Saczko, J.; Kulbacka, J.; Chwiłkowska, A ; Drąg-Zalesińska, M.; Wysocka, T.; Ługowski, M.; & Banaś, T. (2005). The influence of photodynamic therapy on apoptosis in human melanoma cell line. *Folia Histochemica et Cytobiologica*, Vol.43, No.3, pp. 129-132, ISSN 0239-8508

Saczko, J.; Kulbacka, J.; Chwilkowska, A.; Pola, A.; Lugowski, M.; Marcinkowska, A.; Malarska, A. & Banas, T. (2007). Cytosolic superoxide dismutase activity after photodynamic therapy, intracellular distribution of Photofrin II and hypericin, and P-glycoprotein localization in human colon adenocarcinoma. *Folia Histochemica et Cytobiologica*, Vol. 45, No. 2, pp. 93-97, ISSN 0239-8508

Saczko, J.; Kulbacka, L.; Chwiłkowska, A.; Ługowski, M..; Banaś, T. (2007). The response of malignant cells on photodynamic treatment. In: *Aspects of photodynamic medicine*, H. Podbielska, A. Sieroń, W. Stręk (Ed.), 47-56, Kriotechnika Medyczna, Wrocław

Saczko, J.; Mazurkiewicz, M.; Chwilkowska, A.; Kulbacka, J.; Kramer, G.; Lugowski, M.; Snietura, M.; Banas, T. (2007). Intracellular distribution of Photofrin in malignant and normal endothelial cell lines. *Folia Biologica*, Vol.53, No.1, pp. 7-12, ISSN 0015-5500

Saczko, J.; Skrzypek, W.; Chwiłkowska, A.; Choromańska, A.; Poła, A.; Gamian, A.; & Kulbacka, J. (2009). Photo-oxidative action in cervix carcinoma cells induced by HpD-mediated photodynamic therapy. *Experimental Oncology*, Vol.31, No.4, pp. 195-199, ISSN 0204-3564

Santiard, D., Ribiere, C., Nordmann, R., Houee-Levin, C. (1995). Inactivation of Cu,Zn-superoxide dismutase by free radicals derived from ethanol metabolism: a gamma radiolysis study. *Free Radicals in Biology and Medicine*, 19: 121-127, ISSN: 0891-5849

Sheu, SS.; Nauduri, D.; & Anders, M.W. (2006). Targeting antioxidants to mitochondria: A new therapeutic direction. *Biochimica et Biophysica Acta*, Vol.1762, No.2, pp. 256-265, ISSN 0006-3002

Shevchuk, I.N.; Chekulayev, V.A.; & Chekulayeva, L.V. (2002). The role of lipid peroxidation and protein degradation in the photodestruction of Ehrlich ascites carcinoma cells sensitized by hematoporphyrin derivative. *Experimental Oncology*, Vol.24, pp. 216-224, ISSN 0204-3564

Sieroń, A.; & Adamek, M. (1999). Nowe oblicze światłolecznictwa - diagnostyka fluorescencyjna i fotochemoterapia cz.I. *Chirurgia Polska*, 1, 2, 91-99, pp. 91-178, ISSN 1507-5524

Sies, H.; Stahl, W.; & Sundguist, A.R. (1992). Antioxidant functions of vitamins. Vitamin E and C, beta-carotene and other carotenoids. Annals of the New York Academy of Sciences, Vol.669, pp. 7-20, ISSN 0077-8923

Smith, R.P. (2002) Photodynamic therapy. *Current Problems in Cancer*, Vol.26, No.2 (March-April 2002), pp. 67-108, ISSN 0147-027

Szurko, A.; Krämer-Marek, G.; Widel, M.; Ratuszna, A.; Habdas, J.; Kus, P. (2003). Photodynamic effects of two water soluble porphyrins evaluated on human malignant melanoma cells in vitro. *Acta Biochimica Polonica*, Vol. 50, No.4, pp. 1165-1174, ISSN 0001-527X

Tardivo, J.P.; Giglio, A.D.; Oliveira, C.S.; Gabriellib, D.S.; Junqueirab, H.C.; Tadab, D.B.; Severinob, D.; Turchiellob, R.F.; Baptista, M.S. (2005). Methylene blue in photodynamic therapy: from basic mechanisms to clinical applications. *Photodiagnosis and Photodynamic Therapy*, Vol.2, No.3 (November 2005), pp. 175–91, ISSN 1572-1000

Wang, H.P.; Hanlon, J.G.; Rainbow, A.J.; Espiritu, M.; & Singh, G. (2002). Up-regulation of Hsp27 plays a role in the resistance of human colon carcinoma HT29 cells to photooxidative stress. *Photochemistry and Photobiology*, Vol.76, No.1, pp.98-104, ISSN 0031-8655

Wang, X.; Ryter, S.W.; Dai, C.; Tang, Z.L.; Watkins, S.C.; Yin, X.M.; Song, R.; & Choi, A.M. (2003). Necrotic cell death in response to oxidant stress involves the activation of the apoptogenic caspase-8/bid pathway. *Journal of Biological Chemistry*, Vol.278, No.31, pp. 29184-29191, ISSN 0021-9258

Woodburn, K.W.; Fan, Q., Kessel, D.; Luo, Y.; Young, S.W. (1998). Photodynamic therapy of B16F10 murine melanoma with lutetium texaphyrin. *Journal of Investigative Dermatology*, Vol.110 (January 1998), pp. 746–751, ISSN 0022-202X

Woodburn, K.W.; Fan, Q.; Milesm, D.R., Kessel, D.; Luo, Y.; Young S.W. (1998). Localization and efficacy analysis of the phototherapeutic lutetium texaphyrin (PCI-0123) in the murine EMT6 sarcoma model. Photochemistry *and Photobiology*, Vol.65, No.3 (January 2008), pp. 410-415, ISSN 0031-8655

Woods, J.A.; Traynor, N.J.; Brancaleon, L.; & Moseley, H. (2004). The effect of photofrin on DNA strand breaks and base oxidation in HaCaT keratinocytes: a comet assay study. *Photochemistry and Photobiology*, Vol.79, No.1, pp. 105–113, ISSN 0031-8655

Zhang, W.G.; Li, X.W.; Ma, L.P.; Wang, S.W.; Yang, H.Y.; Zhang, Z.Y. (1999). Wild-type p53 protein potentiates phototoxicity of 2-BA-2-DMHA in HT29 cells expressing endogenous mutant p53. *Cancer Letters*, Vol.138, No.1 (April 1999), pp. 189-195, ISSN 0304-3835

Zhen-hui Peng, M.P.; Xiao, S.; Ren, J.; Liu, Y.; Li, X.; Li, Z. (2008). Apoptotic effect and mechanisms of AHPN on human skin malignant melanoma cells. *Journal of Nanjing Medical University*, Vol. 22, No.1 (January 2008), pp. 18-22

Part 6

Clinical Trials

13

Update on Clinical Trials for Malignant Melanoma

Raffaele Califano[1], Ruth Board[2], Aidalena Z Abidin[1], Louise Carter[1], Laura Cove-Smith[1], Bihani Kularatne[3] and Paul Lorigan[1]
[1]*Department of Medical Oncology, The Christie NHS Foundation Trust, Manchester,*
[2]*Rosemere Cancer Centre, Royal Preston Hospital, Sharoe Green Lane, Preston,*
[3]*Department of Medical Oncology, Guy's and St Thomas' NHS Trust, Great Maze Pond, London*
United Kingdom

1. Introduction

After more than 20 years of little improvement in the outcome for patients with malignant melanoma despite a huge international effort spanning basic and clinical research, the last 2 years have shown significant steps forward in treatment options. This year has seen one new drug (Ipilimumab) being licensed and a second (vemurafenib) submitted for approval. This chapter focuses on the key clinical trials in the last 5 years, and gives an indication of the challenges ahead to ensure optimal use of these effective new therapies.

2. Adjuvant treatment

The only agent currently approved in the adjuvant setting for patients with completely resected malignant melanoma is interferon alfa (IFN alfa). A large number of randomised studies evaluating different treatment doses and schedules in a range of American Joint Committee on Cancer (AJCC) stages have been completed.

Despite this, there is still no consensus on the role of IFN as adjuvant treatment and reports have been conflicting in terms of therapeutic efficacy. The majority of studies compared adjuvant IFN to observation alone with a smaller number of studies using vaccines or IFN and chemotherapy as a comparator arm (Kirkwood et al. 2001). This chapter focuses on those studies that have compared interferon to observation only and these are summarised in table 1. Of the 13 published trials, 7 have demonstrated a benefit for IFN over observation in terms of disease free survival (DFS) and 2 have demonstrated an overall survival (OS) benefit (E1684 and DeCOG) (Kirkwood et al. 1996; Garbe et al. 2008)

The Scottish MG trial demonstrated benefits for both DFS and overall survival at 2 years but this diminished with longer follow up and was not statistically significant at 6 years (Cameron et al. 2001).

A meta-analysis of 12 trials was reported in 2003 including 10 trials with IFN compared to observation and 2 studies comparing IFN to a GMK vaccine (Wheatley et al. 2003). This meta-analysis demonstrated a 17% reduction in the risk of recurrence following treatment with IFN compared with control (HR 0.83, $p<0.001$) but no benefit on overall survival (HR 0.93, $p=0.1$).

Trial	Stage	IFN regimen	No	Results
NCCTG (Creagan et al. 1995)	IIA-III	IFN-a 20MU/m^2 im x3/wk x 12wk	IFN=131 Obs=131	DFS: HR 0.83 (0.61-1.13; ns) OS: HR 0.9 (0.64-1.25; ns)
E1684 (Kirkwood et al. 1996)	IIB-III	IFN-a 20MU/m^2 iv x5/wk x4wk then 10MU/ m^2 sc x3/wk x48wk	IFN=147 Obs=140	5yr RFS 37% vs 26% (p=0.0023) 5yr OS 46%vs 37% (p=0.0237)
Austrian MMCG (Pehamberger et al. 1998)	II	IFN-a 3MU sc x7/wk x3wk then 3MU sc x3/wk x49wk	IFN=154 Obs=157	RFS 36% vs 24% (p=0.02) OS 13%vs 11% (ns) Median FU 3.4years
French CGM (Grob et al. 1998)	II	IFN-a 3MU sc x3/wk x18mo	IFN=253 Obs=246	DFS: HR 0.75 (0.57-0.98; p=0.035) OS: HR 0.72 (0.51-1.01; p=0.059)
E1690 (Kirkwood et al. 2000)	IIB-III	High: IFN-a 20MU/m^2 iv x5/wk x4wk then 10MU/ m^2 sc x2/wk x48wk Low: IFN-a 3MU/m^2 sc x3/wk x24mo	IFN High=215 Low=215 Obs=212	DFS: High vs obs: HR 1.28 (1.0-1.65; p=0.05); Low vs Obs: HR 1.19 (0.93-1.53; p=0.17) OS: No differences between the 3 groups.
Scottish MG (Cameron et al. 2001)	IIA-III	IFN-a 3MU sc x3/wk x6mo	IFN=47 Obs=49	Median DFS 22 mo vs 9 mo (ns) Median OS 39mo vs 27mo (ns) Statistically different at 2years but not at 6 years FU
WHO (Cascinelli et al. 2001)	III	IFN-a 3MU sc x3/wk x36mo	IFN=225 Obs=219	5yr DFS 28% vs 28% (p=0.5) 5yr OS 35%vs 37% (p=0.72)
UKCCR (AIMHIGH) (Hancock et al. 2004)	IIB-III	IFN-a 3MU sc x3/wk x24mo	IFN=338 Obs=336	DFS: HR 0.94 (0.75-1.18; p=0.6) OS: HR 0.91 (0.75-1.1; p=0.3)
EORTC18871 (Kleeberg et al. 2004)	IIA-III	IFN-a 1MU sc alt days x12mo	IFN=240 Obs=244	DFS: HR 1.04 (0.84-1.3; ns) OS: HR 0.96 (0.76-1.21; ns)

Trial	Stage	IFN regimen	No	Results
EORTC18952 (Eggermont et al. 2005)	IIB-III	1yr: IFN-a 10MU sc x5/wk x4wk then 10MU sc x3/wk x12mo 2yr: IFN-a 10MU sc x5/wk x4wk then 5MU sc x3/wk x24mo	IFN 1 yr=553 2 yr=556 Obs=279	DFS: 2yr vs obs: HR 0.83 (0.66-1.03; ns); 1yr vs Obs: HR 0.93 (0.75-1.16; ns) OS: No differences between the 3 groups.
DeCOG (Garbe et al. 2008)	III	IFN-a 3MU sc x3/wk x24mo	IFN=148 Obs=148	4yr DFS 59% vs 42% (p=0.0045) 4yr OS 39%vs 27% (p=0.0018)
EORTC18991 (Eggermont et al. 2008)	III	Peg IFN-a 6ug/kg sc x1/wk x8wk then 3mg/kg sc x1/wk x60mo	IFN=627 Obs=629	DFS: HR 0.82 (0.71-0.96; p=0.01) OS: HR 0.98 (0.82-1.16; p=0.78)
Nordic (Mocellin et al. 2010)	IIB-III	1yr: IFN-a 10MU sc x5/wk x4wk then 10MU sc x3/wk x12mo 2yr: IFN-a 10MU sc x5/wk x4wk then 10MU sc x3/wk x24mo	IFN 1 yr=285 2 yr=286 Obs=284	DFS: 2yr vs obs: HR 0.83 (0.68-1.03; p=0.178); 1yr vs Obs: HR 0.77 (0.63-0.96; p=0.034) OS: No differences between the 3 groups.

Abbreviations: IFN-a: interferon alpha; PEG IFN-a: pegylated interferon alpha: DFS, disease free survival; RFS: relapse free survival; OS: overall survival; HR: hazard ratio; wk: week; mo: month; yr: year; sc: subcutaneous; iv: intravenous; im: intramuscular; Obs: observation.

Table 1. Adjuvant studies with Inteferon

An individual patient data (IPD) meta-analysis of 13 trials evaluated efficacy of IFN in high risk melanoma patients (Wheatley 2007). This showed a clear benefit of adjuvant IFN in terms of relapse-free survival (RFS) (HR 0.87, 0.81-0.93; p=0.00004) and an absolute benefit in overall survival of 2% at 10 years (HR 0.9, 0.84-0.97, p=0.008). There was no clear evidence of a difference in outcome by either dose or duration of IFN treatment.

A more recent review and meta-analysis has been published in 2010 and includes 14 trials in total (12 comparing IFN to observation) (Mocellin et al. 2010). This meta-analysis consists of the 12 studies contained in the 2003 report (4 with updated survival data) plus 2 more recent studies (DeCOG and E18991). This demonstrated a relapse-free survival advantage favouring IFN adjuvant treatment (HR 0.82, p<0.001). Original data form 12 of the 14 studies was used to assess overall survival. A statistically significant reduction in risk of death was seen for patients receiving IFN treatment (HR 0.89, p=0.002). No clear differences were identified according to IFN regimen or dose or stage.

Despite the small advantage in OS, the optimal dose and schedule has not been clearly defined. Many of the previous studies used different doses and schedules of IFN and they varied in the inclusion criteria, particularly by stage of disease. The drug itself can have substantial toxicities especially at high doses and can reduce quality of life for the duration of treatment (Bottomley et al. 2009).

Subgroup analyses of adjuvant studies have attempted to define which group of patients who would be most likely to benefit. EORTC 18952 and EORTC 18991 trials stratified patients according to stage of disease and number of lymph nodes involved (Eggermont et al. 2008; Eggermont et al. 2005). Both these studies suggested that the greatest benefit of IFN is seen in stage II or III-N1 disease with reduced advantage of IFN with macroscopic nodal involvement (stage III-N2 disease)

A subgroup analysis of the meta-analysis published in 2007 (Ives et al. 2007) revealed the effect of IFN did not differ according to age, gender, disease site, stage, number of nodes or Breslow thickness. However, patients with ulcerated tumours appeared to have greatest benefit both in terms of disease-free and overall survival ($p<0.03$). Combined post hoc analysis of EORTC 18952 and 18991 studies also demonstrated the greatest reductions in disease-free survival and overall survival in patients with ulcerated tumours (Eggermont 2009). This hypothesis will be tested further in the planned EORTC 18081 trial which will compare PEG-IFNα-2b to observation in patients with ulcerated primary melanoma and a Breslow thickness greater than 1mm.

The subsequent meta-analysis of the EORTC 18952 and 18991 studies showed that the benefit for interferon was confined to patients with ulcerated primary tumours. Conversely, unplanned subgroup analysis of the Nordic trial showed most benefit in patients with highest tumour burden before lymph node dissection and no relationship between benefit of IFN and ulceration of the tumour.

Pegylated interferon (PEG Intron) has been approved as an adjuvant therapy in 2010 on the basis of an improvement in DMFS in patients with resected sentinel node positive disease (Eggermont et al. 2008).

Autoimmunity, as defined by the development of serum autoantibodies and/or clinical vitiligo, has been investigated as a potential predictive factor of efficacy for IFN. In one study, patients receiving high dose IFN who developed autoimmunity (about a quarter of the patients) had an improved DFS and overall survival compared to those patients who did not (Gogas et al. 2006). However, other studies have failed to confirm any associations (Bouwhuis et al. 2009).

Vaccine strategies have also been evaluated in clinical trials, but to date the results have not been encouraging. Three studies (Cancervax stage III, Cancervax stage IV resected and EORTC 18961) have shown a survival disadvantage for these vaccines in this situation, and a further study (ECOG 1694) suggested a survival disadvantage for GMK vaccine. Studies with gp100 vaccines in advanced disease have shown no survival disadvantage (Schwartzentruber et al. 2009; Hodi et al. 2010). It is unclear why these adjuvant studies were negative but it encourages caution in employing long term vaccine based immune stimulation as an adjuvant therapy.

The adjuvant treatment of intermediate and high risk melanoma patients still varies greatly from country to country, with greater use of adjuvant interferon in USA and some North European Countries. Participating in a clinical trial remains the preferred option for these patients and most of randomised studies currently ongoing still include an observation arm.

The DERMA trial (NCT00796445) is currently randomising MAGE-A3 positive patients with high risk (stage III) melanoma to receive a MAGE peptide vaccine plus adjuvant or placebo. A total of 1300 patients are planned to be enrolled. Prespecified subgroup analysis will examine whether apreviously identified genetic classifier can predict those likely to benefit form treatment (Kruit et al. 2008).

The European Organisation for the Research and Treatment of Cancer (EORTC) Melanoma Group is conducting a randomised double-blind phase III trial (EORTC 18071) evaluating Ipilimumab, a blocking antibody to CTLA4, versus placebo in patients with completely resected stage III disease (NCT00636168). Ipilimumab has recently been approved by the FDA for the treatment of advanced disease. A study comparing ipilimumab to high dose IFN in high risk disease is also planned (NCT01274338).

The AVAST-M study is a large randomised study enrolling across the United Kingdom. Patients with completely resected stage IIb-III melanoma are randomised to receive bevacizumab 7.5 mg/kg every 3 weeks for 1 year or observation. The planned sample is 1320 patients and the study aims to identify an 8% difference in overall survival. Relapse-free survival, quality of life, toxicity and biomarkers are secondary end points.

All 3 studies have nearly completed accrual and results will bee available in the next 3-5 years, depending on the mix of risk groups included. The outcomes of these studies, and developments in treatment of advanced disease, will determine the landscape of adjuvant therapy and clinical trials over the next 5-10 years.

3. Advanced disease

The last 20 years have seen a huge body of work trying to improve outcomes for patients with advanced melanoma, with no real benefits. The median survival in recent chemotherapy studies has improved over historical controls, but in the main this has been due to better patient selection and stage migration due to improved imaging techniques. This is now changing very quickly.

Where once we could design clinical trials with an overall survival endpoint, confident that the outcome would not be affected by subsequent treatment, we now have a number of new drugs with either a proven survival benefit, or preliminary data to suggest that this will be the case. Here we review the pivotal clinical trials and their implications for treatment.

3.1 Standard chemotherapy

Single agent dacarbazine (DTIC) became the standard first-line chemotherapy based on a response rate of 10-20% in Phase II studies. No studies have ever been conducted to evaluate single agent chemotherapy against placebo or best supportive care. For this reason, the impact of treatment with DTIC on survival remains unclear.

Temozolamide (TMZ) is an oral alkylating agent and, together with DTIC, a prodrug of the active alkylating agent 5-(3-methyltriazen-1-yl) imidazole-4-carboximide (MTIC). Unlike DTIC, temozolamide spontaneously convert to MTIC.

A large phase III study compared overall survival of 305 chemonaive advanced melanoma patients treated with TMZ (200 mg/m2/d for 5 days every 28 days) or intravenous DTIC (250 mg/m2/d for 5 days every 21 days) (Middleton et al. 2000). The trial was designed to detect a 50% increase in survival compared with the 6 months expected with DTIC. Median progression-free survival (PFS) time was improved for temozolomide (1.9 v 1.5 months; HR 1.37; p=0.012). However, objective response was assessed every two cycles and this could explain the longer PFS interval for the temozolamide arm. Patients in the temozolomide arm experienced longer overall survival, which did not reach statistical significance (7.9 vs 5.7 months; p=0.054). There was no difference in response rates between the two arms (CR rate of 2.6% vs 2.7% and PR rate of 10.9% vs 9.4% for temozolamide and DTIC arm, respectively). Both treatments were well tolerated. Most common grade 3/4 haematological toxicity was thrombocytopenia. Quality of life (QoL) at 12 weeks (QLQ-030 scores) showed a statistically significant difference favouring TMZ for physical functioning, fatigue, and insomnia. This trial demonstrated that TMZ represents an effective alternative to DTIC with potential advantage in QoL. Temozolamide did not receive regulatory approval for use in advanced melanoma, but there is a large use for off-label temozolamide chemotherapy, particularly in patients with brain metastases.

A large study conducted by the European Organization for Research and Treatment of Cancer (EORTC 18032) (Patel et al. 2008), randomized 859 patients with untreated stage IV melanoma, performance status 0-1 and LDH≤ 2x ULN to receive TMZ 150 mg/mg/m2 day 1-7 repeated every 14 days ("week on-week off") or DTIC 1000 mg/m2 every 3 weeks. Both treatments were given until progression. The extended schedule allowed a 2.1 fold higher cumulative dose than the standard 5-days regimen and was thought to prolong depletion of the DNA repair enzyme MGMT, a know mediator of chemoresistance to temozolomide. Overall survival, did not differ between TMZ and DTIC (9.13 vs 9.36 months, p=1.0). There was also no difference in PFS (2.3 vs 2.17 months, p=0.27) and response rate (14% vs 10%, p=0.05) between the two groups. Thrombocytopenia was higher in the TMZ arm but there were no differences in non-haematological toxicities.

Despite well tolerated, the extended schedule temozolamide regimen confers no survival advantage over standard DTIC.

3.2 Biochemotherapy vs chemotherapy

Several randomized trials have evaluated chemotherapy combined with immunotherapy (IFN ± IL-2; ie, biochemotherapy) in an attempt to improve both response rates and overall survival (OS) in the advanced setting. A metaanalysis by Ives et al, evaluated the effect of adding interferon-α (IFNα) ± interleukin-2 (IL-2) to chemotherapy in patients with metastatic melanoma (Ives et al. 2007). Data was extracted from 18 trials with more than 2600 patients. Eleven trials (1395 patients) evaluated chemotherapy ± IFN and seven trials (1226 patients) evaluated chemotherapy ± IFN and IL-2.

Patients treated with biochemotherapy had increased PR (odds ratio = 0.66; 95% CI, 0.53 to 0.82; p=0.0001), CR (odds ratio = 0.50; 95% CI, 0.35 to 0.73; p=0.0003), and overall response rate (odds ratio = 0.59; 95% CI, 0.49 to 0.72; p<0.00001). There was a significant increase in overall response rate (ORR) for both the immunotherapy subgroups; IFN (odds ratio = 0.60; 95% CI, 0.46 to 0.79; p=0.0002) and IFN+IL-2 (odds ratio = 0.58; 95% CI, 0.44 to 0.77; p=0.0001). For PR (test for heterogeneity between subgroups; p=0.08) and CR (p=0.007) there was some evidence of a difference in treatment effect dependent on the type of immunotherapy used (IFN or IFN + IL-2). Biochemotherapy delayed the time to disease progression (odds ratio = 0.80; 95% CI, 0.71 to 0.89; p=0.0001), with no evidence of heterogeneity between individual trials or between the type of immunotherapy used. Despite improvement in response rate and PFS, there was no benefit for biochemotherapy on OS (odds ratio = 0.99; 95% CI, 0.91 to 1.08; p=0.9). Toxicity data was available only from 11 trials. Hematological toxicity was higher in the biochemotherapy arm but the treatment-related deaths rate was similar (0.6% vs 0.9%, p=0.6) for biochemotherapy group and chemotherapy group, respectively. These data suggest no benefit form adding IL-2 or IFN to chemotherapy.

3.3 Single agent vs combination chemotherapy

A number of combination chemotherapies have been evaluated for advanced melanoma. These regimens seemed promising in II trials, but failed to show survival advantage over DTIC alone when tested in randomized phase III trials.

The two most active combinations are the four-drug combination of cisplatin, DTIC, carmustine (BCNU), and tamoxifen (the Dartmouth regimen) and cisplatin, vinblastine, and DTIC (the CVD regimen).

The Dartmouth regimen was initially evaluated in 42 patients and demonstrated a response rate of 54% and overall survival of 412 days (Lattanzi et al. 1995). The Darthmouth regimen was then evaluated against DTIC in a large (n=240) phase III randomized trial (Chapman et al. 1999). Patients receiving the Dartmouth regimens achieved higher response rates, but the difference was not statistically significant (18.5% vs 10.2%, p=0.09). Median survival time from randomization was 7 months and there was no difference in survival time between the two treatment arms. Bone marrow suppression, nausea/vomiting, and fatigue were significantly more common in the Dartmouth arm. This trial demonstrated that polichemotherapy did not improve survival compared to single agent chemotherapy and crowned DTIC as the standard regimen in advanced Melanoma.

The CVD regimen was evaluated in a phase II trial in 52 patients (Legha et al. 1989). Overall response rate was 40% and median survival was 9 months. The treatment was associated with significant nausea, vomiting and diarrhea. On the basis of these promising results, a phase III trial evaluating CVD vs DTIC was conducted and showed a response rate of 24% and 11%, respectively with no difference in median survival between the two groups (6.7 vs 5.2 months) (Buzaid et al. 1993). (Results of the trials evaluating combination chemotherapy are summarized in table 2)

Because of the lack of improvement in overall survival and the worse toxicity achieved with polichemotherapy regimens, DTIC remains the preferred option as first-line chemotherapy in advanced/metastatic melanoma patients.

Author	Regimen	No	Response rate (%)	OS (mos)
Lattanzi (Lattanzi et al. 1995)	DTIC+C+BCNU	16	25	412 days
	DTIC+C+BCNU+ Tam (Dartmouth)	26	54	412 days
Chapman (Chapman et al. 1999)	Dartmouth	119	18.5	7.7
	DTIC	121	10.2	6.3
Legha (Legha et al. 1989)	CVD	52	40	12
Buzaid (Buzaid et al. 1993)	CVD	46	24	6.7
	DTIC	45	11	5.2

Abbreviations: DTIC: Dacarbazine; C: Cisplatin; BCNU: carmustine; Tam: Tamoxifen: CVD: cisplatin, vinblastine, dacarbazine; Dartmouth: dacarbazine + cisplatin + carmustine + tamoxifen; OS: overall survival; mos: months

Table 2. Phase II-III trials of polichemotherapy for advanced melanoma.

4. Immunotherapy

Melanoma cells can express a number of antigens that excite an immune response, as borne out by the better prognosis seen in patients with evidence of immune activation (vitiligo), the occasional case of spontaneous regression, the better outcome for patients with unknown primary (Chang and Knapper 1982; Lee et al. 2008), the increased incidence of melanoma seen in immunocompromised patients, and the response to immunotherapy agents including interferon alpha and interleukin 2.

4.1 Adoptive cell therapy

The ability to isolate and characterize anti-tumor lymphocyte has enabled the identification and characterization of multiple melanoma-associated antigens that can represent target of immunotherapy. Adoptive cell therapy (ACT) describes an immunotherapy approach in which tumor infiltrating lymphocytes (TIL) are harvested form fresh tumour tissue, expanded ex vivo and then reinfused after the patient has been lymphodepleted. Critical components of this complex process include the number, age and type of TILS, the degree of immunosupression of the host, and the use of IL-2 after reinfusion.

Dudley et al, reported on 3 consecutive trials involving 93 patients in total (Dudley et al. 2008). In the first study, 43 patients received non-myeloablative chemotherapy consisting of cyclophosphamide and fludarabine before the TIL transfer. On the two next trials, patients were treated with 2 days of cyclophosphamide (60 mg/kg) plus 5 days of fludarabine (25 mg/m2) followed by a single fraction of 2 Gy of total body irradiation (TBI) (n=25) or 12 Gy of TBI (n=25). On the day following the final dose of TBI, patients received cell infusion with TIL and started high-dose IL-2 consisting of 720,000 IU/kg intravenously every 8 hours to tolerance. One or 2 days after TIL infusion, cryopreserved CD34+ hematopoietic stem cells were infused intravenously. Thirty seven percent of the patients had received previous chemotherapy and 83% had received previous IL-2. The response rates in these 3 studies were 48.8 %, 52% and 72%, respectively. Response of the marker lesions was seen in all visceral and soft tissue sites, including brain. Ten patients achieved a complete response with no relapses at 31-month follow-up. The median follow-up of these trials was 45, 27 and 10 months, respectively and there was no difference in survival between the groups (p=0.13) bearing in mind that the follow-up of the third trial is quite short. These studies demonstrate that ACT has the potential of improve the outcomes of a highly selected patient population, but its use at present should remains strictly as part of clinical trials.

4.2 Cytotoxic T lymphocyte-associated antigen 4 (CTLA 4) blockade

CTLA 4 is a key molecule in T-cell tolerance that serves as a natural braking mechanism for T-cell activation, allowing a return to homeostasis following an immune response. T-cell activation requires engagement of the T-cell receptor to antigen-bound major histocompatibility complex (MHC) on the antigen-presenting cell (APC) as well as engagement of the costimulatory molecule CD28 on the T-cell surface by members of the B7 family on the APC. Following T-cell activation, CTLA 4 cell-surface receptors are upregulated and compete with CD28 for binding to B7 sending an inhibitory signal that downregulates T-cell activation.

This led to the hypothesis that blocking the CTLA 4-B7 interaction would lead to enhanced and prolonged T-cell activation with subsequent more vigorous antitumor immune response.

Two anti-CTLA 4 blocking antibodies have been evaluated in clinical trials: tremelimumab (formerly CP-675,206 or ticilimumab) and ipilimumab (formerly MDX010)

4.3 Tremelimumab

Tremelimumab is a fully human IgG2 monoclonal antibody specific for human CTLA 4. A Phase II study in 251 previously treated paitents with advanced disease reported a median survival of 10 months (Kirkwood et al. 2010)

A phase III trial randomized 655 patients with unresectable stage IIIC and stage IV melanoma without brain metastasis and LDH below twice the upper limit of normal to receive tremelimumab 15 mg/kg every 3 months vs chemotherapy (TMZ 200 mg/m^2 p.o. d1-5 q28d or DTIC 1,000 mg/m^2 IV q21d) (Ribas et al. 2008). The study was stopped early by the data safety monitoring committee after the second interim analysis because of futility. The median OS by was 11.8 months (95% CI 10.4, 13.9) in the tremelimumab arm, and 10.7 months (95% CI 9.3, 12.0) in the chemotherapy arm. Subgroup analysis of this trial has suggested that patients with low baseline C-reactive protein had improved survival (median OS: 19.1 vs 12.7 months, $p = 0.0037$) with tremelimumab compared with chemotherapy. (Marshall, Ribas, and Huang 2010)

4.4 Ipilimumab

Ipilimumab is a fully human monoclonal immunoglobulin (IgG1k) specific for CTLA-4 that was investigated in three phase II trials (study 007, 008, and 022), enrolling a total of 487 treatment-naive and pretreated patients with unresectable stage III or stage IV melanoma. Study 007 randomized 115 pretreated and treatment naive patients to receive ipilimumab (10 mg/kg every 3 weeks, for four doses) with prophylactic budesonide/placebo to prevent colitis (Weber et al. 2009) Budesonide did not affect the rate of grade ≥2 diarrhea and median survival was 17.7 vs 19.3 months for the budesonide and placebo group, respectively. The one-year survival was greater than 55%.

Study 008 was a single-arm phase II trial investigating ipilimumab at the dose of 10 mg/kg in 155 pretreated patients (O'Day et al. 2010). Best overall response rate (BORR) was 5.8% with a disease control rate (DCR) of 27% and a median overall survival of 10.2 months. The 1-year survival rate was 47.2% and ongoing survival analyses showed 18- and 24-month survival rates of 39.4% and 32.8%, respectively. Most common adverse events (AEs) were immune-related, occurring mainly in the skin (grade 3/4: 3.2%) and gastrointestinal tract (grade 3/4: 8.4%). Study 022 was a randomized, double blind, phase 2 trial that assessed three different doses of ipilimumab (0.3 mg/kg, 3.0 mg/kg, or 10 mg/kg) in 217 pretreated patients (Wolchok et al. 2010). Patients were treated with four 3-weekly doses (induction phase), then patients without PD at week 24 were eligible to continue their assigned dose of ipilimumab every 12 weeks (maintenance phase). Only 20 patients received maintenance therapy. Patients progressing after an initial response or stable disease were allowed to undergo reinduction with ipilimumab at the dose of 10 mg/kg. There was a clear dose response with a statistically significant improvement in best overall response rate with the 10 mg/kg dose (BORR 11.1%). Despite the study was not designed to detect differences in survival, there was a trend for improved overall survival favoring the dose of 10 mg/kg that did not reach statistical significance (8.6 vs 8.7 vs 11.4 months). Most common AEs (skin rash and diarrhea) were immune-related and the frequency rose with increasing dose of ipilimumab. The authors concluded that the dose of 10 mg/kg warranted further evaluation.

Phase II trials of ipilimumab in advanced melanoma are summarized in table 3.

Study	Dose (mg/kg)	Population	No	ORR (%)	DCR (%)	MS (mos)	1y-S (%)
007	10 + budesonide	pre-treated and untreated	58	12	31	17.7	55.9
	10 + placebo		57	16	35	19.3	62.4
008	10	pre-treated	155	5.8	27	10.2	47
022	0.3	pre-treated	73	0	13.7	8.6	39.6
	3	pre-treated	72	4.2	26.4	8.7	39.3
	10	pre-treated	72	11.1	29.2	11.4	48.6

Abbreviations: No: number; ORR: overall response rate; DCR: disease control rate; MS: median survival; mos: months; 1y-s: 1-year survival

Table 3. Phase II trials of ipilimumab in advanced Melanoma

A recently published large phase III trial randomized 676 pretreated HLA-A*0201-positive patients with unresectable stage III or IV melanoma to receive, in a 3:1:1 ratio, ipilimumab plus gp100 (n=403 patients), ipilimumab alone (n=137), or gp100 alone (n=136). (Hodi et al. 2010). Ipilimumab was administered at the dose of 3 mg/kg every three weeks, for four cycles. Patients with stable disease for 3 months after week 12 or a confirmed partial or complete response were offered additional courses of therapy (reinduction) with their assigned treatment regimen, at disease progression. The original primary endpoint was the best overall response rate but this was amended to overall survival. Seventy seven (out of 82) patients had central nervous system metastasis at baseline and received at least one dose of ipilimumab. The median overall survival was 10.0 vs 10.1 vs 6.4 months for the ipilimumab-gp100, ipilimumab alone and gp100 alone arms, respectively.

There was no difference in overall survival between the two ipilimumab groups (HR 1.04; p=0.76). The median progression-free survival was 2.76 months in the ipilimumab-gp100 group, 2.86 months in the ipilimumab-alone group, and 2.76 months in the gp100-alone group. One-year survival and 2-year survival for ipilimumab-plus-gp100 group, the ipilimumab-alone group, and the gp100-alone group were 43.6%, 45.6%, 25.3% and 21.6%, 23.5%, 13.7%, respectively. Consistently with phase 2 data, most common adverse events were immune-related and most affected were skin and gastrointestinal tract. Other serious AEs included hepatitis and endocrinopathies. Grade 3/4 colitis occurred in 3-5% of the patients treated in the ipilimumab-gp100 and ipilimumab-alone arm, respectively. There were 14 treatment-related deaths (2.1%), of which 7 were associated with immune-related adverse events. This study was restricted to patients that were HLA-A2 positive, because the vaccine is presented in a HLA restricted fashion. However, CTLA-4 blockade by ipilimumab is independent of HLA status therefore HLA-typing patients who are suitable to receive ipilimumab is not necessary.

This trial is, so far, the only trial showing a survival advantage in the history of melanoma and has set a new standard of care. On the basis of these results, US Food and Drug Administration (FDA) has recently approved ipilimumab for treatment of unresectable or metastatic melanoma.

Bristol Myers Squibb has also announced that a first-line trial (CA180-024) has met its primary end point demonstrating improvement in overall survival with ipilimumab in combination with dacarbazine vs dacarbazine alone. Data will be presented at the forthcoming ASCO Annual Meeting 2011 and are eagerly awaited.

4.5 Immune-related response criteria

The pattern and duration of responses associated with CTLA 4 blockade differ from those associated with cytotoxic agents. Objective responses to ipilimumab may not occur until the post-induction period of therapy and may occur, in some cases, after PD as defined by WHO or RECIST criteria.

Four patterns of response to ipilimumab have been identified: 1) initial response in baseline lesions, 2) stable disease with subsequent slow and steady decline in total tumor volume, 3) response after increase in total tumor volume, 4) reduction in total tumor burden after the appearance of new lesions.

The apparent increase in tumor burden that sometimes happens before an objective response could be either related to continue tumor growth until a sufficient immune response develops or transient immune cells infiltrate that can cause edema.

In order to provide a more comprehensive assessment of clinical activity of these agents, the immune-related response criteria (IrRC) have been developed as a variation of WHO criteria (Wolchok et al. 2009). Using these criteria, new lesions do not always represent progressive disease, and the criteria for calculating response or progression have been modified. The immune-relate response criteria may help to explain why patients with apparent PD by the traditional response criteria go on to experience long-term survival.

5. Targeted agents

The identification of an activating mutation in braf in 50-60% of cutaneous melanoma samples (Davies et al. 2002), and the fact that in this was primarily a single codon mutation, resulting in the V600E mutation in the vast majority of cases, opened up the field to the potential for targeted therapy. Since then, it has been shown that approximately 50-70% of cutaneous melanomas have a mutation in the mAP kinase pathway, either BRAF or NRAS, and approximately 20% of acral lentigenous melanomas have a mutation in c-kit (Curtin et al. 2005; Curtin et al. 2006). The identification of potential targets resulted in the design of a number of targeted therapies, which have been evaluated in clinical trials.

5.1 Sorafenib

Sorafenib (Nexavar®, Bayer Healthcare Pharmaceuticals) is a multikinase inhibitor with potent non-selective action against RAF1, with additional broad-spectrum activity against VEGFR-2, VEGFR-3, PDGFR-β, the tyrosine kinase FLT3 and KIT receptors. It is one of the first small molecules to be tested in the treatment of melanoma.

Its use as a single agent treatment did not seem to confer any meaningful benefit in melanoma patients (Eisen et al. 2006). A phase II trial investigating the combination of sorafenib/placebo and dacarbazine showed promising results, with an improvement in progression-free survival (21.1 weeks vs 11.7 weeks, HR 0.665; p=0.068 for sorafenib and placebo arm, respectively) but no improvement in overall survival (45.6 vs 51.3 weeks HR=1.022; p=0.927, for sorafenib and placebo, respectively) for patients receiving dacarbazine/sorafenib combination (McDermott et al. 2008).

Two large phase III trials investigated sorafenib in combination with carboplatin/paclitaxel chemotherapy.
The PRISM study evaluated carboplatin/paclitaxel (CP) with sorafenib/placebo in a phase III randomized study as a second-line treatment for unresectable stage III or stage IV melanoma patients. There was no improvement in either median PFS (17.9 vs 17.4 weeks, HR=0.91; p=0.49, for CP/placebo and CP/sorafenib, respectively) or median OS (42.0 weeks for both arms, p=0.92) (Hauschild et al. 2009). More recently, results from a first-line phase III trial (E2603 intergroup trial) have been reported. This trial randomized 823 previously untreated patients with metastatic melanoma, to receive sorafenib or placebo in combination with CP. The study crossed the futility boundaries and therefore was stopped and unblinded after 75% of the events required for the final analysis were reached. There was no improvement in median OS (11.0 vs 11.3 months in sorafenib and placebo, respectively, p=N/A), and no difference in median PFS (4.9 vs 4.1 months, p=0.48 for sorafenib and placebo, respectively (Flaherty, Lee et al. 2010).

5.2 BRAF selective inhibitors

Vemurafenib (RG7204, PLX4032), is an orally available inhibitor of mutated BRAF has the most clinical evidence accrued thus far. Preliminary data from the phase I trial of PLX4032 was reported in 2010 in the New England Journal of Medicine (Flaherty, Puzanov et al. 2010). The trial enrolled 55 patients, of which 49 diagnosed with melanoma, in a dose escalation phase and further 32 patients harbouring the BRAF V600E mutation enrolled in an extension phase receiving the recommended dose of 960 mg twice daily. Among the 16 patients with melanoma receiving 240 mg twice a day or more the overall response rate was 69%. Five patients with metastatic melanoma without BRAF mutations were treated with no evidence of tumour response. Notably, in the extension phase, 26 out of 32 (81%) patients treated had an objective response. The estimated median progression-free survival in these patients is 7 months and the estimated median overall survival has not yet been reached. The most common grade 2 or 3 adverse events were arthralgia, fatigue and skin-related toxicity including 18 patients with cutaneous squamous cell carcinomas (keratoacanthoma type) treated with excision without interruption of treatment. Of the adverse events observed, 89% were grade 1 and 2.
The exciting results showed in the phase I trial prompted the design of the phase II trial of RG7204 in previously treated patients with metastatic melanoma harbouring a BRAF V600E mutation (BRIM 2 trial). This data was presented by Sosman and colleagues at The Seventh International Melanoma Research Congress of the Society for Melanoma Research, in November 2010 (Sosman et al. 2010). BRIM 2 (NCT00949702) was a single arm, multicentre, open label phase II trial in which 132 patients received RG7204 until progression. Primary endpoint was overall response rate. The presence of the V600E BRAF mutation was confirmed with the cobas® 4800 BRAF V600 mutation test developed by Roche. The ORR was 52% and 30% of patients achieved stable disease. The median PFS was 6.2 months and, as with the phase I trial, median overall survival has not yet been reached. Consistently to what observed in the phase I trial, most common adverse events observed were arthralgia and skin toxicity, including 26% grade 3 cutaneous squamous cell carcinoma. However, fourteen percent of the patients also experienced grade 3 abnormalities in liver function tests and 10% Grade 3 dysphagia and pancreatitis
The confirmation of clinical efficacy from the phase two trial led to the design of BRIM 3 (NCT01006980), a large phase III randomized trial evaluating RG7204 head to head with

dacarbazine in previously untreated patients with metastatic melanoma harbouring BRAF V600E mutation. This study has recently terminated accrual and a recent press release from Roche has showed that RG7204 met its co-primary endpoints. Patients treated with the BRAF selective inhibitor have achieved longer OS and PFS than the chemotherapy arm. Final data will be presented at the ASCO Annual Meeting 2011(Roche 2011). Since the interim analysis data, the trial protocol has been amended so that patients in the dacarbazine arm who have progressed have now the option to crossover to receive RG7204.
Other BRAF selective inhibitors are now in clinical development. GSK2118436 is a potent oral selective ATP competitive BRAF inhibitor. The results from phase I/II dose escalation study of GSK2118436 in melanoma and other solid tumours were reported at ASCO 2010. When reported, maximum tolerated dose had not been reached but clinical activity with minimal toxicity was seen. The most common grade 3/4 toxicities reported were skin changes, headache, nausea, fatigue and vomiting and low grade squamous cell carcinoma in order of reducing frequency. Notably, 79% of patients with BRAF mutation were shown to have exposure-related decrease in FDG-PET metabolic uptake and 60% had a >20% reduction in tumour size by RECIST at initial restaging (Kefford et al. 2010).
A phase III study is ongoing and will compare GSK2118436 to dacarbazine (DTIC) in previously untreated subjects with BRAF V600E mutation positive advanced (Stage III) or metastatic (Stage IV) melanoma. (NCT01227889). Another phase II trial is evaluating GSK2118436 in BRAF Mutant stage IV melanoma with brain metastases (NCT01266967). The RAS/RAF/MEK/ERK pathway is shown in figure 1.

5.3 MEK inhibitors

MEK 1 and 2 belong to a family of dual specificity kinases which are downstream of RAF in the mitogen activated protein kinase signalling cascade (Crews, Alessandrini, and Erikson 1992; Rosen et al. 1994). ERK1/2 is constitutively active in melanoma cells regardless of their BRAF or NRAS status, presenting a potential target for treatment in this population. Phosphorylated ERK is important for melanoma because it plays key roles in cell cycle entry, invasion, and possibly angiogenesis, as well as in resistance to apoptosis (Smalley 2003). AZD6244 is a highly selective allosteric inhibitor of MEK1/2. Treatment with AZD6244 leads to suppression of pERK levels in melanoma in a manner independent of BRAF and NRAS mutation status (Haass et al. 2008). Single agent therapy of melanoma with AZD6244 has been disappointing.
The interim results from a phase 2 study of the safety and efficacy of AZD6244 versus temozolomide in patients with advanced melanoma were reported in 2008. This was an open label randomised multicentre phase 2 study which randomized 200 patients with untreated stage III or IV melanoma to receive AZD6244 or temozolamide. There was no difference in PFS between the two treatment arms in the overall population (HR 1.07; 80% CI 0.86-1.34) or in the BRAF mutant subgroup (HR 0.85; 80% CI 0.58-1.24). Overall survival data are immature (67 deaths) but the interim analysis showed no difference between the two arms in the overall population (HR 1.23; 80% CI 0.88-1.71). Mutation status was assessed in archival tissue and 67 (50%) cutaneous melanoma patients had a BRAF mutation and 24 (18%) patients had a mutation in NRAS. In BRAF mutant patients, the HR estimate for OS favoured AZD6244 (HR 0.68; 80% CI 0.38-1.21) (Dummer et al. 2008).
A randomised phase II study (AZD Study 6, NCRN063) that randomised 91 BRAF V600E mutant patients to receive DTIC + AZD6244/placebo has completed accrual in 2010 and the results are awaited.

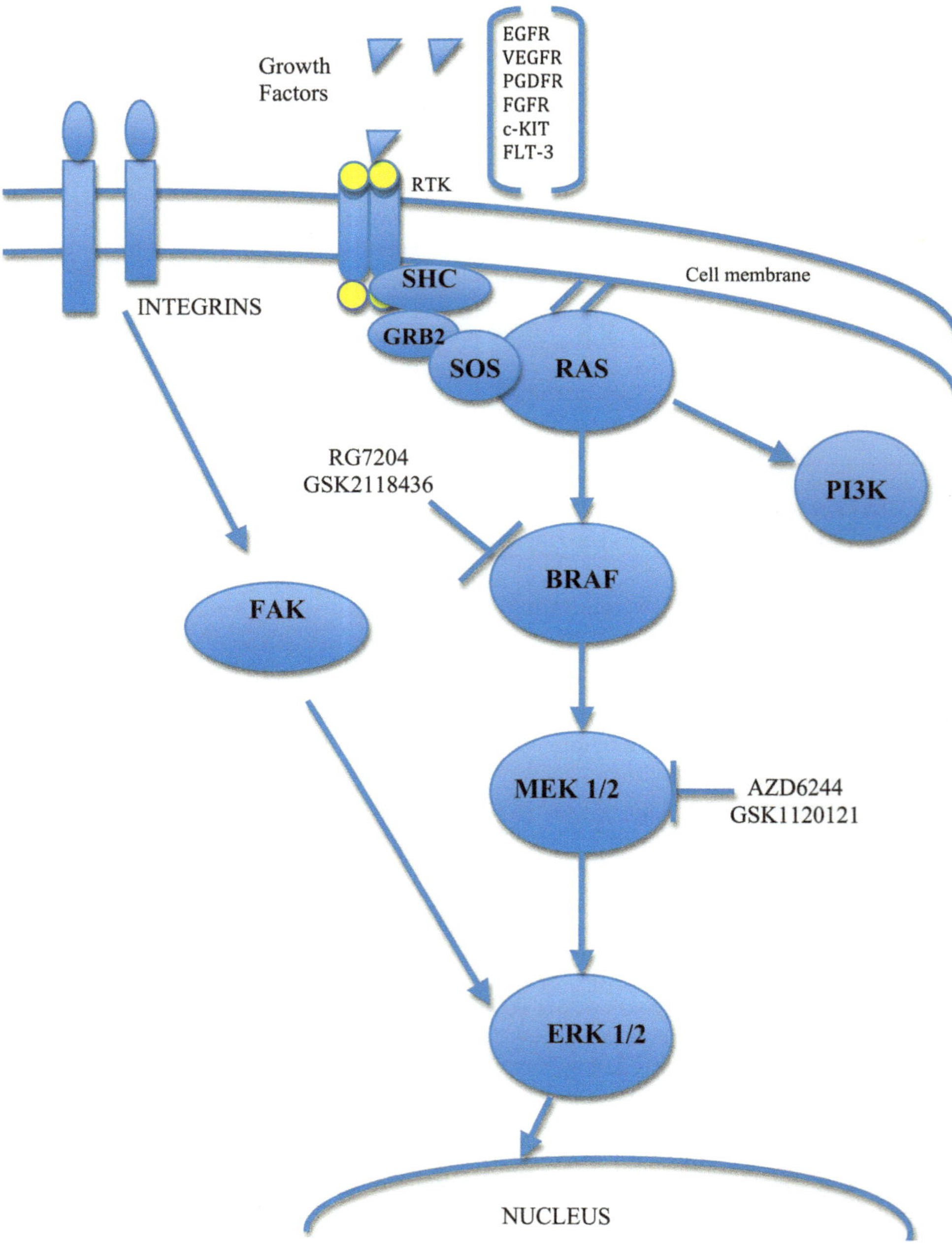

Fig. 1. The RAS/RAF/MEK/ERK pathway

AZD6244 and docetaxel have demonstrated synergy in a variety of animal xenograft models, including melanoma. Furthermore, a patient with wild type BRAF and NRAS treated with AZD6244 showed a response to treatment in the initial study. A phase 1 study of the combination of AZD6244 and docetaxel has been conducted (Astrazeneca study D1532C00004) in 12 patients with melanoma: 1 had a complete response; 1 a partial response; 4 had stable disease beyond 6 cycles of treatment (18+ weeks) indicating clinical activity worthy of further study.
DOC-MEK is a first-line randomised, double-blind placebo controlled phase 2 trial, that randomizes BRAF wild-type stage IV melanoma to receive docetaxel 75mg/m2 IV and placebo/AZD6244.
GSK1120212 is a potent and selective allosteric inhibitor of the MEK1/2 enzymes. A three-part phase I trial evaluating GSK1120212 in 84 patients with advanced solid tumors and lymphoma was reported at ASCO 2010 (Infante et al. 2010). This trial included 29 melanoma and 15 pancreatic cancer patients. The maximum tolerated dose was found to be 3 mg OD and recommended phase II dose (RP2D) chosen was 2 mg OD. At doses ≥ RP2D (n=77), the most common adverse events were rash (30% G2, 5% G3) and diarrhea (9% G2, 3% G3). In the 20 evaluable melanoma patients with known BRAF status, 5 PR were observed, all having ≥ 50% tumor reduction; 3 have stayed ≥ 30 weeks on study, the other 2 are ongoing. In the 11 BRAF mutant melanoma patients, 3 PR, 5 SD (including a patient previously treated with the BRAF inhibitor RG7204), and 3 PD were observed. Two of the 3 PD were due to new brain lesions. In 9 BRAF wild-type patients with melanoma, 2 PR, including a patient with a GNAQ mutation, and 3 SD were achieved.
A Phase II open-label, multi-site study to investigate the objective response rate, safety, and pharmacokinetics of GSK1120212 in subjects with BRAF mutation-positive melanoma who were previously treated with or without a BRAF inhibitor has completed accrual and is ongoing.
The recently initiated METRIC Phase 3 study will compare (2:1 randomisation) GSK1120212 vs DTIC (untreated patients) or paclitaxel (previously treated patients) in advanced or metastatic melanoma harbouring BRAF V600 E/K mutation. The primary endpoint is PFS and subjects who have progression on chemotherapy will be offered the option to cross over to receive GSK1120212.

5.4 Bevacizumab

Bevacizumab is a monoclonal antibody that acts indirectly to prevent angiogenesis by binding the VEGF-A receptors, thus preventing the interaction with VEGFR2. Melanoma cells, when exposed to chemotherapy agents, overproduce VEGF thus encouraging the development of chemoresistant tumour phenotypes. There is evidence of increased production of angiogenic factors with more advanced stage of melanoma (Lev et al. 2004; Ugurel et al. 2001). For this reason bevacizumab was investigated as a treatment for melanoma.
A number of phase II trials with bevacizumab in combination with chemotherapy have been reported so far. The BEAM trial randomized (2:1) 214 patients to carboplatin/taxol + bevacizumab or placebo, in the first-line setting. There was an improvement in progression-free survival (primary endpoint) in the bevacizumab arm compared to placebo (5.6 months vs 4.2 months, HR 0.78, p=0.16), which did not reach statistically significance. Notably there was a non statistically significant improvement in OS (secondary endpoint) (12.3 vs 9.2 months, HR=0.79, P=0.19) (O'Day, Sosman, and Peterson 2009)
A phase II trial evaluated the use of bi-weekly bevacizumab in combination with carboplatin and weekly paclitaxel in 53 previously treated patients. The median PFS and OS were 6 and

12 months, respectively. There was a high incidence of haematological toxicities, most common being grade ≥3 neutropenia (53%), leukopenia (38%) and thrombocytopenia (11%). There were also 40 episodes of bleeding in 31 patients, including two grade 2 bronchopulmonary haemorrhages and one grade 5 central nervous system hemorrhage (Perez et al. 2009).

A Phase II study of temozolomide 150 mg/m2 for 7 days and bevacizumab 10 mg/kg every 2 weeks in 62 patients reported a median PFS of 4.2 months and OS of 9.3 months (Dummer et al. 2010).

5.5 Oblimersen

Oblimersen sodium (Genasense; Genta International Inc, Berkeley Heights, NJ) is a 18-base phosphorothioate antisense oligonucleotide that binds to the first 6 codons of the Bcl-2 mRNA open reading frame (Klasa et al. 2002). Overexpression of Bcl-2 may be partially responsible for the multi drug resistance seen in melanoma (Soengas and Lowe 2003). In a randomised controlled trial reported by Bedikian et al, 771 chemonaive advanced melanoma patients were randomised to receive either dacarbazine (1000 mg/m^2 on day 1) and oblimersen (7 mg/kg/day as a continuous infusion for 5 day) (n=386) or dacarbazine alone (n=385) (Bedikian et al. 2006). There was a trend for longer OS in the oblimersen arm which did not reach the statistical significance (9 vs 7.8 months, HR= 0.87, 95% CI=0.75-1.01, p=0.077). A subgroup analysis for patients with normal LDH showed significantly improved overall survival, PFS and overall response rate in favour of the oblimersen-dacarbazine group. On the basis of these results, a phase III trial (AGENDA trial) has evaluated dacarbazine with or without Genasense in Advanced Melanoma with low LDH level. The initial results showed no impact of the addition of oblimersen to chemotherapy on OS or PFS, but a more mature analysis with longer follow-up is awaited (Genta 2009).

After many years of little or no improvement in outcomes for patients with melanoma, the tides are changing with 2 new agents, either licensed or about to be, showing significant activity in advanced disease. The results of 3 large randomised adjuvant studies will also report in the next few years, hopefully also improving the treatment options for high risk patients. The management algorithm is being rewritten, but is generating more questions than answers. We have little understanding of resistance mechanisms, optimum scheduling, use in combination, long term toxicities etc - these will be the questions addressed in trials over the next 5 years.

Five years ago, we could only have dreamed of being in the position to have to consider these issues. The paradigm of basic scientific research discoveries being explored further in translational studies, then validated in rigorous clinical trials is exemplified by the progress achieved melanoma treatment.

6. References

Bedikian, A. Y., M. Millward, H. Pehamberger, R. Conry, M. Gore, U. Trefzer, A. C. Pavlick, R. DeConti, E. M. Hersh, P. Hersey, J. M. Kirkwood, and F. G. Haluska. 2006. "Bcl-2 antisense (oblimersen sodium) plus dacarbazine in patients with advanced melanoma: the Oblimersen Melanoma Study Group." *J Clin Oncol* no. 24 (29):4738-45.

Bottomley, A., C. Coens, S. Suciu, M. Santinami, W. Kruit, A. Testori, J. Marsden, C. Punt, F. Sales, M. Gore, R. Mackie, Z. Kusic, R. Dummer, P. Patel, D. Schadendorf, A. Spatz, U. Keilholz, and A. Eggermont. 2009. "Adjuvant therapy with pegylated interferon alfa-2b versus observation in resected stage III melanoma: a phase III randomized controlled trial of health-related quality of life and symptoms by the European Organisation for Research and Treatment of Cancer Melanoma Group." *J Clin Oncol* no. 27 (18):2916-23.

Bouwhuis, M. G., S. Suciu, S. Collette, S. Aamdal, W. H. Kruit, L. Bastholt, U. Stierner, F. Sales, P. Patel, C. J. Punt, M. Hernberg, A. Spatz, T. L. ten Hagen, J. Hansson, and A. M. Eggermont. 2009. "Autoimmune antibodies and recurrence-free interval in melanoma patients treated with adjuvant interferon." *J Natl Cancer Inst* no. 101 (12):869-77.

Buzaid A, Legha S, Winn R. 1993. "Cisplatin (C) vinblastine (V), and dacarbazine (D) (CVD) versus dacarbazine alone in metastatic melanoma: preliminary results of a phase III Cancer Community Oncology program (CCOP) trial." *Proc Am Soc Clin Onco* no. 12:389.

Cameron, D. A., M. C. Cornbleet, R. M. Mackie, J. A. Hunter, M. Gore, B. Hancock, and J. F. Smyth. 2001. "Adjuvant interferon alpha 2b in high risk melanoma - the Scottish study." *Br J Cancer* no. 84 (9):1146-9.

Chang, P., and W. H. Knapper. 1982. "Metastatic melanoma of unknown primary." *Cancer* no. 49 (6):1106-11.

Chapman, P. B., L. H. Einhorn, M. L. Meyers, S. Saxman, A. N. Destro, K. S. Panageas, C. B. Begg, S. S. Agarwala, L. M. Schuchter, M. S. Ernstoff, A. N. Houghton, and J. M. Kirkwood. 1999. "Phase III multicenter randomized trial of the Dartmouth regimen versus dacarbazine in patients with metastatic melanoma." *J Clin Oncol* no. 17 (9):2745-51.

Crews, C. M., A. Alessandrini, and R. L. Erikson. 1992. "The primary structure of MEK, a protein kinase that phosphorylates the ERK gene product." *Science* no. 258 (5081):478-80.

Curtin, J. A., K. Busam, D. Pinkel, and B. C. Bastian. 2006. "Somatic activation of KIT in distinct subtypes of melanoma." *J Clin Oncol* no. 24 (26):4340-6.

Curtin, J. A., J. Fridlyand, T. Kageshita, H. N. Patel, K. J. Busam, H. Kutzner, K. H. Cho, S. Aiba, E. B. Brocker, P. E. LeBoit, D. Pinkel, and B. C. Bastian. 2005. "Distinct sets of genetic alterations in melanoma." *N Engl J Med* no. 353 (20):2135-47.

Davies, H., G. R. Bignell, C. Cox, P. Stephens, S. Edkins, S. Clegg, J. Teague, H. Woffendin, M. J. Garnett, W. Bottomley, N. Davis, E. Dicks, R. Ewing, Y. Floyd, K. Gray, S. Hall, R. Hawes, J. Hughes, V. Kosmidou, A. Menzies, C. Mould, A. Parker, C. Stevens, S. Watt, S. Hooper, R. Wilson, H. Jayatilake, B. A. Gusterson, C. Cooper, J. Shipley, D. Hargrave, K. Pritchard-Jones, N. Maitland, G. Chenevix-Trench, G. J. Riggins, D. D. Bigner, G. Palmieri, A. Cossu, A. Flanagan, A. Nicholson, J. W. Ho, S. Y. Leung, S. T. Yuen, B. L. Weber, H. F. Seigler, T. L. Darrow, H. Paterson, R. Marais, C. J. Marshall, R. Wooster, M. R. Stratton, and P. A. Futreal. 2002. "Mutations of the BRAF gene in human cancer." *Nature* no. 417 (6892):949-54. doi: 10.1038/nature00766 nature00766 [pii].

Dudley, M. E., J. C. Yang, R. Sherry, M. S. Hughes, R. Royal, U. Kammula, P. F. Robbins, J. Huang, D. E. Citrin, S. F. Leitman, J. Wunderlich, N. P. Restifo, A. Thomasian, S. G.

Downey, F. O. Smith, J. Klapper, K. Morton, C. Laurencot, D. E. White, and S. A. Rosenberg. 2008. "Adoptive cell therapy for patients with metastatic melanoma: evaluation of intensive myeloablative chemoradiation preparative regimens." *J Clin Oncol* no. 26 (32):5233-9.

Dummer, R., O. Michielin, B. Seifert, A. F. Ochsenbein, R. Cathomas, M. R. Schlaeppi, M. Simcock, S. Gillessen, S. M. Goldinger, R. von Moos, and Swiss Group for Clinical Cancer Research 2010. "First-line temozolomide (TEM) combined with bevacizumab (BEV) in metastatic melanoma (MM): A multicenter phase II trial (SAKK 50/07)." *ASCO Meeting Abstracts* no. 28 (15_suppl):8521.

Dummer, R., C. Robert, P. B. Chapman, J. A. Sosman, M. Middleton, L. Bastholt, K. Kemsley, M. V. Cantarini, C. Morris, and J. M. Kirkwood. 2008. "AZD6244 (ARRY-142886) vs temozolomide (TMZ) in patients (pts) with advanced melanoma: An open-label, randomized, multicenter, phase II study." *ASCO Meeting Abstracts* no. 26 (15_suppl):9033.

Eggermont, A. M., S. Suciu, R. MacKie, W. Ruka, A. Testori, W. Kruit, C. J. Punt, M. Delauney, F. Sales, G. Groenewegen, D. J. Ruiter, I. Jagiello, K. Stoitchkov, U. Keilholz, and D. Lienard. 2005. "Post-surgery adjuvant therapy with intermediate doses of interferon alfa 2b versus observation in patients with stage IIb/III melanoma (EORTC 18952): randomised controlled trial." *Lancet* no. 366 (9492):1189-96.

Eggermont, A. M., S. Suciu, M. Santinami, A. Testori, W. H. Kruit, J. Marsden, C. J. Punt, F. Sales, M. Gore, R. Mackie, Z. Kusic, R. Dummer, A. Hauschild, E. Musat, A. Spatz, and U. Keilholz. 2008. "Adjuvant therapy with pegylated interferon alfa-2b versus observation alone in resected stage III melanoma: final results of EORTC 18991, a randomised phase III trial." *Lancet* no. 372 (9633):117-26.

Eggermont, A., S. Suciu, A. Testori, P. Patel, A. Spatz. 2009. "Ulceration of primary melanoma and responsiveness to adjuvant interferon therapy: Analysis of the adjuvant trials EORTC18952 and EORTC18991 in 2,644 patients." *J Clin Oncol* no. 27:15s (suppl; abstr 9007).

Eisen, T., T. Ahmad, K. T. Flaherty, M. Gore, S. Kaye, R. Marais, I. Gibbens, S. Hackett, M. James, L. M. Schuchter, K. L. Nathanson, C. Xia, R. Simantov, B. Schwartz, M. Poulin-Costello, P. J. O'Dwyer, and M. J. Ratain. 2006. "Sorafenib in advanced melanoma: a Phase II randomised discontinuation trial analysis." *Br J Cancer* no. 95 (5):581-6.

Flaherty, K. T., S. J. Lee, L. M. Schuchter, L. E. Flaherty, J. J. Wright, P. D. Leming, and J. M. Kirkwood. 2010. "Final results of E2603: A double-blind, randomized phase III trial comparing carboplatin (C)/paclitaxel (P) with or without sorafenib (S) in metastatic melanoma." *ASCO Meeting Abstracts* no. 28 (15_suppl):8511.

Flaherty, K. T., I. Puzanov, K. B. Kim, A. Ribas, G. A. McArthur, J. A. Sosman, P. J. O'Dwyer, R. J. Lee, J. F. Grippo, K. Nolop, and P. B. Chapman. 2010. "Inhibition of mutated, activated BRAF in metastatic melanoma." *N Engl J Med* no. 363 (9):809-19.

Garbe, C., P. Radny, R. Linse, R. Dummer, R. Gutzmer, J. Ulrich, R. Stadler, M. Weichenthal, T. Eigentler, U. Ellwanger, and A. Hauschild. 2008. "Adjuvant low-dose interferon {alpha}2a with or without dacarbazine compared with surgery alone: a prospective-randomized phase III DeCOG trial in melanoma patients with regional lymph node metastasis." *Ann Oncol* no. 19 (6):1195-201.

Genta. 2009. New Publication Confirms Critical Link of LDH Biomarker in Genasense® Trials to Overall Survival in Advanced Melanoma, http://www.genta.com/Press_Releases/2009/New_Publication_Confirms_Critical_Link_of_LDH_Biomarker_in_GenasenseÂ®_Trials_to_Overall_Survival_in_Advanced_Melanoma.html.

Gogas, H., J. Ioannovich, U. Dafni, C. Stavropoulou-Giokas, K. Frangia, D. Tsoutsos, P. Panagiotou, A. Polyzos, O. Papadopoulos, A. Stratigos, C. Markopoulos, D. Bafaloukos, D. Pectasides, G. Fountzilas, and J. M. Kirkwood. 2006. "Prognostic significance of autoimmunity during treatment of melanoma with interferon." *N Engl J Med* no. 354 (7):709-18.

Haass, N. K., K. Sproesser, T. K. Nguyen, R. Contractor, C. A. Medina, K. L. Nathanson, M. Herlyn, and K. S. Smalley. 2008. "The mitogen-activated protein/extracellular signal-regulated kinase kinase inhibitor AZD6244 (ARRY-142886) induces growth arrest in melanoma cells and tumor regression when combined with docetaxel." *Clin Cancer Res* no. 14 (1):230-9.

Hauschild, A., S. S. Agarwala, U. Trefzer, D. Hogg, C. Robert, P. Hersey, A. Eggermont, S. Grabbe, R. Gonzalez, J. Gille, C. Peschel, D. Schadendorf, C. Garbe, S. O'Day, A. Daud, J. M. White, C. Xia, K. Patel, J. M. Kirkwood, and U. Keilholz. 2009. "Results of a phase III, randomized, placebo-controlled study of sorafenib in combination with carboplatin and paclitaxel as second-line treatment in patients with unresectable stage III or stage IV melanoma." *J Clin Oncol* no. 27 (17):2823-30.

Hodi, F. S., S. J. O'Day, D. F. McDermott, R. W. Weber, J. A. Sosman, J. B. Haanen, R. Gonzalez, C. Robert, D. Schadendorf, J. C. Hassel, W. Akerley, A. J. van den Eertwegh, J. Lutzky, P. Lorigan, J. M. Vaubel, G. P. Linette, D. Hogg, C. H. Ottensmeier, C. Lebbe, C. Peschel, I. Quirt, J. I. Clark, J. D. Wolchok, J. S. Weber, J. Tian, M. J. Yellin, G. M. Nichol, A. Hoos, and W. J. Urba. 2010. "Improved survival with ipilimumab in patients with metastatic melanoma." *N Engl J Med* no. 363 (8):711-23.

Infante, J.R., L. A. Fecher, S. Nallapareddy, M. S. Gordon, K. T. Flaherty, D. S. Cox, D. J. DeMarini, S. R. Morris, H. A. Burris, W. A. Messersmith; Sarah Cannon 2010. "Safety and efficacy results from the first-in-human study of the oral MEK 1/2 inhibitor GSK1120212." *J Clin Oncol* no. 28 (suppl; abstr 2503).

Ives, N. J., R. L. Stowe, P. Lorigan, and K. Wheatley. 2007. "Chemotherapy compared with biochemotherapy for the treatment of metastatic melanoma: a meta-analysis of 18 trials involving 2,621 patients." *J Clin Oncol* no. 25 (34):5426-34.

Kefford, R., H. Arkenau, M. P. Brown, M. Millward, J. R. Infante, G. V. Long, D. Ouellet, M. Curtis, P. F. Lebowitz, and G. S. Falchook. 2010. "Phase I/II study of GSK2118436, a selective inhibitor of oncogenic mutant BRAF kinase, in patients with metastatic melanoma and other solid tumors." *ASCO Meeting Abstracts* no. 28 (15_suppl):8503.

Kirkwood, J. M., J. G. Ibrahim, J. A. Sosman, V. K. Sondak, S. S. Agarwala, M. S. Ernstoff, and U. Rao. 2001. "High-dose interferon alfa-2b significantly prolongs relapse-free and overall survival compared with the GM2-KLH/QS-21 vaccine in patients with resected stage IIB-III melanoma: results of intergroup trial E1694/S9512/C509801." *J Clin Oncol* no. 19 (9):2370-80.

Kirkwood, J. M., P. Lorigan, P. Hersey, A. Hauschild, C. Robert, D. McDermott, M. A. Marshall, J. Gomez-Navarro, J. Q. Liang, and C. A. Bulanhagui. 2010. "Phase II trial of tremelimumab (CP-675,206) in patients with advanced refractory or relapsed melanoma." *Clin Cancer Res* no. 16 (3):1042-8.

Kirkwood, J. M., M. H. Strawderman, M. S. Ernstoff, T. J. Smith, E. C. Borden, and R. H. Blum. 1996. "Interferon alfa-2b adjuvant therapy of high-risk resected cutaneous melanoma: the Eastern Cooperative Oncology Group Trial EST 1684." *J Clin Oncol* no. 14 (1):7-17.

Klasa, R. J., A. M. Gillum, R. E. Klem, and S. R. Frankel. 2002. "Oblimersen Bcl-2 antisense: facilitating apoptosis in anticancer treatment." *Antisense Nucleic Acid Drug Dev* no. 12 (3):193-213.

Kruit, W. H., S. Suciu, B. Dreno, V. Chiarion-Sileni, L. Mortier, C. Robert, M. Maio, V. G. Brichard, F. Lehmann, and U. Keilholz. 2008. "Immunization with recombinant MAGE-A3 protein combined with adjuvant systems AS15 or AS02B in patients with unresectable and progressive metastatic cutaneous melanoma: A randomized open-label phase II study of the EORTC Melanoma Group (16032- 18031)." *ASCO Meeting Abstracts* no. 26 (15_suppl):9065.

Lattanzi, S. C., T. Tosteson, J. Chertoff, L. H. Maurer, J. O'Donnell, P. J. LeMarbre, L. Mott, S. A. DelPrete, R. J. Forcier, and M. S. Ernstoff. 1995. "Dacarbazine, cisplatin and carmustine, with or without tamoxifen, for metastatic melanoma: 5-year follow-up." *Melanoma Res* no. 5 (5):365-9.

Lee, C. C., M. B. Faries, L. A. Wanek, and D. L. Morton. 2008. "Improved survival after lymphadenectomy for nodal metastasis from an unknown primary melanoma." *J Clin Oncol* no. 26 (4):535-41.

Legha, S. S., S. Ring, N. Papadopoulos, C. Plager, S. Chawla, and R. Benjamin. 1989. "A prospective evaluation of a triple-drug regimen containing cisplatin, vinblastine, and dacarbazine (CVD) for metastatic melanoma." *Cancer* no. 64 (10):2024-9.

Lev, D. C., A. Onn, V. O. Melinkova, C. Miller, V. Stone, M. Ruiz, E. C. McGary, H. N. Ananthaswamy, J. E. Price, and M. Bar-Eli. 2004. "Exposure of melanoma cells to dacarbazine results in enhanced tumor growth and metastasis in vivo." *J Clin Oncol* no. 22 (11):2092-100.

Marshall, M. A., A. Ribas, and B. Huang. 2010. "Evaluation of baseline serum C-reactive protein (CRP) and benefit from tremelimumab compared to chemotherapy in first-line melanoma." *ASCO Meeting Abstracts* no. 28 (15_suppl):2609.

McDermott, D. F., J. A. Sosman, R. Gonzalez, F. S. Hodi, G. P. Linette, J. Richards, J. W. Jakub, M. Beeram, S. Tarantolo, S. Agarwala, G. Frenette, I. Puzanov, L. Cranmer, K. Lewis, J. Kirkwood, J. M. White, C. Xia, K. Patel, and E. Hersh. 2008. "Double-blind randomized phase II study of the combination of sorafenib and dacarbazine in patients with advanced melanoma: a report from the 11715 Study Group." *J Clin Oncol* no. 26 (13):2178-85.

Middleton, M. R., J. J. Grob, N. Aaronson, G. Fierlbeck, W. Tilgen, S. Seiter, M. Gore, S. Aamdal, J. Cebon, A. Coates, B. Dreno, M. Henz, D. Schadendorf, A. Kapp, J. Weiss, U. Fraass, P. Statkevich, M. Muller, and N. Thatcher. 2000. "Randomized phase III study of temozolomide versus dacarbazine in the treatment of patients with advanced metastatic malignant melanoma." *J Clin Oncol* no. 18 (1):158-66.

Mocellin, S., S. Pasquali, C. R. Rossi, and D. Nitti. 2010. "Interferon alpha adjuvant therapy in patients with high-risk melanoma: a systematic review and meta-analysis." *J Natl Cancer Inst* no. 102 (7):493-501.

O'Day, S. J., M. Maio, V. Chiarion-Sileni, T. F. Gajewski, H. Pehamberger, I. N. Bondarenko, P. Queirolo, L. Lundgren, S. Mikhailov, L. Roman, C. Verschraegen, R. Humphrey, R. Ibrahim, V. de Pril, A. Hoos, and J. D. Wolchok. 2010. "Efficacy and safety of ipilimumab monotherapy in patients with pretreated advanced melanoma: a multicenter single-arm phase II study." *Ann Oncol* no. 21 (8):1712-7.

O'Day, S.J., J.A. Sosman, and A.C. Peterson. 2009. "BEAM: A randomized phase II study evaluating the activity of Bevacizumab in combination with carboplatin plus paclitaxel in patients with previously untreated Advanced Melanoma." *Eur J Cancer Supplements* no. 7 (3):13.

Patel P, S. S., Mortier L. 2008. Extended schedule, escalated dose temozolomide versus dacarbazine in stage IV malignant melanoma: Final results of the randomised phase III study EORTC 18032. Paper read at 33rd European Society of Medical Oncology (ESMO) Congress.

Perez, D. G., V. J. Suman, T. R. Fitch, T. Amatruda, 3rd, R. F. Morton, S. Z. Jilani, C. L. Constantinou, J. R. Egner, L. A. Kottschade, and S. N. Markovic. 2009. "Phase 2 trial of carboplatin, weekly paclitaxel, and biweekly bevacizumab in patients with unresectable stage IV melanoma: a North Central Cancer Treatment Group study, N047A." *Cancer* no. 115 (1):119-27.

Ribas, A., A. Hauschild, R. Kefford, J. Gomez-Navarro, D. Pavlov, and M. A. Marshall. 2008. "Phase III, open-label, randomized, comparative study of tremelimumab (CP-675,206) and chemotherapy (temozolomide [TMZ] or dacarbazine [DTIC]) in patients with advanced melanoma." *ASCO Meeting Abstracts* no. 26 (15_suppl):LBA9011.

Roche. 2011. Roche Media Release "Roche Personalised investigational medicine shows survival benefit in advanced skin cancer.
http://www.roche.com/media/media_releases/med-cor-2011-01-19.htm

Rosen, L. B., D. D. Ginty, M. J. Weber, and M. E. Greenberg. 1994. "Membrane depolarization and calcium influx stimulate MEK and MAP kinase via activation of Ras." *Neuron* no. 12 (6):1207-21.

Schwartzentruber, D. J., D. Lawson, J. Richards, R. M. Conry, D. Miller, J. Triesman, F. Gailani, L. B. Riley, D. Vena, and P. Hwu. 2009. "A phase III multi-institutional randomized study of immunization with the gp100: 209-217(210M) peptide followed by high-dose IL-2 compared with high-dose IL-2 alone in patients with metastatic melanoma." *ASCO Meeting Abstracts* no. 27 (18S):CRA9011.

Smalley, K. S. 2003. "A pivotal role for ERK in the oncogenic behaviour of malignant melanoma?" *Int J Cancer* no. 104 (5):527-32.

Soengas, M. S., and S. W. Lowe. 2003. "Apoptosis and melanoma chemoresistance." *Oncogene* no. 22 (20):3138-51.

Sosman, J., K. Kim , L. Schuchter, .R. Gonzalez , A. Pavlick, J. Weber, G.T. McArthur 2010. An open-label, multicentre phase 2 study of continuous oral dosing of RG7204 (PLX4032) in previously treated patients with BRAF V600E mutation- positive metastatic melanoma. Paper read at The Seventh International Melanoma Research Congress of the Society for Melanoma Research at Sydney Australia.

Ugurel, S., G. Rappl, W. Tilgen, and U. Reinhold. 2001. "Increased serum concentration of angiogenic factors in malignant melanoma patients correlates with tumor progression and survival." *J Clin Oncol* no. 19 (2):577-83.

Weber, J., J. A. Thompson, O. Hamid, D. Minor, A. Amin, I. Ron, R. Ridolfi, H. Assi, A. Maraveyas, D. Berman, J. Siegel, and S. J. O'Day. 2009. "A randomized, double-blind, placebo-controlled, phase II study comparing the tolerability and efficacy of ipilimumab administered with or without prophylactic budesonide in patients with unresectable stage III or IV melanoma." *Clin Cancer Res* no. 15 (17):5591-8.

Wheatley, K. , N. Ives, A. Eggermont, J. Kirkwood, N. Cascinelli, S. N. Markovic, B. Hancock, S. Lee, S. Suciu. 2007. "Interferon- as adjuvant therapy for melanoma: An individual patient data meta-analysis of randomised trials." *J Clin Oncol (Meeting Abstracts)* no. 25:18s (June 20 suppl; abstr 8526).

Wheatley, K., N. Ives, B. Hancock, M. Gore, A. Eggermont, and S. Suciu. 2003. "Does adjuvant interferon-alpha for high-risk melanoma provide a worthwhile benefit? A meta-analysis of the randomised trials." *Cancer Treat Rev* no. 29 (4):241-52.

Wolchok, J. D., A. Hoos, S. O'Day, J. S. Weber, O. Hamid, C. Lebbe, M. Maio, M. Binder, O. Bohnsack, G. Nichol, R. Humphrey, and F. S. Hodi. 2009. "Guidelines for the evaluation of immune therapy activity in solid tumors: immune-related response criteria." *Clin Cancer Res* no. 15 (23):7412-20.

Wolchok, J. D., B. Neyns, G. Linette, S. Negrier, J. Lutzky, L. Thomas, W. Waterfield, D. Schadendorf, M. Smylie, T. Guthrie, Jr., J. J. Grob, J. Chesney, K. Chin, K. Chen, A. Hoos, S. J. O'Day, and C. Lebbe. 2010. "Ipilimumab monotherapy in patients with pretreated advanced melanoma: a randomised, double-blind, multicentre, phase 2, dose-ranging study." *Lancet Oncol* no. 11 (2):155-64.

Part 7

Treatment of Oral and Uveal Melanoma

14

Choroidal Melanoma

Raquel Correa, Mario Lobato and José Antonio Medina
Virgen de la Victoria Hospital, Málaga, Spain

1. Introduction

Uveal melanoma is the most common primary ocular malignancy in adults. There are about 0.6-0.8 new patients per 100,000 inhabitants (in Europe). Several studies have demonstrated that complete removal of the tumour by enucleation is not advantageous compared with conservative therapies in terms of metastatic spread and survival.
The primary treatment for uveal melanoma depends on many factors: size, location, extraocular extension, visual function, age and performance status.

2. Enucleation

Enucleation has been the standard treatment since the nineteenth century and is still the treatment of choice in large uveal melanomas.
Enucleation is still required in a significant proportion of patients, either because the tumour is too extensive at presentation or because of the complications of conservative therapy. The procedure is performed in the surgeon's preferred fashion. It is essential to perform binocular indirect ophthalmoscopy after draping the patient to confirm that the correct eye is being removed. The main complication specific to uveal melanoma is orbital tumour recurrence, which is rare. If this occurs, it is treated with local resection and external beam radiotherapy. It was previously believed that surgical manipulations during enucleation disseminated tumour cells into the vascular system, thereby causing metastatic disease; however, as we will see later, COMS-10 study has shown no improvement of survival after pre-enucleation radiotherapy, thereby casting doubt on this hypothesis.
Globe preserving techniques include: laser photocoagulation, transpupillary thermotherapy, local resection, radiotherapy and gammaknife.
Observation without treatment is a modality used for melanomas that are small and have dormant characteristics. Patients managed by this strategy are often asymptomatic and have the lesion picked up on routine ocular examination. Another subgroup of patients who may be managed by observation includes elderly patients with severe systemic health problems or short life expectancy.
Radiotherapy (RT) offers a conservative treatment for those patients who are suitable for visual and motion conservation.

3. Radiobiology

Radiations kills a tumour either by producing free radicals that destroy cellular DNA immediately or by induction of mutations that go on to kill tumour cells over a protracted

period of time. Radiation also induces vascular fibrosis and secondary hypoxia, which again may take time to cause cell death. Thus, RT provides both short- and long-terms effects[1].
There are two main modalities: brachytherapy and external beam radiotherapy (that includes charged particles and special techniques like intensity modulated radiotherapy).

4. Brachytherapy

In the United States, controversies about the appropriate management of choroidal melanoma led to the development of the COMS (Collaborative Ocular Melanoma Study) group, which conducted a series of randomised studies on the use of enucleation, brachytherapy and radiotherapy. To date, their principal results have been that preoperative radiotherapy for large size melanomas does not improve survival compared with enucleation alone, and that there is no difference as regards survival between those patients treated with I-125 seed brachytherapy and those who underwent enucleation. The results of these studies show brachytherapy as an alternative to enucleation.
Various materials for delivering radiation have been investigated in brachytherapy. Iodine-125 is currently the most commonly used isotope for plaque radiotherapy of choroidal melanoma. Although cobalt-60, ruthenium-106, Iridium -196, strontium-90 and palladium-103 have also been used.

Radionuclide	Symbol	Type	Energy	Half-life	Introduced	depth
Cobalt	Co-60	Gamma/beta	1.3MeV/320Kev	5.2 years	1948	
Ruthenium	Ru-106	Beta	293 KeV	373 days	1964	5 mm
Iodine	I-125	Gamma	27-35 KeV	60 days	1975	
Strontium	Sr-90	Beta	546 KeV	29 years	1983	5 mm
Iridium	Ir-192	Gamma/Beta	600KeV/370 KeV	74 days	1983	
Palladium	Pd-102	Gamma	21 KeV	17 days	1986	

Table 1.

Before the COMS trials were initiated in 1986, interest in radiation therapy had increased because of the potential for saving the eye and perhaps some vision.
The COMS-18 trial enrolled 1317 patients with medium size melanomas to enucleation or brachytherapy with iodine-125 (I-125) plaques. Six hundred and sixty were randomly assigned to enucleation and 657 to I-125 brachytherapy (85 Gy). Only 2 patients in the enucleation arm were found to have been misdiagnosed when histopathology was centrally reviewed. All but 17 patients (1.3%) received the assigned treatment. Adherence to the brachytherapy protocol was excellent, with 91% of patients treated per protocol. Based on time since enrolment, 1072 patients (81%) had been followed for mortality at 5 years and 416 (32%) at 10 years. A total of 364 patients had died: 188 (28%) of 660 patients in the enucleation arm and 176 (27%) of 657 patients in the brachytherapy arm. The unadjusted estimated 5-year survival rates were 81% and 82%, respectively; there was no clinically or statistically significant difference in survival rates overall (P =0.48, log-rank test). The

adjusted estimated risk ratio for I-125 brachytherapy vs enucleation was 0.99 (95% confidence interval [CI], 0.80-1.22). Five-year rates of death with histopathologically confirmed melanoma metastases were 11% and 9% following enucleation and brachytherapy respectively; after adjustment, the estimated risk ratio was 0.91 (95% CI, 0.66-1.24). Graphs 1 and 2. They concluded that mortality rates following I-125 brachytherapy did not differ from mortality rates following enucleation for up to 12 years after treatment [2].

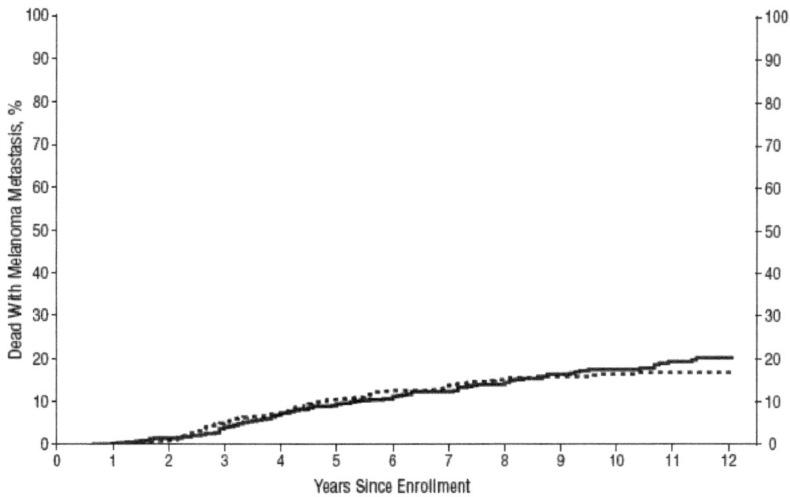

Graph 1. Dead with melanoma metastasis at COMS-18 trial

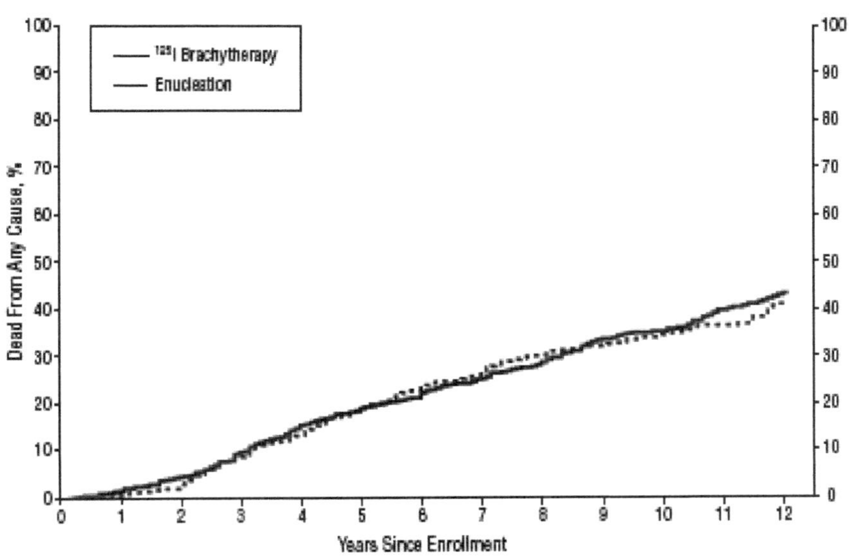

Graph 2. Dead from any cause at COMS-18 trial

Visual acuity declined in a substantial proportion of eyes in the brachytherapy group. There was a quadrupling of the minimum angle of resolution, or loss of 6 or more lines of visual acuity from baseline in 18% of patients at 1 year, 34% at 2 years and 49% at 3 years. The risk of vision loss was associated with a history of diabetes, thick tumours, tumours close to or beneath the macula, tumours with secondary retinal detachments and tumours that were not dome-shaped[3]. Secondary strabismus has also occurred in 5% of patients as a result of moving extraocular muscles in order to properly place the plaque to hold the radioactive seeds (see figure 2).

Tumours with larger basal diameters are more likely to recur. Karlsson et al. found that patients with local tumour recurrence, which is likely to occur at the tumour margin, were at greater risk of life-threatening distant metastasis, having a 5-year survival rate of 58% compared with 82% for those without local recurrence. However, while local control of choroidal melanomas treated with brachytherapy has been reported at more than 90%, many treated eyes develop complications secondary to radiation delivered to adjacent structures. Radiation retinopathy has been identified in up to 43%. Others complications include optic atrophy, cystoid macular edema, cataracts, glaucoma, central retina vein occlusion and scleral necrosis.

In the COMS-10 trial of preoperative radiation, patients with large tumours were randomized to enucleation alone or to enucleation preceded by 20 Gy of external beam radiation. This trial was designed to see if radiation before enucleation (removal of the eye) would prevent metastasis. The idea was to see if pre-operative irradiation would sterilize any cells that might break free during surgery.

The two randomly assigned groups of patients were followed for at least five years or until death and were compared on the basis of length of remaining life and other outcomes. A total of 1,003 patients were enrolled; 506 were assigned to enucleation alone and 497 to pre-enucleation radiation. With 5-year outcome known for 801 patients enrolled (80%), the estimated 5-year survival rates and 95% confidence intervals (CIs) were 57% (95% CI, 52% to 62%) for enucleation alone and 62% (95% CI, 57% to 66%) for pre-enucleation radiation. Among the baseline covariates evaluated, only age and longest basal diameter of the melanoma affected the prognosis for survival to a statistically significant degree. The risk of death among patients treated with pre-enucleation radiation relative to those treated with enucleation alone after adjustment for baseline characteristics of patients, eyes, and tumours was 1.03 (95% CI, 0.85 to 1.25). Of 435 deaths classified by the Mortality Coding Committee, 269 patients had histologically confirmed melanoma metastases at the time of death. Estimated 5-year survival rates for this secondary outcome were 72% (95% CI, 68% to 76%) for enucleation alone and 74% (95% CI, 69% to 78%) for pre-enucleation radiation. The Large-sized Choroidal Melanoma Study concluded that patients who received external irradiation to their eye before it was removed, had an equal chance of developing metastatic disease as compared to those who were treated by enucleation (removal of the eye) alone.

This study did not find any survival difference attributable to pre-enucleation radiation of large choroidal melanoma, using the COMS fractionation Schedule[4].

Accrual to a nonrandomized pilot study to assess the feasibility of a randomized trial for small tumors was halted in 1989. Additional follow-up of these patients was carried out from 1994 to 1996. From December 1986 to August 1989, 204 patients with small choroidal melanoma, not large enough to be eligible for the COMS clinical trials, were offered participation in a nonrandomized prospective follow-up study. Small choroidal melanomas were defined as 1.0 to 3.0 mm in apical height and at least 5.0 mm in basal diameter. A total of 204 patients were enrolled in the study. Patients were followed up annually through August 1989. Two additional assessments of treatment status and mortality were conducted in 1993-1994 and 1995-1996. The median length of follow-up was 92 months. Eight percent of patients were treated at the time of study enrolment and an additional 33% were treated during follow-up. Twenty-seven patients have died; 6 deaths were reported by the clinical center as due to metastatic melanoma. The Kaplan-Meier estimate of 5-year all-cause mortality was 6.0% (95% confidence interval, 2.7%-9.3%) and 8-year all-cause mortality was 14.9% (95% confidence interval, 9.6%-20.2%).

The study concluded that healthy patients, average age of 60 years, without a previous diagnosis of malignant disease who had small choroidal lesions judged to be melanoma had a low risk of dying within 5 years[5].

5. Implant sequence

The procedure is performed thanks to the joint efforts of a multidisciplinary team composed of ophthalmologists, radiation oncologists, anaesthetists, physicists, and specialised radiotherapy technicians.

Patient preparation:

1. Placing of the radioactive plaque. This is carried out with both local and general anaesthetic, depending on each case, but mostly using retrobulbar anaesthesia with akinesis.
2. Gestures: In general, a limbic peritomy is performed, dissecting Tenon's capsule to leave the scleral surface which coincides with the tumour base exposed. If the lesion affects the muscle insertion area, the muscle must be disinserted.
3. CTV (Clinical target volume) Determination: Pupilar transillumination is used for the localization and marking of the base of the melanoma. Various non-absorbable sutures are placed at the scleral level, at positions marked by an inactive phantom, in order to check the correct size of the proposed plaque; the definitive radioactive plaque is then positioned and the sutures,are tied. The diameter of the radioactive applicator should be 2 mm greater than the tumour base, to ensure that the microscopic disease is covered by a safety zone for complete irradiation of its margins. Additional margins are not taken to cover eye movements.
4. Post-operative: Anti-inflammatory drugs and antibiotics are administered subconjuntivally, topically and systemically in theatre. The patient is subsequently transferred to a darkened room.
5. Treatment course: The treatment is given as scheduled and all patients remain admitted to the Brachytherapy Unit. During admission, analgesic and prophylactic antibiotic treatment is prescribed.
6. 6. Implant removal: On extraction of the ophthalmic plaque, the patient is again transferred to the implant room where it is disinserted under anaesthesia and complete removal of the radioactive load is checked. Once the plaque had been extracted, the patient returns to his room where he remains until recovery and discharge. See figure 1, 2 , 3 and 4.

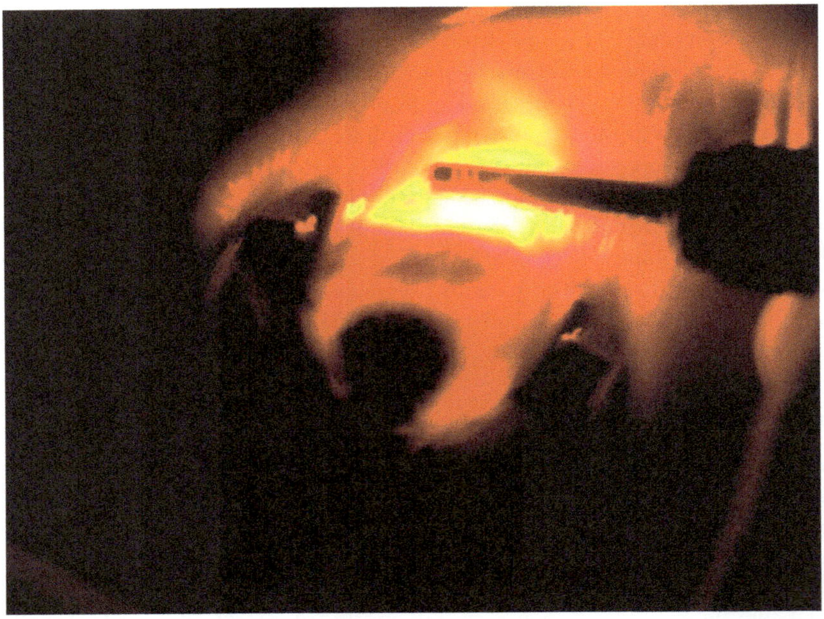

Fig. 1. Pupilar transillumination

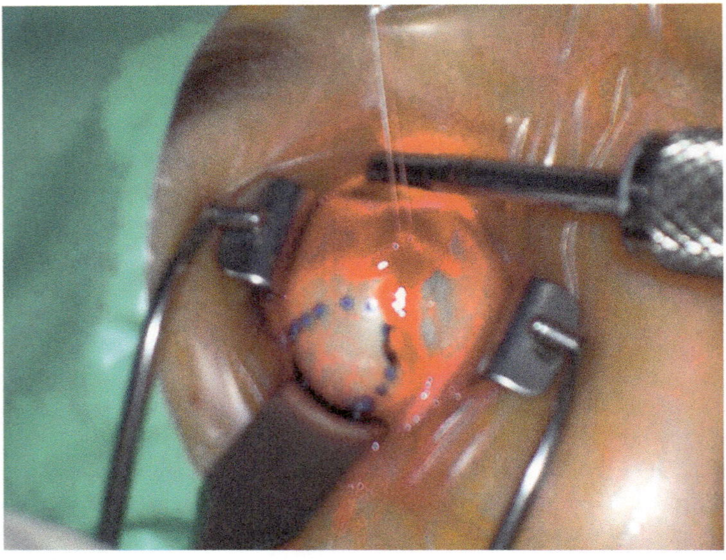

Fig. 2. Target volume delineation

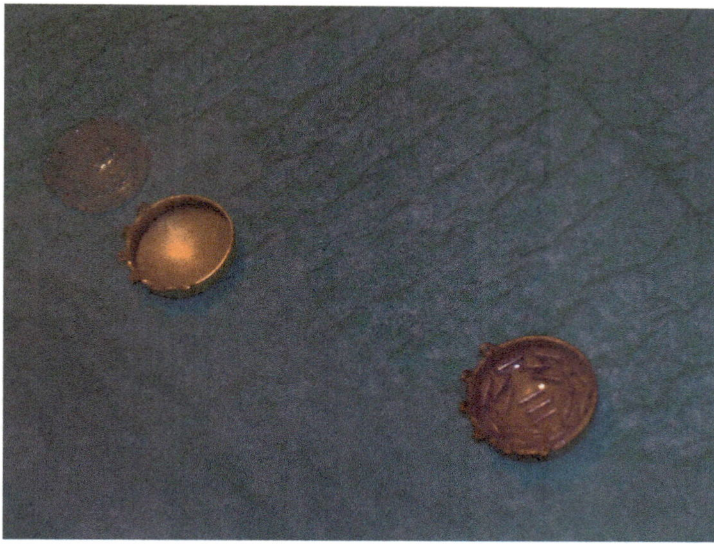

Fig. 3. Plaque with I-125 seeds.

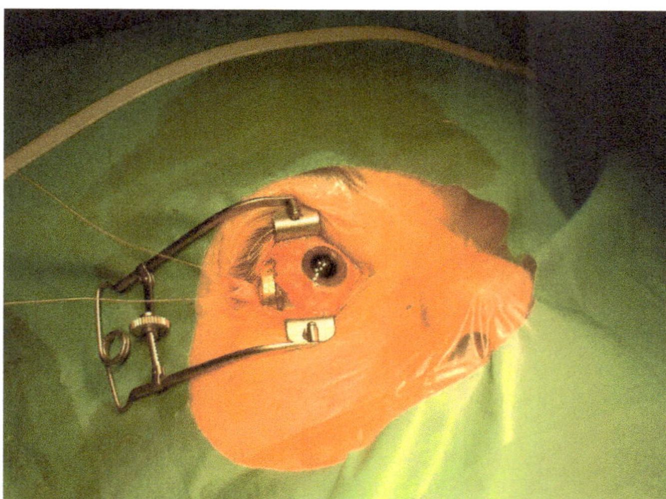

Fig. 4. Eye with the plaque in place.

6. Prescription dose

The prescription point is defined as the tumour apex for tumours measuring 5.0 mm or more in apical height; but for smaller tumours, the prescription point is 5 mm from the interior surface of the sclera. In 1996, the COMS adopted the recommendations of the American Association of Physicists in Medicine Task Group (TG-43) regarding dosimetry of interstitial sources in anticipation of a revised calibration standard for I-125 seeds by the

National Institute for Standards and Technology (NIST). Under the TG-43 formalism, the absorbed dose at the prescription point was 85 Gy delivered at a rate of at least 0.42 Gy/hour, but no more than 1.05 Gy/hour. Before adopting the TG-43 formalism, the prescribed total dose was calculated to be 100 Gy; however, the actual amount of radiation delivered was not affected by the change. All dose data included in the majority of reports were recalculated based on the TG-43 formalism. The actual radiation dose delivered to the prescription point, tumour apex, sclera at the center of the plaque and critical structures within the eye was reported to and confirmed by the COMS Radiologic Physics Center (Houston, TX). Doses were calculated based on presumed plaque location, I-125 seed activity and location in the plaque, and times of plaque insertion and removal.

7. Combined treatment

Combined plaque irradiation and laser photocoagulation or thermotherapy have been used recently to increase the likelihood of complete local tumour destruction, particularly in patients with tumours adjacent to the optic disc. In 1998, Shields et al. published the results of 100 patients treated with plaque and transpupillary thermotherapy and found a recurrence rate of 3% in 8 years.

8. Proton beam radiotherapy

Proton-beam radiotherapy (PBRT) was first utilized in the management of uveal melanoma in 1975[6]. It is now predominantly used for choroidal and ciliary body melanomas. PBRT is an alternative method of delivering radiation to an ocular tumour that uses charged particles, either protons or helium ions (PBRT). Tantalum clips are fixed to the epiescleral surface around the base of the tumour, and charged particles are then directed toward the tumour from an anterior approach. With this technique the dose is delivered in for or five equivalent fractions over a 7-days period. Typically a total dose of 70 Cobalt gray equivalent (CGE) is administered over 5 fractions.

The density of ionization of protons increases markedly near the end of their path (Bragg peak). This characteristic enables accurate treatment, especially important for large lesions close to vital ocular structures. The advantages of charged particles include a uniform dose distribution throughout the treatment zone and a predictable area of treatment, since protons travel in a straight line and stop after a certain distance based on the initial energy imparted. Figure 5

No handling of radioactive material is required by the ophthalmologist or the radiation oncologist dealing with PBRT, in contrast to brachytherapy where handling is required. The highly collimated beam of irradiation includes a 1 mm tumour margin, a 0.5 mm margin for patient movement and a 1 mm margin for de penumbral effect. Seventy percent of the maximum radiation dose is delivered by the entrance beam as it travels through the eye before reaching the tumour. Therefore anterior complications including epiphora, lash loss and neovascular glaucoma occur more frequently with charged particles than with radiation delivered posteriorly[7].

As of December 2002 more than 3000 patients with uveal melanoma have been treated with protons at the Massachusetts General Hospital. The 5-year actuarial local control rate is 96%for all sites within the globe, with an 80% survival rate. The probability of eye retention at 5 years was estimated to be 90% for the entire group and 97%, 93% and 78% for patients

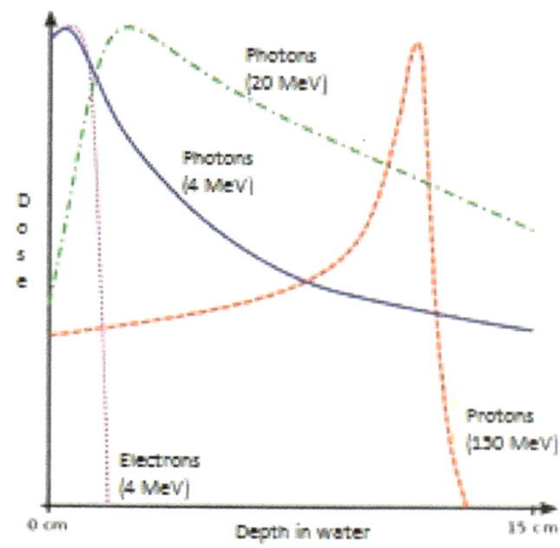

Fig. 5.

with small, intermediate and large tumours respectively. Independent risk factors for enucleation were the involvement of the ciliary body, a tumour height greater than 8 mm and the distance between the posterior tumour edge and the fovea[8]. These results compare favourably with local control rates of 89% reported with protons in Nice, France[9], and similar results from the Paul Scherrer Institute in Villigen, Switzerland.[10]

Because some patients have experienced deteriorating vision after doses of 70 CGE, a randomized trial of 50 versus 70 CGE for small and intermediate-sized lesions located within 6 mm of the optic disc of the macula was conducted. Interim analysis of 188 patients, with a median follow-up of 60 months suggested no reduction in local control or survival. No significant improvement in visual outcomes or complications was observed. However visual field analysis showed a smaller mean defect in the patients randomized to 50 CGE[11].

Egger et al. reported long-term results of eye retention after treatment of uveal melanoma with proton beam radiotherapy[12]. A total of 2645 patients (2648 eyes) were treated at the Paul Scherrer Institute in Switzerland between 1984 and 1999. The overall eye retention rates at 5, 10 and 15 years after treatment were 89, 86 and 83% respectively. Enucleation was related to large tumour size, mainly tumour height, male gender, high intraocular pressure and a large degree of retinal detachment at treatment time.

Gragoudas et al. reported that radiation maculopathy occurred in approximately 75% of tumours within 1 disc diameter of the fovea and in 40% of tumours greater than 1 disc diameter from the fovea treated with PBRT[11].

Wilson and Hungerford found local recurrence of 5.2% with PBRT. Metastatic death rates of 12.8% at 5 years and 20.7% at 10 years were reported following PBRT[13].

9. Stereotactic radiosurgery

Newer techniques like stereotactic radiosurgery and gammaknife radiotherapy are being used at some centres; however, no long-term data is available on the efficacy or complication rates.

Gammaknife radiosurgery (GKR) was initially introduced to successfully treat intracranial lesions such as brain tumours, vascular abnormalities, skull base tumours and neurological functional diseases. Gammaknife radiosurgery has been shown to be an alternative to enucleation for the treatment of large uveal melanomas.

10. Methods

10.1 Extraocular muscle sutures

After the patient receives retrobulbar anesthesia with long-acting agents (5 cm^3 of 1% Ropivacaine) to obtain complete akinesia, two extraocular muscles are sutured through the conjunctiva using 3.0 black silk suture. The two muscles are chosen according to tumour location to optimise globe position during treatment.

10.2 Stereotactic lightweight aluminium frame fixation

The stereotactic frame is attached to the patient's head with four pins lodged in the outer plate of the skull. The frame provides the coordinate system for target determination by magnetic resonance imaging.

10.3 Globe immobilisation and orientation

The threads of the two sutured muscles are fixed to the stereotactic frame to immobilise and orientate the globe. The globe is oriented in order to localise the tumour as closely as possible to the centre of the stereotactic frame. This condition may reduce magnetic resonance image distortion. Correct globe immobilisation is crucial to performing precise GKR.

10.4 Neuroimaging

High-resolution magnetic resonance (2 mm slices) with gadolinium of the brain is performed, and the images are transferred to the gamma knife three-dimensional treatment planning system (Gamma Plan). The use of gadolinium increases the definition of tumour margins in the presence of subretinal fluid and retinal detachment.

Besides the advantages of being non-invasive and easier for the patient to tolerate, radiosurgery provides a single day treatment that can be completed within a few hours[14, 15]. No other technique offers the same convenience for the patient. Although previous studies have shown GKS to be a minimally invasive, eye-saving treatment modality for uveal melanomas, secondary enucleation is still common with this procedure. Tumour volume and tumour location are thought to be major determinants of intraocular complications after GKS. Eagan et al. proposed that tumours of the ciliary body and tumors larger than 8 mm in height are more likely to require secondary enucleation after treatment. Complications of the treatment itself may also lead to enucleation.

For a series of 81 patients who underwent GKS for the treatment of uveal melanoma, Simanová et al. achieved an 84% local tumour control rate at 10 months by applying a minimum dose of 31.4 Gy[16]. Similarly, Modorati and colleagues achieved 91% tumour control in a group of 78 patients treated with 30–50 Gy of radiation at the tumour periphery. However, they observed high complication rates, including enucleation (10.3%), retinal detachment (33.3%) and glaucoma (18.7%). Zehetmayer et al. used one to three fractions of GKS for 62 selected uveal melanoma patients, with a mean follow-up of 28.3 months, achieving a tumour control rate of 98%. In a previous series involving GKS, doses as high as 70 Gy were applied to the immobilized the eye during the procedure; however, it appears that the high intraocular complication rate associated with higher doses may jeopardize the conservative advantages of GKS.

11. Other treatment modalities

11.1 Trans-scleral resection

Local trans-scleral resection has largely been abandoned in favour of more successful treatment methods. In 1986, Foulds and Damato recommended local resection for tumours of 10 to 15 mm in diameter after finding that most of the failures in their series involved tumours larger than 15 mm in diameter. They reported a 19% incidence of retinal detachment as a result of the surgery, only 41% of which responded well to repair[17, 18]. However, 81.1% of the eyes in the COMS showed local invasion of the sclera which the authors stated argued against the advisability of scleral resection as a treatment for choroidal melanoma due to the fact that potentially viable melanoma cells are likely to remain following surgery[19]. Proponents of transcleral resection now recommend adjuvant brachytherapy to irradiate any remaining tumor cells[20].

11.2 Transpupillary Thermotherapy (TTT)

TTT uses a diode laser to deliver a beam of infrared radiation through a dilated pupil into an intraocular tumour in order to induce tumour cell necrosis[21].

The entire surface of the tumour is covered with overlapping treatment areas extending 1.5 mm past the edge of the tumour into normal tissue. The advantages of TTT include immediate necrosis with quickly evident clinical regression, precision of treatment, and ease of treatment on an outpatient basis with local anesthesia. TTT causes less choroidal damage than plaque radiotherapy. However, TTT cannot be performed if the pupil cannot be dilated to allow passage of the beam, if the tumour is so peripheral that the edges are not visible, if opacities prevent a clear view, or if there is more than 3 mm of subretinal fluid. TTT has been used successfully in select cases where plaque brachytherapy has failed. TTT has also been combined with plaque radiotherapy in a technique called sandwich therapy, as TTT is maximally effective at the apex of the tumour and brachytherapy is maximally effective at the base [22, 23, 24]. Moreover, TTT may show benefit in the treatment of hemangiomas and small retinoblastomas in addition to uveal melanomas.

12. References

[1] Finger PT. Radiation therapy for choroidal melanoma. Surv Ophthalmol. 1997; 42: 215-232.

[2] Diener-West M, Earle JD, Fine SLet al. The COMS randomized trial of iodine 125 brachytherapy for choroidal melanoma, III: initial mortality findings. COMS Report No. 18. Arch Ophthalmol. 2001 Jul; 119(7): 969-82

[3] Melia BM, Abramson DH, Albert DM et al. Collaborative ocular melanoma study (COMS) randomized trial of I-125 brachytherapy for medium choroidal melanoma. I. Visual acuity after 3 years COMS report no.16. Ophthalmology. 2001 Feb;108(2):348-66.

[4] The Collaborative Ocular Melanoma Study (COMS) randomized trial of pre-enucleation radiation of large choroidal melanoma II: initial mortality findings. COMS report no. 10. Am J Ophthalmol. 1998 Jun;125(6):779-96.

[5] Mortality in patients with small choroidal melanoma. COMS report N°.4. The Collaborative Ocular Melanoma Study Group. Arch Ophthalmol.1997; 115:886-893.
[6] Gragoudas ES, Goitein M, Koehler AM, et al. Proton irradiation of small choroidal malignant melanomas. Am J Ophthalmol. 1977;83:665–73.
[7] Clinical Radiation Oncology. Gunderson and Tepper. Second edition. Churchill-Livingstone. Elsevier. 2007.
[8] Munzenrider JE: Proton therapy for uveal melanomas and other eye lesions. Strahlenther Onkol 175 (suppl 2): 68, 1999.
[9] Courdi A, CaujolleJP, Grange JD et al: Rasults of proton therapy of uveal melanomas treated in Nice. Int J Radiat Oncol Biol Phys 45: 5-11, 1999.
[10] Egger E, Schalenbourg A, Zografos L, et al: Maximizing local tumor control and survival after proton beam radiotherapy of uveal melanoma. Int J Radiat Oncol Biol Phys 51: 138-147, 2001.
[11] Gragoudas ES, Lane AM, Regan S. A randomized controlled trial of varying radiation doses in the treatment of choroidal melanoma. Arch Ophthalmol. 2000; 118:773-778.
[12] Egger E, Zografos L, Schalenbourg A et al: Eye retention after proton beam radiotherapy for uveal melanomas. Int J Radiat Oncol Biol Phys 55: 867-880, 2003.
[13] Wilson NW, Hungerford JL. Comparison of epiescleral plaque and proton beam radiotherapy for the treatment of choroidal melanoma. Ophthalmology.1999; 106: 1579-1587.
[14] Fakiris AJ, Lo SS, Henderson MA, et al. Gamma-knife-based stereotactic radiosurgery for uveal melanoma. Stereotact Funct Neurosurg 2007;85:106–12.
[15] Modorati G, Miserocchi E, Galli L, et al. Gamma knife radiosurgery for uveal melanoma: 12 years of experience. Br J Ophthalmol 2009;93:40–4.
[16] Simonová G, Novotny´ Jr J, Liscák R, et al. Leksell gamma knife treatment of uveal melanoma. J Neurosurg 2002;97(5 Suppl.):635–9.
[17] Foulds WS, Damato BE. Alternatives to enucleation in the manage- ment of choroidal melanoma. Aust N Z J Ophthalmol. 1986;14: 19-27.
[18] Darren J. Bell, MD, and Matthew W. Wilson, MD. Choroidal Melanoma: Natural History and Management Options. Cancer Control. 2004, Vol. 11, No.5
[19] Histopathologic characteristics of uveal melanomas in eyes enucleated from the Collaborative Ocular Melanoma Study. COMS report No. 6. Am J Ophthalmol. 1998;125:745-766
[20] Damato B, Lecuona K. Conservation of eyes with choroidal melanoma by a multimodality approach to treatment: an audit of 1632 patients. Ophthalmology. 2004;111:977-983
[21] Shields CL, Shields JA, Perez N, et al. Primary transpupillary ther- motherapy for small choroidal melanoma in 256 consecutive cases: outcomes and limitations. Ophthalmology. 2002;109:225-234
[22] Robertson DM, Buettner H, Bennett SR. Transpupillary ther- motherapy as primary treatment for small choroidal melanomas. Arch Ophthalmol. 1999;117:1512-1519
[23] Stoffelns BM. Primary transpupillary thermotherapy (TTT) for malignant choroidal melanoma. Acta Ophthalmol Scand. 2002; 80:25-31.
[24] Journée-de Korver JG, Oosterhuis JA, de Wolff-Rouendaal D, et al. Histopathological findings in human choroidal melanomas after transpupillary thermotherapy. Br J Ophthalmol. 1997;81:234-239.

15

Oral Malignant Melanoma

Thomas Mücke, Anna Borgmann,
Klaus-Dietrich Wolff and David Andrew Mitchell
Department of Oral and Maxillofacial Surgery, Technische Universität München, Klinikum Rechts der Isar
Germany

1. Introduction

It is generally accepted that the outcome of oral malignant melanoma is worse than that of cutaneous and systemic head and neck melanoma. The five-year survival reported in the literature for oral melanomas varies from 0 - 20 % (Liversedge, 1975, Rapidis et al., 2003, Rapini et al., 1985), whereas the overall survival for head and neck melanomas ranges between 20 and 48 % (Guzzo et al., 1993, Patel et al., 2002, Stern and Guillamondegui, 1991, Temam et al., 2005), confirming anatomical site specific variation.

Treatment modalities for primary oral melanoma include surgical resection with or without neck dissection. Adjunctive modalities such as immunotherapy, chemotherapy and radiation therapy may offer a supportive but as yet non curative role. The mainstay of curative treatment is surgery, mandating complete resection of the tumor with clear margins if possible (Rapini et al., 1985, Umeda and Shimada, 1994). Immunotherapy and chemotherapy are techniques which are the subject of controlled trials or palliation (Mendenhall et al., 2005). The rarity of oral malignant melanomas means that to date no randomized clinical trials have been conducted to establish an evidence base in the literature to provide comparisons of treatment modalities. The efficacy of surgery with planned supplementary radiotherapy remain unresolved and continue to generate controversy (Patel et al., 2002).

Due the rarity of this disease, there is a lack of consistency in immunohistochemical confirmation of the diagnosis, staging strategies and treatment planning as diagnostic techniques and treatment have evolved over recent years in melanoma is other body sites and attempts have been made to translate these to the much rarer oral melanoma. This book section would like to aid the reader in understanding the current state of etiology, epidemiology, and treatment modalities of this very rare but aggressive tumor entity.

2. Oral malignant melanoma

The diagnosis of oral malignant melanoma often remains difficult. Differential diagnoses should include benign as well as malignant lesions and exogenous pigmentations can be often found (Figure 1). It also needs to be borne in mind that amelanotic malignant melanoma can affect the mouth, comprising one third of all oral malignant melanomas.

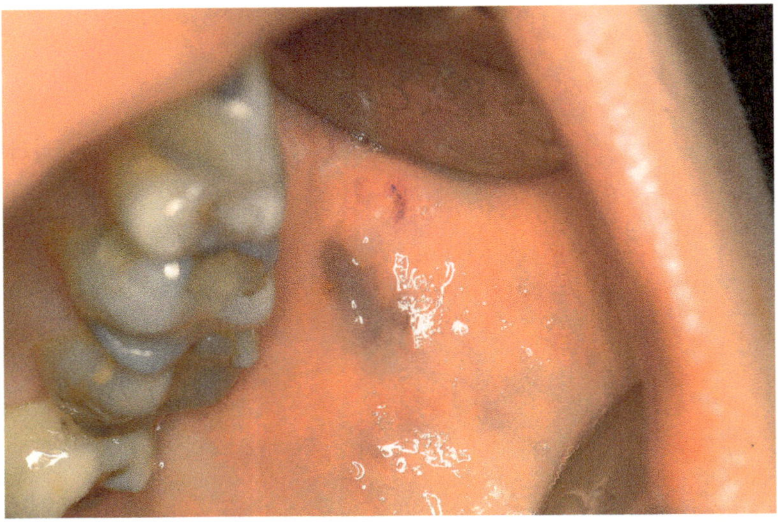

Fig. 1. Oral pigmentation due to inoculation of amalgam after dental treatment in the left buccal mucosa.

The histological spectrum of benign pigmentations is wide: macular hyperpigmentation caused by junctional proliferation with or without cellular atypica, melanocytic naevi (Figure 2), such as junctional, compound, subepithelial, blue and combined naevi. Other causes of oral pigmentation include: race, Peutz-Jeghers syndrome (Daley and Armstrong, 2007), Laugier-Hunziker syndrome (Mowad et al., 1997), Addison´s disease (Lamey et al., 1985), patients with pulmonary diseases, especially in lung cancer (Merchant et al., 1976), and hemosiderosis.

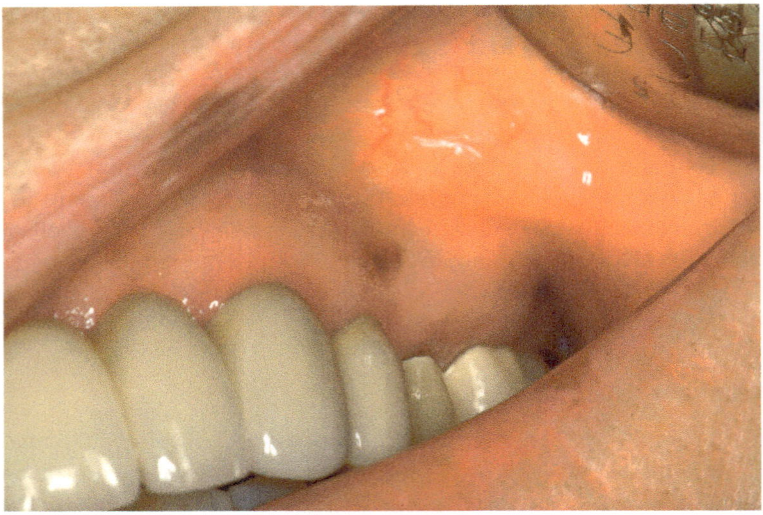

Fig. 2. Melanocytic naevi in the upper left vestibule.

Some authors describe a preexisting oral pigmentation for several month or years in one third of all patients with a primary oral malignant melanoma (Chaudhry et al., 1958, Liversedge, 1975, Rapini et al., 1985), although others found no correlation (Meleti et al., 2007). The appearances of oral malignant melanomas vary and should always be considered in oral lesions without the tendency to heal (Figure 3). Remember that about 1/3 of all oral malignant melanomas are not pigmented (Anneroth et al., 1973, Chaudhry et al., 1958, Greene et al., 1953, Lengyel et al., 2003, Liversedge, 1975, Rapidis et al., 2003).

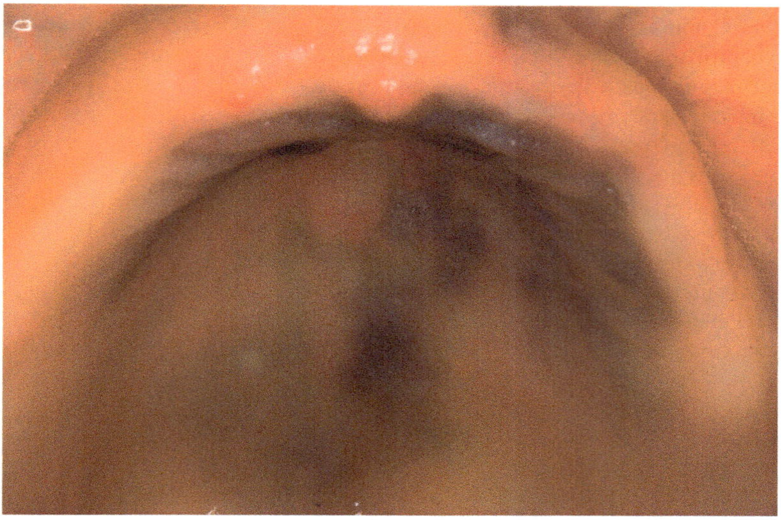

Fig. 3. Intraoral view of a malignant melanoma arising from the palate.

2.1 Etiology

Melanomas are categorized into four different types according to anatomic region and pathological factors: 1. melanomas arising from skin without chronic sun damage, 2. melanomas on skin with chronic sun damage, 3. acral melanomas, and 4. mucosal melanomas (Curtin et al., 2006). The etiology of primary oral malignant melanoma is still unknown. Cigarette smoking, denture irritation and alcohol have been mentioned as possible risk factors, but evidence remains obscure. Intraoral malignant melanomas arise from melanocytic cells of the oral cavity, which represent a minority of all cells of the mucosal membrane. Although just a few melanocytes are present in the oral mucosa the potential to develop malignant melanomas clearly exist. Indeed it is recognized that malignant melanoma can very rarely develop in almost any organ suggesting that circulating melanocytes may be responsible. About 5-30 % of primary malignant melanomas are preceded by oral pigmentations for months or even years. It has been suggested that melanosis represents the initial phase characterized as the radial phase of growth and precedes the invasion of underlying tissues (vertical growth) by years, however the histological spectrum of benign pigmented lesions is wide and a pre-existing pigmented lesion is not usually associated with mucosal melanomas. Most arise as new lesions, from apparently healthy mucosa.

Malignant melanomas develop from melanocytes derived from the neural crest. The most frequently primary sites in the oral cavity are the palate and maxillary gingiva (Barker et al., 1997, Hicks and Flaitz, 2000, Lee et al., 1994). Mucosal melanomas are considered to be more aggressive tumors compared with cutaneous melanomas and they are more inclined to metastasize into regional and distant sites, recur locally or regionally resulting in a high rate of disease specific-death.

2.2 Epidemiology

Malignant melanoma in the head and neck area is rare. Oral cavity primary malignant melanoma comprises 6.3 % of all melanomas in the head and neck area and only about 0.7 - 1.6 % of all melanomas arise in the oral mucosa (Chang et al., 1998, Moore and Martin, 1955). The incidence of primary mucosal melanomas of the head and neck is approximately four per 10 million population per year (Hicks and Flaitz, 2000). The most frequently affected oral sites are the palate and maxillary gingiva (Barker et al., 1997, Hicks and Flaitz, 2000, Lee et al., 1994). The incidence in Japan is much higher than in western countries, in which it occurs with less than 1% (Batsakis, 1982, Brandwein et al., 1997, Umeda and Shimada, 1994). The age of the patients varies between 20 and 80 years, the mean age reported in the literature ranges from 56 to 66.5 years (Gorsky and Epstein, 1998, Hicks and Flaitz, 2000, Patel et al., 2002, Rapidis et al., 2003, Rapini et al., 1985) and a modest male preponderance has been described (Rapini et al., 1985).

2.3 Prognosis

The prognosis is adverse. Due to delayed diagnosis early invasion of surrounding tissue, local lymph node involvement and distant metastasis, the prognosis of oral mucosal melanomas is very poor. The reported 5-year survival rates vary in the literature between 6 and 18 % but also between 45 and 48 % (Enroth CM, 1975, Lee et al., 1994, Lund, 1993, Ravid and Esteves, 1960, Stern and Guillamondegui, 1991). Gingival melanoma has a slightly better 5-year survival rate (18%) than that of palatal melanoma (11%), with a longer median survival period (46 months vs. 22 months). These wide variations are probably due to the fact that comparable classifications are still not agreed internationally. The routine use of tumor thicknessof mucosal melanomas, as described by the Breslow or the Clark levels are not widely performed as a routine method in everyday experience (Prasad et al., 2003, Prasad et al., 2002, Thompson et al., 2003). Therefore an evidence base derived fromhistopathological assessment and subsequent prognosis for malignant mucosal melanomas is lacking.Despite this many reports show a correlation between tumor thickness and prognosis (Mücke et al., 2009, Prasad et al., 2004). Many authors agreed that the survival rate was not only closely related to the stage of the tumor, but the treatment that patients received (Mücke et al., 2009, Prasad et al., 2003, Prasad et al., 2004, Rapidis et al., 2003, Rapini et al., 1985, Tanaka et al., 2004, Temam et al., 2005).

The vast majority of the head and neck mucosal melanomas are Stage 1 at the time of presentation , Prasad et al defined a 3-level-microstaging system, which represents different microanatomical compartments separated by tissue barriers. They found out that this microstaging system is prognostically significant and an independent predictor concerning the 5-year survival rate and the recurrence-free survival (Mücke et al., 2009, Prasad et al., 2004). In 2009, the American Joint Committee on Cancer (AJCC) Melanoma Staging Committee used previously published guidelines and determined criteria which were used in the TNM classification and the stage groupings (Balch et al., 2009). These criteria are established for all kinds of melanomas and are proposed as follows:

1. In patients with localized melanoma, tumor thickness, mitotic rate, tumor burden, and ulceration were the most important prognostic factors.
2. The mitotic rate indicates the level of invasion as a primary criterion for defining T1b melanomas.
3. Components that defined the N category were the presence and number of metastatic nodes of the primary melanoma.
4. All patients with microscopic nodal metastases, regardless of extent of tumor burden, are classified as stage III.
5. On the basis of a multivariate analysis of patients with distant metastases, the two dominant components in defining the M category continue to be the site of distant metastases and an elevated serum lactate dehydrogenase level.

Factors that have been associated with worse disease-specific survival include clinical stage at presentation, thickness of the tumor, tumor burden at the time of staging (microscopic vs. macroscopic), presence or absence of primary tumor ulceration, presence of vascular invasion, melanosis, and development of nodal and distant metastasis ($p < 0.001$) (Balch et al., 2009). Multiple local recurrences are the most common cause of treatment failure and may occur 10-15 years after primary treatment. The most common sites of distant metastases include the lungs, brain, liver and bones.

2.4 Staging

The criteria to verify the presence of a primary intraoral melanoma are:

1. demonstration of clinical and microscopic tumor in the oral mucosa
2. presence of junctional activity in the lesion
3. inability to show any other primary site.

All patients have to fulfill all these criteria to verify the diagnosis of primary oral malignant melanoma (Greene et al., 1953). In addition to the standard staging procedure, patients should be observed by means of: sonography, gastroscopy and bronchoscopy in order to exclude other potential primary sites and confirm by exclusion the diagnosis of primary oral mucosal malignant melanoma (Mücke et al., 2009). It is important to confirm the comparatively rare finding of primary oral mucosal malignant melanoma is supported by exclusion of other potential mucosal sites for example the respiratory and the gastrointestinal tract, which are more frequently found than oral melanomas (Lee et al., 1994, Mendenhall et al., 2005, Prasad et al., 2003).

Patients should be staged according the TNM Melanoma Staging System of the American Joint Committee on Cancer which includes in the staging the extent of the tumor status as well as the extent of the nodal status, but does not provide a specific guideline for oral mucosal melanomas. Therefore a simplified staging system has been established, which classifies tumors in 3 stages: Stage I to localized disease, confined to the primary site, stage II the primary lesion with cervical lymph node metastasis and stage III for distant metastasis.

As previously described there is a 3-level-microstaging system which relates to the prognostic outcome. In this system each level represents a microanatomical compartment, which is defined through tissue barriers.Breach of each barrier correlates with a progressively worse survival rate. Level I is defined as an in situ mucosal melanoma or microinvasion, Level II as an invasion limited to lamina propria and Level III is defined as melanoma with a deep invasion into surrounding tissue such as bone cartilage or skeletal muscles.

2.5 Histopathology

The surface architecture from oral melanomas ranges from macular to ulcerated and nodular. As recommended at the WESTOP (Western Society of Teachers of Oral Pathology) Banff Workshop, oral malignant melanomas should be separately considered from the cutaneous forms and proposed to subclassify them according to the histological pattern into: in situ melanoma, invasive, combined (invasive melanoma with in situ components) and atypical melanocytic proliferation (in case where diagnosis is equivocal) (Barker et al., 1997). In situ melanomas are limited to the epithelium and the epithelial-connective tissue interface, and represent 15% of the oral melanomas. They show a proliferation of atypical melanocytes characterized through hyperchromatic and angular nuclei with infrequent mitotic activity. The melanocytes may be arranged irregularly at the epithel connective tissue-interface or may be distributed in aggregates.

Invasive pattern in which the melanoma extend into the connective tissue is represented in 30% of oral melanoma, showing a wide range of cell types including spindle, plasmocytoid, clear cells and epithelioid, arranged into sheets or organoid/alveolar formation. The large and vesicular nuclei appear frequently with prominent nucleoli and rare mitosis. 55% of oral melanomas having combined pattern, which is typical for advanced lesions (Barker *et al.* 1997, Femiano *et al.* 2008).

In most instances melanomas contain melanin pigmented tumor cells but amelanotic melanoma show a lack of melanin production, which exacerbates the correct diagnosis, because amelanotic melanoma can mimic a variety of poorly differentiated carcinoma or cell lymphoma. For distinguishing these melanomas from other tumors immunohistochemical stains have been proven to be helpful. For differential diagnosis, it should be claimed that immunhistochemical staining of the following markers is mandatory and the basis of the diagnosis of an oral malignant melanoma.

Immunohistochemical markers include S-100 protein, gp100 (HMB-45) and Mart-1 (Melan-A) (Messina et al., 1999). These markers are also used for the identification of micrometastases in lymph nodes (Messina et al., 1999).

The Antibody HMB-45 reacts with the melanosomal glycoprotein gp100, showing a positive staining in active early melanosome formation and showing epithelioid lesions intensily immunoreactive for HMB-45. It is considered as more specific but less sensitive than the S-100 protein, an acidic calcium binding protein, which is a very sensitive marker for nevus and melanoma cells, and even spindled lesions appear intensely immunoreactive for S-100 protein (Blessing et al., 1998, Gazit and Daniels, 1994). Melan-A is considered to be specific for melanoma cell lines, as a product of the MART-1 gene it is a melanocytic differentiation marker which is recognized on melanomas as an antigenic target of T lymphocytes (Kawakami et al., 1994).

In recent years some molecular markers, like the Ki67 antigen emerged as potentially prognostical indicators, however the role of potential therapeutic relevance of KIT inhibitors in mucosal melanoma further needs to be investigated.

2.6 Therapy

Regarding the treatment of the four types of melanomas, melanomas arising from skin without chronic sun damage, melanomas on skin with chronic sun damage, acral melanomas and mucosal melanomas, most authors agree that radical ablative surgery with wide local excision of the primary lesion and dissection of metastatic lymph nodes are the basis of every curative therapy (Curtin et al., 2006). Controversial points are the margin of the excision, the optimal time to dissect the local lymph nodes, and the uncertainty of the extent of lymph nodes dissection. Surgery is the mainstay of treatment but can only be accomplished if vital parts of the body are not affected and therefore anatomical limitations often make a radical excision impossible.

The following protocol refers to the extent of margins:

1. Excision of the primary lesion including at least 1 - 2 cm of healthy tissue based on the primary tumor extent and thickness
2. Lymph node dissection and removal of lymph node metastases
3. Consideration of radiochemotherapy (limited evidence as to the benefit of postoperative radiotherapy exists for other anatomical sites).

2.6.1 Surgery

Principles defined by the first tumor resection in 1857 remain viable today in that the treatment of all melanomas should be performed by wide resection. Cutaneous melanomas are still treated by that principle to avoid local recurrence (Essner, 2003, Hauschild et al., 2003, Veronesi and Cascinelli, 1979). Limited excision of the primary lesion as well as excisional and incisional biopsies are associated with an increased risk of causing accidental dissemination of malignant cells within the adjacent tissues or even into the blood or lymphatic stream with probable devastating consequences (Harter et al., 1992, Kusukawa et al., 2000).

The surgical margin also depends on the thickness of the tumor. In patients with tumors less than 1 mm thickness, a surgical margin of 1 cm has been shown to be adequate, compared with wide tumor margin resections of 3 cm (Veronesi et al., 1988). None of these patients developed local recurrence in the follow-up period revealing an adequate resection extent. In patients with tumor thickness of 1 to 2mm local recurrences were found in both study groups of patients receiving resection margins of 1 cm or 3 cm without significant differences, although more recurrences were found in the 1 cm group (Veronesi et al., 1988). The evidence, that resections of 1 to 2 cm around the tumor are sufficient and show similar results in local control and overall survival, have been also found by other studies comparing the long term results of different resection protocols in varying tumor extent and thicknesses (Balch et al., 1993, Heaton et al., 1998). The local recurrence rate in these studies is 1.7% with 2 cm surgical margin compared with 0.8% with 4 cm after six years without statistically significant differences (Balch et al., 1993, Heaton et al., 1998). The surgical therapy within the oral cavity remains problematic because wide resection margins require also reconstruction techniques after tumor ablation to avoid mutilation, functional impairment and a poor quality of life (Mücke et al., 2009, Mücke et al., 2011, Mücke et al., 2010). In some instances the suggested resection margins would compromise vital structures which mean a compromise between theoretically ideal margins and postoperative function and quality of life must be made.

Regional lymph nodes are the most common sites of metastases for all melanomas. Palpable lymph nodes in the neck or fixed to the adjacent tissues should be suspicious for metastases. Radiologically, lymph nodes larger than 1 cm must also be considered to be involved by metastases. There exists a correlation between the tumor thickness and the occurrence of regional lymph node metastases. Primary lesions less than 1 mm thickness are considered to yield a rate of < 10% lymph node metastases, 1.01 to 2.00 mm are accounting for about 20%, 2.01 to 4.00 mm are accounting for 33%, and >4.00 mm are associated with a risk of lymph node involvement of more than 40% at the time of staging (Morton et al., 2005, Morton et al., 2003, Morton et al., 1993). Another study evaluated an exponential increasing of lymph node metastases if the tumor becomes thicker. A thickness of 0.76 to 1.50 mm was associated with regional lymph node metastases in 2 to 25% of cases. In tumors with a thickness between 1.51 to 4.00 mm the rate of regional lymph node metastases developed to 57%. A tumor thickness larger than 4 mm was associated with microscopic presence of metastases within the lymph nodes (Balch, 1999, Balch et al., 2000, Balch et al., 1996). There has been evidence that lymph node dissection resulted in an increase of overall survival compared to patients receiving palliative treatment to the neck only (Balch, 1999, Balch et al., 2000, Balch et al., 1996, Balch et al., 1993, Cascinelli et al., 1998). Negative lymph nodes are a strong prognostic factor for survival, whereas lymph node metastases yield a 6 times higher relative risk for death (Balch et al., 2009, Gershenwald et al., 1999).

Patients who suffered from oral mucosal malignant melanomas are often diagnosed at an advanced stage followed by ulceration, microsatellites or regional nodal metastases (Chaudhry et al., 1958, Morton et al., 1993, Mücke et al., 2009, Patel et al., 2002, Prasad et al., 2004, Rapidis et al., 2003, Temam et al., 2005). This high rate of regional lymph node metastases means that patients at risk should be considered for therapeutic elective neck dissection with a low threshold for surgery. Although no randomized trials on the treatment of the regional lymph nodes for oral mucosal malignant melanoma exist due to the rarity of this tumor, there is little doubt about this treatment approach. (Balch et al., 2009, Balch et al., 1996, Cascinelli et al., 1998, Chaudhry et al., 1958, Essner, 2003, Hauschild et al., 2003, Medina et al., 2003, Morton et al., 2003, Morton et al., 1993, Mücke et al., 2009, Patel et al., 2002, Tanaka et al., 2004, Temam et al., 2005). As the oral melanoma is very aggressive and the texture of the mucosa is different from the cutis with an earlier occurrence of lymph node metastases, there is actually no role for the sentinel lymph node technique, as the risk of micrometastases has to be excluded by standard therapeutic neck dissection (Prasad et al., 2004, Snow and van der Waal, 1986, Umeda and Shimada, 1994).

2.6.2 Radiotherapy

Radiotherapy has been used to control local recurrence (Balch et al., 1993, Harwood, 1983, Schmidt-Ullrich and Johnson, 1996, Storper et al., 1993). Postoperative, adjuvant radiation therapy results in a lower local recurrence rate in comparison to patients without radiotherapy treated by wide surgical resection only (Harwood, 1983). Hyperfractionated accelerated radiotherapies have appeared most useful (Harwood, 1983, Schmidt-Ullrich and Johnson, 1996, Storper et al., 1993), although the differences were not found to be statistically significant. The adjuvant performance of radiotherapy should be considered in advanced stage malignant melanomas of the oral cavity. There are still no data available from randomized trials regarding the efficacy of adjuvant radiotherapy.

2.7 Adjuvant therapy

Adjuvant therapy modalities vary and include the application of non-specific immunostimulants (Grooms et al., 1977, Morton et al., 1970, Morton et al., 1974, Sondak and Wolfe, 1997), specific immunstimulants (Interferons), vaccination therapy, cytotoxic chemotherapy, and target-therapy.

Non-specific immunstimulants like Bacille Calmette-Guérin (BCG), Cryptosporidium parvum, Levanisole, thymosin, isoprinosine, transfer factor and retinoids, and interleukin had been applied by local injection into the tumor (Grooms et al., 1977, Morton et al., 1970, Morton et al., 1974, Sondak and Wolfe, 1997). Although some authors reported limited evidence that survival was increased by this therapy this adjuvant therapy failed to prove an advantage in comparison with control treatment of any kind. Most studies performed were retrospective studies (Grooms et al., 1977, Morton et al., 1970, Morton et al., 1974, Sondak and Wolfe, 1997).

After non-specific immunostimulants have failed to establish an effect on overall survival or an improvement of symptoms, attention was paid to more specific immunostimulants such as Interferons. These glycoproteins showed a immunmodulatory and anti-tumoral effect, which was thought to be beneficial in melanoma patients. Expression of major histocompatibility complex molecules, enhancing of antigen presentation by dendritic cells, inhibition of angiogenesis, and a directly antiproliferative effect combined with the expression of melanoma-specific antigen and the stimulation of natural killer cells directly affecting the tumor was a promising treatment modality (Ascierto and Kirkwood, 2008, Janku and Kurzrock, 2010, Jonasch and Haluska, 2001, Jonasch et al., 2000, Kalani et al., 2008, Pfeffer et al., 1998). Unfortunaetly early enthusiasm has waned and this strategy is more and more critically debated (Janku and Kurzrock, 2010). The effect of interferon-α (IFN-α) has been well evaluated in different clinical trials in melanoma patients and a dose-dependent and duration-dependent effect has been found, especially in high-risk patients with the presence of lymph node metastases or thick melanoma patients (Kirkwood et al., 2001, Kirkwood et al., 1996, Punt and Eggermont, 2001). In contrast, high-dose IFN-α is often associated with severe toxicity (Eggermont, 2002, Eggermont and Gore, 2002), and the outcome reported by the Southwest Oncology Group revealed no clinical benefit for patients who received adjuvant therapy. Indeed they may have done worse when compared to the patients who received no adjuvant therapy (Barth and Morton, 1995, Taylor et al., 1992).

Another adjuvant method for the therapy of melanoma patients are vaccination therapies. Based on the evidence that the immune system plays a natural role in melanoma progression in the same way that the previous treatment modalities tried to act at the same mechanism, vaccination therapy is designed to activate the host immune response to tumor - associated antigens. In the lack of information about specific tumor antigens, the tumor cell was the best source of antigens for activating the immune system (Hersey et al., 2002, Hersey et al., 1987, Sun et al., 1999). Previous methods of producing vaccines are always based on tumor cell preparations, but there is still no role for vaccination therapies in oral malignant melanomas.

The most established therapy beside surgery combined with radiotherapy remains cytotoxic chemotherapy. Multiple trials about a variety of cytotoxic drugs in adjuvant treatment have been performed but no study demonstrated benefits of adjuvant chemotherapy in melanoma patients at high risk for relapse or affecting overall survival significantly in controlled randomized trials. The mainstay of chemotherapy remains the palliative situation. The mainstays of cytotoxic chemotherapy include; dacarbazine, the nitrosoureas, the vinca alkaloids, cisplatin, paclitaxel, and bleomycin. The use of additional chemotherapeutic agents is still evolving. Single-drug therapy with dacarbazine reported an objective response in 18-22% of patients with measurable metastatic disease (Hill et al., 1979, Hill et al., 1981, Houghton et al., 2006, Houghton et al., 1996, Lee et al., 1995). Some trials describe efficacy of dacarbazine as a postsurgical adjuvant, but suggested no significant clinical benefit in the treatment of patients with high risk melanoma (Hill et al., 1979, Hill et al., 1981, Veronesi et al., 1982). Multiagent cytotoxic therapy is similarly unhelpful in the adjuvant setting. Other trials of multiagent chemotherapy using nitrosoureas, dactinomycin and vincristine present contrary results (1983, Castel et al., 1991, McClay et al., 2000, Pawlik and Sondak, 2003, Wood et al., 1978).

3. Conclusion

The incidence of oral melanoma is very low and results of the treatment are still poor partly due to the advanced stage of tumor at presentation. No single management strategy or guideline can be considered the standard of care on the basis of current data. Within the head and neck the extent of the tumor, spread to the regional lymph nodes, systemic disease and histopathological variables have to be integrated into the disease staging and related to the patients' co-morbidities and personal aims. Radicality of resection has to be balanced against the feasibility of reconstruction of the resected area obtaining form and function as well as the quality of life the patient requires. Treatment of oral mucosal malignant melanoma may not be entirely consistent with the treatment of cutaneous malignant melanoma. The thickness of the primary lesion, stage of regional lymph nodes, sex, age, the reaction of the lesion to treatment are important factors influencing prognosis and treatment choices of the disease. To date, due to the rarity of this tumor entity, no randomized trials exist demonstrating any optimal treatment algorithm.

Multicenter studies collecting data about the treatment strategies and outcomes of patients suffering from oral malignant melanomas are necessary to identify the best treatment algorithm based on patient related clinical work. Oral melanomas are different from cutaneous melanomas and such studies would provide us a far better insight into their behaviour. The tumor thickness is a variable that most accurately determines therapy and prognoses, therefore, the extent of surgery margins should be decided based on the invasive depth of the primary lesion, the neck addressed on the basis of imaging staging but with a low threshold for intervention. Reconstruction follows conventional approaches but adjuvant therapy is currently disappointing.

An increasing understanding of tumour immunology and biology has led to innovative therapies which are necessary if an effective treatment for oral malignant melanomas is to be developed in the future. The application of new or established technologies in experimental tumor models is necessary to increase the potential for such treatments (e.g. proteomics, targeted therapy, vaccination therapy), but is currently still an area of experimentation and hope rather than pragmatic clinical practice.

4. Acknowledgement

The authors would like to thank the patients who gave their pictures for this book chapter.

5. References

(1983) Randomized controlled trial of adjuvant chemoimmunotherapy with DTIC and BCG after complete excision of primary melanoma with a poor prognosis or melanoma metastases. *Can Med Assoc J* 128: 929-933.

Anneroth G, Carlson GO, Eneroth CM & Moberger G (1973) Primary melanoma in the oral mucous membrane. *Sven Tandlak Tidskr* 66: 27-37.

Ascierto PA & Kirkwood JM (2008) Adjuvant therapy of melanoma with interferon: lessons of the past decade. *J Transl Med* 6: 62.

Balch CM (1999) Randomized surgical trials involving elective node dissection for melanoma. *Adv Surg* 32: 255-270.

Balch CM, Gershenwald JE, Soong SJ, Thompson JF, Atkins MB, Byrd DR, Buzaid AC, Cochran AJ, Coit DG, Ding S, Eggermont AM, Flaherty KT, Gimotty PA, Kirkwood JM, McMasters KM, Mihm MC, Jr., Morton DL, Ross MI, Sober AJ & Sondak VK (2009) Final version of 2009 AJCC melanoma staging and classification. *J Clin Oncol* 27: 6199-6206.

Balch CM, Morton DL, Gershenwald JE, McMasters KM, Nieweg OE, Powell B, Ross MI, Sondak VK & Thompson JF (2009) Sentinel node biopsy and standard of care for melanoma. *J Am Acad Dermatol* 60: 872-875.

Balch CM, Soong S, Ross MI, Urist MM, Karakousis CP, Temple WJ, Mihm MC, Barnhill RL, Jewell WR, Wanebo HJ & Harrison R (2000) Long-term results of a multi-institutional randomized trial comparing prognostic factors and surgical results for intermediate thickness melanomas (1.0 to 4.0 mm). Intergroup Melanoma Surgical Trial. *Ann Surg Oncol* 7: 87-97.

Balch CM, Soong SJ, Bartolucci AA, Urist MM, Karakousis CP, Smith TJ, Temple WJ, Ross MI, Jewell WR, Mihm MC, Barnhill RL & Wanebo HJ (1996) Efficacy of an elective regional lymph node dissection of 1 to 4 mm thick melanomas for patients 60 years of age and younger. *Ann Surg* 224: 255-263; discussion 263-256.

Balch CM, Urist MM, Karakousis CP, Smith TJ, Temple WJ, Drzewiecki K, Jewell WR, Bartolucci AA, Mihm MC, Jr., Barnhill R & et al. (1993) Efficacy of 2-cm surgical margins for intermediate-thickness melanomas (1 to 4 mm). Results of a multi-institutional randomized surgical trial. *Ann Surg* 218: 262-267; discussion 267-269.

Barker BF, Carpenter WM, Daniels TE, Kahn MA, Leider AS, Lozada-Nur F, Lynch DP, Melrose R, Merrell P, Morton T, Peters E, Regezi JA, Richards SD, Rick GM, Rohrer MD, Slater L, Stewart JC, Tomich CE, Vickers RA, Wood NK & Young SK (1997) Oral mucosal melanomas: the WESTOP Banff workshop proceedings. Western Society of Teachers of Oral Pathology. *Oral Surg Oral Med Oral Pathol Oral Radiol Endod* 83: 672-679.

Barth A & Morton DL (1995) The role of adjuvant therapy in melanoma management. *Cancer* 75: 726-734.

Batsakis JG (1982) The pathology of head and neck tumors: the lymphoepithelial lesion and Sjogren's syndrome, Part 16. *Head Neck Surg* 5: 150-163.

Blessing K, Sanders DS & Grant JJ (1998) Comparison of immunohistochemical staining of the novel antibody melan-A with S100 protein and HMB-45 in malignant melanoma and melanoma variants. *Histopathology* 32: 139-146.

Brandwein MS, Rothstein A, Lawson W, Bodian C & Urken ML (1997) Sinonasal melanoma. A clinicopathologic study of 25 cases and literature meta-analysis. *Arch Otolaryngol Head Neck Surg* 123: 290-296.

Cascinelli N, Morabito A, Santinami M, MacKie RM & Belli F (1998) Immediate or delayed dissection of regional nodes in patients with melanoma of the trunk: a randomised trial. WHO Melanoma Programme. *Lancet* 351: 793-796.

Castel T, Estape J, Vinolas N, Mascaro JM, Castro J, Vilalta A, Gratacos R, Daniels M, Palou J, Grau JJ & et al. (1991) Adjuvant treatment in stage I and II malignant melanoma:

a randomized trial between chemoimmunotherapy and immunotherapy. *Dermatologica* 183: 25-30.

Chang AE, Karnell LH & Menck HR (1998) The National Cancer Data Base report on cutaneous and noncutaneous melanoma: a summary of 84,836 cases from the past decade. The American College of Surgeons Commission on Cancer and the American Cancer Society. *Cancer* 83: 1664-1678.

Chaudhry AP, Hampel A & Gorlin RJ (1958) Primary malignant melanoma of the oral cavity: a review of 105 cases. *Cancer* 11: 923-928.

Curtin JA, Busam K, Pinkel D & Bastian BC (2006) Somatic activation of KIT in distinct subtypes of melanoma. *J Clin Oncol* 24: 4340-4346.

Daley TD & Armstrong JE (2007) Oral manifestations of gastrointestinal diseases. *Can J Gastroenterol* 21: 241-244.

Eggermont AM (2002) Critical appraisal of IFN-alpha-based adjuvant therapy in stage II-III malignant melanoma. *Expert Rev Anticancer Ther* 2: 563-569.

Eggermont AM & Gore M (2002) European approach to adjuvant treatment of intermediate- and high-risk malignant melanoma. *Semin Oncol* 29: 382-388.

Enroth CM LC (1975) Mucosal malignant melanoma of the head and neck. *Acta Otolaryngol* 80: 452-458.

Essner R (2003) Surgical treatment of malignant melanoma. *Surg Clin North Am* 83: 109-156.

Gazit D & Daniels TE (1994) Oral melanocytic lesions: differences in expression of HMB-45 and S-100 antigens in round and spindle cells of malignant and benign lesions. *J Oral Pathol Med* 23: 60-64.

Gershenwald JE, Thompson W, Mansfield PF, Lee JE, Colome MI, Tseng CH, Lee JJ, Balch CM, Reintgen DS & Ross MI (1999) Multi-institutional melanoma lymphatic mapping experience: the prognostic value of sentinel lymph node status in 612 stage I or II melanoma patients. *J Clin Oncol* 17: 976-983.

Gorsky M & Epstein JB (1998) Melanoma arising from the mucosal surfaces of the head and neck. *Oral Surg Oral Med Oral Pathol Oral Radiol Endod* 86: 715-719.

Greene GW, Haynes JW, Dozier M, Blumberg JM & Bernier JL (1953) Primary malignant melanoma of the oral mucosa. *Oral Surg Oral Med Oral Pathol* 6: 1435-1443.

Grooms GA, Eilber FR & Morton DL (1977) Failure of adjuvant immunotherapy to prevent central nervous system metastases in malignant melanoma patients. *J Surg Oncol* 9: 147-153.

Guzzo M, Grandi C, Licitra L, Podrecca S, Cascinelli N & Molinari R (1993) Mucosal malignant melanoma of head and neck: forty-eight cases treated at Istituto Nazionale Tumori of Milan. *Eur J Surg Oncol* 19: 316-319.

Harter LP, Curtis JS, Ponto G & Craig PH (1992) Malignant seeding of the needle track during stereotaxic core needle breast biopsy. *Radiology* 185: 713-714.

Harwood AR (1983) Melanomas of the head and neck. *J Otolaryngol* 12: 64-69.

Hauschild A, Rosien F & Lischner S (2003) Surgical standards in the primary care of melanoma patients. *Onkologie* 26: 218-222.

Heaton KM, Sussman JJ, Gershenwald JE, Lee JE, Reintgen DS, Mansfield PF & Ross MI (1998) Surgical margins and prognostic factors in patients with thick (>4mm) primary melanoma. *Ann Surg Oncol* 5: 322-328.

Hersey P, Coates AS, McCarthy WH, Thompson JF, Sillar RW, McLeod R, Gill PG, Coventry BJ, McMullen A, Dillon H & Simes RJ (2002) Adjuvant immunotherapy of patients with high-risk melanoma using vaccinia viral lysates of melanoma: results of a randomized trial. *J Clin Oncol* 20: 4181-4190.

Hersey P, Edwards A, Coates A, Shaw H, McCarthy W & Milton G (1987) Evidence that treatment with vaccinia melanoma cell lysates (VMCL) may improve survival of patients with stage II melanoma. Treatment of stage II melanoma with viral lysates. *Cancer Immunol Immunother* 25: 257-265.

Hicks MJ & Flaitz CM (2000) Oral mucosal melanoma: epidemiology and pathobiology. *Oral Oncol* 36: 152-169.

Hill GJ, 2nd, Metter GE, Krementz ET, Fletcher WS, Golomb FM, Ramirez G, Grage TB & Moss SE (1979) DTIC and combination therapy for melanoma. II. Escalating schedules of DTIC with BCNU, CCNU, and vincristine. *Cancer Treat Rep* 63: 1989-1992.

Hill GJ, 2nd, Moss SE, Golomb FM, Grage TB, Fletcher WS, Minton JP & Krementz ET (1981) DTIC and combination therapy for melanoma: III. DTIC (NSC 45388) Surgical Adjuvant Study COG PROTOCOL 7040. *Cancer* 47: 2556-2562.

Houghton AN, Coit DG, Daud A, Dilawari RA, Dimaio D, Gollob JA, Haas NB, Halpern A, Johnson TM, Kashani-Sabet M, Kraybill WG, Lange JR, Martini M, Ross MI, Samlowski WE, Sener SF, Tanabe KK, Thompson JA, Trisal V, Urist MM & Walker MJ (2006) Melanoma. *J Natl Compr Canc Netw* 4: 666-684.

Houghton AN, Meyers ML & Chapman PB (1996) Medical treatment of metastatic melanoma. *Surg Clin North Am* 76: 1343-1354.

Janku F & Kurzrock R (2010) Adjuvant interferon in high-risk melanoma: end of the era? *J Clin Oncol* 28: e15-16; author reply e17-18.

Jonasch E & Haluska FG (2001) Interferon in oncological practice: review of interferon biology, clinical applications, and toxicities. *Oncologist* 6: 34-55.

Jonasch E, Kumar UN, Linette GP, Hodi FS, Soiffer RJ, Ryan BF, Sober AJ, Mihm MC, Tsao H, Langley RG, Cosimi BA, Gadd MA, Tanabe KK, Souba W, Haynes HA, Barnhill R, Osteen R & Haluska FG (2000) Adjuvant high-dose interferon alfa-2b in patients with high-risk melanoma. *Cancer J* 6: 139-145.

Kalani AD, Jack A, Montenegro G, Degliuomini J & Wallack MK (2008) Immunotherapy as an adjuvant therapy in the management of advanced, surgically resected, melanoma. *G Ital Dermatol Venereol* 143: 59-70.

Kawakami Y, Eliyahu S, Delgado CH, Robbins PF, Rivoltini L, Topalian SL, Miki T & Rosenberg SA (1994) Cloning of the gene coding for a shared human melanoma antigen recognized by autologous T cells infiltrating into tumor. *Proc Natl Acad Sci U S A* 91: 3515-3519.

Kirkwood JM, Ibrahim JG, Sosman JA, Sondak VK, Agarwala SS, Ernstoff MS & Rao U (2001) High-dose interferon alfa-2b significantly prolongs relapse-free and overall survival compared with the GM2-KLH/QS-21 vaccine in patients with resected stage IIB-III melanoma: results of intergroup trial E1694/S9512/C509801. *J Clin Oncol* 19: 2370-2380.

Kirkwood JM, Strawderman MH, Ernstoff MS, Smith TJ, Borden EC & Blum RH (1996) Interferon alfa-2b adjuvant therapy of high-risk resected cutaneous melanoma: the Eastern Cooperative Oncology Group Trial EST 1684. *J Clin Oncol* 14: 7-17.

Kusukawa J, Suefuji Y, Ryu F, Noguchi R, Iwamoto O & Kameyama T (2000) Dissemination of cancer cells into circulation occurs by incisional biopsy of oral squamous cell carcinoma. *J Oral Pathol Med* 29: 303-307.

Lamey PJ, Carmichael F & Scully C (1985) Oral pigmentation, Addison's disease and the results of screening for adrenocortical insufficiency. *Br Dent J* 158: 297-298.

Lee SM, Betticher DC & Thatcher N (1995) Melanoma: chemotherapy. *Br Med Bull* 51: 609-630.

Lee SP, Shimizu KT, Tran LM, Juillard G & Calcaterra TC (1994) Mucosal melanoma of the head and neck: the impact of local control on survival. *Laryngoscope* 104: 121-126.

Lengyel E, Gilde K, Remenar E & Esik O (2003) Malignant mucosal melanoma of the head and neck. *Pathol Oncol Res* 9: 7-12.

Liversedge RL (1975) Oral malignant melanoma. *Br J Oral Surg* 13: 40-55.

Lund VJ (1993) Malignant melanoma of the nasal cavity and paranasal sinuses. *Ear Nose Throat J* 72: 285-290.

McClay EF, McClay ME, Monroe L, Baron PL, Cole DJ, O'Brien PH, Metcalf JS & Maize JC (2000) The effect of tamoxifen and cisplatin on the disease-free and overall survival of patients with high risk malignant melanoma. *Br J Cancer* 83: 16-21.

Medina JE, Ferlito A, Pellitteri PK, Shaha AR, Khafif A, Devaney KO, Fisher SR, O'Brien CJ, Byers RM, Robbins KT, Pitman KT & Rinaldo A (2003) Current management of mucosal melanoma of the head and neck. *J Surg Oncol* 83: 116-122.

Meleti M, Mooi WJ, Casparie MK & van der Waal I (2007) Melanocytic nevi of the oral mucosa - no evidence of increased risk for oral malignant melanoma: an analysis of 119 cases. *Oral Oncol* 43: 976-981.

Mendenhall WM, Amdur RJ, Hinerman RW, Werning JW, Villaret DB & Mendenhall NP (2005) Head and neck mucosal melanoma. *Am J Clin Oncol* 28: 626-630.

Merchant HW, Hayes LE & Ellison LT (1976) Soft-palate pigmentation in lung disease, including cancer. *Oral Surg Oral Med Oral Pathol* 41: 726-733.

Messina JL, Glass LF, Cruse CW, Berman C, Ku NK & Reintgen DS (1999) Pathologic examination of the sentinel lymph node in malignant melanoma. *Am J Surg Pathol* 23: 686-690.

Moore ES & Martin H (1955) Melanoma of the upper respiratory tract and oral cavity. *Cancer* 8: 1167-1176.

Morton D, Eilber FR, Malmgren RA & Wood WC (1970) Immunological factors which influence response to immunotherapy in malignant melanoma. *Surgery* 68: 158-163; discussion 163-154.

Morton DL, Cochran AJ, Thompson JF, Elashoff R, Essner R, Glass EC, Mozzillo N, Nieweg OE, Roses DF, Hoekstra HJ, Karakousis CP, Reintgen DS, Coventry BJ & Wang HJ (2005) Sentinel node biopsy for early-stage melanoma: accuracy and morbidity in MSLT-I, an international multicenter trial. *Ann Surg* 242: 302-311; discussion 311-303.

Morton DL, Eilber FR, Holmes EC, Hunt JS, Ketcham AS, Silverstein MJ & Sparks FC (1974) BCG immunotherapy of malignant melanoma: summary of a seven-year experience. *Ann Surg* 180: 635-643.

Morton DL, Hoon DS, Cochran AJ, Turner RR, Essner R, Takeuchi H, Wanek LA, Glass E, Foshag LJ, Hsueh EC, Bilchik AJ, Elashoff D & Elashoff R (2003) Lymphatic mapping and sentinel lymphadenectomy for early-stage melanoma: therapeutic utility and implications of nodal microanatomy and molecular staging for improving the accuracy of detection of nodal micrometastases. *Ann Surg* 238: 538-549; discussion 549-550.

Morton DL, Wen DR, Foshag LJ, Essner R & Cochran A (1993) Intraoperative lymphatic mapping and selective cervical lymphadenectomy for early-stage melanomas of the head and neck. *J Clin Oncol* 11: 1751-1756.

Mowad CM, Shrager J & Elenitsas R (1997) Oral pigmentation representing Laugier-Hunziker syndrome. *Cutis* 60: 37-39.

Mücke T, Hölzle F, Kesting MR, Loeffelbein DJ, Robitzky LK, Hohlweg-Majert B, Tannapfel A & Wolff KD (2009) Tumor size and depth in primary malignant melanoma in the oral cavity influences survival. *J Oral Maxillofac Surg* 67: 1409-1415.

Mücke T, Hölzle F, Wagenpfeil S, Wolff KD & Kesting M (2011) The role of tumor invasion into the mandible of oral squamous cell carcinoma. *J Cancer Res Clin Oncol* 137: 165-171.

Mücke T, Wolff KD, Wagenpfeil S, Mitchell DA & Hölzle F (2010) Immediate microsurgical reconstruction after tumor ablation predicts survival among patients with head and neck carcinoma. *Ann Surg Oncol* 17: 287-295.

Patel SG, Prasad ML, Escrig M, Singh B, Shaha AR, Kraus DH, Boyle JO, Huvos AG, Busam K & Shah JP (2002) Primary mucosal malignant melanoma of the head and neck. *Head Neck* 24: 247-257.

Pawlik TM & Sondak VK (2003) Malignant melanoma: current state of primary and adjuvant treatment. *Crit Rev Oncol Hematol* 45: 245-264.

Pfeffer LM, Dinarello CA, Herberman RB, Williams BR, Borden EC, Bordens R, Walter MR, Nagabhushan TL, Trotta PP & Pestka S (1998) Biological properties of recombinant alpha-interferons: 40th anniversary of the discovery of interferons. *Cancer Res* 58: 2489-2499.

Prasad ML, Busam KJ, Patel SG, Hoshaw-Woodard S, Shah JP & Huvos AG (2003) Clinicopathologic differences in malignant melanoma arising in oral squamous and sinonasal respiratory mucosa of the upper aerodigestive tract. *Arch Pathol Lab Med* 127: 997-1002.

Prasad ML, Patel S, Hoshaw-Woodard S, Escrig M, Shah JP, Huvos AG & Busam KJ (2002) Prognostic factors for malignant melanoma of the squamous mucosa of the head and neck. *Am J Surg Pathol* 26: 883-892.

Prasad ML, Patel SG, Huvos AG, Shah JP & Busam KJ (2004) Primary mucosal melanoma of the head and neck: a proposal for microstaging localized, Stage I (lymph node-negative) tumors. *Cancer* 100: 1657-1664.

Punt CJ & Eggermont AM (2001) Adjuvant interferon-alpha for melanoma revisited: news from old and new studies. *Ann Oncol* 12: 1663-1666.

Rapidis AD, Apostolidis C, Vilos G & Valsamis S (2003) Primary malignant melanoma of the oral mucosa. *J Oral Maxillofac Surg* 61: 1132-1139.

Rapini RP, Golitz LE, Greer RO, Jr., Krekorian EA & Poulson T (1985) Primary malignant melanoma of the oral cavity. A review of 177 cases. *Cancer* 55: 1543-1551.

Ravid JM & Esteves JA (1960) Malignant melanoma of the nose and paranasal sinuses and juvenile melanoma of the nose. *Arch Otolaryngol* 72: 431-444.

Schmidt-Ullrich RK & Johnson CR (1996) Role of radiotherapy and hyperthermia in the management of malignant melanoma. *Semin Surg Oncol* 12: 407-415.

Snow GB & van der Waal I (1986) Mucosal melanomas of the head and neck. *Otolaryngol Clin North Am* 19: 537-547.

Sondak VK & Wolfe JA (1997) Adjuvant therapy for melanoma. *Curr Opin Oncol* 9: 189-204.

Stern SJ & Guillamondegui OM (1991) Mucosal melanoma of the head and neck. *Head Neck* 13: 22-27.

Storper IS, Lee SP, Abemayor E & Juillard G (1993) The role of radiation therapy in the treatment of head and neck cutaneous melanoma. *Am J Otolaryngol* 14: 426-431.

Sun Y, Paschen A & Schadendorf D (1999) Cell-based vaccination against melanoma--background, preliminary results, and perspective. *J Mol Med* 77: 593-608.

Tanaka N, Mimura M, Ogi K & Amagasa T (2004) Primary malignant melanoma of the oral cavity: assessment of outcome from the clinical records of 35 patients. *Int J Oral Maxillofac Surg* 33: 761-765.

Taylor CW, Chase EM, Whitehead RP, Rinehart JJ, Neidhart JA, Gonzalez R, Bunn PA & Hersh EM (1992) A Southwest Oncology Group Phase I study of the sequential combination of recombinant interferon-gamma and recombinant interleukin-2 in patients with cancer. *J Immunother (1991)* 11: 176-183.

Temam S, Mamelle G, Marandas P, Wibault P, Avril MF, Janot F, Julieron M, Schwaab G & Luboinski B (2005) Postoperative radiotherapy for primary mucosal melanoma of the head and neck. *Cancer* 103: 313-319.

Thompson LD, Wieneke JA & Miettinen M (2003) Sinonasal tract and nasopharyngeal melanomas: a clinicopathologic study of 115 cases with a proposed staging system. *Am J Surg Pathol* 27: 594-611.

Umeda M & Shimada K (1994) Primary malignant melanoma of the oral cavity--its histological classification and treatment. *Br J Oral Maxillofac Surg* 32: 39-47.

Veronesi U, Adamus J, Aubert C, Bajetta E, Beretta G, Bonadonna G, Bufalino R, Cascinelli N, Cocconi G, Durand J, De Marsillac J, Ikonopisov RL, Kiss B, Lejeune F, MacKie R, Madej G, Mulder H, Mechl Z, Milton GW, Morabito A, Peter H, Priario J, Paul E, Rumke P, Sertoli R & Tomin R (1982) A randomized trial of adjuvant chemotherapy and immunotherapy in cutaneous melanoma. *N Engl J Med* 307: 913-916.

Veronesi U & Cascinelli N (1979) Surgical treatment of malignant melanoma of the skin. *World J Surg* 3: 279-288.

Veronesi U, Cascinelli N, Adamus J, Balch C, Bandiera D, Barchuk A, Bufalino R, Craig P, De Marsillac J, Durand JC & et al. (1988) Thin stage I primary cutaneous malignant melanoma. Comparison of excision with margins of 1 or 3 cm. *N Engl J Med* 318: 1159-1162.

Wood WC, Cosimi AB, Carey RW & Kaufman SD (1978) Randomized trial of adjuvant therapy for "high risk" primary malignant melanoma. *Surgery* 83: 677-681.

Permissions

The contributors of this book come from diverse backgrounds, making this book a truly international effort. This book will bring forth new frontiers with its revolutionizing research information and detailed analysis of the nascent developments around the world.

We would like to thank Rachael Morton, for lending her expertise to make the book truly unique. She has played a crucial role in the development of this book. Without her invaluable contribution this book wouldn't have been possible. She has made vital efforts to compile up to date information on the varied aspects of this subject to make this book a valuable addition to the collection of many professionals and students.

This book was conceptualized with the vision of imparting up-to-date information and advanced data in this field. To ensure the same, a matchless editorial board was set up. Every individual on the board went through rigorous rounds of assessment to prove their worth. After which they invested a large part of their time researching and compiling the most relevant data for our readers. Conferences and sessions were held from time to time between the editorial board and the contributing authors to present the data in the most comprehensible form. The editorial team has worked tirelessly to provide valuable and valid information to help people across the globe.

Every chapter published in this book has been scrutinized by our experts. Their significance has been extensively debated. The topics covered herein carry significant findings which will fuel the growth of the discipline. They may even be implemented as practical applications or may be referred to as a beginning point for another development. Chapters in this book were first published by InTech; hereby published with permission under the Creative Commons Attribution License or equivalent.

The editorial board has been involved in producing this book since its inception. They have spent rigorous hours researching and exploring the diverse topics which have resulted in the successful publishing of this book. They have passed on their knowledge of decades through this book. To expedite this challenging task, the publisher supported the team at every step. A small team of assistant editors was also appointed to further simplify the editing procedure and attain best results for the readers.

Our editorial team has been hand-picked from every corner of the world. Their multi-ethnicity adds dynamic inputs to the discussions which result in innovative outcomes. These outcomes are then further discussed with the researchers and contributors who give their valuable feedback and opinion regarding the same. The feedback is then collaborated with the researches and they are edited in a comprehensive manner to aid the understanding of the subject.

Apart from the editorial board, the designing team has also invested a significant amount of their time in understanding the subject and creating the most relevant covers. They scrutinized every image to scout for the most suitable representation of the subject and create an appropriate cover for the book.

The publishing team has been involved in this book since its early stages. They were actively engaged in every process, be it collecting the data, connecting with the contributors or procuring relevant information. The team has been an ardent support to the editorial, designing and production team. Their endless efforts to recruit the best for this project, has resulted in the accomplishment of this book. They are a veteran in the field of academics and their pool of knowledge is as vast as their experience in printing. Their expertise and guidance has proved useful at every step. Their uncompromising quality standards have made this book an exceptional effort. Their encouragement from time to time has been an inspiration for everyone.

The publisher and the editorial board hope that this book will prove to be a valuable piece of knowledge for researchers, students, practitioners and scholars across the globe.

List of Contributors

Paola Savoia, Paolo Fava and Maria Grazia Bernengo
Department of Biomedical Sciences and Human Oncology, Section of Dermatology, University of Turin, Italy

James H F Shaw and Michael Fay
Auckland Hospital, Great Mercury Island, New Zealand

Justin Kelly and MJ Kerin
Dept of Academic Surgery, UCHG /NUIG, Galway, Ireland

Khan K. Chaichana and Kaisorn L. Chaichana
Johns Hopkins University School of Medicine, Department of Neurosurgery, Baltimore, USA

Aylin Türel Ermertcan, Ferdi Öztürk and Kamer Gündüz
Celal Bayar University, Faculty of Medicine, Department of Dermatology, Turkey

Paul Howell and Hung Khong
Mitchell Cancer Institute, University of South Alabama, Mobile, United States of America

Soroosh Radfar
Dana-Farber Cancer Institute, Boston, United States of America

Yixiang Wang
Central Laboratory, Peking University School and Hospital of Stomatology, Beijing, China

Jianli Dong and Chet L. Schwab
University of Texas Medical Branch, Galveston Texas, USA

Bently P. Doonan, Jessica D. Hathaway and Azizul Haque
Medical University of South Carolina, United States of America

Bao Lam, Patrick A. Ott and Anna C. Pavlick
New York University School of Medicine, USA

Stephen J. Beebe, Wentia E. Ford, Wei Ren and Xinhua Chen
Old Dominion University / Frank Reidy Research Center for Bioelectrics Norfolk, Virginia, USA

Mecker G. Möller
Division of Surgical Oncology, Department of Surgery, University of Miami, Miller School of Medicine, Miami, Florida, USA

Slawomir Salwa, Declan M. Soden and Gerald C. O'Sullivan
Cork Cancer Research Centre, Leslie C. Quick Laboratory, BioSciences Institute, University College Cork and Department of Surgery, Mercy University Hospital, Cork, Ireland

Anna Choromańska, Julita Kulbacka, Agnieszka Chwiłkowska, Nina Skołucka, Andrzej Gamian and Jolanta Saczko
Wroclaw Medical University, Department of Medical Biochemistry, Wroclaw, Poland

Raffaele Califano, Aidalena Z Abidin, Louise Carter, Laura Cove-Smith and Paul Lorigan
Department of Medical Oncology, The Christie NHS Foundation Trust, Manchester, United Kingdom

Ruth Board
Rosemere Cancer Centre, Royal Preston Hospital, Sharoe Green Lane, Preston, United Kingdom

Bihani Kularatne
Department of Medical Oncology, Guy's and St Thomas' NHS Trust, Great Maze Pond, London, United Kingdom

Raquel Correa, Mario Lobato and José Antonio Medina
Virgen de la Victoria Hospital, Málaga, Spain

Thomas Mücke and Anna Borgmann,
Klaus-Dietrich Wolff and David Andrew Mitchell, Department of Oral and Maxillofacial Surgery, Technische Universität München, Klinikum Rechts der Isar, Germany